IMMUNOPHARMACOLOGY
IN AUTOIMMUNE DISEASES
AND TRANSPLANTATION

IMMUNOPHARMACOLOGY IN AUTOIMMUNE DISEASES AND TRANSPLANTATION

Edited by

Hans Erik Rugstad

Rikshospitalet
Oslo, Norway

Liv Endresen

Rikshospitalet
Oslo, Norway

and

Øystein Førre

Oslo Sanitetsforening Rheumatism Hospital
Oslo, Norway

Plenum Press • New York and London

Library of Congress Cataloging-in-Publication Data

Immunopharmacology in autoimmune diseases and transplantation / edited
  by Hans Erik Rugstad and Liv Endresen and Øystein Førre.
      p.   cm.
  Includes bibliographical references and index.
  ISBN 0-306-43994-8
    1. Autoimmune diseases--Immunotherapy. 2. Transplantation of
organs, tissues, etc. 3. Immunopharmacology.   I. Rugstad, Hans
Erik.   II. Endresen, Liv.   III. Førre, Øystein.
    [DNLM: 1. Autoimmune Diseases--immunology. 2. Autoimmune
Diseases--therapy. 3. Immunosuppressive Agents--pharmacology.
4. Immunosuppressive Agents--therapeutic use. 5. Immunotherapy.
6. Transplantation Immunology.   WD 305 I334]
RC600.I48 1992
616.97'8061--dc20
DNLM/DLC
for Library of Congress   92-49484
                                                                 CIP

RC
600
.I48
1992

ISBN 0-306-43994-8

©1992 Plenum Press, New York
A Division of Plenum Publishing Corporation
233 Spring Street, New York, N.Y. 10013

Printed in the United States of America

CONTRIBUTORS

D. Adu   Department of Nephrology, Queen Elizabeth Hospital, Birmingham B15 2TJ, England

Dagfinn H. Albrechtsen   Surgical Department, The National Hospital, University of Oslo, 0027 Oslo 1, Norway

O. Baadsgaard   Department of Dermatology, University of Michigan Medical Center, 1910 A. Taubman Center, Ann Arbor, Michigan 48109

Jean-François Bach   Immunology Clinic, Necker Hospital, 75743 Paris Cedex 15, France

P. A. Bacon   Department of Rheumatology, The University of Birmingham, The Medical School, Birmingham B15 2TT, England

Knut J. Berg   Section for Nephrology, Department of Medicine, The National Hospital, University of Oslo, 0027 Oslo 1, Norway

David C. Blakey   ICI Pharmaceuticals, Macclesfield SK10 4TG, Cheshire, England

Marc D. Brown   Department of Dermatology, University of Michigan Medical Center, Ann Arbor, Michigan 48109

Lucienne Chatenoud   Immunology Clinic, Necker Hospital, 75743 Paris Cedex 15, France

Kevin D. Cooper   Department of Dermatology, University of Michigan Medical Center, Ann Arbor, Michigan 48109

A. M. Denman   Division of Immunological Medicine, Clinical Research Centre, Northwick Park Hospital, Harrow, Middlesex HA1 3UJ, England

D. J. Denman   Division of Immunological Medicine, Clinical Research Centre, Northwick Park Hospital, Harrow, Middlesex, HA1 3UJ, England

J. Dupre   University Hospital, The University of Western Ontario, London, Ontario N6A 5A5, Canada

Charles N. Ellis   Department of Dermatology, University of Michigan Medical Center, Ann Arbor, Michigan 48109

Liv Endresen   Institute of Clinical Biochemistry, The National Hospital, University of Oslo, 0027 Oslo 1, Norway

Gilles Feutren Clinical Research/Immunology, Sandoz Pharma Ltd., CH-4002 Basle, Switzerland

Marie L. Foegh Department of Surgery, Georgetown University Medical Center, Washington, D.C. 20007

Øystein Førre Oslo Sanitetsforening Rheumatism Hospital, N-0172 Oslo 1, Norway

Mark S. Fradin Department of Dermatology, University of Michigan Medical Center, Ann Arbor, Michigan 48109

Leif Gjerstad Department of Neurology, The National Hospital, University of Oslo, 0027 Oslo 1, Norway

Sudhir Gupta Division of Basic and Clinical Immunology, University of California, Irvine, Irvine, California 92717

Graham Robert Vivian Hughes Lupus Arthritis Research Laboratory, The Rayne Institute, St. Thomas' Hospital, London SE1 7EH, England

Catherine Kalvenes Institute of Immunology and Rheumatology, The National Hospital, N-0172 Oslo 1, Norway

Munther Andrawes Khamashta Lupus Arthritis Research Laboratory, The Rayne Institute, St. Thomas' Hospital, London SE1 7EH, England

Bruce W. Kirkham Rheumatology Unit, United Medical and Dental Schools, Guy's Hospital, London SE1 9RT, England

Jens Kjeldsen-Kragh Institute of Immunology and Rheumatology, The National Hospital, N-0172 Oslo 1, Norway

Lars Klareskog Department of Clinical Immunology, Uppsala University Hospital, S-751 85 Uppsala, Sweden

Robert L. Kormos Department of Surgery, University Health Center of Pittsburgh, University of Pittsburg, and the Veterans Administration Medical Center, Pittsburgh, Pennsylvania 15213

Martin Lombard Institute of Liver Studies, King's College School of Medicine, London SE5 8RX, England

R. A. Luqmani Department of Rheumatology, The University of Birmingham, The Medical School, Birmingham B15 2TT, England

J. L. Mahon University Hospital, The University of Western Ontario, London, Ontario N6A 5A5, Canada

Leonard Makowka Department of Surgery, University Health Center of Pittsburgh, University of Pittsburgh, and the Veterans Administration Medical Center, Pittsburgh, Pennsylvania 15213. *Present address*: Department of Surgery, Cedar Sinai Medical Center, Los Angeles, California 90048

Ove J. Mellbye Institute of Immunology and Rheumatology, The National Hospital, N-0172 Oslo 1, Norway

Luis Mieles Department of Surgery, University Health Center of Pittsburgh, University of Pittsburgh, and the Veterans Administration Medical Center, Pittsburgh, Pennsylvania 15213

Alfonso Monereo Department of Internal Medicine, La Paz Hospital, 28002 Madrid, Spain

Jacob B. Natvig Institute of Immunology and Rheumatology, The National Hospital, N-0172 Oslo 1, Norway

Robert B. Nussenblatt National Eye Institute, National Institutes of Health, Bethesda, Maryland 20892

Rolf Nyberg-Hansen Department of Neurology, The National Hospital, University of Oslo, 0027 Oslo 1, Norway

Monika Østensen Department of Rheumatology, University Hospital of Trondheim, 7006 Trondheim, Norway

R. G. Palmer Division of Immunological Medicine, Clinical Research Centre, Northwick Park Hospital, Harrow, Middlesex HA1 3UJ, England. *Present address:* Solihull Hospital, Solihull, West Midlands B91 2JL, England

Gabriel S. Panayi Rheumatology Unit, United Medical and Dental Schools, Guy's Hospital, London SE1 9RT, England

Alison Quayle Institute of Immunology and Rheumatology, The National Hospital, N-0172 Oslo 1, Norway

Hans Erik Rugstad Department of Clinical Pharmacology, The National Hospital, University of Oslo, N-0027 Oslo 1, Norway

D. G. I. Scott Norfolk and Norwich Hospital, Norfolk, Norwich NR1 3SE, England

Dag Sørskaar Oslo Sanitetsforening Rheumatism Hospital, N-0172 Oslo 1, Norway

Thomas E. Starzl Department of Surgery, University Health Center of Pittsburgh, University of Pittsburgh, and the Veterans Administration Medical Center, Pittsburgh, Pennsylvania 15213

C. R. Stiller University Hospital, The Unviersity of Western Ontario, London, Ontario N6A 5A5, Canada

Norman Talal Clinical Immunology Section, Audie L. Murphy Memorial Veterans Hospital, and the Department of Medicine, The University of Texas Health Science Center at San Antonio, San Antonio, Texas 78284

T. Talseth Section for Nephrology, Department of Medicine, The National Hospital, University of Oslo, 0027 Oslo 1, Norway

Morten H. Vatn Medical Department A, The National Hospital, University of Oslo, N-0027 Oslo 1, Norway

Juan José Vazquez Department of Internal Medicine, La Paz Hospital, 28002 Madrid, Spain

Eric M. Veys Department of Rheumatology, Ghent University Hospital, University of Ghent, B-9000 Ghent, Belgium

Beat von Graffenried Clinical Research/Immunology, Sandoz Pharma Ltd., CH-4002 Basle, Switzerland

John J. Voorhees Department of Dermatology, University of Michigan Medical Center, Ann Arbor, Michigan 48109

Kristian Waalen Department of Animal Genetics, National College of Veterinary Medicine, and the Institute of Immunology and Rheumatology, The National Hospital, 0033 Oslo 1, Norway. *Present Address*: Vaccine Department, National Institute of Public Health, N-0472 Oslo 4, Norway

Roger Williams Institute of Liver Studies, King's College School of Medicine, London SE5 8RX, England

Robert Winchester Department of Pediatrics, Division of Autoimmune and Molecular Diseases, Columbia University College of Physicians and Surgeons, New York, NY 10032

Yejun Zhao Department of Surgery, Georgetown University Medical Center, Washington, D.C. 20007

PREFACE

This book incorporates the latest advances in immunopharmacological treatment. One objective has been to provide appropriate bridges between the basic sciences of immunology and pharmacology on the one hand and clinical medicine on the other. A further intention has been to emphasize those advances in immunology and pharmacology that are of clinical importance while retaining those facts that, while not new, remain clinically useful.

The immunology section provides the necessary background for immunopharmacological treatment. The chapters on individual cell types include normal surface markers, mode of activation, and activation markers and functions in health and disease.

The chapters on pharmacology give comprehensive information on immunosuppressive drugs in regular use today, their biochemical and cellular mechanisms of action, pharmacokinetics, dosage regimens, therapeutic responses, adverse reactions, and drug interactions and tolerance. In addition, certain therapeutic principles that are still in an experimental phase are described, for example, immunotoxins, thymic hormones, and interleukins.

The book presents comprehensive information on various autoimmune diseases, the etiopathogenetic immune mechanisms where these are known, and the current possibilities for immunopharmacological intervention. The specific disease section also covers rare situations, fluctuations in disease patterns, and subgroups of patients and immunopharmacological treatment in these situations. Altogether, the book represents a practical textbook for clinicians and advanced students who want to be updated on therapeutic principles with regard to autoimmune diseases and transplantation.

The editors have made particular efforts to include references that were published recently. The group of outstanding authors from the United States, Canada, and Europe have each made a major commitment to present the very best literature in his or her field.

CONTENTS

PART I. IMMUNOLOGY AND PATHOGENETIC MECHANISMS

Chapter 1
Human Immune Response Genes
Robert Winchester

Chapter 2
Accessory Cells
Kristian Waalen and Øystein Førre

Chapter 3
B Cells in Autoimmunity
Øystein Førre, Kristian Waalen, Jens Kjeldsen-Kragh, Dag Sørskaar, Ove J. Mellbye, and Jacob B. Natvig

Chapter 4
T Lymphocytes in Autoimmunity and Transplantation
Jens Kjeldsen-Kragh, Alison Quayle, Catherine Kalvenes, and Øystein Førre

Chapter 5
Natural Killer Cells in Autoimmune Diseases: Function and Markers
Dag Sørskaar and Øystein Førre

Chapter 6
Interleukins: Molecular and Biological Properties
Sudhir Gupta

Chapter 7
The Immunologic Network: Possibilities for a New Immunopharmacology
Norman Talal

PART II. PHARMACOLOGY AND GENERAL THERAPEUTIC PRINCIPLES OF IMMUNOMODULATING DRUGS

Chapter 8
Steroids
Bruce W. Kirkham and Gabriel S. Panayi

Chapter 12
Cyclosporin A: Pharmacology and Therapeutic Use in Autoimmune Diseases
Gilles Feutren and Beat von Graffenried

PART III. IMMUNOTHERAPY IN AUTOIMMUNE DISEASE

Chapter 20
Systemic Lupus Erythematosus and Related Syndromes
Alfonso Monereo, Munther Andrawes Khamashta, Juan José Vazquez, and Graham Robert Vivian Hughes

Chapter 21
Immunopharmacology of Vasculitic Syndromes
P. A. Bacon, R. A. Luqmani, D. G. I. Scott, and D. Adu

Chapter 25
Disorders of Neuromuscular Transmission
Rolf Nyberg-Hansen and Leif Gjerstad

Chapter 26
Immune Therapy for Autoimmune Uveitis
Robert B. Nussenblatt

Chapter 27
Cyclosporine A in the Treatment of Dermatologic Diseases
*Mark S. Fradin, Marc D. Brown, Charles N. Ellis, Kevin D. Cooper,
and John J. Voorhees*

Chapter 28
Immunotherapy in Kidney Diseases
Knut J. Berg and Tore Talseth

Chapter 29
Mechanisms Involved in Immunomodulatory Treatment of Rheumatoid Arthritis
Lars Klareskog

PART IV. IMMUNOTHERAPY IN ORGAN AND BONE MARROW TRANSPLANTATION

Chapter 30
Immunotherapy in Organ Transplantation
Luis Mieles, Robert L. Kormos, Leonard Makowka, and Thomas E. Starzl

Chapter 31
Bone Marrow Transplantation
Dagfinn H. Albrechtsen

Part I

IMMUNOLOGY AND PATHOGENETIC MECHANISMS

Chapter 1

HUMAN IMMUNE RESPONSE GENES

Robert Winchester

Directly stated, the function of the immune system is to eliminate intruding microorganisms or certain large molecules that enter the milieu of the body. Immunity is the successful outcome of this mechanism and its failure is progressive infection. Apart from the overt congenital or acquired immune deficiencies, there are also more subtle variations in the "resistance" of individuals to specific components of microorganisms that are under the control of alternative genes coding for functionally different molecules involved in immune recognition. There inherited elements are the "immune response genes," and their study is "immunogenetics."

In addition to the role of the immune response genes in avoiding progressive infections, alterations in the appropriate operation of the immune mechanism involving these genes result in a variety of allergic and autoimmune diseases. These disorders reflect a dysfunction in the distinction the immune response must make between "self" and "nonself." The differences among the immune response genes found among individuals are generally referred to as "polymorphisms" because they are present in the population at a frequency greater than expected by random mutation, suggesting that under certain circumstances they have survival value.

1. CLONES AND REPERTOIRES

The unit of function in the immune system is the lymphocyte. It operates by expression of a receptor specific for a given antigen. The specificity of the receptor depends on its distinctive primary amino acid sequence that arose through selective expression of combinations of gene segments determined by somatic genetic events. The progeny of such a lymphocyte all share the same distinctive receptor for a given antigen and the ensemble is termed a "clone." The collection of all clones with different receptors for different peptides constitutes a repertoire. The repertoire is a set of a very large number of clones endowing an individual with the ability to recognize a vast but not limitless number of antigen

Robert Winchester • Department of Pediatrics, Division of Autoimmune and Molecular Diseases, Columbia University College of Physicians and Surgeons, New York, NY 10032.

Immunopharmacology in Autoimmune Diseases and Transplantation, edited by Hans Erik Rugstad *et al.* Plenum Press, New York, 1992.

conformations. Repertoires, especially those of the T cells, differ from individual to individual as a result of self-tolerance to different major histocompatibility complex (MHC) polymorphisms and other allelic products that, in combination, make up each person's nearly unique immunologic self.

2. MOLECULAR INTERACTIONS IN THE IMMUNE RESPONSE

To initiate an immune response, an antigen fragment, usually a peptide, interacts with several different types of molecules, all of which are derived from the evolutionarily ancient immunoglobulin family (Figure 1.1) (Williams and Barclay, 1988). Members of this family have long antedated the immunoglobulin molecule itself and almost all have the general function of binding to ligands and being involved in cell-to-cell interactions. This trait is

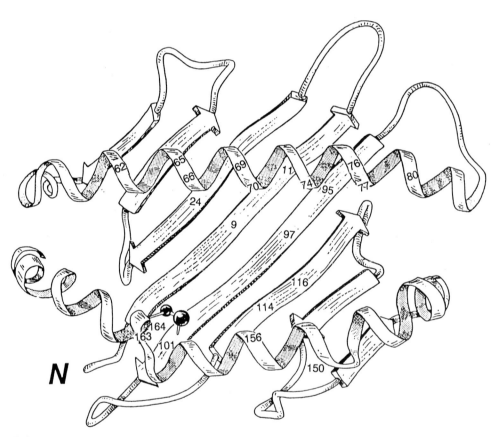

FIGURE 1.1.   The conformation of the antigen-binding cleft of the class I HLA molecule as determined by x-ray crystallography. The position of the peptide backbone is shown. The numbered amino acid residues are the principal polymorphic sites that distinguish the different allelic products. The chemical and physical differences in size, shape, charge, and hydrophobicity of these amino acid side chains determine specific complementary interactions with the amino acid side chains of foreign peptides that are being presented. (Reprinted from Bjorkman *et al.*, 1989; by permission from *Nature*. Copyright MacMillan Journals, Ltd.)

exemplified by each of the receptors involved in immune recognition, such as the Ig molecule itself which directly binds antigen.

The clonal T-cell receptor for antigen is a member of this family but has a more complex process of recognition in that it does not directly bind usual antigens but depends on prior binding of the peptide antigen to an antigen-presenting molecule. The occurrence of an immune response is critically dependent on both the T cell and the antigen-presenting structure. As shown in gene transfer experiments, the alpha and beta chains of the T-cell receptor confers both antigen specificity and specificity for self-MHC molecules, or MHC restriction, on the responding T cell (Saito et al., 1987).

Because they were first recognized as barriers to transplantation, the antigen-presenting structures are designated major histocompatibility (MHC) molecules, but it is their role as immune response genes that will concern us in this chapter. The MHC molecules are also members of the Ig family. Thus, there are two specific complementary interactions in T-cell recognition involving members of the Ig family: the binding of the peptide to the MHC molecule and the subsequent binding of the T-cell antigen receptor to the complex of antigen in the context of MHC molecule in a trimolecular interaction.

Accordingly, to the extent that the binding property of an allelic product influences the nature of the peptides that can be bound, individuals with different alleles have different capacities to bind one or another of the antigens that a person encounters. There are currently two views that have been advanced to explain why T cells only recognize antigen in the context of self-MHC molecules, and that the particular MHC alleles an individual receives control whether they will respond to a given antigen. In one theory, "determinant selection," proposed by Alan Rosenthal, the central role is played by the affinity or specificity with which the antigen fragment binds to a particular MHC allelic product (Rosenthal, 1978). In the second, the "hole in the T-cell repertoire" theory of Jan Klein, all antigenic fragments are viewed as equally likely to bind to the MHC molecule, but because of the requirement to delete autoreactive T-cell clones, each individual with a different MHC has deleted different T-cell clones with a consequential loss of the ability to recognize certain antigens (Klein, 1982). Extensive support for both views exists (Paul, 1984; Babbitt et al., 1985; Buus et al., 1986), and recent studies provide evidence that each mechanism is probably operating in the same animal in the immune response to a single antigen (Schaeffer et al., 1989). Thus, it is visualized that a necessary but not sufficient condition for a T-cell immune response is specific binding of the peptide to the MHC allelic product, but that the T-cell repertoire must contain a clone with a receptor complementary to the peptide displayed in the context of that MHC allelic product for the response to occur. The formation of the T-cell repertoire is one aspect of the process of tolerance. Since the generation of the T-cell clonal diversity is achieved by random non-germ line events during early T-cell development while the T cells are still in the thymus, in principle all possible types of T-cell receptors are generated. T cells with receptors that yield unsatisfactory combinations are eliminated in the thymus. The thymic selective mechanism is necessary to encourage only the propagation of T-cell clonal progenitors with receptors that recognize the autologous MHC molecules that a person chanced to inherit sufficiently well to present the foreign antigen, but not with such vigor that autoimmune self-recognition results. The still incompletely understood task of the thymus is to forge a working immune system from material provided to it largely through chance processes, namely, the random generation of T-cell receptors and the random inheritance of MHC alleles. There is evidently a fine balance between the discrimination of self from non-self. The more closely the distinction is drawn, the less likely is the possibility that a microorganism can exploit a gap in recognition; however, conversely, it would appear that the possibility of an autoimmune reaction becomes more likely.

3. STRATEGIES FOR RECEPTOR DIVERSITY

Whereas in principle the repertoires of B-cell and T-cell antigen receptors are immense and present in each individual, with certain critical adjustments, an entirely different strategy is followed by the MHC system. Here it is the species that has the repertoire for all varieties of MHC molecules, with each individual having only a small proportion of all potentially reactive polymorphic receptors. Yet it is the particular MHC allele that an individual receives that is responsible for the way in which he sees the universe of molecular conformations. This polymorphism has a special evolutionary significance.

4. MHC POLYMORPHISM AS AN ADAPTIVE RESPONSE

The forging of the T-cell repertoire has a major consequence that is apparently at the root of the necessity for the polymorphisms of the MHC: namely, the deleted or inactivated T-cell clones that are removed to avoid autoreactivity leave "holes" in the T-cell repertoire (Kappler *et al.*, 1987, 1988; Vidovic and Matzinger, 1988). This is potentially a catastrophic situation. However, as a species, and because of the MHC polymorphisms, these "holes" in one's immune repertoire vary from individual to individual and from generation to generation in a person's offspring, making it quite unlikely that a microorganism could systematically exploit the constantly changing target to threaten the species by a process of adaptation, although a certain fraction of individuals may succumb to an infection. The immense diversity of the MHC that frustrates the transplantation surgeon has its converse in the biologic individuality of the T-cell receptor repertoire and in its diversity within the species. Accordingly, the result of the nested set of requirements—control of B-cell differentiation by T helper cells and recognition of antigen by these T cells in the context of MHC molecules, with the attendant process of tolerance—requires a genetically poly- morphic MHC. Simply put, if each individual had a complete repertoire of MHC molecules, the available evidence is that he would lose an unacceptably large proportion of his T-cell repertoire to avoid autoreactivity.

5. AUTOIMMUNITY AND T-CELL REGULATION

Autoimmunity is most commonly recognized by the presence of autoantibodies in serum. A considerable proportion, perhaps a third or more, of the normal B-cell Ig receptor repertoire is directed to the production of antibodies reactive with "self" antigens. This is readily evident in the polyclonal B-cell activation that occurs in infection by the Epstein- Barr virus, especially when the infection is done *in vitro* under situations when the B-cell progeny can be cloned (Nakamura *et al.*, 1988). However, the requirement that helper T cells induce the differentiations of B cells to plasma cells means that the autoreactive B-cell clones will usually remain inert, perhaps accounting for the fact that autoantibody-mediated autoimmune diseases are uncommon. Much of autoimmunity therefore depends on the presence and subsequent amplifications of T-cell clones that perceive autoantigens in the context of self-MHC, and which then provide T-cell help to the differentiation of B cells with antigen receptors directed to self-molecules. In this limited sense, the immune re- sponse in autoimmunity is "normal," although highly inappropriate for the individual's well- being. What is abnormal is the loss of tolerance for self at the level of the T cell. There appears little likelihood that autoimmune disease results from the *de novo* proliferation of "forbidden" B-cell clones or failure of a general T-cell suppressor mechanism, ideas that were formerly popular explanations.

6. STRUCTURE OF MHC MOLECULES

The overall structure of a MHC molecule consists of a superdomain that contains a groove or cleft created by the amino acid side chains that binds specific peptide antigens through complementary conformational interactions with the side chains of the antigen (Figure 1.1). The superdomain is approximately 200 amino acids in size and is formed by a curving, almost saddlelike floor of some eight strands of β-pleated sheet and demarcated by two arching strands of α helix that are pursed together at either end of the ovoid cleft (Bjorkman *et al.*, 1987). A foreign peptide of 10–15 amino acids can be contained in the cleft. It is this complex of MHC molecule and bound peptide that is recognized by the T cell. This superdomain is supported by two domains highly homologous to the domains in the constant region of the MHC. A transmembrane segment and a small intracytoplasmic portion attaches the molecule to the cell membrane. This structure has been precisely determined for the class I molecule in an exciting series of x-ray crystallographic structures (Bjorkman *et al.*, 1987). Because of homologies with the primary and inferred secondary structure of the class II molecule, it is currently visualized that structure of the class II molecule is highly similar to that of the class I molecule. This implies that the immune recognition event determined by the trimolecular interaction of antigenic fragment, MHC molecule, and T cell receptor are highly similar if not identical in the instance of either class I or class II molecules.

7. FUNCTIONAL DIFFERENCES OF CLASS I AND CLASS II MOLECULES

Although class I and class II molecules bind and present antigen to T cells, both the type of antigen and the lineage and function of the T cell differs for each class. The class I and II molecules have a differential tissue distribution, with the former on virtually every cell type and the latter on the classic antigen-presenting cells (Winchester and Kunkel, 1979). Moreover, in addition to their differential tissue distribution, the intracellular traffic pattern of the class I molecule differs from that of class II. The class I molecules transit directly from the Golgi to the surface and primarily present fragments of endogenously synthesized molecules such as components of a virus infecting a cell. The class I molecules contains a site in the α_3 domain involving residue 245 that binds the CD8 (T8) accessory molecule present on cytotoxic T cells (Parham *et al.*, 1989). This results in a cytotoxic attack on the cell presenting the antigen and is a critical defense system against certain types of viral infection and allogeneic cells.

In contrast, the class II molecule, perhaps by its specific association with the invariant chain, complexes with exogenous antigen fragments that result from endocytosis and acid hydrolysis of the antigen in the endosome. In this way, the class II molecules effectively present exogenous antigens. The class II molecule has a site that binds to the CD4 accessory molecule expressed on helper T cells. The peptides presented in the class II CD4 lineage T-cell system primarily are soluble exogenous antigens that elicit the delayed hypersensitivity type of cell-mediated immunity or an antibody response. As might be anticipated from their function, class I molecules are found on virtually every nucleated cell while class II molecules are restricted to the so-called professional antigen-presenting cells. Under conditions of activation, however, a variety of cells express class II molecules. In the presentation of antigens by a class II molecule on a macrophage, we are presumably looking at the phylogenetically oldest step in the response, where the specific recognition structures of the immune system in its most direct manner aids the otherwise non-antigen-specific actions of the mononuclear phagocytic system by a variety of amplication loops.

8. GENETIC ORGANIZATION OF THE MHC

The genes present in the MHC are located on the sixth chromosome in what is termed the HLA complex (Bodmer, 1989). There are three class I MHC genes responsible for encoding the α chains of three highly homologous varieties of class I MHC molecule, designated HLA-A, -B, and -C. The much smaller, light- or β-chains, which is β_2 microglobulin, is an extrinsic membrane component encoded by genes located on a different chromosome. It is nonpolymorphic.

The class II MHC gene products, or Ia molecules, consist of three closely related isotypic varieties of molecules designated DR, DQ, and DP (Figure 1.2). In terms of history, the allelic series of genes encoding the class II molecules was originally designated the DR series. It was naively assumed to be a simple system of one locus. Indeed, some still use this term to refer to all class II molecules, a usage that leads to some confusion. The current picture of the class II region of the MHC is more complex. Homologous duplicated genes are grouped into three subregions: DP, DQ, and DR. Each subregion contains at least two genes that encode an α and a β chain that specifically bind to one another. The α and β chains differ appreciably from subregion to subregion in terms of amino acid sequence, each defining an isotypic class II molecule. The DR subregion includes the genes encoding one or,

GENE ORGANIZATION OF THE HLA CLASS II REGION

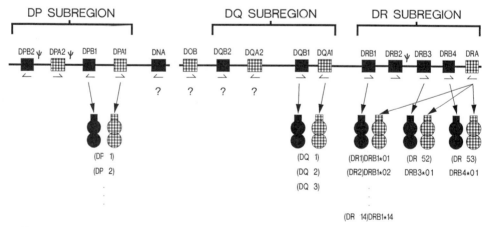

FIGURE 1.2. The currently recognized sequence of class II (Ia) genes on the sixth chromosome. The class II genes are situated to the left and are centromeric to the class III genes. The DP, DQ, and DR products of these genes are shown below, along with designations of alternative alleles or serologic specificities.

sometimes, two expressed polymorphic β chains, designated β_1 (B1) and β_2 (B3, B4, or B5), and the nonpolymorphic α chain. These interact to yield two types of DR molecules, $DR\beta_1$ and $DR\beta_2$.

The result of this gene duplication is that there are usually six distinct class I molecular conformations for antigen presentation and six to eight II conformations in an individual. Class I structures are found on all cells capable of significant DNA synthesis and thus of supporting viral replication. All of the class II structures are expressed on mononuclear phagocytes and B cells, although there are quantitative variations. Since DQ and DP genes encoding both α and β chains are polymorphic, the possibility arises that *trans* combinations can occur, creating up to four additional conformations for antigen presentation by class II molecules. Thus, because of their codominant expression, all nucleated cells have from three to six conformations with which to bind antigen and specialized antigen-presenting cells have an additional 6 to 12 conformations. In addition, a variety of other structurally unrelated genes are found in the MHC. These include the related set of genes encoding the complement components C2, C4, and fB of the classic and alternative pathways forming part of the C3 convertase activity, the genes that encode tumor necrosis factor, molecules expressed on B cells, and the genes encoding the P450 functions of steroid 21 hydroxylation. This chapter will not be concerned with these latter genes.

8.1. DR Polymorphisms Define Haplotypes

Rather fixed haplotypes of class II genes result because the gene situated in tandem from *DR* A to *DQ* A, for all practical purposes, do not exhibit recombination, and recombination is very infrequent between *DQ* B and *DQ* A and between *HLA* −B and *DR* A. The haplotypes are primarily defined, and in practice designated, by the highly polymorphic DR B1 chain alleles, which maintains the historical usage of the DR terminology. Three major families of DR polymorphisms can be identified by examining the DR β and DQ α chains (Figure 1.2). *DR1*, *DR2*, and *DR10* constitute one family in that, except for DR2, they lack the β_2 chain gene and all share similar *DQ* B chain genes. The second family is serologically identified as DR52 (MT2). In this family, the $DR\beta_2$ chains are all nearly identical, as are the DQ α chains. It includes the *DR3*, *DR5*, *DR6*, and *DR8* haplotypes. This family also exhibits the most marked similarities among DR B chain sequences. The DR53 family (MT3) is characterized by identical DR β_2 chains and a set of highly similar DQ A chains. It includes the *DR4*, *DR7*, and *DR9* haplotypes. The serologic DR53 specificity is borne on the DR β_2 molecule encoded by each haplotype. The DRβ chains of this group are dissimilar.

Certain DQ β chains are commonly associated with haplotypes defined by DR B chain polymorphisms. However, there are three main types of DQ B chains. As described above, *DR1*, *DR2*, and *DR10* haplotypes have nearly identical DQ B chains that bear the DQ1 specificity. The *DR3* haplotype has the second variety of DQ B chain that bears the DQ2 specificity. However, despite the similarity of DR3 and DR5 haplotypes, the *DR5* haplotypes commonly express a third type of DQ β chain that bears the DQ3 specificity. Less frequently, *DR5* haplotypes are found encoding the DQ1 β chain. DR4 haplotypes express the DQ3 β chain, as do a small proportion of DR7 haplotypes recognized by a distinctive mixed lymphocyte culture (MLC) type (Dw11) and the absence of the $DR\beta_2$ gene product. The common DR7 haplotypes express the DQ2 β chain. These DQ combinations are stable characteristics of populations, and examples of recombination are exceedingly rare.

Haplotypes also exist among the *HLA-A*, *-B*, and *-C* of the class I genes and extended haplotypes are found embracing all three classes of MHC genes. *HLA-A1-B8-DR3* is perhaps the best known of these haplotypes, which includes a deletion for one of the C4 complement genes and is associated with susceptibility to several different autoimmune diseases.

8.2. Location of Allelic Differences

The nature of the structural differences that distinguish the various alleles of both class I and class II MHC molecules—and ultimately determine their property of combining with particular antigens—is due to the presence of multiple amino acid substitutions that characterize each allelic product. These amino acid substitutions are clustered in three or four regions of diversity or "hypervariability" in a manner that resembles those in the Ig variable region, although it should be emphasized that they do not exhibit the somatic hypervariability of the Ig variable genes (Parham et al., 1989). Table I illustrates certain of

TABLE I. Major Sites of Sequence Polymorphism Among DR β Chain Alleles Illustrating Patchwork Pattern of Developing Variability from Recombination of a Smaller Number of Antecedent Genes[a]

	Amino acid positions in DR β chain diversity regions										
	First			Second				Third			
	9	11	13	26	28	30	37	67	70	71	74
DR1 β1	W	L	F	L	E	C	S	L	Q	R	A
DR1 Cetus	W	L	F	L	E	C	S	I	D	E	A
DR2 Dw2βI	Q	D	Y	F	H	D	D	F	D	R	A
DR2 Dw12βI	Q	D	Y	F	H	G	N	F	D	R	A
DR2 AZHβI	Q	D	Y	F	H	G	N	I	Q	R	A
DR3 βI	E	S	S	Y	D	Y	H	L	Q	K	R
DR3 DQWa	E	S	S	F	E	Y	H	L	Q	K	R
DR4 Dw4	E	V	H	F	D	Y	Y	L	Q	K	A
DR4 Dw14	E	V	H	F	D	Y	Y	L	Q	R	A
DR4 Dw15	E	V	H	F	D	Y	Y	L	Q	R	A
DR4 Dw10	E	V	H	F	D	Y	Y	I	D	E	A
DR5 Dw5βI	E	S	S	F	D	Y	Y	F	D	R	A
DR5 JVM	E	S	S	F	D	Y	Y	I	D	E	A
DR6a βI	E	S	S	F	D	Y	N	I	D	E	A
DR6b βI	E	S	S	F	D	Y	F	L	R	E	E
DR6 Amala	E	S	S	F	E	Y	N	L	Q	R	A
DR7 βI	W	G	Y	F	E	L	F	I	D	R	Q
DR8 βI	E	S	G	F	D	Y	Y	F	D	R	L
DR9 βI	K	D	F	Y	H	G	N	F	R	R	E
DR10 βI	E	V	F	L	E	R	Y	L	R	R	A
DW2 βIII	W	P	R	F	D	Y	S	I	Q	A	A
AZH βIII	W	P	R	F	D	Y	S	F	D	R	A
DR52aβIII	E	R	S	Y	D	H	F	L	Q	K	R
DR52bβIII	E	R	S	F	E	H	Y	L	Q	K	R
DR52cβIII	E	R	S	F	E	Y	L	L	Q	K	R
DR53βIII	E	A	C	N	I	Y	Y	L	R	R	E

[a]Gene conversion or intragenic recombination, methods of lateral gene transfer, appears to be the way in which the current repertoire of alleles was assembled from portions of antecedent genes. The serologic specificities correlate well with the sequence of the first diversity region shown in single letter amino acid code. A family of structurally related sequences include the DR3, 5, and 6 alleles. In the case of the second diversity region, DR4 shares a sequence with members of this family. The third diversity region is of greatest interest because it is completely dissociated from the first two regions. Seven basic patterns are used for the 26 genes. For example, I D E A is found in DR1 Cetus, DR4, Dw10, and DR6aβI. The sharing of L Q R/K A is found in DR1 β1, DR4, Dw4, Dw14, Dw15, and DR6 Amala, the presence of which are all associated with susceptibility to rheumatoid arthritis.

these for the DR β locus (Gregersen et al., 1989). The intervening framework stretches of amino acids are constant among all the alleles of a specific locus and, in fact, define the isotypic characteristics of the locus. Recent studies of the exact conformation of two HLA-A products reveals that the ten amino acid differences that distinguish HLA-A2 and Aw68.1 are principally located at sites that define the margins and shape of the antigen-binding cleft or the region where the T-cell receptor is thought to bind (Garrett et al., 1989). The polymorphism between the two molecules is responsible for the creation of distinctive pockets and subsites positioned to maximize interactions with different kinds of side chains on peptide antigens. In this way, the polymorphisms are the direct structural basis of the allele specific binding of antigen that is the molecular basis of the genetic regulation of immune responsiveness. This is now seen to reside in the allele-determined overall shape of the cleft and particular considerations of charge and hydrophobicity of its constituent amino acids. From Table I it is evident that several different alleles encode the same DR specificity and are equivalently recognized in standard HLA typing.

For example, both MLC typing using the discrimination of the T-cell receptor and DNA sequence studies distinguish several subtypes of DR4, including those designated Dw4 and Dw10, Dw13, Dw14, and Dw15. These alleles are highly similar but differ with respect to several critical amino acids in the third hypervariable region as well as, most strikingly, in their disease associations (Gregersen et al., 1987; Winchester, 1990). The findings emphasize the importance of particular conformations in the hypervariable regions of the MHC molecules encoded by different alleles as determinants of antigen responsiveness.

9. IMMUNE RECOGNITION EVENTS IN CLASS I MHC DISEASES

In determining susceptibility to autoimmune diseases, we see one of the several important consequences of the polymorphism of MHC molecules in the biology of human disease. It appears likely that most of the associations reflect the existence of a specific immune recognition event that underlies a critical step in the early events that result in autoimmunity. Susceptibility to certain diseases such as ankylosing spondylitis, Reiter's syndrome, and psoriasis is associated with HLA and I alleles, notably HLA-B27 or Cw6. These disorders have little or no evidence of delayed hypersensitivity like cell-mediated immunity or serologic autoantibodies. That certain of these disorders occur in individuals with AIDS where the CD4 lineage of T cells is not properly functional suggests that the critical immune recognition event in this group of disorders involves presentation of a cellularly derived antigen by class I MHC molecules to T cells of the CD8 linage (Winchester and Gregersen, 1988).

10. IMMUNE RECOGNITION EVENTS IN CLASS II MHC DISEASE

In contrast, diseases with associations to particular class II alleles such as rheumatoid arthritis, systemic lupus erythematosus, and myasthenia gravis are characterized by the presence of autoantibodies and sometimes a considerable lymphoid response. In the case of rheumatoid arthritis, the association of susceptibility with DR1 and DR4 and the lack of association with the DR4 subtypes Dw10 and Dw13, taken together with both the sequences of the relevant genes and differences in the susceptibility in various ethnically distinct populations, led to the formulation of the "epitope hypothesis," or the "conformational equivalence hypothesis" (Gregersen et al., 1987; Winchester and Gregersen, 1988; Winchester, 1990). The pattern of distribution of DR specificities among individuals with rheumatoid arthritis suggests that the mode of inheritance is one of dominant susceptibility. The interpretation of the data that gives rise to the notion of conformational equivalence concludes that the molecular basis of susceptibility to rheumatoid arthritis can be mapped to a consensus sequence of Gln–Arg/Lys–Arg–Ala–Ala in the third diversity (hypervariable) region of the DR β chain beginning at position 70. This sequence occupies a position on the α helical portion of the DR β chain that apparently is readily accessible to the T-cell antigen receptor (Figure 1.3). It is encoded by all of the haplotypes that confer susceptibility to rheumatoid arthritis, including DR1 and the Dw4, Dw14, and Dw15 varieties of DR4 (see Table I). However, the DR β chains of the DR4 haplotypes that are not associated with susceptibility contain significant differences in amino acid sequence in the third diversity region. These include the presence of negatively charged residues at position 70–71 (Dw10) or at position 74 (Dw13) which are contiguous in view of the fact that each turn of the helix requires 3.6 residues as shown by modeling conformation on an Edmundson wheel (Figure 1.3) (Winchester and Dwyer, 1990). Taken together, these data suggest that a unitary immune recognition event encoded by class II molecules underlies the molecular basis of susceptibility to rheumatoid arthritis. Here the existence of a critical immune recognition event is based on the conformationally equivalent structures that imply either presentation of an antigen by class II MHC molecules to CD4 lineage T cells with the subsequent opportunity for the provision of B cell help for autoantibody production or a more direct superantigen type of interaction with the T-cell receptor (Kappler et al., 1989).

Each of these disorders involve two hypothetical events: first, specific complexing of an antigen with a particular MHC molecule capable of binding the antigen with high avidity in a determinant selection mechanism, and, second, recognition of the antigen by a reactive

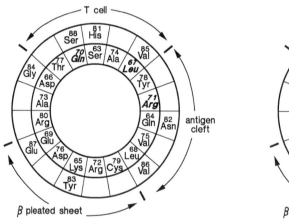 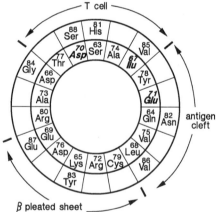

DR4 Dw 14, DR 1
associated with RA

DR4 Dw 10
NOT associated with RA

FIGURE 1.3.   Edmundson wheel image of the α helical portion of the DR β chain from residue 63 to 86, including the third diversity region. This is a view from the right end of the DR β chain looking along the axis of the α helix with the antigen-binding cleft to the right and the portion of the α helix that presumably contacts the T cell on the top of the diagram. The diagram shows the inferred position of the residues that make up a strip of helix on each face. Note that all DR alleles not associated with susceptibility to rheumatoid arthritis have negatively charged residues at position 70 or 74 which are contiguous on the same strip of helix facing toward the T cell.

clone of the T-cell repertoire not deleted in self-tolerance. Such a clonal deletion could be induced by an otherwise irrelevant HLA molecule accounting for a lowered penetrance of the trait for an autoimmune response. But it is possible that certain diseases also can result from the absence of effective recognition by either of these elements. Lyme disease is a possible example of the latter type of disorder. Susceptibility to chronic arthritis is associated with DR4 and DR2. Here one can hypothetically view the immune response to certain individuals to the *Borrelia* as excessive but ineffective and incapable of eliminating the organism, perhaps through a "hole" in the T-cell repertoire induced by the presence of DR4 or DR2 (Steere *et al.*, 1989).

11. SUMMARY

Immune response genes and their role in autoimmunity have been reviewed with emphasis on considering the interdependent repertoires of recognition structures involved in an antigen response. Issues of the purpose and consequences of MHC polymorphisms were discussed. The structure of MHC molecules and the genes encoding them was summarized. Emphasis was placed on conceptualizing these molecules an antigen-presenting structures. Autoimmune responses were classified into two categories: (1) those involving susceptibility determined by type I MHC molecules with a paucicellular T-cell response primarily involving the CD8 lineage; and (2) those diseases involving susceptibility determined by type II molecules that have their interactions with CD4 cells involved in a delayed hypersensitivity type cell-mediated immunity and in providing help to B cells for the production of autoantibodies. Central immune recognition events appear to underlie autoimmune responses involving either type I or II molecules.

REFERENCES

Babbitt, B., Allen, P., Matsueda, G., Haber, E., and Unanue, E., 1985, Binding of immunogenic peptides to Ia histocompatibility molecules, *Nature* 317:359–361.
Bjorkman, P. J., Saper, M. A., Samraoui, B., Bennett, W. S., Strominger, J. L., and Wiley, D. C., 1987, Structure of the human class I histocompatibility antigen, HLA-A2, *Nature* 329:506–512.
Bodmer, W. F., 1989, HLA 1987, in: *Immunobiology of HLA*, Volume II: *Immunogenetics and Histocompatibility* (B. Dupont, ed.), Springer-Verlag, New York, p. 1.
Buus, S., Sette, A., Colon, S. M., Jenis, D. M., and Grey, H. M., 1986, Isolation and characterization of antigen-Ia complexes involved in T cell recognition, *Cell* 47:1071–1077.
Garrett, T. P. J., Saper, M. A., Bjorkman, P. J., Strominger, J. L., and Wiley, D. C., 1989, Specificity pockets for the side chains of peptide antigens in HLA-Aw68, *Nature* 342:692–696.
Gregersen, P. K., Silver, J., and Winchester, R. J., 1987, The shared epitope hypothesis—an approach to understanding the molecular genetics of rheumatoid arthritis susceptibility, *Arthritis Rheum.* 30:1205–1213.
Gregersen, P. K., Todd, J. A., Erlich, H. A., Long, E., Servenius, B., Choi, E., Kao, H. T., and Lee, J. S., 1989, First domain sequence diversity of DR and DQ subregion alleles, in: *Immunobiology of HLA*, Volume I: *Histocompatibility Testing 1987* (B. Dupont, ed.), Springer-Verlag, New York, p. 1027.
Kappler, J. W., Roehm, N., and Marrack, P., 1987, T cell tolerance by clonal elimination in the thymus, *Cell* 49:273–280.
Kappler, J. W., Staerz, U., White, J., and Marrack, P. C., 1988, Self-tolerance eliminates T cells specific for Mls-modified products of the major histocompatibility complex, *Nature* 332:35–40.
Kappler, J., Kotzin, B., Herron, L., Gelfand, E. W., Bigler, R. D., Boylston, A., Carrel, S., Posnett, D. N., Choi, Y., and Marrack, P., 1989, Vβ-specific stimulation of human T cells by staphylococcal toxins, *Science* 244:813.
Klein, J., 1982, *Immunology*, Wiley, New York.
Nakamura, M., Burastero, S. E., Ueki, Y., Larrick, J. W., Notkins, A. L., and Casali, P., 1988, Probing the normal and autoimmune B cell repertoire with EBV. High frequency of B cells producing monoreactive high affinity autoantibodies in patients with Hashimoto's disease and SLE, *J.Immunol.* 141:4160.
Parham, P., Lawlor, D. A., Salter, R. D., Lomen, C. E., Bjorkman, P. J., and Ennis, P. D., 1989, HLA-A,B,C: Patterns of polymorphism in peptide-binding proteins, in: *Immunobiology of HLA*, Volume II: *Immunogenetics and Histocompatibility* (B. Dupont, ed), Springer-Verlag, New York, p. 10.
Paul, W., 1984, in: *Fundamental Immunology* (W. Paul, ed.), Raven, New York, p. 439.

Rosenthal, A. S., 1978, Determinant selection and macrophage function in genetic control of the immune response, *Immunol. Rev.* 40:136.

Saito, T., Weiss, A., Miller, J., Norcross, M. A., and Germain, R. N., 1987, Specific antigen-Ia activation of transfected human T cells expressing murine Ti alpha beta-human T3 receptor complexes, *Nature* 325:125–130.

Schaeffer, E. B., Sette, A., Johnson, D. L., Bekoff, M. C., Smith, J. A., Grey, H. M., and Buus, S., 1989, Relative contribution of "determinant selection" and "holes in the T-cell repertoire" to T-cell responses. *Proc. Natl. Acad. Sci. USA* 86:4649–4653.

Steere, A. C., Dwyer, E., and Winchester, R., 1990, Association of chronic Lyme arthritis with HLA-DR4 and HLA-DR2 alleles, *N. Engl. J. Med.* 323:219–223.

Vidovic, D., and Matzinger, P., 1988, Unresponsiveness to a foreign antigen can be caused by self-tolerance, *Nature* 336:222–225.

Williams, A. F., and Barclay, A. N., 1988, The immunoglobulin superfamily—domains for cell surface recognition, *Annu Rev. Immunol.* 6:381–406.

Winchester, R., 1990, Mapping susceptibility to rheumatoid arthritis into a conformationally equivalent region of MHC class II molecules encoded by different alleles, in: *Molecular Aspects of Autoimmunity* (N. R. Farid, ed.), Academic Press, Orlando, pp. 241–263

Winchester, R., and Dwyer, E., 1991, MHC and autoimmune diseases: Susceptibility to rheumatoid arthritis associated with a hydrophobic strip of α helix encoded by several MHC alleles , in: *Molecular Immunobiology of Self Reactivity* (C. A. Bona and A. Kaushik, eds.), Marcel Dekker, New York.

Winchester, R., and Gregersen, P. K., 1988, The molecular basis of susceptibility to rheumatoid arthritis: The conformational equivalence hypothesis, *Springer Semin. Immunopathol.* 10:119–139.

Winchester, R., and Kunkel, H. G., 1979, The human Ia system, *Adv. Immunol.* 28:221–292.

Chapter 2

ACCESSORY CELLS

Kristian Waalen and *Øystein Førre*

1. INTRODUCTION

An accessory cell is a cell that can present antigens and activate T lymphocytes and/or B lymphocytes. For many years the macrophage has been regarded as the main accessory cell for the various immune responses (Unanue, 1984). Later, however, it has become evident that a variety of other lymphoid cells like dendritic cells, resting and immune B cells, B cell lines or tumors, and major histocompatibility (MHC) class II-positive T cells also can act as accessory cells (Waalen et al., 1988). Recent observations have also disclosed that other cells like human thyroid epithelial cells and vascular endothelial cells expressing MHC class II molecules may act as accessory cells that probably have local immunoregulatory function. The accessory functions for activation of T cells involve (1) processing of antigen, (2) binding of processed antigen to MHC molecules, and (3) presentation of antigenic fragments.

2. PROCESSING OF ANTIGENS BY ACCESSORY CELLS

Induction of antigen-specific T-lymphocyte immune responses requires that the antigen (microbes/autoantigens) is processed and fragmented to small peptides by proteolytic processes by the accessory cell (Lanzavecchia, 1990). The antigens are usually divided into two groups, exogenous and endogenous. Exogenous antigens are processed in the endosomal compartment and presented for CD4-positive helper or cytotoxic T lymphocytes in association with MHC class II molecules. Endogenous antigens, processed in the endoplasmic reticulum, are presented in association with MHC class I molecules for CD8-positive cytotoxic T lymphocytes (CTL) (Germain, 1986; Yewdell and Bennink, 1990). The dichotomy between these two antigen-presenting pathways may be regulated by the invariant chain (I). This suggests that I chains may be of importance in autoimmune diseases (Teyton et al., 1990). However, recent data also indicate that some antigens may enter both processing pathways (Nuchtern et al., 1990).

Kristian Waalen • Department of Animal Genetics, National College of Veterinary Medicine, and the Institute of Immunology and Rheumatology, The National Hospital, 0033 Oslo 1, Norway. *Present Address:* Vaccine Department, National Institute of Public Health, N-0472 Oslo 4, Norway. *Øystein Førre* • Oslo Sanitetsforening Rheumatism Hospital, N-0172 Oslo 1, Norway.

Immunopharmacology in Autoimmune Diseases and Transplantation, edited by Hans Erik Rugstad et al. Plenum Press, New York, 1992.

The processing of antigens has been studied extensively in macrophages (Allen, 1987). These cells phagocytose foreign and possibly self-molecules, which are fragmented by proteolytic enzymes in the lysosomes (Mills, 1986; Allen, 1987). The other types of accessory cells are nonphagocytic and have few lysosomes (Watts and Howard, 1986). Alternative routes for antigen processing have been proposed (Allen, 1987). By these mechanisms the antigens are either intact, unfolded, or internalized in endosomes and processed by other proteolytic systems than that in lysosomes or by proteolysis of the antigens at the cell membrane surface. Recently it has been shown that lymphoid dendritic cells also process soluble antigens by a nonlysosomal pathway (Chain et al., 1986). The presentation of the antigen was in other respects similar or identical to that of macrophages.

3. THE IMPORTANCE OF MHC MOLECULES FOR ACCESSORY CELL FUNCTION

After processing, the antigenic fragments are transported to the cell surface and are then noncovalently bound to specific cell membrane complexes, the MHC molecules, on the accessory cell. Very recently a new gene in the MHC gene region has been described that possibly is important in the intracellular transport and presentation of peptide antigens and is related to a superfamily of genes involved in ATP-dependent transport of a variety of substrates across cell membranes (Deverson et al., 1990; Monaco et al., 1990). The complex consisting of fragmented antigenic peptide and MHC class I or MHC class II molecules will constitute a specific ligand for the antigen receptor (TCR) on the responding CD4-positive or CD8-positive T lymphocyte (Table I) (Braciale et al., 1987). In addition to the antigen-specific accessory cell and T-cell interaction, various nonspecific adhesion molecules are also involved (Table I) (McMichael et al., 1989; King and Katz, 1990).

The MHC molecules are highly polymorphic. This polymorphism is located at the putative site for binding of fragments of processed antigen. Recent x-ray crystallographic studies (Bjørkman et al., 1987; Garret et al., 1989) of the purified MHC class I molecules HLA-A2 and HLA-Aw68 have revealed that HLA class I molecules have an antigen-binding cleft consisting of the two N-terminal domains of the α-chain, the α_1 and α_2 (Bjørkman et al., 1987). It is also evident that these two MHC class I alleles have a very similar overall structure, except for 13 amino acids. These studies show that the polymorphic sites are mainly located in a groove or pocket providing a site for binding of the processed antigen. In

TABLE I. Membrane Adhesion Molecules Involved in the Specific and Nonspecific Interaction between Accessory Cells and T Cells during Activation of T Cells

Molecule	Accessory cell	T cell
Specific:	MHC class I + antigen	TCRαβ-CD3/CD8
	MHC class II + antigen	TCRαβ-CD3/CD4
Nonspecific:	CD11a/CD18	CD54 (ICAM1)
	CD54 (ICAM1)	CD11a/CD18
	CD58 (LFA3)	CD2

Abbreviations: MHC, major histocompatibility complex; TCR, T-cell antigen receptor; CD, cluster of differentiation; ICAM1, Intercellular adhesion molecule 1; LFA3, Leukocyte functional antigen 3.

HLA-A2 and HLA-Aw68, 10 of the 13 amino acid differences are faced into the putative antigen-binding pocket. From these studies it is assumed that the comparison of the three-dimensional structure of HLA-A2 and HLA-Aw68 provides a representative model of the polymorphic changes within the site for antigen binding in MHC class I molecules. Based on amino acid sequence homology between MHC class I and class II molecules and the general secondary molecular conformations predicted by computer, it is reasonable to assume that the three-dimensional structure of the MHC class II molecules resemble the MHC class I structure quite closely (Brown et al., 1988). It thus appears that the class II MHC molecules, like the MHC class I molecules, have an antigen-binding cleft that is built up by the N-terminal parts of the α and β chains, the α_1 and β_1 domain. MHC class II molecules have also recently been shown to bind small peptides (Buus et al., 1987; Brown et al., 1988).

4. ACCESSORY CELL HETEROGENEITY

Accessory cells are widely distributed in lymphoid and nonlymphoid organs and are a heterogeneous population of cells. Among these, dendritic cells and macrophages are regarded as the most predominant accessory cell types, although resting B cells and other MHC class II-positive cells also can act as accessory cells. MHC class II molecules can be induced on many different cell types by interferon-gamma (IFN-gamma), tumor necrosis factor (TNF), and granulocyte—macrophage colony-stimulating factor (GM-CSF). The accessory cells can be further subdivided based on histological localization, marker expression, function, and degree of activation. However, dendritic cells seem to be required for the activation of resting T cells, while sensitized T cells can be activated by other MHC class II-positive cells (macrophages, resting B cells) as well (Werb et al., 1986; Waalen, 1988). The dominant markers and characteristics displayed by monocytes/macrophages, the various dendritic cell types, and B cells are shown in Table II. In Table III CD-defined membrane molecules expressed by accessory cells are shown (McMichael et al., 1989).

TABLE II. Markers and Characteristics of the Various Types of Dendritic Cells, Monocytes/Macrophages (Mo/Ma), and B Cells

Marker/characteristic	LDC[a]	IDC	LC	FDC	Mo/Ma	B cells
MHC class I	+	+	+	+	+	+
MHC class II	+	+	+	+/−	+/−	+
T-cell antigens (CD3)	−	−	−	−	−	−
B-cell antigens (CD19)	−	−	−	−	−	+
Mo/Ma antigens	−	−/+	−/+	−	+	−
CD11b (CR3, C3$_{bi}$R)	−	nd	+/−	−	+	−
CD16 (FcRIII)	−	nd	+	+	+	−
CD35 (CR1, C3bR)	−	nd	+	+	+	+
CD45	+	nd	+	+	+	+
Birbeck granules	−	(+)	+	−	−	−
Pox/NSE	−	nd	−	nd	+	−
Phagocytosis	−	−	−/+	−/+	+	−
IL-1 production	+/−	nd	+	nd	+	+
Accessory activity	+	nd	+	nd	+/−	+/−

[a]Including blood and rheumatoid synovial dendritic cells.
Abbreviations: Pox/NSE, peroxidase/nonspecific esterase; nd, not demonstrated.

TABLE III. CD Molecules Expressed by Accessory Cells

Molecule	Accessory cell	Other cells	Membrane component
CD1a,b,c	LC, B subset	Thymocytes	gp49,45,43
CD9	M	Pre-B cells	p24
CD11a	M	Leukocytes	LFA1 (gp180/95)
b	M	G, NK cells	C3b$_i$, receptor
c	M, B subset	G, NK cells	gp150/95
CD12	M	G, platelets	p(90–120)
CD16	M, LC, FDC	NK cells, G	FcRIII, gp50–65
CD18		Leukocytes	β-chain to CD11a,b,c
CD23	M(act.) B subset		Fc$_\epsilon$RIII, gp45–50
CDw32	M, B	G	FcRIII, gp40
CD45	M,DC,B	Leukocytes	LCA, T200
CD45RA	M, B	T subset, G	Restricted T200, gp200
CD45RB	M, B	T subset, G	Restricted T200
CD45RO	M, B	T subset, G	Restricted T200, gp180
CDw49	M, LC, B	T, Thymocytes	VLA-α4, gp150
CD58		Leukocytes	LFA-3,gp40–65
CD64	M		FcRI,gp75
CD68	M		gp110
CD71	Mac	Prolif. cells	Transferrin receptor
CD74	M, B		Class II associated invariant chain

Abbreviations: LC, Langerhans cells; B, B cells; M, monocytes; DC, dendritic cells; Mac, macrophages; G, granulocytes; T, T cells.

4.1. Monocytes and Macrophages

Monocytes are bone marrow-derived cells in the circulation that develop into macrophages after migration into various tissues (van Furth, 1981). Inflammatory conditions will increase the turnover of monocytes with augmented proliferation of progenitors in the bone marrow. This production has been shown to be regulated by circulating enhancing and inhibitory factors produced at inflammatory sites, while very few activated macrophages will proliferate at the inflammatory sites (van Furth, 1981). Blood monocytes are less mature than tissue macrophages. Macrophages can be divided into subpopulations (e.g., peritoneal macrophages, tissue macrophages) based on localization and different properties, like MHC class II expression and microbiocidal capacity. Macrophages can phagocytose and degrade foreign material in the lysozomes. This property was previously regarded as a prerequisite for accessory cell function (Mills, 1986; Allen, 1987). However, new data indicate that the processing and presentation of antigenic molecules may be regarded as separate processes (Watts and Howard, 1986; Allen, 1987). Macrophages can produce a large variety of biologically active substances. Among these are cytokines, enzymes, and prostaglandins (Werb et al., 1986).

4.2. Dendritic Cells

Dendritic cells (DC) were first described in mouse spleen (Steinman and Cohn, 1973). Later dendritic cells from many different lymphoid (spleen, lymph nodes, thymus, afferent lymph) and nonlymphoid (circulation, skin, heart, liver, kidney, inflamed synovial tissue, synovial fluid) organs and from different species (mouse, rat, human) have been isolated and characterized (Austyn, 1987; Waalen, 1988). From these studies it appears that dendritic cells comprise a heterogeneous group of cells which in most respects differ from classic monocytes/macrophages (VanVoorhis et al., 1982; Unkeless and Springer, 1986). The dendritic cells have an irregular shape both when adhering to glass or plastic surfaces and after culture for one day in suspension (Førre et al., 1985; Steinman et al., 1986). Viable, adherent dendritic cells continuously form and retract processes, while nonadherent dendritic cells have active banding and wavelike movements which are quite distinct from the behavior of phagocytic cells (Førre et al., 1985). Apart from macrophages, the dendritic cells are mainly nonphagocytic. Dendritic cells are very potent accessory and antigen-presenting cells for lymphocytes (King and Katz, 1990; Waalen et al., 1988).

4.2.1. Classification of Dendritic Cells

Based on anatomical localization and other features, dendritic cells are usually classified in the following way (see Table II):

1. *Lymphoid dendritic cells (LDC)* have been identified in suspensions of cells from lymphoid organs, peripheral blood, and chronic inflammatory sites. They strongly express MHC class I and class II antigens and the common leukocyte (CD45) determinant, which indicates that they are bone marrow derived. The lymphoid dendritic cells lack IgG-Fc receptors (CD16) and C3b receptors (CR1, CD35), as well as the majority of macrophage-specific surface antigens (Kuntz-Crow and Kunkel, 1982; VanVoorhis et al., 1982; Unkeless and Springer, 1986; Waalen et al., 1986a; Waalen et al., 1987a) The lymphoid dendritic cells are efficient accessory cells for various immune responses (Steinman et al., 1986; Waalen, 1988).

2. *Interdigitating cells (IDC)* can be identified in sections from lymphoid tissues. They are primarily localized in the T-cell-dependent areas (paracortical areas) of the spleen, lymph nodes, and thymus. They express MHC class II antigens and have some surface determinants in common with macrophages. It is not known whether these cells express the CD16, the CD35, or the CD45 surface determinants (Unkeless and Springer, 1986). Studies on MHC class II (HLA-DR) positive human thymic dendritic cells in culture suggest that these cells are identical with the interdigitating dendritic cells studied *in situ* (Pelletier et al., 1986). A monoclonal antibody, RFD1, has been reported to be specific for interdigitating dendritic cells (Poulter et al., 1986). It has not yet been clarified whether the interdigitating dendritic cells have accessory activities for various types of immune responses.

3. *Langerhans cells (LC)* have been identified in cell suspensions obtained from skin epidermis. These cells strongly express MHC class II antigens and have typical Birbeck granules. They also express the CD16, CD35, and CD45 determinants on their surface and are thus bone marrow derived. The LC also express the CD1a (T6) thymocyte marker, a property that has been used to purify these cells. The LC also have some surface markers in common with macrophages and have been shown to exhibit accessory activities in several immune reactions (Bjercke et al., 1984; Unkeless and Springer, 1986).

4. *Follicular dendritic cells (FDC, sometimes denoted dendritic reticulum cells)* have been identified in sections in lymphoid follicles. In contrast to the interdigitating dendritic cells, the follicular dendritic cells are localized in close contact with B cells. The follicular dendritic cells are probably accessory cells for B cells and may exert their function through trapping of immune complexes on their surface (Humphrey et al., 1984). These cells express MHC class II antigens, CD16, CD21 (C3d complement

receptors, CR2), and CD45 antigens, but are negative for macrophage-specific antigens and are nonphagocytic and nonadherent. Follicular dendritic cells have also recently been isolated and studied in suspension (Schnitzlein *et al.*, 1985).

5. MARKERS AND CHARACTERISTICS OF ACCESSORY CELLS (DENDRITIC CELLS, MACROPHAGES, AND B CELLS)

The most characteristic features of dendritic cells, monocytes/macrophages, and B cells are outlined in Table II. Dendritic cells strongly express CD45 and MHC class II molecules (HLA-DP, -DQ, -DR), but they otherwise lack most markers expressed by monocytes/ macrophages and B cells. Even after three to five days in culture, the lymphoid dendritic cells still express MHC class II antigens. Dendritic cells lack markers expressed by T cells, NK cells, and fibroblasts, nor do they express CD35 except for LC and FDC or CD71 (Waalen *et al.*, 1987a; King and Katz, 1990).

6. FUNCTIONAL CHARACTERISTICS OF DENDRITIC CELLS IN CHRONIC INFLAMMATION

The chronic inflammatory process in rheumatoid arthritis has previously been intensively studied with respect to the active involvement of T lymphocyte and B lymphocyte systems (Natvig and Winchester, 1988). In contrast, until a few years ago, much less was known about accessory cells in the rheumatoid inflammatory process. In light of the importance of accessory cells for the activation of lymphocytes, such cells could be one of the driving forces of the chronic inflammatory processes seen in rheumatoid arthritis.

In a series of studies (Waalen, 1988a) dendritic cells from rheumatoid synovial tissue and synovial fluid as well as from normal peripheral blood have been intensively characterized. When dendritic cells from both compartments are incubated with autologous T cells, characteristic cell clusters are observed (Figures 2.1 and 2.2). The binding of T lymphocytes to dendritic cells are mediated by various adhesion molecules (Table I). Clusters of rheumatoid synovial or blood dendritic cells and T cells could be separated from nonclustered cells (Waalen *et al.*, 1988b). The clustered cells had five to ten times higher proliferation ([³H]thymidine incorporation) than nonclustered cells. This observation indicates that cell adhesion and direct contact between dendritic cells and T cells are of vital importance for the activation of resting T cells. The *in vitro* clustering phenomenon may thus have its counterpart in the nodular aggregates found *in vivo* in the inflamed synovial tissue of patients with rheumatic disease and at the inflammatory sites of other autoimmune diseases.

6.1. T-Cell Activation Antigens Induced by Dendritic Cells *in Vitro*

In agreement with the potent accessory properties of the dendritic cells for the various T-cell responses, it is also found that dendritic cells are able to induce activation antigens on T cells during autologous MLR cultures (Waalen, 1988). These activation markers include MHC class II (HLA-DR) molecules, receptors for transferrin (CD71), and receptors for interleukin-2 (IL-2) (Tac, CD25). Interestingly, the number of T cells expressing these activation markers after stimulation by dendritic cells were very similar to the number of T cells from rheumatoid synovial tissue and synovial fluid expressing these markers (Waalen *et al.*, 1987b). In addition, the synovial T cells also express the activation markers TLiSA1

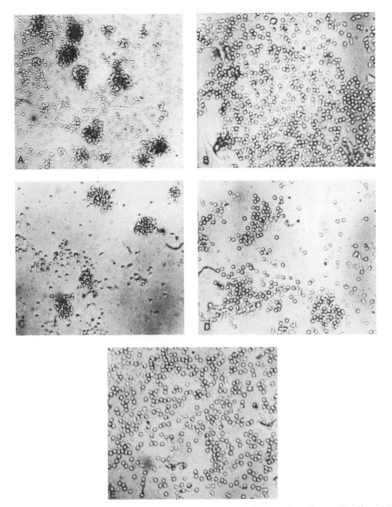

FIGURE 2.1.   Cluster formation between (A) synovial dendritic cells (DC) and autologous T cells and (C) blood DC and autologous T cells. (B) and (D) show the inhibition of cluster formation with MHC class II (anti-HLA-DR) antibody (0.5 μg/ml). In (E) is shown T cells alone (Waalen *et al.*, 1987b).

and VLA1 (Førre *et al.*, 1988). Synovial dendritic cells may thus be involved in the activation process seen in the rheumatoid synovitis.

6.2. Activation of T Cells and B Cells by Accessory Cells

After the accessory cell and the T cells have attached to each other by various adhesion molecules, the T cells can react with the antigen/MHC molecular complexes on the accessory cell via their receptor for antigen, the TCR–CD3 complex. CD8-positive T cells react with antigen–MHC class I molecular complexes, while CD4-positive T cells recognize antigens bound to MHC class II molecules (Parnes, 1986). The antigen presentation for B cells is less well characterized. B cells outside lymphoid follicles are most probably activated

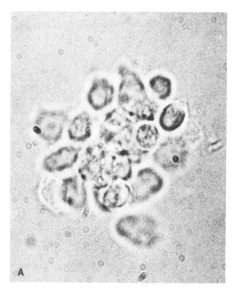
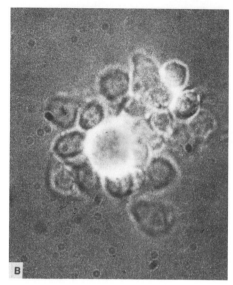

FIGURE 2.2. (A) A dendritic cell (DC) T-cell cluster in light microscopy and (B) in combined light and fluorescence microscopy after staining with anti-MHC class II (anti-HLA-DR) antibody. A HLA-DR-positive DC is seen in the middle of the cluster (Waalen *et al.*, 1988a).

by a T-cell-dependent activation pathway, while B cells in the follicles seem to be activated by follicular dendritic cells (MacLennan *et al.*, 1988).

In recent studies purified peripheral blood monocytes and dendritic cells from blood and rheumatoid synovial tissue and fluid were compared for various accessory cell functions. These studies clearly showed that dendritic cells both from normal PB and from rheumatoid synovial compartments were superior to monocytes as accessory cells for antigen (PPD, HSV) and mitogen (PHA and Con A) induced T-cell responses and to induce autologous as well as allogeneic T-cell responses (MLR). However, when *Chlamydia trachomatis* particles were used, a somewhat different picture was seen. Thus, a mixture of monocytes and dendritic cells gave an enhanced T-cell response, indicating a possible cooperation between the monocytes and dendritic cells (Waalen, 1988; Waalen *et al.*, 1986a). Monoclonal antibodies to MHC class II molecules (HLA-DR and HLA-DQ) also inhibited the specific antigen activation of T cells to PPD, HSV, and *C. trachomatis*, indicating that the sites on the MHC molecules for antigen binding were blocked by these antibodies. Interestingly, it has also been shown that dendritic cells can present autoantigens like collagen type II and IgG Fc fragments to autologous T cells (Waalen *et al.*, 1988b).

7. CYTOKINE PRODUCTION BY ACCESSORY CELLS

The current interpretation of T-cell activation is that an accessory cell presents antigens to the T cells in the context of class II MHC molecules. In addition, interleukin-1 (IL-1) is produced by the accessory cell and acts as a comitogenic signal in the activation process (Oppenheim *et al.*, 1986; Weaver and Unanue, 1990). These stimuli then trigger the T cells to produce and become responsive to IL-2. In the mouse, recent data indicate that mainly T_h2 T cells express receptors for IL-1.

Dendritic cells from inflamed synovial tissue have been shown to produce high amounts of IL-1-like activity both spontaneously and after stimulation with lipopolysaccharide (LPS), while the blood dendritic cells produce some, although much less, of this substance (Waalen *et al.*, 1986b). The enhanced release of IL-1 by dendritic cells thus seem to be restricted to the synovial inflammatory compartment. In addition, it is shown (Waalen and Førre, 1990) that rheumatoid synovial dendritic cells also express mRNA for both IL-1 alpha and beta as well as IL-6. In contrast, the mouse dendritic cells have not been shown to produce IL-1 (Koide and Steinman, 1987). The cytokines produced by accessory cells (monocytes, dendritic cells and B cells) are shown in Table IV. The molecular and biological properties of the various cytokines are outlined elsewhere (Akira *et al.*, 1990; Chapter 6, this volume).

8. ACCESSORY CELL ADHESION MOLECULES AND HOMING TO SITES OF INFLAMMATION

Migration of leukocytes is essential for their maturation and their distribution in various lymphoid tissues, as well as their homing to inflammatory sites. Accessory cells like Langerhans cells seem to migrate from the periphery, where they have picked up antigens, to lymphoid tissues to initiate immune responses. During migration and recirculation, the cells bind to endothelial cells of the postcapillary venules in lymphoid tissues (Austyn and Larsen, 1990). The binding is mediated by specialized homing receptors on the endothelial cells. These receptors are organ-specific and are essential for the migration of cells into the tissues.

At sites of inflammation the endothelial cells of microvessels develop into high endothelial venules (HEV), exerting enhanced adhesion for leukocytes. This process is regulated by cells and factors in the immediate environment of the postcapillary venules. Three inflammatory cytokines, IFN-gamma, IL-1, and TNF-alpha, have been shown to stimulate increased receptor-mediated adhesiveness of leukocytes to HEV, resulting in increased migration of leukocytes to sites of tissue inflammation. At least two sets of adhesion molecules are induced or up-regulated, the intercellular adhesion molecule (ICAM-1, CD54) and ELAM-1. ICAM-1 can be induced by IL-1 and TNF-alpha, while ELAM-1 can be induced by IL-1 and TNF-alpha as well as bacterial lipopolysaccharides. ICAM-1 is the ligand for LFA1 (CD11a/CD18), which is involved in many cell–cell adhesive interactions (Albelda and Buck, 1990). IFN-gamma also induces the expression of MHC

TABLE IV. Cytokines Produced by Accessory Cells

Cytokine	Accessory cells			Other cells	Detected in RA[a]
	Mo/Ma	DC	B cells		
Interleukin-1 (IL-1 alpha and beta)	+	+	+	+	+
Interleukin-6 (IL-6)	+	+	−	+	+
Interleukin-8 (IL-8)	+	nd	nd	+	nd
Tumor necrosis factor (TNF-alpha)	+	−	−	+	+
Lymphotoxin (TNF-beta)	+	−	+	+	nd
Interferon (IFN-alpha)	+	−	−	+	+/−
Transforming growth factor (TGF-beta)	+	−	−	+	+
G-CSF	+	−	−	+	nd
M-CSF	+	−	−	+	+

[a]Detected in the rheumatoid synovial compartments.
Abbreviations: RA, rheumatoid arthritis; nd, not demonstrated.

class II molecules on endothelial cells, which results in augmented numbers of lymphocyte-binding receptors at inflammatory sites (Lipsky *et al.*, 1989). Interaction between the endothelial cell MHC class II antigen complex and CD4-positive T helper cells might thus be important in directing the traffic of specialized cell populations to the tissues. Another molecule, CD44 (p80), (including the Hermes class of lymphocyte homing receptors), is also involved in leukocyte binding to HEV during normal leukocyte circulation and at sites of tissue inflammation. A recently described endothelial cell molecule, vascular addressin, has been shown to mediate the binding of lymphocytes and has been proposed to be a ligand on HEV for the CD44 molecule in normal lymphoid tissues and at inflammatory sites (Hayes *et al.*, 1989). Human endothelial cells activated by IL-1, TNF-alpha, or LPS also starts to secrete a soluble factor (leukocyte adhesion inhibitor, LAI), which is able to attenuate the hyperadhesive interaction with leukocytes. LAI has been identified as endothelial inter-leukin 8 (IL-8) (Gimbrone *et al.*, 1989). "Natural" inhibitors like endothelial-derived IL-8 or other soluble factors, like IL-1 inhibitors, with anti-inflammatory effects may be of potential therapeutic importance in the future.

In the rheumatoid synovium, there is high spontaneous production of several potent inflammatory mediators like IL-1, IFN-gamma, and TNF-alpha. These factors can thus induce changes in the vascular endothelial cell morphology resembling HEV in normal lymphoid organs and increase the binding and the migration of leukocytes to inflamed tissues. Therefore, in the future, homing receptors and addressins might also be possible targets for therapeutic interventions in rheumatoid arthritis.

9. ACCESSORY CELLS AS TARGET FOR IMMUNE MODULATION

The pivotal role of accessory cells in immune reactions and inflammatory processes may be of importance with regard to design of therapeutic drugs and possibilities for intervention in certain autoimmune diseases such as rheumatoid arthritis (Adorini *et al.*, 1990). Different strategies have been suggested as outlined in Table V, and described as follows.

9.1. Immunomodulating Drugs

Two of the most important immunomodulatory drugs used today in autoimmunity and transplantation are corticosteroids and cyclosprine A. The main action of these two drugs is inhibition of lymphokine production in early steps in T-cell activation. Cyclosporine A seems to inhibit the transcription and production of all T-cell-derived lymphokines. Recent data also indicate that corticosteroids might have some action on accessory cells as it has been shown that the production and transcription of IL-1, IL-6, and TNF by monocytes are

TABLE V. Possible Approaches for Modulation of Accessory Cells in Autoimmune Diseases

Immunomodulating drugs	Specific inhibitors of cytokines
Monoclonal antibodies to:	Natural inhibitors
MHC molecules	Soluble receptors
Cytokines	Cytokine–toxin chimeras
Adhesion molecules	Cytokines
Peptide competition	Vaccination

blocked. Corticosteroids and cyclosporine A also down-regulate the expression of MHC class II molecules, which might be of importance in autoimmune diseases where overexpression of MHC molecules is seen at inflammatory sites, and in preventing allograft rejections (Dupont, 1988; Førre et al., 1988). Drugs like cyclophosphamide, azathioprine, and methotrexate are also currently used for the treatment of autoimmune diseases and transplantation rejection. These drugs interfere with the immune system in various ways. It is therefore also possible that they can modulate function of accessory cells (Fox and McCune, 1989).

9.2. Monoclonal Antibodies

In animals, promising results have been obtained in some spontaneous and experimentally induced autoimmune diseases, including collagen type-II–induced arthritis, after treatment with monoclonal and polyclonal anti-MHC class II antibodies (Sany, 1988). Treatment with anti-MHC class II antibodies significantly delayed the onset of the disease. The effector mechanism in anti-MHC class II treatment is not clear. It may result in inhibition of antigen presentation by blocking the binding of immunogenic peptides to the MHC molecules on the accessory cells, thus preventing activation of the T lymphocytes. MHC class II molecules expressed on accessory cells are of great importance in autoimmune diseases since they also are usually overexpressed at inflammatory sites. Autoimmune diseases are usually linked to certain MHC (HLA) types. In rheumatoid arthritis (RA), the MHC class II (HLA) types DR1 and DR4 (the subtypes Dw4, Dw14, and Dw15) predominate. The genetic linkage of HLA allotypes to autoimmune diseases could be useful in therapeutic approaches using specific antiallotype monoclonal antibodies. Treatment of autoimmune diseases in humans, including RA, with anti-MHC class II antibodies has not yet been carried out, and more data concerning efficacy and safety are needed (Sany, 1988). Monoclonal antibodies against adhesion molecules might also be a way of inducing effective immunosuppression.

Monoclonal antibodies covalently conjugated with plant or bacterial toxins (immunotoxins), that is, A-chains of ricin, have been shown to be effective in eradicating certain tumors (Thorpe et al., 1988). This approach could also be used for the treatment of autoimmune diseases like rheumatoid arthritis. In the rheumatoid synovium, most of the T cells are activated (Waalen, 1988; Waalen et al., 1988a). They constitute more than 80% of the inflammatory cells. So far, experiments using immunotoxins have been designed to eliminate the activated T cells in the rheumatoid synovium (Blakely and Thorpe, 1988). However, accessory cells like dendritic cells and macrophages at the inflammatory sites might also be useful target for immunotoxin treatment. These cells might be selectively eliminated by using immunotoxins and monoclonal antibodies against MHC class II molecules or other specific molecules expressed on the cell membrane. The monoclonal antibodies used so far have been mouse or rat antibodies. New principles for creating recombinant human monoclonal antibodies by genetic engineering, however, have greatly enhanced the possibilities for the use of specific human antibodies in the treatment of rheumatic diseases (Huse et al., 1989). Selective removal of accessory cells from the inflamed site might thus reduce the continuous stimulation/activation of reactive T lymphocytes.

9.3. Peptide Competition

T-cell immunity relies on the specific recognition of linearized peptide fragments bound to self-MHC class I or class II molecules by the T-cell antigen receptor (Møller, 1987). The interaction between peptides and purified MHC class II molecules has been shown to have unusual kinetics. The rate of association is very slow, but after the complexes have formed, they are very stable (Buus *et al.*, 1986, 1987). In experimental models it has been shown that, under physiological conditions, exchanges of different peptides in the MHC binding site can take place. It has also been shown that most MHC-binding peptides share structural motifs detectable at the level of the primary amino acid sequence. This might predict that competition occurs between peptides of unrelated sequences for the same MHC binding site. Thus it might be possible to modulate T-cell activation by interfering with the binding of antigenic peptides to MHC class II molecules (Adorini *et al.*, 1990). When peptides responsible for self-destructive autoimmune processes are characterized, this approach might be used for treatment of autoimmune diseases and also to prevent graft rejection in transplantation.

9.4. Specific Inhibitors of Cytokines (Anticytokine Antibodies, Soluble Receptors)

Recent work (Eisenberg *et al.*, 1990) reports on identification and cloning of a protein with interleukin-1 receptor antagonistic activity. The protein was cloned from human monocytes after stimulation with adherent IgG and acts as a pure receptor antagonist since it has no effect on the activity of IL-1 itself. Monocytes and dendritic cells are two of the main producers of IL-1, and high levels of IL-1 are produced at local inflammatory sites in rheumatoid arthritis (Waalen, 1988). The IL-1 receptor antagonist may thus be a useful therapeutic agent that blocks the biochemical cascade causing chronic inflammation. Preliminary studies in rats with induced experimental arthritis indicate that the inhibitor blocks swelling and cartilage degeneration in the joints (Eisenberg *et al.*, 1990). Anticytokine antibodies and soluble receptors might also be worthwhile evaluating in autoimmunity and transplantation.

9.5. Cytokine–Toxin Chimeras

In the same way as with antibody–toxin conjugates, it is possible to use cytokines with covalently bound toxins for specific elimination of cells causing inflammation in autoimmune diseases. In this way it might be possible to eliminate accessory cells or other inflammatory cells expressing receptors for the actual cytokine.

9.6. Cytokines

It is also possible that naturally occurring cytokines with immunosuppressive effects like TGF beta might be effective in the treatment of autoimmune diseases. However, studies are needed to show this.

9.7. Vaccination

Vaccination might be a new approach for treatment of autoimmune diseases. In rats it has been shown that experimental allergic encephalomyelitis (EAE) is prevented after immunization with a synthetic peptide representing residues 72–89 of a hypervariable region of a T-cell receptor (TCR) V beta 8 molecule identified on a T cell specific for the major encephalogenic epitope of the myelin basic protein (Vandenbark *et al.*, 1989). T cells specific for the TCR V beta 8 peptide also conferred passive protection against the disease on naive rats. Recent studies on the preferential use of certain TCR V region families by rheumatoid T cells might indicate that induction by accessory cells of T cells and antibody-producing B cells specific for TCR V epitopes characteristic of rheumatoid T cells could be a selective approach to the prevention of autoimmune diseases like rheumatoid arthritis (Førre and Sioud, 1991).

10. CONCLUSION

Accessory cells have important functions in mediating lymphocyte immune responses. In autoimmune diseases the accessory cells may be the driving force in perpetuating chronic reactions at inflammatory sites. Interference with and modulation of accessory cells by drugs, monoclonal antibodies, or specific peptides may thus turn out to be an interesting way in the future of treating autoimmune diseases and of preventing graft rejection after transplantation.

ACKNOWLEDGMENTS. This work was supported by grants from Norma and Leon Hess' Foundation for Research on Rheumatological Diseases, Norwegian Women's Public Health Organization, Grethe Harbitz Legacy, and the Norwegian Research Council for Science and the Humanities.

REFERENCES

Adorini, L., and Nagy, Z. A., 1990, Peptide competition for antigen presentation, *Immunol. Today* **11**:21–24.

Adorini, L., Barnaba, V., Bona, C., Celada, F., Lanzavecchia, A., Sercarz, E., Suciu-Foca, N., and Werkerle, H., 1990, New perspective on immunointervention in autoimmune diseases, *Immunol. Today* **11**:383–385.

Akira, S., Hirano, T., Taga, T., and Kishimoto, T., 1990, Biology of multifunctional cytokines: IL-6 and related molecules (IL 1 and TNF), *FASEB J.* **4**:2860–2867.

Albeda, S. M., and Buck, C. A., 1990, Integrins and other cell adhesion molecules, *FASEB J.* **4**:2868–2880.

Allen, P. M., 1987, Antigen processing at the molecular level, *Immunol. Today* **8**:270–273.

Austyn, J. M., 1987, Lymphoid dendritic cells, *Immunology* **62**:161–170.

Austyn, J. M., and Larsen, C. P., 1990, Migration pattern for dendritic leucocytes. Implications for transplantation, *Transplantation* **49**:1–7.

Bjercke, S., Lea, T., Braathen, L. R., and Thorsby, E., 1984, Enrichment of human epidermal Langerhans cells, *Scand. J. Immunol.* **11**:255–264.

Bjørkman, P. J., Saper, M. A., Samraoui, B., Bennett, W. S., Strominger, J. L., and Wiley, D. C., 1987, The foreign antigen binding site and T cell recognition regions of class I histocompatibility antigens, *Nature* **329**:512–518.

Blakely, D. C., and Thorpe, P. E., 1988, Treatment of malignant disease and rheumatoid arthritis using ricin A-chain immunotoxins, *Scand. J. Rheumatol.*, (Suppl.) **76**:279–287.

Braciale, T. J., Morrison, L. A., Sweetser, M. T., Sambrook, J., Gething, J.-J., and Braciale, V. L., 1987, Antigen presentation pathways to class I and class II MHC-restricted T lymphocytes, *Immunol. Rev.* **98**:95–114.

Brown, J. H., Jardetzky, T., Saper, M. A., Samraoui, B., Bjørkman, P. J., and Wiley, D. C., 1988, A hypothetical model of the foreign antigen binding site of class II histocompatibility molecules, *Nature* **332**:845–849.

Buus, S., Colon, S., Smith, C., Freed, J. H., Miles, C., and Grey, H. M., 1986, Interaction between a "processed" ovalbumin peptide and Ia molecules, *Proc. Natl. Acad. Sci. USA* **83**:3968–3973.

Buus, S., Sette, A., and Grey, H. M., 1987, The interaction between protein-derived immunogenetic peptides and Ia, *Immunol. Rev.* **98**:115–142.

Chain, B. M., Kay, P. M., and Feldman, M., 1986, The cellular pathway of antigen presentation: Biochemical and functional analysis of antigen in dendritic cells and macrophages, *Immunology* **58**:271–277.

Deverson, E. V., Gow, I. R., Coadwell, J., Monaco, J. J., Butcher, G. W., and Howard, J. C., 1990, MHC class II related region encoding proteins related to the multidrug resistance family of transmembrane transporters, *Nature* **348**:738–741.

Dupont, E., 1988, Immunological actions of corticosteroids and cyclosporine A, *Curr. Opin. Immunol.* **1**(2):253–256.

Eisenberg, S. P., Evans, R. J., Arend, W. P., Verderber, E., Brewer, M. T., Hannum, C. H., and Thompson, R. C., 1990, Primary structure and functional expression of a human interleukin-1 receptor antagonist, *Nature* **343**:341–346.

Førre, O., and Sioud, M., 1991, Immunosuppression therapy in rheumatoid arthritis, in: *Advances in Rheumatology and Inflammation: Trends in RA-Research* (P. Hedqvist, J. R. Kalden, R. Muller-Peddinghaus, and D. R. Robinson, eds.), *EULAR* Publishers, Basel, pp. 129–137.

Førre, Ø., Waalen, K., Thoen, J., and Hovig, T., 1985, Macrophages and dendritic cells in rheumatic diseases, in: *Immunology of Rheumatic Diseases* (S. Gupta, and N. Talal, eds.), Plenum Press, New York, pp. 543–545.

Førre, Ø., Waalen, K., Rugstad, H. E., Berg, K. J., Solbu, D., and Kåss, E., 1988, Cyclosporine and rheumatoid arthritis, *Springer Semin. Immunopathol.* **10**:263–277.

Fox, D. A., and McCune, W. J., 1989, Immunological and clinical effects of cytostatic drugs used in the treatment of rheumatoid arthritis and systemic lupus erythematosus, in: *Therapy of Autoimmune Diseases* (Concepts in Immunopathology series, Volume 7) (J. M. Cruse and R. E. Lewis, eds.), Karger, Basel, pp. 20–78.

Garrett, T. P. J., Saper, M. A., Bjørkman, P. J., Strominger, J. L., and Wiley, D. C., 1989, Specificity pockets for the side chains of peptide antigens in HLA-Aw68, *Nature* **342**:692–696.

Germain, R. N., 1986, The ins and outs of antigen processing and presentation, *Nature* **322**:687–689.

Gimbrone, M. A., Obin, M. S., Brock, A. F., Luis, E. A., Hass, P. E., Hebert, C. A., Yip, Y. K., Leung, D. W., Lowe, D. G., Kohr, W. J., Darbonne, W. C., Bechtol, K. B., and Baker, J. B., 1989, Endothelial interleukin-8: A novel inhibitor of leukocyte–endothelial interactions, *Science* **246**:1601–1603.

Haynes, B. F., Hale, L. P., Denning, S. M., Le, P. T., and Singer, K. H., 1989, The role of leukocyte adhesion molecules in cellular interactions: Implications for the pathogenesis of inflammatory synovitis, *Springer Semin. Immunopathol.* **11**:163–185.

Humphrey, J. H., Grennan, D., and Sundarm, V., 1984, The origin of follicular dendritic cells in the mouse and the mechanism of trapping immune complexes on them, *Eur. J. Immunol.* **14**:859–864.

Huse, W. D., Sastry, L., Iverson, S. A., Kang, A. S., Alting-Mees, M., Burton, D. R., Benkovic, S. J., and Lerner, R. A., 1989, Generation of a large combinatorial library of the immunoglobulin repertoire in phage lambda, *Science* **246**:1275–1281.

King, P. D., and Katz, D. R., 1990, Mechanisms of dendritic cell function, *Immunol. Today* **11**:206–211.

Koide, S. L., and Steinman, R. M., 1987, Induction of murine interleukin 1: Stimuli and responsive primary cells, *Proc. Natl. Acad. Sci. USA* **84**:3802–3806.

Kuntz-Crow, M., and Kunkel, H. G., 1982, Human dendritic cells: Major stimulators of the autologous and allogeneic mixed leukocyte reactions, *Clin. Exp. Immunol.* **49**:338–346.

Lanzavecchia, A., 1990, Receptor-mediated antigen uptake and its effect on antigen presentation to class II-restricted T lymphocytes, *Annu. Rev. Immunol.* **8**:773–793.

Lipsky, P. E., Davies, L. S., Cush, J. J., and Oppenheimer-Marks, N., 1989, The role of cytokines in the pathogenesis of rheumatoid arthritis, *Springer Semin. Immunopathol.* **11**:123–162.

MacLennan, I. M. C., Oldfield, S., Liu, Y-J., and Lane, P. J. L., 1988, Regulation of B-cell population, in: *The Cell Kinetics of the Inflammatory Reaction. Current Topics in Pathology*, Vol. 79 (O. H. Iversen, ed.), Springer Verlag, New York, pp. 37–57.

McMichael, A. J., Beverly, P. C. L., Cobbold, S., Crumpton, M. J., et al., 1989, *Leucocyte Typing III: White Blood Cell Differentiation Antigens*, Oxford University Press, Oxford.

Mills, K. H. G., 1986, Processing of viral antigens and presentation to class II-restricted T cells, *Immunol. Today* **7**:260–263.

Monaco, J. J., Cho, S., and Attaya, M., 1990, Transport protein genes in the murine MHC: Possible implications for antigen processing, *Science* **250**:1723–1726.

Møller, G., ed., 1988, Antigen processing, *Immunol. Rev.* **106**:1–187.

Natvig, J. B., and Winchester, R. eds., 1988, Immunopathology of rheumatoid inflammation, *Springer Semin. Immunopathol.* **10**:115–277.

Nuchtern, J. G., Biddison, W. E., and Klausner, R. D., 1990, Class II MHC molecules can use the endogenous pathway of antigen presentation, *Nature* **343**:74–76.

Oppenheim, J. J., Kovacs, E. J., Matsushima, K., and Durum, S. K., 1986, There is more than one interleukin 1, *Immunol. Today* **7**:45–47.

Parnes, J. R., 1986, T cell differentiation antigens: Proteins, genes and function, *BioAssays* **4**:255–259.

Pelletier, M., Tautu, C., Landry, D., Montplaisir, S., Chartrand, C., and Perreault, C., 1986, Characterization of human thymic dendritic cells in culture, *Immunology* **58**:263–270.

Poulter, L. W., Campbell, D. A., Munro, C., and Janossy, G., 1986, Discrimination of human macrophages and dendritic cells by means of monoclonal antibodies, *Scand. J. Immunol.* **24**:351–357.

Sany, J., 1988, Treatment of rheumatoid arthritis by antibodies directed against class II MHC antigens, *Scand. J. Rheumatol.* (Suppl.) **76**:289–295.

Schnitzlein, C. T., Kosco, M. H., Szakal, A. K., and Tew, J. G., 1985, Follicular dendritic cells in suspension: Identification, enrichment and initial characterization indicating immune complex trapping and lack of adherence and phagocytic activity, *J. Immunol.* **134**:1360–1368.

Steinman, R. M., and Cohn, Z. A., 1973, Identification of a novel cell type in peripheral lymphoid organs of mice. I. Morphology, quantitation and tissue distribution, *J. Exp. Med.* **137**:1142–1162.

Steinman, R., VanVoorhis, W. C., and Spalding, D. M., 1986, Dendritic cells, in: *Handbook of Experimental Immunology*, 4th ed. (D. M. Weir, C. Blackwell and L. A. Herzenberg, eds.), Blackwell Scientific Publications, Oxford, pp. 49.1–49.9.

Teyton, L., O'Sullivan, D., Dickerson, P. W., Lotteau, V., Sette, A., Fink, P., and Peterson, P. A., 1990, Invariant chain distinguishes between the exogenous and endogenous antigen presentation pathways, *Nature* **348**:39–44.

Thorpe, P. E., Wallace, P. M., et al., 1988, Improved antitumor effects of immunotoxins prepared with deglycosylated ricin A-chain and hindered disulphide-linkages, *Cancer Res.* **48**:6396–6403.

Unanue, E. R., 1984, Antigen presenting function of the macrophage, *Annu. Rev. Immunol.* **2**:385–428.

Unkeless, J. C., and Springer, T. A., 1986, Macrophages, in: *Handbook of Experimental Immunology*, 4th ed. (D. M. Weir,

C. Blackwell and L. A. Herzenberg, eds.), Blackwell Scientific Publications, Oxford, pp. 118.1–118.17.

Van Voorhis, W. C., Hair, L. S., Steinman, R. M., and Kaplan, G., 1982, Human dendritic cells: Enrichment and characterization from peripheral blood, *J. Exp. Med.* **155:**1172–1187.

Vandenbark, A. A., Hashim, G., and Offner, H., 1989, Immunization with a synthetic peptide protects against experimental autoimmune encephalomyelitis, *Nature* **341:**541–544.

van Furth, R., 1981, The origin of phagocytic cells in the joint and bone, *Scand. J. Rheumatol.* (Suppl.) **40:**13–20.

Waalen, K., 1988, Lymphoid dendritic cells in the rheumatoid inflammation, Thesis, University of Oslo.

Waalen, K., and Førre, Ø., 1992, Rheumatoid synovial dendritic cells spontaneously express mRNA for interleukin 1 and interleukin 6 (manuscript in preparation).

Waalen, K., Thoen, J., Førre, Ø., Hovig, T., Teigland, J., and Natvig, J. B., 1986a, Rheumatoid synovial dendritic cells as stimulators in allogeneic and autologous mixed leukocyte reactions—Comparison with autologous monocytes as stimulator cells, *Scand. J. Immunol.* **23:**233–243.

Waalen, K., Duff, G., Førre, Ø., Dickens, E., Kvarnes, L., and Nuki, G., 1986b, Interleukin 1 activity produced by human rheumatoid and normal dendritic cells, *Scand. J. Immunol.* **23:**365–371.

Waalen, K., Førre, Ø., Pahle, J., Natvig, J. B., and Burmester, G. R., 1987a, Characteristics of human rheumatoid synovial and normal blood dendritic cells. Retention of class II MHC antigens and accessory function during short-term culture, *Scand. J. Immunol.* **26:**525–533.

Waalen, K., Førre, Ø., Linker-Israeli, M., and Thoen, J., 1987b, Evidence of an activated T-cell system with augmented turnover of interleukin 2 in rheumatoid arthritis. Stimulation of human T lymphocytes by dendritic cells as a model for rheumatoid T-cell activation, *Scand. J. Immunol.* **25:**367–373.

Waalen, K., Førre, Ø., and Natvig, J. B., 1988a, Rheumatoid lymphoid dendritic cells—Characteristics and functions, *Scand. J. Rheumatol.*, (Suppl.) **76:**47–60.

Waalen, K., Førre, Ø., and Natvig, J. B., 1988b, Lymphoid dendritic cells in rheumatoid tissue and normal blood—Characteristics and functions, in: *Histophysiology of the Immune System: The Life, Organization and Interactions of its Cell Population* (S. Fossum, and B. Rolstad, eds.), Plenum Press, New York, pp. 761–765.

Watts, C., and Howard, J. C., 1986, Membrane recycling and antigen presentation, *BioAssays* **4:**265.

Weaver, C. T., and Unanue, E. R., 1990, The costimulatory function of antigen-presenting cells, *Immunol. Today* **11:**49–55.

Werb, Z., Banda, M. J., Takemura, R., and Gordon, S., 1986, Secreted proteins of resting and activated macrophages, in: *Handbook of Experimental Immunology*, 4th ed, (D. M. Weir, C. Blackwell and L. A. Herzenberg, eds.), Blackwell Scientific Publications, Oxford, pp. 47.1–47.29.

Yewdell, J. W., and Bennink, J. R., 1990, The binary logic of antigen processing and presentation to T cells, *Cell* **62:**203–206.

Chapter 3

B CELLS IN AUTOIMMUNITY

Øystein Førre, Kristian Waalen, Jens Kjeldsen-Kragh,
Dag Sørskaar, Ove J. Mellbye, and Jacob B. Natvig

1. INTRODUCTION

The antibody production by cells of the B-cell lineage have an intricate connection with antigen-presenting cells and T cells, the mediators of cell-mediated immunity. This means that to a large extent the antibody production is T-cell dependent. Many soluble products of both T helper cells and antigen-presenting cells (APC) (interleukins) have stimulatory effects on the proliferation and maturation of B cells.

There is a fundamental difference in the manner by which B cells and T cells recognize antigens, foreign or self. The immunoglobulin molecules (receptors) of B cells are capable of binding native antigen alone in solution. Since B cells recognize primarily intact protein, antibody–antigen interactions are often dependent on three-dimensional conformation. T cells are blind to intact native antigen molecules; antigen must be processed (cleaved into peptide fragments) and the peptide fragments are then presented on the surface of specialized antigen-presenting cells in association with class II or class I major histocompatibility complex (MHC) molecules that serve as the target for CD4+ and CD8+ T cells, respectively.

Low levels of nonpathologic "natural" autoantibodies are found in the normal state. Although autoantibodies are a predominant feature of many diseases, the factors that lead to their production and their role in pathogenesis remain largely unresolved. In many cases, autoantibodies may simply be epiphenomena, appearing as a result of, rather than being responsible for, the primary autoimmune process. For example, type I diabetes seems to be primarily mediated by T cells, even though a large majority of patients develop antibodies to pancreatic beta cells. Autoantibodies may be involved in effecting or perpetuating tissue damage rather than initiating it (Sinha *et al.*, 1990). Cells of the B-cell lineage and their

Øystein Førre and *Dag Sørskaar* • Oslo Sanitetsforening Rheumatism Hospital, N-0172, Oslo 1, Norway. *Kristian Waalen* • Department of Animal Genetics, National College of Veterinary Medicine, and the Institute of Immunology and Rheumatology, The National Hospital, 0033 Oslo 1, Norway. *Present Address:* Vaccine Department, National Institute of Public Health, N-0472 Oslo 4, Norway. *Jens Kjeldsen-Kragh, Ove J. Mellbye,* and *Jacob B. Natvig* • Institute of Immunology and Rheumatology, The National Hospital, N-0172 Oslo 1, Norway.

Immunopharmacology in Autoimmune Diseases and Transplantation, edited by Hans Erik Rugstad *et al.* Plenum Press, New York, 1992.

products (autoantibodies) seem, however, to play an important role for the pathogenesis of autoimmune diseases like systemic lupus erythematosus (SLE) and rheumatoid arthritis (RA) and vasculitis syndromes.

Although autoantibodies can clearly be involved in the effector phase of autoimmunity, the induction of disease most likely involves T cells. Because B cells require T cell help, most immune responses begin with the activation of $CD4^+$ T helper cells in a ternary complex with MHC and peptide. Thus, the control of self–nonself discrimination is largely the responsibility of the T-cell compartment. Multispecific antibodies in response to previous transfusions or previous transplantation and isohemagglutinins may also cause acute and hyperacute rejection of transplanted organs.

2. ORGANIZATION AND EXPRESSION OF IMMUNOGLOBULIN GENES

Important for understanding the B-cell biology is the fact that the B-cell repertoire (the capacity to recognize a myriad of different antigens) is formed in an antigen-independent fashion. Thus long before encountering antigen, individually distinct immunoglobulin molecules are assembled in developing B cells and subsequently expressed at the cell surface of mature B cells as complete membrane-bound immunoglobulin molecules. The organization of immunoglobulin (Ig) genes, like that of T-cell receptor genes, involves recombination between genes and encoding of the variable and constant parts of the receptor molecule (Tonegawa, 1983; Hood *et al.*, 1985).

The variable region of the heavy (H) chain of the Ig molecule is encoded by three germ line DNA segments: A V_H, which is hooked up to a D (diversity) segment, which in turn is linked to a J_H (joining segment). These V_H, D_H, and J_H segments are encoded in three separate gene clusters in the Ig locus on chromosome 14 of humans.

The variable region of the kappa and lambda light chain are encoded by two germ line DNA segments: V_L and J_L. Genes encoding human kappa and lambda light chain regions are located on chromosome 2 and 22, respectively (Alt *et al.*, 1986). The rearrangements of the Ig heavy chain genes and the kappa light chain genes are shown in Figure 3.1.

The different germ line elements are separated by noncoding regions of varying lengths. The different gene segments are coupled to each other during B-cell differentiation by a controlled recombination process (Alt *et al.*, 1986).

The usage of V, D, and J segments creates a large number of different possibilities. Additional variability of antigen-binding regions is created by imprecision in the joining process leading to loss or gain of nucleotides of the gene segments (Alt *et al.*, 1986). The exact number of VDJ heavy and VJ light segments in the human genome is not known at present, but the situation is closely analogous to that in the mouse. In the mouse there are 500 V_H, 15 D_H, and 4 J_H segments, in addition to 200 V_L kappa and four V_J kappa segments (Goverman *et al.*, 1986). In the mouse, in contrast to humans, lambda light chains contribute only little to the repertoire.

Assembled variable region genes are transcribed and eventually fused to a constant region encoding sequence to form the complete heavy or light chain messenger RNA (Fig. 3.1). The first constant region gene available to the heavy chain variable gene transcript is the C *my* gene. The complete mRNA for the *my* chain of the IgM is thus generated and the *my* chain synthesis can start. By recombination of V_H transcripts to constant H chain genes further downstream (class switching), other classes of immunoglobulin heavy chain are produced in the following sequence: μ, δ, γ_3, γ_1, α_1, γ_2, γ_4, ϵ, α_2. The class switching has been shown to be regulated by cytokines like interferon-γ (IFN-γ), interleukin-4 (IL-4) (Paliard *et al.*, 1988), and transforming growth factor β (TGF-β) (Kehrl

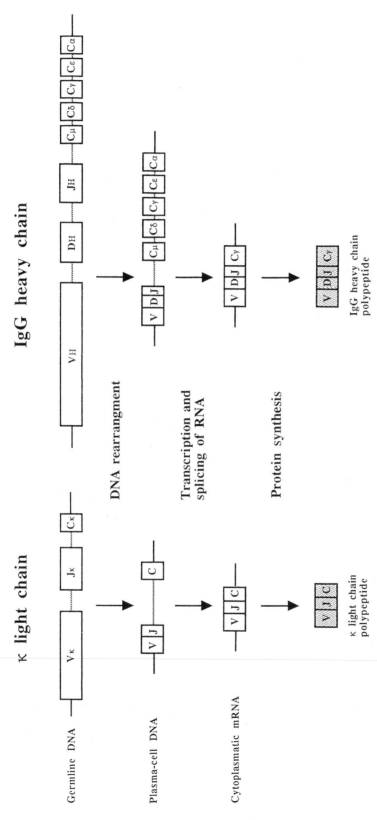

FIGURE 3.1. Schematic presentation of the sequence of events from rearrangement of the germ line DNA before birth to the production of a light chain polypeptide (exemplified by κ-light chain) and a heavy chain polypeptide (exemplified by IgG heavy chain) in the mature plasma cell. There are approximately 50–300 different V_κ gene segments, 5 J_κ segments, and only one C_κ segment. The heavy chain loci are comprised of 10^2–10^3 V_H gene segment, 10–20 D_H segments, 6 J_H segments, 4 $C\gamma$ segments, 2 $C\alpha$ segments, and one segment each of $C\mu$, $C\epsilon$, and $C\delta$. The final immunoglobulin molecule consists of two identical light chains (κ- or γ chains) and two identical heavy chains.

et al., 1986). Recent experiments have shown that cytokine-induced immunoglobulin class switching is accomplished by intramolecular DNA deletion (Matsuoka *et al.*, 1990).

3. ACTIVATION OF B CELLS

Only a few antigens are able to elicit antibody production without a need for T helper cell assistance. Principally, antibody production and regulation result from cooperation and interactions between accessory cells (macrophages, monocytes, and dendritic cells), T lymphocytes, and B lymphocytes (Melchers and Andersson, 1986). B-cell activation is a result of binding of antigen to surface immunoglobulin and influence of soluble T-cell products (cytokines) (Melchers and Andersson, 1986; Lipsky *et al.*, 1988).

A typical T-cell-dependent antibody response can be described in the following way: The T-cell receptor (TCR) (alpha/beta and possibly also gamma/delta) on CD4+ T helper cells react with a complex consisting of antigen bound to HLA class II molecules (HLA-DP, -DQ, and -DR) on accessory cells. Signals are transduced via the TCR-associated CD_3 polypeptides to the interior of the T cell, leading via many events to induction of genes. This in turn, leads to expression of activation markers, secretion of lymphokines, and T cell proliferation. The activated T helper cells start the production of cytokines such as interleukin-2 (IL-2), IFN-γ, IL-4, interleukin-5 (IL-5), and interleukin-6 (IL-6), which all have stimulatory effects on the B-cell maturation and proliferation (Table I) (Jelinck and Lipsky 1987; Gupta, 1988; Chapter 6, this volume). In addition to these T-cell-derived cytokines, there are also other cytokines produced by stromal cells of bone marrow and of lymphoid organs (Henney, 1989) and by monocytes/macrophages (Gupta, 1988) and dendritic cells (Waalen *et al.*, 1986; Førre *et al.*, 1989), which stimulate B-cell/antibody production. These are IL-1β, IL-6, IL-7, and tumor necrosis factor-α (TNF-α). In contrast with these activities, TGF-β inhibits B-cell proliferation and B-cell differentiation (Wahl *et al.*, 1989) (Table I).

4. MATURATION OF B LYMPHOCYTES AS REFLECTED BY EXPRESSION OF CELL SURFACE MARKERS

Cytoplasmatic μ chain is the first Ig gene product to become expressed during B-cell maturation (Jellinck and Lipsky, 1987). The cell at this stage is called a pre-B cell. Pre-B cells express the CD10 surface marker (common ALL antigen, CALLA) and the CD19 antigen, which is also a specific differentiation marker for B cells. Pre-B cells also express HLA class II antigen and terminal transferase (TdT) activity in the cytoplasm.

The CD19 and HLA class II markers remain expressed during the maturation and activation process of the B cells. During maturation of pre-B cells to B cells, Ig light chains are synthesized, allowing surface expression of IgM/IgD. The CD20 marker is pan-B-specific and is expressed on surface Ig+ B cells. Like the CD19 marker, the CD20 marker remains expressed up to the plasma cell stage. At that stage both the CD19, the CD20 markers, and the HLA class II antigens are lost. TdT is only expressed in early B cells, probably because this enzyme is involved in the Ig gene assembly. The CD10 marker is lost slightly later than the TdT activity (Alt *et al.*, 1986).

Another functionally interesting surface structure is the receptor for the C3d fragment of complement (CR2). This receptor is B-cell-specific and also known as the CD21 antigen of B cells. Polyclonal and monoclonal anti-CR2 antibodies stimulate B cells to proliferate

TABLE I. Effects of Various Cytokines on Antigen-Specific B Cells

	Interleukin alone		Interleukin + antigen	
	Proliferation	Antibody formation	Proliferation	Antibody formation
IL-1	−	±	+ +	+ +
IL-2	−	±	+ +	+ +
IL-3	+	−	±	±
IL-4	+ +	±	+ + +	±
IL-5	−	±		+ +
IL-6	−	+		
IL-7[a]	+ +	−	−	−
TGF$_\beta$	I		I	
γIFN	−		+ +	

[a]IL-7 stimulate the proliferation of pre-β/pro β cells but not the proliferation of mature B cells (Henney, 1989).
+, Stimulation; −, no effect; I, inhibition.
This table is based on Henney (1989), Wahl et al. (1989), Di Giovine et al. (1988), and Chapter 6, this volume.

and differentiate in the presence of T cells or T-derived soluble factors (Frade et al., 1985; Wilson et al., 1985; Melchers and Andersson, 1986). CR2 also serves as the receptor for Epstein-Barr virus (EBV) on human B cells (Fingeroth et al., 1984). Recently it has also been reported that a monoclonal antibody that functionally blocks CR2 can inhibit antibody production (Heyman et al., 1990).

Binding of EBV to the receptor may be one of the signals causing B-cell proliferation by EBV, but clearly not the only one (Golay, 1986; Melchers and Andersson, 1986; Zola, 1987). The complement receptor CR1, the C3b receptor, may also be involved in human B-cell triggering (Daha et al., 1984). In the mouse, C3b or C3d, either aggregated or Sepharose-bound, can replace accessory cell factors in the B-cell cycle (Melchers and Andersson, 1986).

The B cell markers in relation to the maturation step are shown in Tables II and III. Follicular dendritic cells have been identified in sections of lymphoid follicles. These cells are localized in close contact with B cells. The follicular dendritic cells are probably accessory cells for B cells and may exert their function through trapping of immune complexes on their surface (Humphrey et al., 1984).

TABLE II. B-Cell Differentiation and Immunoglobulin Expression

				B lymphocyte		
Cell type	Pluripotential stem cell	Committed progenitor	Pre-B cell	Immature/ resting	Mature/ activated	Plasma cell
Immunoglobulin genes	Germ line	V_H rearranged	V_H transcribed	V_H and V_L rearranged and subject to mutation		
Immunoglobulin expression	Nil	Nil	Cytoplasmic μ	Membrane IgM	Membrane IgM/D/G etc.	Cytoplasmic and secreted
	Maturation independent of antigen			Maturation driven by antigen		

TABLE III. Expression of B-Cell Markers, Relation to the Maturation Step of B Cells

| | Cell type | | | | | |
| | | | | B lymphocyte | | |
Markers	Pluripotential stem cell	Committed progenitor	Pre-B cell	Immature/ resting	Mature/ activated	Plasma
MHC class II		————————————————————————				
CD10 (CALLA)			————————			
CD19 (p95)		———————————————————————				
CD20 (p35)		———————————————————————				
CD21 (p140)				————————————		
CR1				————————————		
Terminal transferase		———————————————				

Note: Solid lines in columns indicate the presence of marker during B-cell maturation.

5. B CELLS, AUTOANTIBODIES, AND IMMUNE COMPLEXES

Besides producing antibodies, another important function of the B cells is probably to act as antigen-presenting cells *in vivo* (Ashwell, 1988). Thus, the B cells are involved in T-cell activation. The B lymphocytes are also involved in the pathogenesis of various diseases through their production of autoantibodies and through the subsequent formation of immune complexes. In mice, B lymphocytes can be divided into two populations of distinct lineages: the conventional bone marrow-derived B-cell subset and the self-renewing peripheral subset. B lymphocytes of the latter lineage express an antigen initially described as T-cell-specific: the Ly-1 (mice) or the CD5 antigen (Maini and Plater-Zyberk, 1988).

It has been shown that both in rheumatoid arthritis and in primary Sjögren's syndrome there is an increase in circulating CD5+ B cells (Plater-Zyberk *et al.*, 1985; Youinou *et al.*, 1988). Furthermore, a high percentage of the CD5+ B cells appear to develop into plasma cells that produce IgM rheumatoid factor and other autoantibodies (Dighiero *et al.*, 1983; Logtenberg *et al.*, 1987). One hypothesis is that the persistence of a high number of CD5+ B cells in adulthood may predispose to chronic inflammatory arthritis due to the reactivity of their antigen receptor with a variety of autoantigens in the joint (Maini and Plater-Zyberk, 1988).

However, recent experiments indicate that CD5+ B lymphocytes are committed to the production of a discrete type of antibody that is polyreactive. Polyreactive antibodies appear to use selected V gene segments—mostly in an unmutated configuration—and generally display relatively low affinity for different antigens (Randen *et al.*, 1990). They are often part of the primary response to a defined antigen. Polyreactive antibodies probably play a major role *in vivo* as a first line of defense against infectious agents: they would help to temporarily prevent invasion by microorganisms at the onset of the infection, but their relatively poor fit for the antigenic determinants on the invading agents would not usually suffice to completely eradicate these pathogens. Only the high-affinity antibodies (mainly IgG) that appear late in the antibody response could accomplish this.

Experiments have clearly established that the "autoantibodies" normally produced by CD5+ B cells (polyreactive and low affinity) differ functionally from the autoantibodies that are characteristic of various autoimmune diseases (monoreactive and high affinity). These monoreactive high-affinity autoantibodies are produced by cells that are consistently detectable only in autoimmune patients. As in the case of the maturation of the response to an exogenous antigen, these cells are probably the progeny of lymphocytes that underwent an antigen-driven process of somatic point mutation and positive selection (Randen et al., 1989; Casali and Notkins 1990).

Antibodies are also involved in hyperacute rejection after organ transplantation. This can be caused by preformed isohemagglutinins (anti-A and anti-B) that are circulating in the plasma of the recipient. The rejection can also be due to circulating antibodies that are caused by presensitization (pregnancy, blood transfusion, previous organ transplantation).

Many types of organ-specific and organ-nonspecific autoantibodies have been characterized. However, in this book we will concentrate on three types of autoantibodies, namely, the rheumatoid factors, the antinuclear autoantibodies, and antimitochondrial antibodies.

5.1. Rheumatoid Factor

Rheumatoid factor (RF) is the major B-cell response seen in the rheumatoid synovial inflammation. These autoantibodies belong to most of the Ig classes, but IgG and IgM predominate. However, IgA rheumatoid factor has also frequently been seen. The RF antibodies bind to IgG (its antigen) and make complexes that can build up lattice and thus form the complexes seen in the rheumatoid synovial tissue (Natvig et al., 1989). The large complement-binding complexes in the tissues are found both in the intracellular spaces and inside the macrophages. Similarly, both intracellular and soluble complexes with strong complement-binding ability are seen in the joint fluid. In serum the complexes are small and mostly non-complement-fixing (Pope et al., 1975; Winchester, 1975; Mannik et al., 1988).

Concerning immune complexes in the various compartments in rheumatoid arthritis (RA), there appears to be a gradient with the largest complexes in the synovial tissue (Table III). Many of these complexes move into the joint fluid, while only the smallest and most soluble complexes, which are probably the least pathogenetic, spill over into the general circulation. The RF-containing complexes, particularly those containing IgG1 and IgG3 RF, are probably an important part of the pathogenetic mechanism in RA because of their efficient activation of complement and because of their ability to form complexes even inside the plasma cells where they are produced (Munthe and Natvig, 1972; Natvig and Munthe, 1975) (Table IV).

At least two pathogenetic mechanisms that might aggravate the disease process in RA emerge from the observation presented above:

1. When the Ig products of the plasma cells are secreted in a complexed form, this may prevent the normal feedback mechanisms that are important for the down-regulation of the antibody response.
2. The immune complexes may represent a fresh antigen stimulation for B cells producing RF. The IgG complexes are probably taken up by macrophages, degraded, and presented by accessory cells for T helper cells, which are supporting the help for RF-producing B cells.

TABLE IV. Immune Complexes and Rheumatoid Factors (RF) in Rheumatoid Arthritis (RA)

	Immune complexes	RF
Joint tissue	Large, insoluble; bind complement	Mostly IgG, some IgM
Joint fluid	Large, mostly soluble; bind complement	Mostly IgG, some IgM
Serum	Small ("intermediate"); mostly not complement-binding	Mostly IgM, some IgG

One important challenge in understanding the rheumatoid inflammatory process is the question of why and how RF antibodies constitute a pathogenetic mechanism in RA, whereas they are a physiological response in normal individuals upon antigenic stimulation, for example, vaccination. Patients with M-components with RF activity are in a different group again, because these patients have no signs of RA. Some clear differences have now been found between RF antibodies in RA, those in normal individuals, and those in diseases like mixed cryoglobulinemia and Waldenström's macroglobulinemia, where RF antibodies occur spontaneously within M-components (Natvig *et al.*, 1989) (Table V):

1. In RA and normal individuals, the RF production is T cell-dependent, antigen-driven, and polyclonal. On the other hand, in patients with M-components with RF, the response is T cell-independent, not antigen-driven, and monoclonal and malignant.
2. In RA, RF antibodies are produced to a large extent locally in the synovial tissues and have their main pathogenetic effects there. In normal individuals and patients with M-component RF, the RF antibodies are produced in the ordinary lymphoid tissues and RF-producing cells do not home to the joints.
3. In normal individuals virtually all RF antibodies are of the IgM type. In M-components they may be both IgM and IgG, but the IgG type, which appears to be the more pathogenic, produces circulating immune complexes that primarily affect the kidneys and not the joints. In RA, the RF antibodies are both IgM and IgG, and here, too, the IgG type seems to be the more pathogenic and primarily causes arthritis. IgM appears to escape into the circulation and probably does not cause much harm.
4. There also appear to be differences in the structure of the variable regions of the different types of RF antibodies. We and others have found similar cross-idiotypic groups in RF from RA patients and RF M-components in other diseases and also clear differences (Førre *et al.*, 1979; Crowley *et al.*, 1988). For example, the majority of the RF M-component proteins express the same cross-idiotype and belong to the V_k III variable region subgroup. They commonly utilize two variable light chain genes, V 325 and V 328, related to the 17.109 and 6B6.6 idiotypic groups, respectively (Carson *et al.*, 1987; Crowley *et al.*, 1988). In contrast, the 17.109 subgroup represents only 5% or less of the RF in a panel of RA sera (Carson *et al.*, 1987; Crowley *et al.*, 1988). In a recent study, only 3 of 14 human monoclonal IgM RFs derived from the polyclonal repertoire of rheumatoid synovial tissue expressed the 17.109 cross-idiotype (Thompson *et al.*, 1990).

Rheumatoid factor autoantibodies reacting with the constant regions of IgG heavy chains are also often produced in patients with SLE and Sjögren's syndrome and in other autoimmune diseases, as well as in various infectious diseases like subacute bacterial endocarditis (Fong *et al.*, 1985). They most probably participate in the pathogenesis of autoimmune diseases by forming immune complexes.

TABLE V. Comparison of Rheumatoid Factor (RF) Antibodies in Various Conditions

	RF antibodies in M-components	RA	Normal immunization
Antigen-driven	−	+	+
T cell-dependent	−	+	+
Clonality	Monoclonal	Polyclonal	Polyclonal
Ig class	IgG and IgM	IgG and IgM	IgM
Character	Malignant	Benign, chronic, self-perpetuating	Benign, self-limiting

5.2. Antinuclear Antibodies

B cells also have been shown to be in an activated state in the peripheral blood of SLE patients (Ginsberg *et al.*, 1979). It has also been shown that there is an increased production of cytokines that promote B-cell maturation in this disease (Alarcon-Segovia, 1988). Autoantibodies demonstrated in SLE and other autoimmune diseases such as drug-induced autoimmunity, mixed connective tissue disease (MCTD), Sjögren's syndrome, dermatomyositis, and scleroderma range from antibodies reactive with nucleic acids to antibodies reactive with nucleic acid-binding proteins (Tan, 1989) (Table VI).

The autoantibodies in SLE may be deleterious and cause disease by different mechanisms:

1. The autoantibodies can participate in the formation of immune complexes leading to immune-mediated tissue damage after complement activation.
2. The autoantibodies can interact with self-antigens and cause antibody-dependent cytotoxicity often mediated by complement or Fc-receptor-bearing cytotoxic cells.
3. The autoantibodies may also interact in various ways with cells of the immune system and accentuate or modulate their dysregulation.

5.3. Antimitochondrial Antibodies

Antimitochondrial antibodies are closely associated with primary biliary cirrhosis (PBC), a chronic liver disease characterized by spontaneous destruction of bile ducts, which often ends in liver failure. In PBC there are striking B-cell abnormalities, including high levels of serum immunoglobulins with a relative IgG3 subclass restriction, several types of autoantibodies including antimitochondrial antibodies, circulating immunocomplexes containing the relevant mitochondrial antigens, increased complement consumption and activation, and occasionally anticentromeric antigen (MacKay and Gershwin, 1989). Therefore, PBC has been considered as a "model" in autoimmune disease, although the relevance of the antimitochondrial antibodies to the pathogenesis of PBC is still unknown.

Recently, considerable progress has been made in the characterization of the molecular basis of the mitochondrial autoreactivity in PBC. The antimitochondrial antibodies recognize a cluster of four major mitochondrial inner membrane proteins, called M2, of approx-

TABLE VI. Antinuclear Antibodies and Main Disease Associations

Antibody specificity	Primary disease associations
DNA	Systemic lupus erythematosus (SLE)
Histone	SLE, drug-induced LE
RNP	Mixed connective tissue disease, overlapping syndromes, SLE
Sm	SLE
SSA (Ro)	Primary Sjögren's
SSB (Ha, La)	Primary Sjögren's
SSC (RANA)	Rheumatoid arthritis
Centromere	Primary biliary cirrhosis
PM1	Myositis
Sc170	Systemic sclerosis
Jo1	Myositis and pulmonary fibrosis
SL (Ki)	SLE

imately 74, 52, 45, and 39 kDa, which are found in mitochondria of mammals and microorganisms (Frazer et al., 1985). The cloning of the cDNA for mitochondrial antigens has led to the identification of the antigens as three enzymes of the t-oxo-acid dehydrogenase family. The autoantigens are associated with the so-called E2 subunit of these enzymes (Gershwin et al., 1988; MacKay and Gershwin, 1989). The autoepitope was identified as a decapeptide.

If the antimitochondrial antibodies are pathogenetically important, it is still unknown how such antibodies, directed against an epitope on an intracellular organelle, can get access to its antigen. It is also difficult to understand why the disease predominantly affects cells of the bile duct, although the antigen is present in all cells in the body. It has been claimed, though, that the antigens may also be present on the surface of cells under certain circumstances (MacKay and Gershwin, 1989), and it has also been suggested that bile duct cells may be especially vulnerable to antibody penetration because of an abnormality in the composition of bile.

Although the antigen for antimitochondrial antibodies has been well characterized, there is evidence that primary antigenic stimulants for production of such antibodies may be in bacteria. It seems that the relevant antigens are expressed in gram-negative bacteria (Stemerowicz et al., 1988). It has previously been suggested that since the structure and metabolism of mitochondria are similar to those of aerobic bacteria, the mitochondria may have evolved from free-living prokaryotes taken up by amoeboid cells, with a subsequent integration of mitochondrial metabolism.

5.4. Other Antibodies and Circulating Immune Complexes

Systemic lupus erythematosus patients also often have autoantibodies that react with surface antigens on lymphocytes, other leukocytes, erythrocytes, platelets, neurons, or with antigenic molecules present in various cell population such as HLA class II antigens (Alarcon-Segovia, 1988). Another clinically important autoantibody is the anti-glomerular basement membrane (anti-GBM) antibody, which causes the glomerular and pulmonary damage and nephrotoxic nephritis in Goodpasture's syndrome. The studies of the GBM antigen involved in anti-GBM nephritis have been complicated by the complex and highly cross-linked organization of the basement membrane. The epitope, however, has been localized to a small peptide on a globular domain termed M2, probably on a kidney-specific collagen IV chain (Butkowski et al., 1985). The primary antigenic stimulus causing the B cells to produce this antibody is still unknown.

The autoantibodies to formed elements of the blood and to GBM are examples of autoantibodies that can directly cause disease. In other instances the pathogenetic effect of both autoantibodies and other antibodies is mediated via the formation of immune complexes, complexes causing complement activation and thereby secondary tissue damage. Circulating immune complexes and local deposition of immune complexes in tissues have been demonstrated in a number of clinical conditions, primarily in SLE, RA, and various forms of nephritis.

6. DRUG-INDUCED AUTOIMMUNITY

Drug-induced autoimmunity is of special interest since the etiologic agent is known. The most frequent observation of this type of autoimmunity is the production of antinuclear antibodies after use of procainamide, more rarely by hydralazine, quinidine, and several other classes of drugs. Usually antibodies to denatured DNA and histones are found, but in contrast to SLE there are usually no antibodies to native DNA or extractable nuclear antigens (ENA) antigens. Another characteristic is that only 15–20% of patients with these autoantibodies will develop clinical symptoms. This depends partly on genetic factors, but there is also a clear difference in the distribution of specificities to various types of histones between patients with clinical symptoms and patients without.

Another example is D-penicillamine, which can cause production of anti-glomerulus basement membrane (GBM) leading to Goodpasture's disease, anti-skin antibodies leading to pemphigus, and other autoantibodies related to serious clinical conditions (Smith and Hammarström, 1985). Autoantibodies induced by drugs should represent a good model for studying the abnormalities in B cells related to autoimmunity.

7. IMMUNE INTERVENTION

7.1. Glucocorticoids

Proliferation of and antibody formation by B cells in the presence of appropriate growth and differentiation factors are relatively resistant to glucocorticoids (Paavonen, 1985; Chapter 8, this volume). However, it has been shown that these drugs inhibit in vivo Ig production while they may have both stimulatory and inhibitory effects on in vitro Ig production. Glucocorticoids can also inhibit B-cell responses indirectly via effects on T cells (Chapter 8, this volume) and on accessory cells (Chapter 2, this volume).

7.2. Cytotoxic Drugs

7.2.1. Alkylating Drugs

Cyclophosphamide taken orally often results in a marked B- and T-cell lymphopenia and decreased serum Ig levels (Cubbs et al., 1982). It also seems that B lymphocytes are more sensitive to cyclophosphamide treatment than T lymphocytes (Cubbs et al., 1982).

7.2.2. Folic Acid Antagonists

Methotrexate (MTX) is commonly used for the treatment of rheumatoid arthritis, juvenile rheumatoid arthritis, and psoriasis. Low-dose MTX treatment is reported to reduce IgM rheumatoid factor synthesis during the first 24 hr of treatment (Olsen et al., 1987). Decreases in total IgM production have also been noted in RA patients on MTX treatment (Olsen et al., 1987) as well as decreases in serum IgG levels (Andersen et al., 1985). It is not known whether the suppressive effect of MTX is exerted directly on the B cells or indirectly via actions on regulatory T cells or on accessory cells like macrophages and dendritic cells.

7.2.3. Thiopurines (Azathiopurine, 6-Mercaptopurine)

A selective suppressive effect on B cells by these drugs has been suggested (Dimitriu and Fauci, 1978). It has been shown that azathiopurine selectively affects the sensitivity of B cells to signals produced by helper T cells in vitro (Duclos et al., 1982). However, most experimental data both in man and animals favor a preferential effect on T lymphocytes

(Chapter 9, this volume). Thus, T cell-dependent responses are more affected than those of B cells alone both *in vivo* and *in vitro*.

7.2.4. Cyclosporine A

Cyclosporine A can suppress antibody production indirectly by suppressing T helper cell activity (Carmistuli, 1981). Cyclosporine also indirectly inhibits B-cell function and early B-cell activation by direct effect on B cells (Muraguchi *et al.*, 1983).

7.2.5. Monoclonal Antibodies

Theoretically, one way of eradicating harmful B cells would be to treat patients with monoclonal anti-idiotype antibodies coupled to toxins or radioactive isotypes. Such anti-idiotype reagents have been produced against both rheumatoid factor and antinuclear antibodies (Carson *et al.*, 1987; Schoenfeld, 1990).

ACKNOWLEDGMENTS. The Norma and Leon Hess Foundation for Rheumatology Research, the Norwegian Woman's Health Organization, and the Grethe Harbitz Legacy are gratefully acknowledged for financial support, and Bente Brenna and Suzanne Garman-Vik for secretarial assistance.

REFERENCES

Alarcon-Segovia, D., 1988, Systemic lupus erythematosus, in: *Immunopathogenetic Mechanisms of Arthritis* (J. Gordacre and W. Carson Dick, eds.), MTP Press Limited, Lancaster, pp. 198–210.

Alt, F. W., Blackwell, T. K., De Pinho, R. A., Reth, M. G., and Yancopoulos, G. D., 1986, Regulation of genome rearrangement events during lymphocyte differentiation, *Immunol. Rev.* **89**:5–30.

Andersen, P. A., West, S. G., O'Dell, J. R., Via, C. S., Claypool, R. G., and Kotzin, B. L., 1985, Weekly pulse methotrexate in rheumatoid arthritis. Clinical and immunological effects in a randomized double-blind study, *Ann. Intern. Med.* **103**:489–496.

Ashwell, G. D., 1988, Are B lymphocytes the principal antigen presenting cells *in vivo? J. Immunol.* **140**:3697–3700.

Butowski, R., Wieslander, J., Wisdom, B., Barr, J., Noelken, M., and Hudson, B., 1985, Properties of the globular domain of type IV collagen and its relationship to the Goodpasture antigen, *J. Biol. Chem.* **260**:3739–3747.

Carmistuli, S., 1981, Inhibition of a secondary humoral immune response by cyclosporin A, *Transplant. Clin. Immunol.* **13**:15–20.

Carson, D. A., Chen, P. P., Kipps, T. J., Rodaux, V., Jirik, F., Goldfien, R. D., Fox, R. I., Silverman, G. J., and Fong, S., 1987, Molecular basis of the cross-reactive idiotypes on human anti-IgG autoantibodies (rheumatoid factors), *Ciba Found. Symp.* **129**:123–132.

Casali, P., and Notkins, A. L., 1990, CD5+ B lymphocytes, polyreactive antibodies and the human B cell repertoire, *Immunol. Today* **10**:364–368.

Crowley, J. J., Goldfien, R. D., Schrohenloher, R. E., Spiegelberg, H. L., Silverman, G. T., Mageed, R. A., Jefferis, R., Koopman, W. J., Carson, D. A., and Fong, S., 1988, Incidence of three cross-reactive idiotypes on human rheumatoid factor paraproteins, *J. Immunol.* **140**:3411–3419.

Cubbs, T. R., Edgar, L. C., and Fauci, A. S., 1982, Suppression of human B-lymphocyte function by cyclophosphamide, *J. Immunol.* **128**:2453–2457.

Daha, M. A., Bloem, A. C., and Ballieux, R. E., 1984, Immunoglobulin production by human peripheral lymphocytes induced by anti-C3 receptor antibodies, *J. Immunol.* **132**:1197–1201.

Dighiero, G., Lymburi, P., Mazie, G. C., Rouyre, S., Butler-Browne, G. S., Whalen, R. T., and Armameas, S., 1983, Murine hybridomas secreting natural monoclonal antibodies reacting with self antigens, *J. Immunol.* **131**:2267–2272.

Di Giovine, F. D., Symons, G. A., Manson, J., and Duff, G., 1988, Soluble mediators of immunity. Interleukins, in: *Immuno-pathogenetic Mechanisms of Arthritis* (G. Goodacre and W. Carson Dick, eds.) MTP Press Limited, Lancaster, pp. 102–121.

Dimitriu, A., and Fauci, A. S., 1978, Activation of human B lymphocytes. XI. Differential effect of azathioprine on B lymphocytes and lymphocyte subpopulations regulating B cell function, *J. Immunol.* **121**:2335–2342.

Duclos, H., Maillof, M. C., and Galanaud, P., 1982, Differential effects of azathioprine on T cells regulating murine B cell function, *Immunology* **46**:595–602.

Fingeroth, J. D., Weis, G. G., Tedder, T. F., Strominger, J. L., Biro, P. A., and Fearon, D. T., 1984, Epstein-Barr virus receptor of human B-lymphocytes is the C3d receptor CR2, *Proc. Natl. Acad. Sci. USA* **81**:4510–4513.

Fong, S., Carson, D. A., and Vaughan, J., 1985, Rheumatoid factor, in: *Immunology of Rheumatic Diseases* (S. Gupta and N. Talal, eds.) Plenum Press, New York, pp. 167–196.

Førre, Ø., Dobloug, J. H., Michaelsen, T. E., and Natvig, J. B., 1979, Evidence of similar idiotype determinants on different rheumatoid factor populations, *Scand. J. Immunol.* **9**:281–289.

Førre, Ø., Waalen, K., and Natvig, J. B., 1989, Evidence for lymphoid dendritic cells as the driving force in rheumatoid inflammation, in: *Proceedings of the ILAR'89 Congress* (W. H. Chadade, R. D. Giorgi, E. M. Hirose-Pastor, and E. I. Sato, eds.), Rio de Janeiro, Sao Paulo, Brazil: Companhia Mellhoramentos de Sao Paulo, pp. 354–358.

Frade, R., Crevon, M. C., Marell, M. Vazquez, A., Krikorian, L., Charriaut, C., and Galavant, P., 1985, Enhancement of human B cell proliferation by antibody to the C3d receptor, the gp 140 molecule, *Eur. J. Immunol.* **15**:73–76.

Frazer, I. H., MacKay, I. R., Jordan, T. W., *et al.*, 1985, Reactivity of anti-mitochondrial autoantibodies in primary bilary cirrhosis: Definition of two novel mitochondrial polypeptide autoantigens, *J. Immunol.* **135**:1739–1745.

Gershwin, M. E., MacKay, I. R., Sturgess, A., *et al.*, 1988, Identification and specificity of a cDNA encoding 70 kD mitochondrial antigen recognized in primary biliary cirrhosis, *J. Immunol.* **138**:3525–3531.

Ginsburg, W. W., Finkelman, F. D., and Lipsky, P. E., 1979, Circulating and pokeweed mitogen-induced immunoglobulin-secreting cells in systemic lupus erythematosus, *Clin. Exp. Immunol.* **35**:76–88.

Golay, F. T., 1986, Functional B-lymphocyte surface antigens, *Immunology* **59**:1–5.

Goverman, J., Hunkapillar, T., and Hood, L., 1986, A speculative view of the multicomponent nature of T cell antigen recognition, *Cell* **45**:475–484.

Gupta, S., 1988, Cytokines: Molecular and biological characteristics, *Scand. J. Rheumatol. (Suppl.)* **76**:189–201.

Henney, C. S., 1989, Interleukin 7: Effects on early events in lymphopoiesis, *Immunol Today* **10**:170–173.

Heyman, B., Wiersma, E. J., and Kinoshita, T., 1990, *In vivo* inhibition of the antibody response by a complement receptor-specific monoclonal antibody, *J. Exp. Med.* **172**:665–668.

Hood, L., Kronenberg, M., and Hunkarpillar, T., 1985, T cell antigen receptor and the immunoglobulin supergene family, *Cell* **40**:225–229.

Humphrey, J. H., Grennan, D., and Sundarm, V., 1984, The origin of follicular dendritic cells in the mouse and the mechanism of trapping immune complexes on them, *Eur. J. Immunol.* **14**:859–864.

Jelinck, D. F., and Lipsky, P. E., 1987, Regulation of human B lymphocyte activation, proliferation and differentiation, *Adv. Immunol.* **40**:1–59.

Kehrl, J. H., Roberts, A. B., Wakefield, L. M., Jakowlew, S., Sporn, M. B., and Fauci, A. S., 1986, Transforming growth factor β is an important immunomodulatory protein for human B lymphocytes, *J. Immunol.* **137**:3855–3864.

Lipsky, P. E., Hirohata, S., Jelinck, D. F., McAnally, L. F., and Splawski, J. B., 1988, Regulation of human B lymphocyte responsiveness, *Scand. J. Rheumatol. (Suppl.)* **76**:229–235.

Logtenberg, T., Kroon, A., Gmelig-Meyling, F. J. H., and Ballieux, R. E., 1987, Analysis of the human tonsil B cell repertoire by somatic hybridization: Occurrence of both "monospecific" and "multispecific" (auto) antibody-secreting cells, *Eur. J. Immunol.* **17**:855–859.

MacKay, I. R., and Gershwin, M. E., 1989, Molecular basis of mitochondrial autoreactivity in primary biliary cirrhosis, *Immunol. Today* **10**:315–318.

Maini, R. N., and Plater-Zyberk, C., 1988, The significance of CD5+ B cells in rheumatic diseases, *Scand. J. Rheumatol. (Suppl.)* **76**:237–242.

Mannik, M., Nardella, F. A., and Sasso, E. H., 1988, Rheumatoid factors in immune complexes of patients with rheumatoid arthritis, *Springer Semin. Immunopathol.* **10**:215–230.

Matsuoka, M., Yoshida, K., Maeda, T., Usuda, S., and Sakano, H., 1990, Switch circular DNA formed in cytokine-treated mouse splenocytes: Evidence for intramolecular DNA deletion in immunoglobulin class switching, *Cell* **62**:135–142.

Melchers, F., and Andersson, J., 1986, Factors controlling the B-cell cycle, *Annu. Rev. Immunol.* **4**:13–36.

Munthe, E., and Natvig, J. B., 1972, Complement-fixing intracellular complexes of IgG rheumatoid factor in rheumatoid plasma cells, *Scand. J. Immunol.* **1**:217–222.

Muraguchi, A., Butler, J. L., Kehrl, J. H., Falkoff, R. J., and Fauci, A. S., 1983, Selective suppression of an early step in human B cell activation by cyclosporin A, *J. Exp. Med.* **158**:690–702.

Natvig, J. B., and Munthe, E., 1975, Self-associating IgG rheumatoid factor represents a major response of plasma cells in rheumatoid inflammatory tissue, *Ann. NY Acad. Sci.* **256**:88–99.

Natvig, J. B., Randen, I., Thompson, K., Førre, Ø., and Munthe, E., 1989, The B-cell system in the rheumatoid inflammation. New insights into the pathogenesis of rheumatoid arthritis using synovial B cell hybridoma clones, *Springer Semin. Immunopathol.* **11**:301–314.

Olson, N. J., Callahan, L. F., and Pincus, T., 1987, Immunologic studies of rheumatoid arthritis patients treated with methotrexate, *Arthritis Rheum.* **30**:481–488.

Paavonen, T., 1985, Glucocorticoids enhance the *in vitro* Ig synthesis of pokeweed mitogen-stimulated human B cells by inhibiting the suppression effect of T8+ T cells *Scand. J. Immunol.* **21**:67–71.

Paliard, X., de Waal Malefyt, R., Yssel, H., Blanchard, D., Chrétient, J., Abrahams, J., de Vries, J. E., and Spits, H., 1988, Simultaneous production of IL-2, IL-4, and IFN-γ by activated human CD4+ and CD8+ T cell clones, *J. Immunol.* **141**:849–855.

Plater-Zyberk, C., Maini, R. N., Lam, K., Kennedy, T. D., and Janossy, G. A., 1985, Rheumatoid arthritis B cell subset expresses a phenotype similar to that in chronic lymphocytic leukemia, *Arthritis Rheum.* **28**:971–976.

Pope, R. M., Teller., D. C., and Mannik, M., 1975, Intermediate complexes formed by self-association of IgG-rheumatoid factors, *Ann. NY. Acad. Sci.* **256**:82–90.

Randen, I., Thompson, K. M., Natvig, J. B., Førre, Ø., and Waalen, K., 1989, Human monoclonal rheumatoid factors from the polyclonal repertoire of rheumatoid synovial tissue: Production and characterization, *Clin. Exp. Immunol.* **78**:13.

Schoenfeld, Y., 1990, Idiotypes and autoimmunity, *Immunology* **2**(4):593–597.

Sinha, A. A., Lopez, M. T., and McDevitt, H. O., 1990, Autoimmune diseases: The failure of self-tolerance, *Science* **248**:1378–1387.

Smith, C. I. E., and Hammarström, L., 1985, Immunologic abnormalities induced by D-pencillamine, in: *PAR: Pseudo-Allergic Reactions* (P. Dukor, P. Kallós, H. D. Schlumberger, and G. B. West, eds.), Karger, Basel, pp. 139–180.

Stemerowicz, R., Möller, B., Rodloff, A., Freudenberg, M., Hopf, U., Wittenbrink, C., Reinhardt, R., and Galanos, C., 1988, Are antimitochondrial antibodies in primary biliary cirrhosis induced by R(rough)-mutants of enterobacteriaceae? *Lancet* **II**:1166–1170.

Tan, E., 1989, Antinuclear antibodies: Diagnostic markers for autoimmune diseases and probes for cell biology, *Adv. Immunol.* **44**:93–138.

Thompson, K. M., Randen, I., Natvig, J. B., Mageed, R. A., Jefferis, R., Carsson, D. A. Tighe, H., and Førre, Ø., 1990, Human monoclonal rheumatoid factors derived from the polyclonal repertoire of rheumatoid synovial tissue: Incidence of cross-reactive idiotypes and expression of V_H and V_k subgroups, *Eur. J. Immunol.* **20**:863–868.

Tonegawa, S., 1983, Somatic generation of antibody diversity, *Nature* **302**:575–581.

Waalen, K., Duff, G. W., Førre, Ø., Dickens, E., Kvarnes, L., and Nuki, P., 1986, Interleukin-1 activity produced by human rheumatoid and normal dendritic cells, *Scand J. Immunol.* **23**:365–371.

Wahl, S. M., McCartney-Francis, N., and Mergen-Hagen, S. E., 1989, Inflammatory and immunomodulatory roles of TGF-β, *Immunol. Today* **10**:258–261.

Wilson, B. S., Platt, G. L., and Kay, N. E., 1985, Monoclonal antibodies to the 140,000 molecular weight glycoprotein on B lymphocyte membranes (CR2 receptor) initiate proliferation of B cells *in vitro*, *Blood* **66**:824–829.

Winchester, R. J., 1975, Characterization of IgG complexes in patients with rheumatoid arthritis, *Ann. NY Acad. Sci.* **256**:73–82.

Youinou, P., Mackenzie, L., Broker, B. M., Isenberg, D. I., DrogouLelong, A., Gentric, A., and Lydyard, P., 1988, The importance of CD5 positive B cells in nonorgan-specific autoimmune diseases, *Scand. J. Rheumatol. (Suppl.)* **76**:243–249.

Zola, H., 1987, The surface antigens of human B lymphocytes, *Immunol. Today* **8**:308–315.

Chapter 4

T LYMPHOCYTES IN AUTOIMMUNITY AND TRANSPLANTATION

Jens Kjeldsen-Kragh, Alison Quayle, Catherine Kalvenes, and Øystein Førre

1. INTRODUCTION

Approximately 80% of circulating lymphocytes are thymus-derived T cells, and these play an essential role in the regulation of humoral and cellular immune responses. The antigen recognition structure of T cells is the T-cell receptor (TCR). The majority of T cells express a TCR that consists of two disulfide-linked chains, the α and the β chain, which have two extracellular domains, one variable and the other constant, with a joining segment between. These TCRα/β-positive cells recognize antigen that is processed and expressed in the context of major histocompatibility complex (MHC) gene products on the membrane of accessory cells (Zinkernagel and Doherty, 1974). A small proportion of cells express γ and δ chains (Triebel and Hercend, 1989) instead of α and β chains. The function of the γδ TCR, and the identity of its ligand, is as yet unclear.

The αβ and γδ TCRs are expressed on the surface of lymphocytes in association with the CD3 proteins that are present on all peripheral T cells. For membrane expression of a functional receptor, both CD3 and TCR are required (Weiss and Stobo, 1984).

2. THE T-CELL REPERTOIRE

The T-cell antigen receptor is encoded by dispersed variable (V), joining (J), diversity (D), and constant (C) gene segments. They undergo somatic rearrangement, and following RNA transcription and splicing, they give rise to the functional TCR (Yanagi *et al.*, 1984; Hedrick *et al.*, 1984) (Figure 4.1). The great diversity of the αβ TCR gene repertoire is

Jens Kjeldsen-Kragh, Alison Quayle, and *Catherine Kalvenes* • Institute of Immunology and Rheumatology, The National Hospital, N-0172 Oslo 1, Norway. *Øystein Førre* • Oslo Sanitetsforening Rheumatism Hospital, N-0172 Oslo 1, Norway.

Immunopharmacology in Autoimmune Diseases and Transplantation, edited by Hans Erik Rugstad *et al.* Plenum Press, New York, 1992.

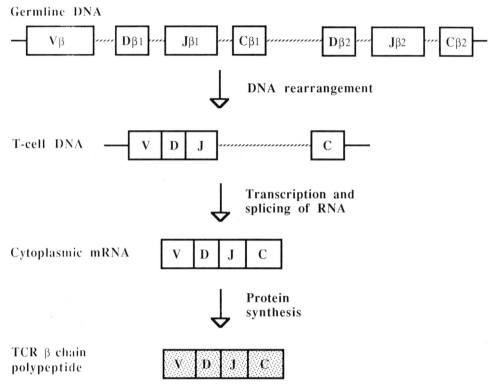

FIGURE 4.1.   Genetic basis for the synthesis of the TCR β chain. The germ line TCR β chain DNA consists of a group of 50–100 variable (V_β) region gene segments and a tandem duplication of DNA containing one diversity (D_β) region gene segment, a cluster of joining (J_β) region gene segments, and one constant (C_β) region gene segment. The $J_{\beta1}$ and the $J_{\beta2}$ clusters contains six and seven functional gene segments, respectively. Rearrangement first occurs between one D_β and one J_β segment followed by addition of one V_β segment. The fully rearranged gene is then transcribed, the mRNA is spliced, and finally translated to a TRC β chain polypeptide.

generated by the random utilization of multiple germ line gene segments for the variable regions V, D, and J. Additional diversity is provided by junctional variability in VJ or VDJ joining, and nucleotide (N) addition at VDJ joints (for review, see Davis and Bjorkman, 1988). The TCR γ and δ chains have a relatively limited germ line gene repertoire with the majority of their potential sequence diversity provided by junctional flexibility between gene segments and the addition of N region sequences (Takihara *et al.*, 1989).

Once a developing T cell expresses a TCR on its surface, it then passes through a positive and a negative cellular selection process in the thymus. Negative selection enables the immune system to distinguish self from nonself (that is, to react to foreign antigens yet be tolerant to self-antigens), and involves recognition of thymic (self) MHC antigens (Bevan and Fink, 1978). T cells with a high affinity for self-MHC antigens, which could cause autoimmunity, are clonally deleted at this stage (Kappler *et al.*, 1987). Positive selection is assumed to favor the development of T cells expressing TCRs that preferentially recognize foreign antigens in association with self-MHC molecules (for review, see Fowlkes and Pardoll, 1989).

3. ANTIGEN RECOGNITION

Protein antigens must be physically altered or "processed" by antigen-presenting cells (APCs) such as macrophages before they can be recognized by T cells. Models of the interaction between antigen–MHC–TCR contain distinct functional sites on the MHC for antigen and TCR binding. The crystalline structure of the MHC class I HLA-A2 molecule shows a single antigen recognition site present as a groove (Bjorkman *et al.*, 1987). The polymorphic amino acids of the different class I alleles are located almost entirely in the antigen-binding site. Modeling of the α1 and β1 domains of the MHC class II to the same structure as HLA-A2 also positions the polymorphic residues in the proposed antigen recognition site.

4. T-CELL ACTIVATION

The interactions between an antigen-specific T cell and an antigen-presenting cell plus antigen transduce cell surface events into intracellular biochemical second messengers, and these influence specific targeted genes that can become transcriptionally active or inactive. This can ultimately produce an "activated" T cell whose characteristics include expression of the new cell surface proteins, production of growth factors, and acquirement of effector function (Figure 4.2).

4.1. The TCR–CD3 Complex

The CD3 complex consists of four integral membrane proteins which are the γ, δ, ε and the disulfide-linked ζ chains. In the absence of the CD3 complex, the TCR heterodimer cannot be expressed. As cross-linking of CD3 mimics the antigen–MHC stimulation of T cells (resulting in, for example, protein kinase C activation and a rise in intracellular calcium) and because the CD3 polypeptide chains have long intracellular domains, it is believed that the CD3 complex mediates signal transduction on antigen recognition by the TCR (Clevers *et al.*, 1988).

4.2. Accessory Cell Markers

Although the TCR–CD3 complex confers specificity to a T-cell response, a number of accessory molecules are also intimately involved in the regulation of T-cell activation. These nonpolymorphic molecules include CD2, CD4, and CD8, which all belong to the immuno-globulin superfamily, and LFA-1, which is a member of the integrin superfamily. These molecules have all been demonstrated to play a role in cellular adhesion and more recently to transduce intracellular signals that synergize with those generated by the TCR/CD3 complex.

CD4 and CD8 molecules are cell surface glycoproteins that are expressed on mutually exclusive subpopulations of peripheral T cells. CD4-positive cells generally exhibit helper function while CD8 cells have a predominantly cytotoxic or suppressor function. A much stricter correlation is found between CD4 or CD8 expression and the class of MHC protein recognized by the T cell. Thus CD4 cells only recognize antigen in the context of MHC class II and CD8 cells in the context of MHC class I. There is a direct binding between CD4 or

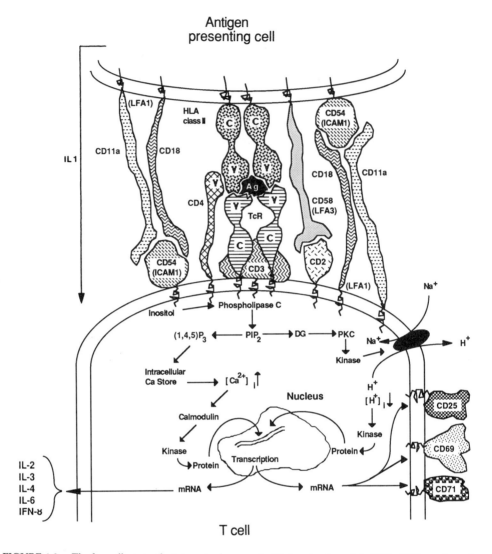

FIGURE 4.2. The figure illustrates the interaction between the HLA molecules and the TCR–CD3 complex and other accessory molecules involved in cell-to-cell contact that are essential for T-cell activation. Transmembrane signaling via the TCR–CD3 complex leads to a cascade of intracellular events culminating in expression of activation antigens, secretion of lymphokines, and cell proliferation. Abbreviations: C/V, constant/variable region; Ag, antigen; PIP_2, phosphatidylinositol biphosphate; DG, diacylglycerol; $(1,4,5)P_3$, inositol 1,4,5-triphosphate; PKC, protein kinase C; $[Ca^{2+}]$, intracellular free calcium concentration; IL, interleukin; IFN, interferon; $[H^+]$, intracelular proton concentration.

CD8 and the relatively nonpolymorphic regions of the appropriate MHC proteins (Doyle and Strominger, 1987; Rosenstein *et al.*, 1989).

In resting T cells the TCR–CD3 complex and CD4/CD8 molecules are well separated, but on TCR engagement with antigen, they physically associate (Fig. 4.2) (Emmrich *et al.*, 1987; Rivas *et al.*, 1988). While CD4/CD8 may play a stabilizing or strengthening role in TCR binding to MHC, there is recent evidence that they are also involved in signal transduction. Veillette *et al.* (1988) have recently provided evidence that CD4/CD8 molecules are physically connected to a tyrosine protein kinase. As the ϵ chain of CD3 is a putative substrate (Marth *et al.*, 1985), Mustelin and Altman (1989) have suggested that CD4/CD8 regulate T-cell activation by controlling the mobility of the tyrosine protein kinase.

The ligand for CD2 (LFA-2, sheep red blood cell receptor) is the ubiquitous molecule, leukocyte function-associated antigen 3 (LFA-3). Monoclonal antibodies to CD2 indicate that CD2–LFA-3 interactions are essential in antigen-specific and nonspecific conjugate formation (Krensky *et al.*, 1984; Shaw *et al.*, 1986). *In vivo* pairs of anti-CD2 monoclonal antibodies stimulate T-cell proliferation and effector function (Meuer *et al.*. 1984) without a concurrent signal by the TCR. It is unclear if this "alternative activation" pathway is relevant *in vivo*, but it is clear that LFA-3 binding to CD2 provides a partial activation signal that is also dependent on the T-cell receptor complex (Hunig *et al.*, 1987; Bockenstedt *et al.*, 1988).

LFA-1 is a heterodimer with a unique α chain (CD11a) and a β chain (CD18) common to other leukocyte integrins (the $\beta2$ family). Intercellular adhesion molecule 1 (ICAM-1, CD54) (Marlin and Springer, 1987) and ICAM-2 (Staunton *et al.*, 1989) are the ligands for LFA-1, and it is known that ICAM-1 is only highly expressed on most cell types after activation or induction with inflammatory lymphokines (Dustin *et al.*, 1989). Recent elegant studies by Dustin and Springer (1989) have demonstrated that 5–10 min after TCR stimulation, LFA-1 is converted to a high avidity state, returning to a low avidity state by 30 min to 2 hr. By this sequence of events, T cells achieve a balance between the opposite needs for sensitive antigen recognition and stable cell–cell adhesion. The authors also demonstrated that the TCR and LFA-1 are coupled by intracellular signaling pathways.

4.3. T-Cell Activation Markers

Activation antigens are defined as those molecules that are absent or expressed in very low levels on resting T cells, but following T-cell activation are induced or up-regulated, suggesting they may play a role in the activation process itself. Expression of these activation antigens follows a distinct order of kinetics; antigens such as the activation-inducer molecule (CD69), the interleukin-2 receptor (IL-2R, CD25), the transferrin receptor (CD71), the insulin receptor, 4F2, EA1, and TLISA1 are molecules that appear early in activation, before DNA synthesis occurs (Helderman and Strom, 1978; Haynes *et al.*, 1981; Trowbridge and Omary, 1981; Leonard *et al.*, 1982; Burns *et al.*, 1985; Hara *et al.*, 1986; Cebrián *et al.*, 1988). Others such as TP103, Ta1, Ki-1 (CD30), T10 (CD38), HLA-DR, VLA-1, and Act 1, appear later (Hercend *et al.*, 1981; Fox *et al.*, 1984; Lazarovits *et al.*, 1984; Hemler *et al.*, 1985; Beverley, 1987; Fleischer, 1987). Although the biological function of many of these antigens is not well understood, a number of them, including the IL-2R, are well characterized. IL-2Rs appear on CD4 and CD8 cells within hours of activation and are the ligands for the growth factor interleukin-2 (IL-2), which is primarily produced by CD4-positive cells (Palacois, 1982). IL-2 released from the cells binds to the IL-2R, leading to proliferation. IL-2 and IL-2R mRNA and protein synthesis are induced following TCR engagement or binding of mitogen to their ligands and are dependent on protein kinase C stimulation (Smith and Cantrell, 1985). The time course of IL-2R expression parallels proliferation, and induction and down-regulation play a role in controlling responses (Cantrell and Smith, 1983, 1984).

5. T CELLS IN TRANSPLANTATION

If cells or a whole organ are introduced into a genetically different recipient, an immune response is elicited. In principle, this response is of the same nature as if the host were infected by a microorganism. In infection the host T cells recognize a complex of an antigenic peptide and a self-HLA molecule, and subsequently the T cell is activated. In transplantation some of the host T cells recognize foreign HLA molecules on donor cells as if they were foreign peptides bound to self-HLA molecules. Helper T cells (CD4-positive) are activated, and they provide help both for activation of specific cytotoxic T cells and for production of anti-HLA antibodies by B cells (plasma cells). Generation of cytotoxic T cells and antibodies against the donor cells ultimately results in killing of the foreign cells and/or rejection of the transplanted organ (for review, see Mason and Morris, 1986).

The rejection of a transplant can occur within the first 24 hr. Hyperacute rejection is always mediated by anti-HLA antibodies already present in the host. Such antibodies can appear in patients who have been sensitized after receiving multiple blood transfusions. In accelerated or acute rejection, as well as in chronic rejection, both humoral and cellular mechanisms are thought to be involved. However, it has not been settled yet whether the cellular mechanism of rejection is of delayed-type hypersensitivity or whether cytotoxic T cells play the main role (Mason and Morris, 1986).

If a bone marrow recipient is severely immunosuppressed, there is a considerable risk that T cells from the donor will be activated by the HLA molecules of the recipient. This serious complication, called graft versus host disease (GVHD), can have a deadly outcome if not treated (Chapter 31, this volume).

In order to prevent organ rejection or GVHD, the donor must carry the same or nearly the same HLA haplotypes as the recipient. However, even in transplantations between HLA-identical siblings, rejection or GVHD can occur. This triggering of T cells on either the host or donor is poorly understood, but is probably due to other non-HLA molecules, which have not yet been identified. For this reason it is necessary to give the recipient immunosuppressive therapy in order to increase the chances for a successful transplantation.

6. T CELLS IN AUTOIMMUNITY

It is assumed that T cells play a central role in the pathogenesis of autoimmune diseases. This is based on the fact that the many different autoantibodies produced in autoimmunity are dependent on T cell help (Natvig *et al.*, 1989). Furthermore, in many autoimmune diseases there is an infiltration of T cells at the inflammatory site and many of these exhibit properties attributed to activation. For example, T cells isolated from the rheumatoid synovium have a high spontaneous proliferation, they express both early and late activation antigens, and they have a high production and consumption of IL-2 (Førre *et al.*, 1982; Waalen *et al.*, 1987; Quayle *et al.*, 1989). The causes of T-cell activation in autoimmune diseases is not known, but at a certain stage tolerance to self-antigens breaks down.

6.1. Breakdown of T-Cell Tolerance to Self-Antigens

A number of hypotheses have been launched to explain this. In the first, autoreactive T cells are thought to arise from a breakthrough of "forbidden clones" due to insufficient deletion of self-reactive T cells during thymic education. This theory alone cannot explain why T cells specific for self-antigens do not always cause autoimmune disease. Autoreactive T cells have been isolated from peripheral blood from normal individuals. T cells specific for myelin basic protein, the antigen causing experimental autoimmune encephalitis, can also be isolated from the T-cell repertoire of healthy mice (Schluesener and Wekerle, 1984).

In the second, it is proposed that self-antigens, which previously have been "hidden" from the immune system, are presented in the correct context for the T cells. Such antigens may have been physically sequestered from the immune system as in the case of the collagen type II in normal cartilage or by the blood–brain or blood–testis barrier. Another possibility is that self-antigens could be "protected" from the immune system by the mere absence of antigen-presenting cells. In a physiological situation only macrophages, dendritic cells, and B cells express MHC class II molecules, but after appropriate stimulation (e.g., interferon γ), many other cell types can be stimulated to express these proteins as well. Such "ectopic" MHC expression is thought to contribute to the presentation of sequestered antigens in autoimmune diseases (Bottazzo et al., 1986).

In a third hypothesis, T cells against epitopes on foreign antigens are thought to cross-react with certain self-antigens. Finally, in cases of insufficient clonal deletion of autoreactive T cells, autoimmune disease may be prevented by the action of suppressor T cells. In certain mouse strains antigen-specific T suppressor cells have been identified that suppress the function of autoreactive T cells (Jensen and Kapp, 1985). If the host is infected by a microorganism that has epitopes closely resembling the self-antigen, one can imagine that the autoreactive T cells that previously were suppressed now become activated. Thus the homeostasis between T cell help contra T cell suppression is disturbed in favor of T cell help. In rheumatoid arthritis, the T cells have been shown to exert diminished suppressor function compared with T cells from normal controls (Chattopadhyay et al., 1979).

None of these four hypotheses alone explain why T cells react with self-antigens, but since they are not mutually exclusive together, they may reflect some of the fundamental mechanisms involved. To further increase our understanding of the autoimmune phenomenon, one has to look into the molecular triad formed between antigen, MHC, and TCR molecules.

6.2. The Role of MHC Genes in Autoimmunity

The susceptibility or resistance to the development of autoimmune disease is to some extent determined genetically. Expression of certain MHC gene products have been shown to render the person more susceptible. Most autoimmune diseases are associated with certain MHC class II alleles, but association with MHC class I alleles is involved in a few diseases, like ankylosing spondylitis (HLA-27) and psoriasis vulgaris (HLA-Cw6) (Svejgaard et al., 1983).

In rheumatoid arthritis (RA), 80–90% of the patients carry either the HLA-DR1 haplotype or three variants of the HLA-DR4 haplotype (Dw4, Dw14, or Dw15). The Dw10 variant of the HLA-DR4 haplotype is not associated with RA (Todd et al., 1988a). A comparison of the sequences of the β_1 chains of these haplotypes shows that a stretch of six amino acids (from 65–71) in the third hypervariable region is identical. It has been suggested that this particular part of the HLA molecule is of crucial importance for presentation of antigen to the inflammatory T cells in the joint (Winchester and Gregersen, 1989).

Recently it has been reported that a polymorphism in the HLA-DQ β chain at position 57 appears to be the major determinant of susceptibility and resistance to insulin-dependent diabetes mellitus (IDDM). Aspartic acid at this position confers protection against the disease, while a neutral amino acid such as alanine, serine, or valine is associated with increased susceptibility (Todd *et al.*, 1988b). However, while this holds true for Caucasians, IDDM in Japanese and Chinese has been shown to occur in patients with aspartic acid at position 57 in the HLA-DQ β chain (Dotta and Eisenbarth, 1989). This suggests that other residues may also contribute to susceptibility.

Susceptibility to autoimmune diseases is not only conferred to the MHC genes. Studies of monozygotic twins show a much higher concordance rate for disease in monozygotic twins than in HLA-identical siblings (Gorsuch *et al.*, 1982; Johnston *et al.*, 1983). Genetic factors contributing to susceptibility might involve the TCR, immunoglobulin, lymphokines, and hormones, and expression of self-antigens.

6.3. Antigens Involved

In a few autoimmune diseases like myasthenia gravis and Graves' disease, the triggering antigen is known. However, in most of the other human autoimmune diseases the main self-antigens responsible for T-cell activation is unknown. In one RA patient, three T-cell clones specific for collagen type II have been isolated from the joints on two different occasions (Londei *et al.*, 1989). However, we and Feldmann's group have tested many T-cell clones from the joints of RA patients and so far only the aforementioned clones appear to be specific for this antigen. Thus collagen type II might be a relevant antigen in only a few patients with RA (Quayle *et al.*, 1989).

Recently it has been suggested that a mycobacterial antigen may play an important role in inflammatory arthritides. More than ten years ago, Abrahamsen *et al.* (1978) showed that the proliferative response against PPD was much higher in T cells from the joint compared to T cells from the blood. During the last years interest has focused on the 65-kDa heat-shock protein from *Mycobacterium tuberculosis*. Heat-shock proteins are produced in all eukaryotic cells when they are subjected to many kinds of stress, such as increased temperature, virus infection, and exposure to free oxygen radicals (Lindquist, 1986). These proteins have been highly conserved during evolution and the 65-kDa protein from *M. tuberculosis* has a high degree of sequence homology with a human heat-shock protein. In many arthritis patients, especially in those patients with a short disease duration, T cells from the inflammatory compartment have a much higher response against this antigen than peripheral blood T cells (Res *et al.*, 1988). Furthermore, in our laboratory we have found *in vivo*-activated T cells in the joint that are specific for the 65-kDa protein from *M. tuberculosis*, which suggests that this antigen is of some pathogenic importance.

It has been suggested that a T-cell response against bacterial-specific epitopes confers protection of the host against the microorganism, while a T-cell response against epitopes homologous with the human analogue initiates an autoimmune process (Young *et al.*, 1988). This hypothesis still lacks experimental proof, but it is interesting to note that rat T cells specific for the 65-kDa protein from *M. tuberculosis* have been shown to be cytotoxic against autologous monocytes "stressed" with interferon-γ or infected with cytomegalovirus (Koga *et al.*, 1989). In the inflamed joint there are many "stressed" macrophages, and it will be of great interest to see if *in vivo*-activated synovial T cells specific for the 65-kDa heat-shock protein can lyse autologous *in vivo*-activated synovial macrophages.

6.4. Restriction of TCR Gene Usage

It is conceivable that germ line alterations in the T-cell receptor gene repertoire might influence the immune regulatory balance and thereby impose susceptibility to autoimmune diseases. In murine experimental autoimmune encephalomyelitis (EAE) there is a marked limited heterogeneity of TCR gene usage in T cells from the inflammatory site. Almost all of the T cells specific for the etiological agent use the Vβ8 gene (Acha-Orbea *et al.*, 1988).

In human autoimmune diseases, such as IDDM, Graves' disease, multiple sclerosis, and myasthenia gravis, the germ line TCR gene repertoire has been studied by many groups (Demaine *et al.*, 1987; Millward *et al.*, 1987; Oksenberg *et al.*, 1989). Some reports have claimed that characteristic restriction fragment length polymorphisms (RFLP) produced with different TCR probes are found in patients with these autoimmune diseases but not in healthy controls. Other groups have not been able to confirm these results, and the reported association between a marker allele and a disease may simply reflect the population stratification. Only careful scrutiny of multiplex families with sibling-pair analysis can tell us whether certain RFPLs are associated with the disease. Furthermore, studies of the germ line TCR gene repertoire will not necessarily give us information about the T cells at the inflammatory site, those which are supposed to be of pathogenic importance.

In RA one has a unique possibility to study the inflammatory T cells. Many investigators have looked for clonal dominance among the synovial T cells in RA by studying the pattern of TCR β gene rearrangement, but the results are conflicting. In some studies synovial T cells have been expanded *in vitro* in order to raise enough cells for the experiments, and the conclusion in all these studies is that clonal dominance is present (Stamenkovic *et al.*, 1988; Miltenburg *et al.*, 1990). Other studies looking at clonality of T-cell clones have reached the opposite conclusion (Cooper *et al.*, 1989; Kroczek *et al.*, 1989).

So far, a restricted TCR gene usage does not seem to be a typical feature in autoimmune diseases apart from a few exceptions. This is in contrast to the close linkage to certain MHC alleles. Perhaps this difference reflects the difference by which MHC and TCR molecules attain their diversity: multiple loci and allelic diversity in the case of MHC and multiple germ line VDJ gene segments coupled with gene rearrangement in the case of the TCR.

7. IMMUNE INTERVENTION

Most of the immunosuppressive agents so far used in autoimmune diseases and transplantation give a nonspecific suppression of the immune system. Commonly used drugs are alkylating agents (cyclophosphamide and chlorambucil), antimetabolites (azathioprine and methotrexate), glucocorticoids, and cyclosporine A (Table I).

The alkylating agents and antimetabolites probably kill dividing cells by blocking cell replication by alkylating DNA or interfering with DNA synthesis, respectively (Fox and McCune, 1989). This mechanism results in suppression of humoral and cellular immunity, but also gives rise to many of the side effects of these drugs. Furthermore, some immunomodulatory effects have also been ascribed to these drugs (Fox and McCune, 1989). However, in the treatment of autoimmune diseases the mechanism of action of methotrexate is probably mainly due to an anti-inflammatory effect of this drug. The very low doses of methotrexate used in these diseases do not have a profound cytotoxic or immunomodulatory effect (Fox and McCune, 1989).

Glucocorticoids are probably the most powerful immunosuppressants known. They reduce the number of circulating lymphocytes and monocytes, and suppress the production of IL-1, IL-2, prostaglandins, and leukotrienes (Cruse and Lewis, 1989). These drugs are commonly used in autoimmune diseases and transplantation.

The mode of action of cyclosporine A is completely different from the aforementioned

TABLE I. Possible Modes of Immune Intervention

Immunosuppression by drugs	
Drugs	**Therapeutic usage:**
Corticosteroids	AD (Rugstad, 1988), organ TX (Chapter 30, this volume), BMTX (Chapter 31, this volume)
Alkylating agents	Severe AD (Chapter 11, this volume), BMTX (Chapter 31, this volume)
Anti-metabolites	AD (Fox and McCune, 1989), organ TX (Chapter 30, this volume), BMTX (Chapter 31, this volume)
Cyclosporin A	AD (Forre *et al*, 1988), organ TX (Chaper 30, this volume), BMTX (Chapter 31, this volume)
Monoclonal antibodies against T-cell membrane molecules	
MAbs	**Therapeutic usage:**
Anti-CD2	MS (Weiner *et al.*, 1986)
Anti-CD3	Renal TX (Norman *et al.*, 1987), GVHD (Prentice *et al.*, 1982)
Anti-TCR$_{\alpha\beta}$	Renal TX (Smely *et al.*, 1989)
Anti-TCR V$_{\beta 8}$	The murine model of MS, EAE (Acha-Orbea *et al.*, 1988)
Anti-CD4	Renal TX (Morel *et al.*, 1989), RA (Herzog *et al.*, 1989a), MS (Weiner *et al.*, 1986)
Anti-CD6	Renal TX (Kirkman *et al.*, 1983), GVHD (Reinherz *et al.*, 1982), MS (Hafler *et al.*, 1988)
Anti-CD7	RA (Kirkham *et al.*, 1988)
Anti-CD8	BMTX (Favrot *et al.*, 1987)
Anti-CD11a/CD18	BMTX (Fischer *et al.*, 1987)
Anti-CD25	Renal TX (Cantarovish *et al.*, 1989), GVHD (Hervé and Wijdenes, 1989)
Anti-CD5 linked ricin	GVHD (Blakey and Thorpe, 1988)
Monoclonal antibodies against MHC molecules on the antigen-presenting cell	
Anti-MHC class II	The murine model of MS, EAE (Wraith *et al.*, 1989)
Synthetic peptides competing with antigen for binding to the MHC molecules on the antigen-presenting cell	
	The murine model of MS, EAE (Wraith *et al.*, 1989)

Abbreviations: AD, autoimmune disease; TX, transplantation; BMTX, bone marrow transplantation; MS, multiple sclerosis; GVHD, graft versus host disease; EAE, experimental autoimmune encephalomyelitis; RA, rheumatoid arthritis.

drugs. It primarily affects the T helper cell subset by inhibiting production of IL-2 and other lymphokines (Førre *et al.*, 1988; Herzog *et al.*, 1989b).

Many of the serious adverse effects of these immunosuppressive drugs are caused by their general immunosuppression. Thus there is an obvious need for more specific immunosuppressive treatment. Our present knowledge of the antigen recognition and activation of T cells opens up completely new principles for immune intervention. Although these methods have not yet been applied to any great extent in humans, they deserve a brief discussion.

Blocking of T-cell recognition by monoclonal antibodies (mAbs) against the CD4 molecule has been used successfully in a number of experimentally induced autoimmune diseases (Wraith *et al.*, 1989). Since the anti-CD4 blocking is nonspecific, one could suspect a general immune suppression during this therapy. However, serious side effects have not been noticed in the few clinical trials so far carried out on patients with RA (Herzog *et al.*, 1989a; Reiter *et al.*, 1989) and recipients of renal cadaver allografts (Morel *et al.*, 1989).

Treatment with anti-MHC mAbs has been effective in experimental animal models of autoimmune diseases (Wraith *et al.*, 1989) but has not yet been tried in humans. Efforts are also being put into construction of specially designed peptides that can compete with antigen for binding to the MHC molecule. The big advantage of "attacking" the MHC side of T-cell activation is that all the other MHC isotypes are left free for presentation of foreign antigens.

The anti-CD3 monoclonal antibody OKT-3 has been shown to have potent immunosuppressive effects in kidney transplantation and allogeneic bone marrow recipients (Prentice *et al.*, 1982; Norman *et al.*, 1987). Unfortunately, this treatment results in many side effects, some of which can be ascribed to the activation of the T cells by the mAb (Chatenoud *et al.*, 1989). However, the pan-anti-TCR$_{\alpha\beta}$ mAb BMA-031 has recently been tried in renal transplantation, and so far it seems to be very well tolerated by these patients (Weschka *et al.*, 1989).

General immunosuppression can be prevented if the anti-TCR mAb is specific for only a limited proportion of the TCR molecules. In EAE the pathogeneic T cells use only $V_{\beta}8$, and this disease has been successfully treated with mAbs against $V_{\beta}8$ (Acha-Orbea *et al.*, 1988). In human autoimmune diseases no clear evidence has so far been presented for the existence of clonal dominance of the inflammatory T cells or for a restricted TCR gene usage. Until such evidence is obtained, this strategy of therapy does not seem to be applicable to human autoimmune diseases.

Other approaches include treatment with anti-CD25 (IL-2 receptor) mAbs and lymphotoxins, which has recently been tried in renal transplantation (Cantarovish *et al.*, 1989; Hervé and Wijdenes, 1989), and GVHD, respectively (Blakey and Thorpe, 1988). Lymphotoxins are mAbs that are covalently linked to a cytotoxic drug such as risin. If the specificity of the mAb is directed against a T-membrane molecule, the drug coupled to the antibody will ensure that cells carrying this particular antigen are killed.

Treatment strategies using mAbs are still in their infancy. One important problem is the generation of anti-mouse immunoglobulin antibodies, especially anti-idiotypic antibodies, upon repeated injections of the therapeutic antibody. These anti-idiotypic antibodies will neutralize the therapeutic effect of the injected antibody, and they are potentially able to trigger a life-threatening anaphylactic response in the patient. To circumvent this problem, efforts are being made to produce antibodies through recombinant DNA technology where the antigen-binding sites are from the mouse, whereas the remainder of the antibody is human. However, if such antibodies can be produced on a large scale, the hazards of long-term administration need to be assessed.

REFERENCES

Abrahamsen, T. G., Frøland, S. S., and Natvig, J. B., 1978, In vitro mitogen stimulation of synovial fluid lymphocytes from rheumatoid arthritis and juvenile rheumatoid arthritis patients: Dissociation between the response to antigen and polyclonal mitogens. *Scand. J. Imunol.* **7:**81–90.

Acha-Orbea, H., Mitchell, D. J., Timmermann, L., Wraith, D. C., Tausch, G. S., Waldor, M. K., Zamvil, S. S., McDevitt, H. O., and Steinman, L., 1988, Limited heterogeneity of T cell receptors from lymphocytes mediating autoimmune encephalomyelitis allows specific immune intervention, *Cell* **54:**263–273.

Bevan, M. J., and Fink, P., 1978, The influence of the thymus H-2 antigens on the specificity of maturing killer and helper T cells, *Immunol. Rev.* **42:**3–19.

Beverley, P., 1987, Activation antigens: New and previously defined clusters, in: *Leucocyte Typing III. White Cell Differentiation Antigens* (A. J. McMichael, P. Beverley, S. Cobbold, M. J. Crumpton, W. Gilks, F. M. Gotch, N. Hogg, M. Horton, N. Ling, I. C. M. MacLennan, D. Y. Mason, C. Milstein, D. Spiegelhalter, and H. Waldmann, eds.), Oxford University Press, Oxford, pp. 516–524.

Bjorkman, P. J., Saper, M. A., Samraoui, B., Bennett, W. S., Strominger, J. L., and Wiley, D. C., 1987, Structure of the human class I histocompatibility antigen, HLA-A2, *Nature* **329:**506–512.

Blakey, D. C., and Thorpe, P. E., 1988, Treatment of malignant disease and rheumatoid arthritis using ricin A-chain immunotoxins, *Scand. J. Rheumatol. (Suppl.)* **76:**279–287.

Bockenstedt, L. K., Goldsmith, M. A., Dustin, M., Olive, D., Springer, T. A., and Weiss, A., 1988, The CD2 ligand LFA-3 activates T cells but depends on the expression and function of the antigen receptor, *J. Immunol.* **141:**1904–1911.

Bottazzo, G. F., Todd, I., Mirakian, R., Belfiore, A., and Pujol-Borrell, R., 1986, Organ-specific autoimmunity: A 1986 overview, *Immunol. Rev.* **94:**137–169.

Burns, G. F., Triglia, T., Werkmeister, J. A., Begley, C. G., and Boyd, A. W., 1985, TLiSA, a human T lineage-specific antigen involved in the differentiation of cytotoxic cells and anomolous killer cells from their precursors. *J. Exp. Med.* **161:**1063–1078.

Cantarovish, D., Jacques, Y., Le Mauff, B., Giral, M., Hourment, M., Hirn, M., and Soulilou, J.-P., 1989, A randomized controlled trial of anti-interleukin 2 receptor monoclonal antibody (33B3.1) immunosuppression in human renal transplantation, in: *7th International Congress of Immunology*, Berlin (West), July 30–August 5, 1989 (Abstract), Gustav Fischer, Stuttgart, p. 886.

Cantrell, D. A., and Smith, K. A., 1983, Transient expression of interleukin 2 receptors. Consequences for T cell growth, *J. Exp. Med.* **158**:1895–1911.

Cantrell, D. A., and Smith, K. A., 1984, The interleukin 2 T cell system: A new cell growth model, *Science* **224**:1312–1316.

Cebrián, M., Yagüe, E., Rincón, M., López-Botet, M., de Landázuri, M. O., and Sánchez-Madrid, F., 1988, Triggering of T cell proliferation through AIM, an activation inducer molecule expressed on activated human lymphocytes, *J. Exp. Med.* **168**:1621–1637.

Chatenoud, L., Ferran, C., Legendre, C., Kreis, H., and Bach, J.-F., 1989, In vivo use of anti-CD3/Ti murine monoclonal antibodies in renal allograft recipients, in: *7th International Congress of Immunology*, Berlin (West), July 30–August 5, 1989 (Abstract), Gustav Fischer, Stuttgart, p. 886.

Chattopadhyay, C., Chattopadhyay, H., Natvig, J. B., Michaelsen, T. E., and Mellbye, O. J., 1979, Lack of suppressor cell activity in rheumatoid synovial lymphocytes, *Scand. J. Immunol.* **10**:309–316.

Clevers, H., Alarcon, B., Wileman, T., and Terhorst, C., 1988, The T cell receptor/CD3 complex: A dynamic protein ensemble, *Annu. Rev. Immunol.* **6**:629–662.

Cooper, S. M., Roessner, K. D., and Dier, D. L., 1989, Diversity of rheumatoid synovial tissue T cells by T cell receptor analysis, in: *7th International Congress of Immunology*, Berlin (West), July 30–August 5, 1989 (Abstract), Gustav Fischer, Stuttgart, p. 552.

Cruse, J. M., and Lewis, R. E., Jr., 1989, Cyclosporin therapy of autoimmune diseases, in: *Therapy of Autoimmune Diseases. Concepts in Immunopathology*, Volume 7 (J. M. Cruse and R. E. Lewis, Jr., eds.), Karger, Basel, pp. 1–19.

Davis, M., and Bjorkman, P. J., 1988, T cell antigen receptor genes and T cell recognition, *Nature* **334**:395–402.

Demaine, A., Welsh, K. I., Hawes, B. S., and Farid, N. R., 1987, Polymorphism of the TCR β chain in Grave's disease, *J. Clin. Endocrinol. Metab.* **65**:643–646.

Dotta, F., and Eisenbarth, G. S., 1989, Type I diabetes mellitus: A predictable autoimmune disease with interindividual variation in the rate of β cell destruction, *Clin. Immunol. Immunopathol.* **50**:S85–S95.

Doyle, C., and Strominger, J. L., 1987, Interaction between CD4 and class II MHC molecules mediates cell adhesion, *Nature* **330**:256–259.

Dustin, M. L., and Springer, T. A., 1989, T cell receptor cross-linking transiently stimulates adhesiveness through LFA-1, *Nature* **341**:619–624.

Dustin, M. L., Singer, K. H., Tuck, D. T., and Springer, T. A., 1988, Adhesion of T lymphoblasts to epidermal keratinocytes is regulated by interferon gamma and is mediated by intracellular adhesion molecule 1 (ICAM-1), *J. Exp. Med.* **167**:1323–1340.

Emmrich, F., Kanz, L., and Eichmann, K., 1987, Cross-linking of the T cell receptor complex with the subset-specific differentiation antigen stimulates interleukin 2 receptor expression in human CD4 and CD8 T cells, *Eur. J. Immunol.* **17**:529–534.

Favrot, M. C., Philip, T., Combaret, V., *et al.*, 1987, In vivo therapy by CD8 monoclonal antibody for delays to hematological recovery after autologous bone marrow transplantation, *Immunobiology* **3**(Suppl.):217.

Fischer, A., Blanche, S., Le Deist, F., *et al.*, 1987, Prevention of graft failure by an anti-LFA-1 monoclonal antibody in HLA mismatched bone marrow transplantation, in: *Clinical Applications of Anti-leucocyte Monoclonal Antibodies. Symposium Satellite de la 18ème Conférence Internationale sur les Cultures de Leucocytes* (J. F., Bach, G. Laurent, and G. Mawas, eds.), La Grand Motte, France, p. 56.

Fleischer, B., 1987, A novel pathway of human T cell activation via a 103 kD T cell activation antigen, *J. Immunol.* **138**:1346–1350.

Førre, Ø., Dobloug, J. H., and Natvig, J. B., 1982, Augmented numbers of HLA-DR positive T lymphocytes in synovial fluid and synovial tissue of patients with rheumatoid arthritis and juvenile rheumatoid arthritis, *Scand. J. Immunol.* **15**:227–231.

Førre, Ø., Waalen, K. Rugstad, H. E., Berg, K., Solby, D., and Kaas, E., 1988, Cyclosporine and rheumatoid arthritis, *Springer Semin. Immunopathol.* **10**:263–277.

Fowlkes, B. J., and Pardoll, D. M., 1989, Molecular and cellular events of T cell development, *Adv. Immunol.* **44**:207–264.

Fox, D. A., and McCune, W. J., 1989, Immunologic and clinical effects of cytotoxic drugs used in the treatment of rheumatoid arthritis and systemic lupus erythematosus, in: *Therapy of Autoimmune Diseases. Concepts in Immunopathology*, Volume 7 (J. M. Cruse and R. E. Lewis, Jr., eds.), Karger, Basel, pp. 20–78.

Fox, D. A., Hussey, R. E., Fitzgerald, K. A., Acuto, O., Poole, C., Palley, L., Daley, J. F., Schlossman, S. F., and Reinherz, E. L., 1984, Ta₁, a novel 105 KD human T cell activation antigen defined by a monoclonal antibody, *J. Immunol.* **133**:1250–1256.

Gorsuch, A. N., Spencer, K. M., Lister, J., Wolf, E., Bottazzo, G. F., and Cudworth, A. G., 1982, Can future type I diabetes be predicted? A study in families of affected children, *Diabetes* **31**:862–866.

Hafler, D. A., Fallis, R. J., Dawson, D. M., Schlossman, S. F., Reinherz, E. L., and Weiner, H. L., 1988, Immunologic responses of progressive multiple sclerosis patients treated with an anti-T-cell monoclonal antibody anti-T12, *Neurology* **36**:777–784.

Hara, T., Jung, L. K. L., Bjorndahl, J. M., and Fu, S. M., 1986, Human T cell activation. III. Rapid induction of a phosphorylated 28KD/32KD disulfide-linked early activation antigen (EA1) by 12-O-tetradecanoyl phorbol-13 acetate, mitogens and antigens, *J. Exp. Med.* **164**:1988–2005.

Haynes, B. F., Hemler, M. E., Mann, D. L., Eisenbarth, G. S., Shelhamer, J., Mostowski, H. S., Thomas, C. A., Strominger, J. L., and Fauci, A. S., 1981, Characterization of a monoclonal antibody (4F2) that binds to human monocytes and to a subset of activated lymphocytes, *J. Immunol.* **126**:1409–1414.

Hedrick, S. M., Nielsen, E. A., Kavaler, J., Cohen, P. J., and Davies, M. M., 1984, Sequence relationships between putative T cell receptor polypeptides and immunoglobulins, *Nature* **308**:153–158.

Helderman, J. H., and Strom, T. B., 1978, Specific insulin binding sites on T and B lymphocytes as a marker of cell activation, *Nature* **274**:62–63.

Hemler, M. E., Jascobson, J. G., Brenner, M. B., Mann, D., and Strominger, J. L., 1985, VLA-1: A T cell surface antigen which defines a novel late stage of human T cell activation, *Eur. J. Immunol.* **15**:502–508.

Hercend, T., Ritz, J., Schlossman, S. F., and Reinherz, E. L., 1981, Comparative expression of T9, T10, and Ia antigens on activated human T cells subsets, *Hum. Immunol.* **3**:247–259.

Hervé, P., and Wijdenes, J., 1989, In vivo treatment of steroid resistant acute GvHD with a monoclonal antibody for the IL-2 receptor (B-B10, in: *7th International Congress of Immunology*, Berlin (West), July 30–August 5, 1989 (Abstract), Gustav Fischer, Stuttgart, p. 888.

Herzog, C., Walker, C., Moser, B., Stockinger, H., Knapp, W., Rieber, P., Rietmüler, G., Müller, W., and Pichler, W. J., 1989a, Therapy of rheumatoid arthritis with anti-CD4 monoclonal antibodies, in: *7th International Congress of Immunology*, Berlin (West), July 30–August 5, 1989 (Abstract), Gustav Fischer, Stuttgart, p. 524.

Herzog, C., Walker, C., and Pichler, W. J., 1989b, New therapeutic approaches in rheumatoid arthritis, in: *Therapy of Autoimmune Diseases. Concepts in Immunopathology*, Volume 7 (J. M. Cruse and R. E. Lewis, Jr., eds.), Karger, Basel, pp. 79–105.

Hunig, T., Tiefenthaler, G., Meyer, Z. U. M., Buschenfeld, E. K. H., and Meuer, S. C., 1987, Alternative pathway activation of T cells by binding of CD2 to its cell-surface ligand, *Nature* 326:298–301.

Jensen, P. E., and Kapp, J. A., 1985, Genetics of insulin-specific helper and suppressor T cells in non-responder mice, *J. Immunol.* 135:2990–2995.

Johnston, C., Pyke, D. A., Cudworth, A. G., and Wolf, E., 1983, HLA-DR typing in identical twins with insulin diabetes: Difference between concordant and disconcordant pairs, *Br. Med. J.* 286:253–255.

Kappler, J. W., Roehm, N., and Marrack, P., 1987, T cell tolerance by clonal elimination in the thymus, *Cell* 49:273–280.

Kirkham, B., Chikanaza, I., Pitzalis, C., Kingsley, G. H., Grahame, R., Gibson, T., and Panayi, G. S., 1988, Response to monoclonal CD7 antibody in rheumatoid arthritis (letter), *Lancet* 1:589.

Kirkman, R. L., Araujo, J. L., Busch, G. J., Carpenter, C. B., Milford, E. L., Reinherz, E. L., Schlossman, S. F., Strom, T. B., and Tilney, N. L., 1983, Treatment of acute renal allograft rejection with monoclonal anti-T12 antibody, *Transplantation* 36:620–626.

Koga, T., Wand-Wurttenberger, A., DeBruyn, J., Munk, M. E., Schoel, B., and Kaufmann, S. H., 1989, T cell against a bacterial heat shock protein recognize stressed macrophages, *Science* 245:1112–1115.

Krensky, A. M., Robbins, E., Springer, T. A., and Burakoff, S. J., 1984, LFA-1, LFA-2, and LFA-3 antigens are involved in CTL target conjugation, *J. Immunol.* 132:2180–2182.

Kroczek, R. A., Hennerkes, B., Burmester, G., Menninger, W., Zacher, J., and Emmrich, F., 1989, Analysis of clonal heterogeneity in T cells from synovial fluid and synovial membrane of patients with rheumatoid arthritis, in: *7th International Congress of Immunology*, Berlin (West), July 30–August 5, 1989 (Abstract), Gustav Fischer, Stuttgart, p. 526.

Lazarovits, A. I., Moscicki, R. A., Kurnick, J. T., Carmerini, D., Bhan, A. K., Baird, L. G., Erikson, M., and Colvin, R. B., 1984, Lymphocyte activation antigens. I. A monoclonal antibody, anti-Act I, defines a new late lymphocyte activation antigen, *J. Immunol.* 133:1857–1862.

Leonard, W. J., Depper, J. M., Uchiyama, T., Smith, K. A., Waldmann, T. A., and Greene, W. C., 1982, A monoclonal antibody appears to recognize the receptor for human T cell growth factor; partial characterization of the receptor, *Nature* 300:267–269.

Lindquist, S., 1986, The heat-shock response, *Annu. Rev. Biochem.* 55:1151–1191.

Londei, M., Savill, C. M., Verhoeff, A., Brennan, F., Leech, Z. A., Duance, V., Maini, R. N., and Feldmann, M., 1989, Persistence of collagen type II-specific T cell clones in the synovial membrane of a patient with rheumatoid arthritis, *Proc. Natl. Acad. Sci. USA* 86:636–640.

Marlin, S. D., and Springer, T. A., 1987, Purified intracellular adhesion molecule 1 (ICAM 1) is a ligand for lymphocyte function associated antigen 1 (LFA-1), *Cell* 51:813–819.

Marth, J. D., Peet, R., Krebs, E. G., and Perlmutter, R. M., 1985, A lymphocyte-specific protein-tyrosine kinase gene is rearranged and overexpressed in the murine T cell lymphoma LSTRA, *Cell* 43:393–404.

Mason, D. W., and Morris, P. J., 1986, Effector mechanisms in allograft rejection, *Annu. Rev. Immunol.* 4:119–145.

Meuer, S. C., Hussey, R. E., Fabbi, M., Fox, D., Acuto, Fitzgerald, K. A., Hodgdon, J. C., Protentis, J. P., Schlossman, S. F., and Reinhertz, E. L., 1984, An alternative pathway of T cell activation: A functional role for the 50 KD T11 sheep erythrocyte receptor protein, *Cell* 36:897–906.

Millward, B. A., Welsh, K. I., Leslie, R. D. G., Pyke, D. A., and Demaine, A. G., 1987, T cell receptor beta chain polymorphisms are associated with insulin dependent diabetes, *Clin. Exp. Immunol.* 70:152–157.

Miltenburg, A. M. M., Laar, J. M., Daha, M. R., DeVries, R. R. P., Van den Elsen, P. J., and Breedveld, F. C., 1990, Dominant T cell receptor (TCR) beta-chain gene rearrangements indicate clonal expansion in the rheumatoid joint, *Scand. J. Immunol.* 31:121–125.

Morel, P., Cordier, G., Vincent, C., Traeger, J., Carosella, E., and Revillard, J.-P., 1989, Anti-CD4 monoclonal antibody therapy in humans, in: *7th International Congress of Immunology*, Berlin (West), July 30–August 5, 1989 (Abstract), Gustav Fischer, Stuttgart, p. 890.

Mustelin, T., and Altman, A., 1989, Do CD4 and CD8 control T cell activation via a specific tyrosine protein kinase? *Immunol. Today* 10:189–191.

Natvig, J. B., Randen, I., Thompson, K., Førre, Ø., and Munthe, E., 1989, The B cell system in the rheumatoid inflammation. New insights into the pathogenesis of rheumatoid arthritis using synovial B cell hybridoma clones, *Springer Semin. Immunopathol.* 11:301–314.

Norman, D. J., Shield, C. F., Barry, J. M., Henell, K., Funnell, M. B., and Lemon, J., 1987, Therapeutic use of OKT3 monoclonal antibody for acute renal allograft rejection, *Nephron* 46(Suppl.):41–47.

Oksenberg, J. G., Sherritt, M., Begovich, A. B., Erlich, H. A., Bernard, C. C., Cavalli-Sforze, L. L., and Steinman, L., 1989, T cell receptor Vα and Cα alleles associated with multiple sclerosis and myasthenia gravis, *Proc. Natl. Acad. Sci. USA* 86:988–992.

Palacois, H., 1982, Mechanism of T cell activation: Role and functional relationship of HLA-DR antigens and interleukins, *Immunol. Rev.* 63:73–110.

Prentice, H. G., Blacklock, H. A., Janossy, G., Bradstock, K. F., Skeggs, D., Goldstein, G., and Hoffbrand, A. V., 1982, Use of anti-T-cell monoclonal antibody OKT3 to prevent acute graft-versus-host disease in allogeneic bone marrow transplantation for acute leukaemia, *Lancet* 1:700–703.

Reinherz, E. L., Geha, R., Rappeport, J. M., Wilson, M., Penta, A. C., Hussey, R. E., Fitzgerald, K. A., Daley, J. K., Levine, H., Rosen, F. S., and Schlossman, S. F., 1982, Reconstitution after transplantation with T lymphocyte depleted HLA haplotype-mismatched bone marrow for severe combined immunodeficiencies, *Proc. Natl. Acad. Sci. USA* **79:**6047–6051.

Reiter, C., Kruger, K., Schattenkirchner, M., Rietmüller, G., and Rieber, P., 1989, Treatment of rheumatoid arthritis with a monoclonal anti-CD4-body, in: *7th International Congress of Immunology*, Berlin (West), July 30–August 5, 1989 (Abstract), Gustav Fischer, Stuttgart, p. 891.

Res, P. C. M., Schaar, C. G., Breedveld, F. C., van Eden, W., van Embden, J. D. A., Cohen, I. R., and deVries, R. R. P., 1988, Synovial fluid T cell reactivity against 65 kD heat shock protein of mycobacteria in early chronic arthritis, *Lancet* **2:**478–480.

Rivas, A., Takada, S., Koide, J., Sonderstrup-McDevitt, G., and Engleman, E. G., 1988, CD4 molecules are associated with the antigen receptor complex on activated but not resting T cells, *J. Immunol.* **140:**2912–2918.

Rosenstein, Y., Ratnovsky, S., Burakoff, S., and Herrmann, S. H., 1989, Direct evidence for binding of CD8 to HLA class I antigens, *J. Exp. Med.* **169:**149–160.

Rugstad, H. E., 1988, Antiinflammatory and immunomodulatory effects of glucocorticoids: Mode of action, *Scand. J. Rheumatol.* (Suppl.)**76:**257–64.

Quayle, A., Kjelden-Kragh, J., Førre, Ø., Waalen, K., Sioud, M., Kalvenes, C., and Natvig, J. B., 1989, Immunoregulatory T cell subsets and T cell activation in rheumatoid arthritis. A need for analysis on the clonal and molecular level, *Springer Semin. Immunopathol.* **1989:**273–288.

Schluesener, H. J., and Wekerle, H., 1984, In vivo selection of permanent T lymphocyte lines with receptors for myelin basic protein (MBP), *Prog. Clin. Biol. Res.* **146:**285–290.

Shaw, S., Luce, G. E., Quinones, R., Gress, R. E., Springer, T. A., and Sanders, M. E., 1986, Two antigen-independent pathways used by human cytotoxic T cell clones, *Nature* **323:**262–264.

Smely, S., Weschka, M., Dendorfer, U., Hillebrand, G., Kurrle, R., Land, W., and Hammer, C., 1989, Prophylactic use of the new monoclonal antibody BI 51.013 (BMA 031) in clinical kidney transplantation: Phenotypic evaluation of the lymphocytic target cells, in: *7th International Congress of Immunology*, Berlin (West), July 30–August 5, 1989 (Abstract), Gustav Fischer, Stuttgart, p. 892.

Smith, K. A., and Cantrell, D. A., 1985, Interleukin 2 regulates its own receptors, *Proc. Natl. Acad. Sci. USA* **82:**864–868.

Stamenkovic, I., Stegano, M., Wright, K. A., Krane, S. M., Amento, E. P., Colvin, R. B., Duquesnoy, R. J., and Kurnick, J. T., 1988, Clonal dominance among T-lymphocyte infiltrates in arthritis, *Proc. Natl. Acad. Sci. USA* **85:**1179–1183.

Staunton, D. E., Dustin, M. L., and Springer, T. A., 1989, Functional cloning of ICAM-2, a cell adhesion ligand for LFA-1 homologous to ICAM-1, *Nature* **339:**61–64.

Svejgaard, A., Platz, P., and Ryder, L. P., 1983, HLA and disease 1982–A survey, *Immunol. Rev.* **70:**193–218.

Takihara, Y., Reiman, J., Michalpoulis, E., Ciccone, E., Moretta, L., and Mak, T. W., 1989, Diversity and structure of human T cell receptor chain genes in peripheral blood-bearing T lymphocytes, *J. Exp. Med.* **169:**393–405.

Todd, J. A., Acha-Orbea, H., Bell, J. I., Chao, N., Fronek, Z., Jacob, C. O., McDermott, M., Sinha, A. A., Timmerman, L., Steinman, L., and McDevitt, H. O., 1988a, A molecular basis for MHC Class II-associated autoimmunity, *Science* **240:**1003–1009.

Todd, J. A., Bell, J. I., and McDevitt, H. O., 1988b, A molecular basis for genetic susceptibility to insulin dependent diabetes mellitus, *Trends Genet.* **4:**129–134.

Triebel, F., and Hercend, T., 1989, Subpopulations of human peripheral T gamma delta lymphocytes, *Immunol. Today* **10:**186–188.

Trowbridge, I. S., and Omary, M. B., 1981, Human cell surface glycoprotein related to cell proliferation is receptor for transferrin, *Proc. Natl. Acad. Sci. USA* **78:**3039–3043.

Veillette, A., Bookman, M. A., Horak, E. M., and Bolen, J. B., 1988, The CD4 and CD8 T cell surface antigens are associated with the internal membrane tyrosine-protein kinase p56lck, *Cell* **55:**301–308.

Waalen, K., Førre, Ø., Linker-Israeli, M., and Thoen, J., 1987, Evidence of an activated T cell system with augmented turnover of interleukin 2 in rheumatoid arthritis, *Scand. J. Immunol.* **25:**367–373.

Weiner, H. L., Fallis, R. J., Aoun, M., et al., 1986, Immunologic effects in progressive MS patients treated with anti-T11 and T4 monoclonal antibodies, *Neurology* **36**(Suppl. 1):284.

Weiss, A., and Stobo, J. D., 1984, Requirement for the coexpression of T3 and the T cell antigen receptor on a malignant human T cell line, *J. Exp. Med.* **160:**1284–1299.

Weschka, M., Smely, S., Dendorfer, U., Hillebrand, G., Kurrle, R., Land, W., and Hammer, C., 1989, Prophylactic use of the new monoclonal antibody BI 51.013 (BMA 031) in clinical kidney transplantation: Pharmacokinetics, antibody response, and cytokine release, in: *7th International Congress of Immunology*, Berlin (West), July 30–August 5, 1989 (Abstract), Gustav Fischer, Stuttgart, p. 893.

Winchester, R., and Gregersen, P., 1989, The molecular basis of susceptibility the rheumatoid arthritis: The conformational equivalence hypothesis, *Springer Semin. Immunopathol.* **10:**119–139.

Wraith, D. C., McDevitt, H. O., Steinman, L., and Acha-Orbea, H., 1989, T cell recognition as the target for immune intervention in autoimmune disease, *Cell* **57:**709–715.

Yanagi, T., Yoshikai, Y., Legget, K., Clark, S. P., Aleksander, I., and Mak, T. W., 1984, A human T cell specific cDNA clone encodes a protein having an extensive homology to immunoglobulin chains, *Nature* **308:**145–149.

Young, D. B., Mehlert, A., Bal, V., Mendez-Samperio, P., Ivanyi, J., and Lamb, J. R., 1988, Stress proteins and the immune response to mycobacterial antigens as virulence factors? *Antonie van Leeuwenhoek* **54:**431–439.

Zinkernagel, R. M., and Doherty, P. C., 1974, Restriction of in vitro T cell mediated cytotoxicity in lymphocyte choriomeningitis within a syngeneic or semiallogeneic system, *Nature* **248:**701–702.

Chapter 5

NATURAL KILLER CELLS IN AUTOIMMUNE DISEASES

Function and Markers

Dag Sørskaar and *Øystein Førre*

1. INTRODUCTION

Natural killer cell activity was first recognized around 1970 (McCoy *et al.*, 1973; Takasugi *et al.*, 1973). This activity can be demonstrated without the apparent previous sensitization of the effector cells. It has therefore been termed either spontaneous or natural cell-mediated cytotoxicity (Takasugi *et al.*, 1977), spontaneous lymphocyte-mediated or mononuclear cell cytotoxicity (Pross and Baines, 1977), and now usually natural killer (NK) cell activity. The effector cells responsible for this activity are called natural killer cells (NK cells). They are considered to be distinct from other cells capable of mediating spontaneous cytotoxicity such as cytotoxic T lymphocytes and monocytes (Ritz *et al.*, 1988). *In vitro* lymphokine-activated killer (LAK) cells are interleukin-2 (IL-2)-stimulated lymphocytes with the ability to lyse NK resistant target cells *in vivo* (Grimm *et al.*, 1982). However, LAK cells have so far not been shown to represent a distinct effector cell population. They mostly appear to represent IL-2-stimulated NK cells with enhanced cytolytic activity (Ritz *et al.*, 1988; Lotzová and Ades, 1989).

The NK cells are heterogeneous subsets of lymphocytes (Hercend *et al.*, 1983) capable of spontaneous cytotoxicity against tumor cells (Herberman *et al.*, 1979), and virally infected cells (Biron *et al.*, 1989) in the absence of any prior sensitization. Currently, NK cells are identified with an increasingly broader set of functions as they participate in the rejection of bone marrow grafts (Lotzová *et al.*, 1983), undergo activation in mixed leukocyte reaction cultures (Seeley and Golub, 1978), and act as suppressor cells (Tilden *et al.*, 1983) or as accessory cells (Scala *et al.*, 1985). The NK cells also recognize and lyse normal cells (Hansson *et al.*, 1982). Recently Garcia-Penarrubia *et al.* (1989) have demonstrated the antibacterial activity of human NK cells. Increasing evidence for a role of NK cells in

Dag Sørskaar and *Øystein Førre* • Oslo Sanitetsforening Rheumatism Hospital, N-0172 Oslo 1, Norway.

Immunopharmacology in Autoimmune Diseases and Transplantation, edited by Hans Erik Rugstad *et al.* Plenum Press, New York, 1992.

autoimmune diseases has been put forward (Ortaldo and Herberman, 1984; Whiteside and Herberman, 1989).

Numerous attempts have been made to characterize these cells. Despite this, no single definition of NK cells has so far emerged. The present view is that NK cells are phenotypically and functionally heterogeneous lymphocyte subpopulations, sharing no common trait except for lysis of the human erythroleukemia K562 cell line (Ortaldo and Herberman, 1984). Their cytolytic reactions do not require either class I or class II major histocompatibility complex (MHC) expression on the target cells (Hercend and Schmidt, 1988; Lotzová and Ades, 1989).

2. PHENOTYPE OF NK CELLS

Morphologically, human NK cells have been described as large granular lymphocytes with a high cytoplasm-to-nucleus ratio. The cytoplasm is pale and contains 6–12 azurophilic granules together with an eccentric and reniform nucleus (Timonen et al., 1979). Human NK cells bear Fc receptors (Bakacs et al., 1977). Some of the human NK cells possess a number of T-cell-associated antigens such as CD2 (E receptors) (Zarling et al., 1981) and antigens detected with anti-CD8 (OKT8) and anti-CD38 (OKT10) (Ortaldo et al., 1981) (Table I).

Several monoclonal antibodies reacting more or less specifically with human NK cells have been described (Knapp et al., 1989). One of these is a monoclonal IgM antibody to a membrane antigen CD57 (HNK-1 or Leu-7), which is present on 15% of normal blood lymphocytes (Abo and Balch, 1981). CD57-positive cells include both E rosetting and non-E-rosetting cells, but no cells expressing surface immunoglobulin. Most of the CD57-positive cells also express the Fcγ receptor. Three different Fc receptors (FcR) for IgG have been characterized: CD64 (FcRI), CDw32 (FcRII), and CD16 (FcRIII) (Anderson and Looney, 1986). CD16 is found on large granular lymphocytes (Anderson and Looney, 1986) and on NK cells (Perussia et al., 1984). The monoclonal antibody to human NK cells, anti-CD16 (Leu-11), detects approximately 15% of peripheral blood lymphocytes (Lanier et al., 1983). A variable number of CD16-positive cells coexpress the CD57 antigen and to some extent also the CD8 antigen, but none of the other T-cell antigens, such as CD5, CD4, or CD3. By far most of the NK cell function is mediated by the CD16-positive and CD57-

TABLE I. Surface Markers of Human NK Cells

Cluster	Antibodies
CD2	OKT11, Leu-5b (E-receptor)
CD7	3AI, Leu-9
CD8	OKT8, Leu-2
CD11a	LFA-1
CD11b	OKM1 (CR3)
CD11c	Leu-M5
CD16	3G8, B73.1, Leu-11 (FcRIII)
CD18	β chain of CD11
CD25	TAC (IL-2 receptor)
CD38	OKT10, Leu-17
CD56	NKH-1, Leu-19
CD57	HNK-1, Leu-7
CD71	OKT9, transferrin receptor

positive cells. The CD16-positive, CD57-negative cell subset was found to have the most NK cell activity, whereas the CD16-negative, CD57-positive cells only showed weak lytic activity (Lanier *et al.*, 1983). CD16-positive cells might also coexpress the pan-NK cell antigen CD56 (NKH1 and Leu 19) (Knapp *et al.*, 1989; Morio *et al.*, 1989).

3. LYSIS BY NK CELLS

Santoli *et al.* (1976) found that human peripheral blood lymphocytes preferentially lysed human target cells, and of all human cell lines, tumor cells were killed with the highest efficiency. However, the functions of NK cells have been found to be as diverse as the phenotypic markers.

The molecular mechanisms leading to NK cell recognition and cytolysis of tumor targets are still poorly understood. The NK cell-mediated cytolysis proceeds through several stages: (1) effector target cell recognition and binding followed by (2) triggering and activation of the NK cells, (3) release and binding of the lethal substance on the target cell surface, and finally (4) target cell death (Bonavida and Wright, 1986). Ucker (1987) and Golstein (1987) have proposed that the target cell itself may actively play a role in the killing event. According to this endogenous suicide model, the target cell can be activated by several different stimuli, resulting in induced target cell death. This may apply to both cytotoxic T-lymphocyte and NK cell-mediated lysis.

An interesting finding is the recycling capacity of the NK cells. Ullberg and Jondal (1981) demonstrated that NK cells after lysing a target cell could dissociate from that cell and thereafter bind to and kill another target cell.

Several studies have shown that interferon, or interferon inducers, can mediate the augmentation of normal NK cells (Gidlund *et al.*, 1978; Ortaldo *et al.*, 1981). This can be achieved by different mechanisms: (1) by increasing the number of target-binding NK cells (Perussia *et al.*, 1983), (2) by accelerating the kinetics of lysis (Targan and Dorey, 1980), and (3) by increasing the recycling capacity of NK cells (Timonen *et al.*, 1982a). NK cells have also been shown to proliferate (Timonen *et al.*, 1982b) and augment their cytolytic activity in response to IL-2.

As mentioned, there is increasing evidence that NK cells are a part of the host defense system. Numerous studies on the NK cell activity in patients with various diseases have been published. However, the studies of the NK cell cytotoxic profile in patients with autoimmune diseases are still relatively few.

4. NK CELL ACTIVITY IN AUTOIMMUNE DISEASES

Although abnormalities of the immune system play an important role in the pathogenesis of rheumatoid arthritis, the primary cause of the disease remains unknown. Rheumatoid arthritis is characterized by the presence of autoantibodies and chronic inflammation in the synovial membranes. The classic histological picture of rheumatoid synovitis emerges with the progress of the disease (Pope and Talal, 1985), with hyperplasia of the synovial lining layer and infiltration of the sublining layer by large numbers of different cell subpopulations such as lymphocytes, plasma cells, and macrophages (Førre *et al.*, 1985). Also, the NK cells might participate in this process.

Interestingly, it has been shown in an animal model that NK-like cells from the spleens of mice have spontaneous natural cytotoxicity against autologous chondrocytes, but not against fibroblasts (Malejczyk *et al.*, 1985).

4.1. Rheumatoid Arthritis and Juvenile Rheumatoid Arthritis

Some disagreement exists about the NK cell function in patients with rheumatoid arthritis. Several reports have found normal NK cell activity in peripheral blood from rheumatoid arthritis patients (Neighbour et al., 1982; Silver et al., 1982). One report claims enhanced NK cell function in rheumatoid arthritis (Goto et al., 1981) while others have described reduced NK activity (Russell and Miller, 1984). In our own studies (Thoen et al., 1987), we have demonstrated reduced NK cell activity in peripheral blood from patients with rheumatoid arthritis and in IgM rheumatoid factor-positive polyarticular juvenile rheumatoid arthritis, which probably represents a different expression of the same disorder (Førre et al., 1983) (Table II). Reduced NK cell activity against adenovirus-infected target cells has been reported in systemic juvenile rheumatoid arthritis (Still's disease) (Luder et al., 1989).

The NK activity in mononuclear cells from synovial fluids of rheumatoid arthritis patients has been found to be of the same level as that of the blood (Thoen et al., 1987). However, this is not in agreement with a report of Burmester et al. (1978), who found increased NK cell activity in rheumatoid synovial fluid, whereas Silver et al. (1982) have claimed decreased NK cell activity in rheumatoid synovial fluid. These conflicting results might be due to differences in the NK cell assays used or rely on differences in disease activity of unselected seropositive patients. In peripheral blood from patients with rheumatoid arthritis, impaired NK cell activity has been described in active disease, whereas patients in remission had normal NK cell function.

Mononuclear cells from rheumatoid synovial membranes have been found almost devoid of NK cell activity simultaneously with very few CD57-positive cells (Thoen et al., 1987). In patients with rheumatoid arthritis the number of CD57-positive cells in synovial fluid do not differ from that in the peripheral blood.

A possible role for the NK cells in the pathogenesis of rheumatoid diseases has not yet been clarified. An impairment of NK cell activity might result in an inefficient control of virus-infected target cells and also in uncontrolled B-cell activity (Pistoia et al., 1985). The NK cells might thus have immunoregulatory properties in antibody production (Tilden et al., 1983).

Interestingly, Taylor et al. (1989) have found evidence for an increased incidence of chronic lymphatic leukemia in patients with rheumatoid arthritis. These patients had significantly lower NK cell activity compared to patients with rheumatoid arthritis or normal controls.

4.2. Systemic Lupus Erythematosus

Numerous studies have demonstrated reduced NK cell activity in systemic lupus erythematosus (SLE) (Hoffman, 1980; Katz et al., 1982; Sibbitt et al., 1983; Struyf et al., 1990). Most investigators agree that the deficiency of NK cells activity is most pronounced in active and untreated disease. However, one study by Goto et al. (1980) was not in agreement with this. The reason for the impaired NK cell function in SLE patients is highly controversial. Several mechanisms might be involved. Suppression of the NK cell-mediated cytotoxicity in SLE patients by antibodies reacting with NK cells has been demonstrated (Goto et al., 1980), although this could not be corroborated by others (Gonzalez-Amaro et al., 1988). Decreased IL-2 production by peripheral mononuclear cells from SLE patients has been reported (Linker-Israeli et al., 1983; Miyasaka et al., 1984b). IL-2 is essential for the growth and culture of NK cells, and without sufficient IL-2 the NK cell function will decrease

TABLE II. NK Cell Activity[a]
in Peripheral Blood of Patients
with Autoimmune Diseases

Rheumatoid arthritis	↓ ↔ ↑
Juvenile rheumatoid arthritis	↓
Ankylosing spondylitis	↔
Psoriatic arthropathy	↔
Systemic lupus erythematosus	↓
Sjögren's syndrome	↓

[a] ↓, Deceased; ↑, increased; ↔, normal.

(Miyasaka et al., 1984a). Sibbitt et al. (1983) demonstrated a marked increase in NK cell activity when mononuclear cells from SLE patients were treated with IL-2. However, the NK activity did not reach the same level as in cells from normal controls, indicating that the impaired IL-2 production in patients with SLE is not the only reason for the decreased NK cell activity in these patients.

The effect of IL-1 on NK cell activity has not been extensively studied. Probably IL-1 does not affect the NK cell function directly, but might act together with IL-2 or other cytokines to increase NK cell cytotoxicity against certain tumor cells (Dinarello et al., 1986). Decreased IL-1 production reported in SLE patients (Linker-Israeli et al., 1983) might thus partly be responsible for the impaired NK cell activity.

On the contrary, the interferon levels in SLE patients are elevated (Ytterberg and Schnitzer, 1982). Human NK cells express high-affinity receptors for all types of interferon (Faltynek et al., 1986). Accordingly, interferons of both alpha, beta, and gamma types are found to enhance the NK activity (Perussia et al., 1980). However, prestimulation of NK cells from SLE patients with interferon revealed reduced ability to augment cytotoxicity of the NK cells (Neighbour et al., 1982). Less than 50% of SLE patients showed any increase of NK cell cytotoxicity after interferon stimulation. The interferon production in patients with SLE might already be about maximal and cannot be further augmented. Whether the unusual interferon profile with interferon-γ deficiency and interferon-α augmentation found in SLE patients has any relation with the impaired NK cell cytotoxicity in SLE remains uncertain.

Interferon can inhibit cytotoxicity of the NK cells in long-term cultures containing IL-2 (Riccardi et al., 1983), indicating that interferon might inhibit IL-2-dependent growth and maturation of NK effectors. In support of this is that SLE patients treated with interferon-α showed reduction of NK cell activity (Maluish et al., 1983).

An interesting observation is that the potential NK cells from patients with SLE bind normally to the target cells and recycle frequently (Katz et al., 1982). However, they do not lyse as efficiently as NK cells from normal donors. The reason for this could be an impaired release of NK cells as suggested by Sibbitt et al. (1984). Decreased numbers of NK cells as defined by anti-CD57 and simultaneous impaired NK cell activity have been observed in SLE patients (Egan et al., 1983).

4.3. Sjögren's Syndrome

Patients with Sjögren's syndrome are not usually treated with immunomodulating agents that may influence NK cell activity. Sjögren's syndrome patients therefore represent an interesting patient group to study the NK cell function in autoimmune diseases. Several studies have demonstrated decreased cytotoxic activity of the NK cells in Sjögren's syndrome (Goto et al., 1981; Pedersen et al., 1986; Struyf et al., 1990). Miyasaka et al. (1983) have reported that reduced NK cell activity is more commonly found in patients with secondary Sjögren's syndrome than in patients with primary Sjögren's syndrome. There might be several reasons for this reduced NK cell activity. One model suggests that suppressive mechanisms involving prostaglandin, hydrogen peroxide, and endogenous circulating serum factors are associated with the impaired NK cell function in Sjögren's syndrome patients (Miyasaka et al., 1983). In another study by Miyasaka et al. (1984), five of eight patients with Sjögren's syndrome had lower IL-2 production than any of the 19 control subjects. IL-2 receptors have been recognized on NK cells, and IL-2 stimulation of NK cells restored the reduced NK cell activity in patients with Sjögren's syndrome (Pedersen et al., 1986). This indicates that the impaired NK cell activity in these patients might be functional since the total number of NK cells was normal. Taken together, the impaired NK cell function might partly be due to a defect in IL-2 production in Sjögren's syndrome as in SLE. Also, interferon stimulation of NK cells from patients with Sjögren's syndrome leads to increased NK cell activity, but the interferon-enhanced NK activity was significantly reduced in comparison to that of the normal controls (Pedersen et al., 1986).

The incidence of lymphoproliferative malignancies has been estimated to be increased 44-fold in Sjögren's syndrome (Manthorpe et al., 1981). The reduced NK cell activity might be related to the high risk of lymphoma and pseudolymphoma seen in these patients. The observation of highly reduced NK cell activity in both peripheral blood and bone marrow cells from patients with preleukemia support this (Sørskaar et al., 1986).

However, the status of NK cell function in Sjögren's syndrome is still controversial. The impaired NK cell activity demonstrated in Sjögren's syndrome is only one of several cellular immunity disturbances, such as defective IL-1 and IL-2 synthesis (Enk et al., 1986; Enk and Oxholm, 1988), depressed lymphocyte proliferation to lectins, defective T-cell activation (Gerli et al., 1989), and reduced autologous mixed lymphocyte reaction (Miyasaka et al., 1981).

5. EFFECT OF ANTIRHEUMATIC DRUGS ON NK CELL FUNCTION

In vitro, disease-modifying drugs have been shown to have various effects on NK cell function. However, an effect on NK cell function in vitro does not necessarily lead to an in vivo effect (Table III). Corticosteroids suppress NK cell activity both in vitro (Pedersen et al., 1986) and in vivo (Pedersen et al., 1984) during methylprednisolone pulse therapy in rheumatoid arthritis patients. In healthy individuals, however, the NK cell activity against K562 cells seem to be corticosteroid-resistant (Onsrud and Thorsby, 1981).

It has been demonstrated that D-penicillamine markedly inhibits NK cell activity in vitro (Lipsky, 1984). In our studies, six months of D-penicillamine treatment did not alter the function of circulating NK cells in patients with rheumatoid arthritis (Thoen et al., 1987, 1988), confirming previous results of Pedersen et al. (1984).

The antimalarial chloroquine has been shown to lower the NK cell activity both in vitro (Thiele and Lipsky, 1985) and in vivo (Ausiello et al., 1986).

Low concentrations of auranofin in vitro augments NK cell activity, whereas higher concentrations lead to reduced NK cell function (Pedersen and Abom, 1986). Conflicting results have been put forward regarding NK cell function after in vivo administration of oral gold (auranofin). Russel and Miller (1984) have demonstrated depressed NK cell activity in rheumatoid arthritis patients after administration of auranofin, while others have found

TABLE III. Drug Influence on NK Cell Activity[a]

	NK cell activity	
	In vitro	In vivo
Corticosteroid	↓	↓ ↔
D-penicillamine	↓ ↔	↔
Chloroquine	↓	↓
Auranofin	↓	↔
Sodium thiomalate	↔	↑
Azathioprine	↔	↓
6-Mercaptopurine	↓	
Methotrexate	↑	
Cyclosporine		↓
Piroxicam		↓
Indomethacin		↑

[a] ↓ , Decreased; ↑ , increased; ↔, no change.

normal NK cytotoxicity (Abom and Pedersen, 1987). In contrast, sodium aurothiomalate had no effect on NK killing *in vitro* (Pedersen and Abom, 1986). However, parenteral gold increased NK cell activity (Goto *et al.*, 1981).

The purine analogues azathioprine and 6-mercaptopurine both depress the NK cell function *in vivo* as shown in several studies of patients with rheumatoid arthritis (Abom and Pedersen, 1987; Cseuz and Panayi, 1990). *In vitro* no such influence on NK cell activity was demonstrated (Pedersen and Beyer, 1986b). Azathioprine may decrease the number of NK precursor cells (Shih *et al.*, 1982). However, Cseuz *et al.* (1990) did not find any consistent drop of NK cells as detected by the use of the monoclonal anti-CD57 and anti-CD16.

Methotrexate enhances NK cell function *in vitro* at concentrations that are easily achieved with oral therapy (Kremer *et al.*, 1986). Methotrexate improves the synthesizing deficiency of IL-2 in rheumatoid arthritis patients (Combe *et al.*, 1985), which in turn also may improve NK cell function.

Cyclosporine has become an important therapeutic tool in autoimmune diseases. Cyclosporine-treated patients are shown to have only a slight reduction of NK cell cytotoxicity compared to normal subjects (Versluis *et al.*, 1988). In contrast, clinical responders on cyclosporine treatment had increased levels of CD57-positive NK cells compared with control subjects (Yocum *et al.*, 1990).

Finally, nonsteroidal anti-inflammatory drug (NSAID) treatment probably does not alter NK cell activity in patients with rheumatoid arthritis (Russell and Miller, 1984). However, indomethacin has been demonstrated to enhance NK cell activity. In a study of Thoen *et al.* (1988) it was shown that NSAID piroxicam reduced NK cell activity, but this might be due to an increase in disease activity during piroxicam treatment.

6. SUMMARY

Most investigators report decreased NK cell activity in rheumatoid arthritis, juvenile rheumatoid arthritis, systemic lupus erythematosus, and Sjögren's syndrome. Normal NK activity was found in ankylosing spondylitis and psoriatic arthropathy. Except for sodium thiomalate and indomethacin, antirheumatic drugs have a down-modulating effect on NK cell function *in vivo*.

There is no unifying cause for the impaired NK cell function in autoimmune diseases.

So far it has not been clarified whether the impaired NK cell function in autoimmune diseases is primary or secondary to the pathological condition as such.

ACKNOWLEDGMENTS. This work was supported by the Norwegian Women's Public Health Organization, Grete Harbitz Legacy, Norma and Leon Hess Foundation for Research on Rheumatological Diseases, and the Norwegian Cancer Society. The expert secretarial assistance of Kari Bertelsen is greatly appreciated.

REFERENCES

Abo, T., and Balch, C. M., 1981, A differentiation antigen of human NK and K cells identified by a monoclonal antibody (HNK-1), J. Immunol. 127:1024–1029.

Abom, B., and Pedersen, B. K., 1987, The in vivo effect of triethylphosphine gold (auranofin), sodium aurothiomalate and azathioprine on natural killer cell activity of patients with rheumatoid arthritis, Clin. Exp. Rheumatol. 5:47–52.

Anderson, C. L., and Looney, J. R., 1986, Human leukocyte IgG Fc receptors, Immunol. Today 7:264–266.

Ausiello, C. M., Barbieri, P., Spagnoli, G. C., Ciompi, M. L., and Casciani, C. U., 1986, In vivo effects of chloroquine treatment on spontaneous and interferon-induced natural killer activities in rheumatoid arthritis patients. Clin. Exp. Rheum. 4:255–259.

Bakacs, T., Gergely, P., and Klein, E., 1977, Characterization of cytotoxic human lymphocyte subpopulations: The role of Fc-receptor-carrying cells, Cell. Immunol. 32:317–328.

Biron, C. A., Byron, K. S., & Sullivan, J. L., 1989, Severe herpesvirus infections in an adolescent without natural killer cells, N. Engl. J. Med. 320:1731–1735.

Bonavida, B., and Wright, S. C., 1986, Role of natural killer cytotoxic factors in the mechanism of target-cell killing by natural killer cells, J. Clin. Immunol. 6:1–8.

Burmester, G. R., Kalden, J. R., Peter, H. H., Schodel, I., Beck, P., and Wittenberg, A., 1978, Immunological and functional characteristics of peripheral blood and synovial fluid lymphocytes from patients with rheumatoid arthritis. Scand. J. Immunol. 7:405–417.

Combe, B., Pope, R. M., Fischbach, M., Darnell, B., Baron, S., and Talal, N., 1985, Interleukin-2 in rheumatoid arthritis: Production of and response to interleukin-2 in rheumatoid synovial fluid, synovial tissue and peripheral blood, Clin. Exp. Immunol. 59:520–528.

Cseuz, R., and Panayi, G. S., 1990, The inhibition of NK cell function by azathioprine during the treatment of patients with rheumatoid arthritis, Br. J. Rheumatol. 29:358–362.

Cseuz, R., Barnes, P., and Panayi, G. S., 1990, Natural killer cells in the blood of patients with rheumatoid arthritis treated with azathioprine, Br. J. Rheumatol. 29:284–287.

Dinarello, C. A., Conti, P., and Mier, J. W., 1986, Effects of human interleukin-1 on natural killer cell activity: Is fever a host defense mechanism for tumor killing? Yale J. Biol. Med. 59:97–106.

Egan, M. L., Mendelsohn, S. L., Abo, T., and Balch, C. M., 1983, Natural killer cells in systemic lupus erythematosus. Abnormal numbers and functional immaturity of HNK-1+ cells, Arthritis Rheum. 26:623–629.

Enk, C., and Oxholm, P., 1988, Decreased interleukin-1 responsiveness of blood lymphocytes in patients with primary Sjøgren's syndrome, Clin. Exp. Rheumatol. 6:67–69.

Enk,C., Oxholm, P., Tvede, N., and Bendtzen, K., 1986, Blood mononuclear cells in patients with primary Sjøgren's syndrome: Production of interleukins, enumeration of interleukin-2 receptors, and DNA synthesis, Scand. J. Rheumatol. 615:131–138.

Faltynek, C. R., Princler, G. L., and Ortaldo, J. R., 1986, Expression of IFN-alpha and IFN-gamma receptors on normal human small resting T lymphocytes and large granular lymphocytes, J. Immunol. 136:4134–4139.

Førre, Ø., Dobloug, J. H., Heyeraal, H. M., and Thorsby, E., 1983, HLA antigens in juvenile arthritis. Genetic basis for the different subtypes, Arthritis Rheum. 26:35–38.

Førre, Ø., Waalen, K., Thoen, J., and Hovig, T., 1985, Macrophages and dendritic cells in rheumatic diseases, in: Immunology of Rheumatic Diseases (S. Gupta and N. Talal, eds.), Plenum Press, New York, pp. 543–562.

Garcia-Penarrubia, P., Koster, F. T., Kelley, R. O., McDowell, T. D., and Bankhurst, A. D., 1989, Antibacterial activity of human natural killer cells, J. Exp. Med. 169:99–133.

Gerli, R., Bertotto, A., Cernetti, C., Agea, E., Crupi, S., Arcangeli, C., Spinozzi, F., Galandrini, R., and Rambotti, P., 1989, Anti-CD3 and anti-CD2-induced T-cell activation in primary Sjøgren's syndrome, Clin. Exp. Rheum. 7/S-3:129–134.

Gidlund, M., Orn, A., Wigzell, H., Senik, A., and Gresser, I., 1978, Enhanced NK cell activity in mice injected with interferon and interferon inducers, Nature 273:759–761.

Golstein, P., 1987, Cytotoxic T-cell melodrama, Nature 327:12.

Gonzalez-Amaro, R., Alcocer-Varela, J., and Alarcon-Segovia, D., 1988, Natural killer cell activity in the systemic connective tissue diseases, J. Rheum. 15:1223–1228.

Goto, M., Tanimoto, K., and Horiuchi, Y., 1980, Natural cell mediated cytotoxicity in systemic lupus erythematosus: Suppression by antilymphocyte antibody, Arthritis Rheum. 23(11):1274–1281.

Goto, M., Tanimoto, K., Chihara, T., and Horiuchi, Y. I., 1981, Natural cell-mediated cytotoxicity in Sjøgren's syndrome and rheumatoid arthritis, Arthritis Rheum. 24:1377–1382.

Grimm, E. A., Mazumder, A., Zhang, H. Z., and Rosenberg, S. A., 1982, Lymphokine-activated killer cell phenomenon. Lysis of natural killer-resistant fresh solid tumor cells by interleukin-2-activated autologous human peripheral blood lymphocytes, *J. Exp. Med.* **155**:1823–1841.

Hansson, M., Beran, M., Andersson, B., and Kiessling, R., 1982, Inhibition of *in vitro* granulopoiesis by autologous allogeneic human NK cells, *J. Immunol.* **129**:126–132.

Herberman, R. B., Djeu, J. Y., Kay, H. D., Ortaldo, J. R., Riccardi, C., Bonnard, G. D., Holden, H. T., Fagnani, R., Santoni, A. S., and Puccetti, P., 1979, Natural killer cells: Characteristics and regulation of activity, *Immunol. Rev.* **44**:43–70.

Hercend, T., and Schmidt, R. E., 1988, Characteristics and uses of natural killer cells, *Immunol. Today* **9**:291–293.

Hercend, T., Reinherz, E. L., Meuer, S., Schlossman, S. F., and Ritz, J., 1983, Phenotypic and functional heterogeneity of human cloned natural killer cell lines, *Nature* **301**:158–160.

Hoffman, T., 1980, Natural killer function in systemic lupus erythematosus, *Arthritis Rheum.* **23**:30–35.

Katz, D., Zatoun, A., Lee, J. A., Punush, R. S., and Longley, S., 1982, Abnormal killer cell activity in systemic lupus erythematosus: An intrinsic defect in the lytic event, *J. Immunol.* **129**:1966–1971.

Knapp, W., Rieber, P., Dörken, B., Schmidt, R. E., Stein, H., and v. d. Borne, A. E. G., Kr., 1987, Towards a better definition of human leucocyte surface molecules, *Immunol. Today* **10**:253–258.

Kremer, J. M., Galivan, J., Streckfuss, A., and Kamen, B., 1986, Methotrexate metabolism analysis in blood and liver of rheumatoid arthritis patients: Association with hepatic folate deficiency and formation of polyglutamates, *Arthritis Rheum.* **29**:832–835.

Lanier, L. L., Le, A. M., Phillips, J. H., Warner, N. L., and Babcock, G. F., 1983, Subpopulations of human natural killer cells defined by expression of the Leu-7 (HNK-1) and Leu-11 (NK-15) antigens, *J. Immunol.* **131**:1789–1796.

Linker-Israeli, M., Bakke, A. C., Kitridou, R. C., Gendler, S., Gillis, S., and Horwitz, D. A., 1983, Defective production of interleukin 1 and interleukin 2 in patients with systemic lupus erythematosus (SLE), *J. Immunol.* **130**:2651–2655.

Lipsky, P. E., 1984, Immunosuppression by D-penicillamine *in vitro*. Inhibition of human T lymphocyte proliferation by copper- or ceruloplasmin-dependent generation of hydrogen peroxide and protection by monocytes, *J. Clin. Invest.* **73**:53–65.

Lotzová, E., and Ades, E. W., 1989, Natural killer cells: Definition, heterogeneity, lytic mechanism, functions and clinical application. Highlights of the Fifth International Workshop on Natural Killer Cells, Hilton Head Island, N.C., *Nat. Immun. Cell Growth Regul.* **8**:1–9.

Lotzová, E., Savary, C. A., and Pollack, S. B., 1983, Prevention of rejection of allogeneic bone marrow transplants by NK 1.1 antiserum, *Transplantation* **35**:490–494.

Luder, A. S., Naphtali, V., Porat, E. B., and Lahat, N., 1989, Still's disease associated with adenovirus infection and defect in adenovirus directed natural killing, *Ann. Rheum. Dis.* **48**:781–786.

Malejczyk, J., Kaminiski, M. J., Malejczyk, M., and Majewski, S., 1985, Natural cell-mediated cytotoxic activity against isolated chondrocytes in the mouse, *Clin. Exp. Immunol.* **59**:110–116.

Maluish, A. E., Ortaldo, J. R., Conlon, J. C., Sherwin, S. A., Leawitt, R., Strong, D. M., Weirnik, P., Oldham, R. K., and Herberman, R. B., 1983, Depression of natural killer cytotoxicty after in vivo administration of recombinant leukocyte interferon, *J. Immunol.* **131**:503–507.

Manthorpe, R., Frost-Larsen, K., Isager, H., and Prause, J. U., 1981, Sjøgren's syndrome. A review with emphasis on immunological features, *Allergy* **36**:139–153.

McCoy, J. L., Herberman, R. B., Rosenberg, E. B., Donnelly, F. C., Levine, P. H., and Alford, C., 1973, 51Chromium-release assay for cell-mediated cytotoxicity of human leukemia and lymphoid tissue-culture cells, *Natl. Cancer Inst. Monogr.* **37**:59–67.

Miyasaka, N., Sauvezie, B., and Pierce, D., 1981, Decreased autologous mixed lymphocyte reaction in Sjøgren's syndrome, *J. Clin. Invest.* **66**:928–932.

Miyasaka, N., Seaman, W., Bakshi, A., Sauvezie, B., Strand, V., Pope, R., and Talal, N., 1983, Natural killing activity in Sjøgren's syndrome. An analysis of the defective mechanisms, *Arthritis Rheum.* **26**:954–960.

Miyiasaka, N., Darnell, B., Baron, T., and Talal, N., 1984a, Interleukin 2 enhances natural killing of normal lymphocytes, *Cell. Immunol.* **84**:154–162.

Miyasaka, N., Nakamura, T., Russell, I. J., and Talal, N., 1984b, Interleukin 2 deficiencies in rheumatoid arthritis and systemic lupus erythematosus, *Clin. Immunol. Immunopathol.* **31**:109–117.

Morio, T., Nonoyama, S., and Yata, J., 1989, Suppression of *in vitro* immunoglobulin synthesis by CD16 (Leu 11a)+ CD56 (NKH1, Leu 19)+ non-T lineage cells; lack of suppression of cells from immunodeficient patients, *Clin. Exp. Immunol.* **78**:159–165.

Neighbour, P. A., Grayzel, A. I., and Miller, A. E., 1982, Endogenous and interferon-augmented natural killer cell activity of human peripheral blood mononuclear cells in vitro. Studies of patients with multiple sclerosis, systemic lupus erythematosus or rheumatoid arthritis, *Clin. Exp. Immunol.* **49**:11–21.

Onsrud, M., and Thorsby, E., 1981, Influence of in vivo hydrocortisone on some human blood lymphocyte populations, *Scand. J. Immunol.* **13**:573–579.

Ortaldo, J. R., and Herberman, R. B., 1984, Heterogeneity of natural killer cells, *Annu. Rev. Immunol.* **2**:359–394.

Ortaldo, J. R., Sharrow, S. O., Timonen, T., and Herberman, R. B., 1981, Determination of surface antigens on highly purified human NK cells by flow cytometry with monoclonal antibodies, *J. Immunol.* **127**:2401–2409.

Oshimi, K., Oshimi, Y., Motoji, T., Kobayashi, S., and Mizoguchi, H., 1983, Lysis of leukemia and lymphoma cells by autologous and allogeneic interferon-activated blood mononuclear cells, *Blood* **61**:790–798.

Pedersen, B. K., and Abom,B. 1986, Characterization of the in vitro effects of triethylphosphine gold (Auranofin) on human NK cell activity, *Clin. Exp. Rheum.* **4**:249–253.

Pedersen, B. K., and Beyer, J. M., 1986a, Characterization of the in vitro effects of glucocorticosteroids on NK cell activity, *Allergy* **41**:220–224.

Pedersen, B. K., and Beyer, J. M., 1986b, A longitudinal study on the influence of azathioprine on natural killer (NK) cell activity, *Allergy* **41**:286–289.

Pedersen, B. K., Beyer, J. M., Rasmussen, A., Klarlund, K., Pedersen, B. N., and Helin, P., 1984, Methylprednisolone pulse therapy induced fall in natural killer cell activity in rheumatoid arthritis, *Acta Pathol. Microbiol. Immunol. Scand. (C)* **92:**319–323.

Pedersen, B. K., Oxholm, P., Manthorpe, R., and Andersen, V., 1986, Interleukin 2 augmentation of the defective natural killer cell activity in patients with primary Sjøgren's syndrome, *Clin. Exp. Immunol.* **63:**1–7.

Perussia, B., Santoli, D., and Trinchieri, G., 1980, Interferon modulation of natural killer cell activity, *Ann. NY Acad. Sci.* **350:** 55–62.

Perussia, B., Starr, S., Abraham, S., Fanning, V., and Trinchieri, G., 1983, Human natural killer cells analyzed by B73.1, a monoclonal antibody blocking Fc receptor functions. I. Characterization of the lymphocyte subset reactive with B73.1, *J. Immunol.* **130:**2133–2141.

Perussia, B., Trinchieri, G., Jackson, A., Warner, N. L., Faust, J., Rumpold, H., Kraft, D., and Lanier, L. L., 1984, The Fc receptor for IgG on human natural killer cells: Phenotypic, functional and comparative studies with monoclonal antibodies, *J. Immunol.* **133:**180–189.

Pistoia, V., Cozzalino, F., and Ferrarini, M., 1985, More about NK cells and regulation of B cell activity, *Immunol. Today* **6:** 287–288.

Pope, R. M., and Talal, N., 1985, Autoimmunity in rheumatoid arthritis, *Concepts Immunpathol.* **1:**219–250.

Pross, H. F., and Baines, M. G., 1977, Spontaneous human lymphocyte-mediated cytotoxicity against tumor target cells. VI. A brief review, *Cancer Immunol. Immunother.* **3:**75–85.

Riccardi, C., Vose, B. M., and Herberman, R. B., 1983, Modulation of IL-2-dependent growth of mouse NK cells by interferon and T lymphocytes, *J. Immunol.* **130:**228–232.

Ritz, J., Schmidt, R. E., Michon, J., Hercend, T., and Schlossman, S. F., 1988, Characterization of functional surface structures on human natural killer cells, *Adv. Immunol.* **42:**181–211.

Russell, A. S., and Miller, C., 1984, The activity of natural killer cells in patients with rheumatoid arthritis: I. The effect of drugs used in vivo, *Clin. Exp. Rheumatol.* **2:**227–229.

Santoli, D., Trinchieri, G., Zmijewski, C. M., and Koprowski, H., 1976, HLA-related control of spontaneous and antibody-dependent cell-mediated cytotoxic activity in humans, *J. Immunol.* **117:**765–770.

Scala, G., Allavena, P., Ortaldo, J. R., Herberman, R. B., and Oppenheim, J. J., 1985, Subsets of human large granular lymphocytes (LGL) exhibit accessory cell functions, *J. Immunol.* **134:**3049–3055.

Seeley, J. K., and Golub, S. H., 1978, Studies on cytotoxicity generated in human mixed lymphocyte cultures. II. Time course and target spectrum of several distinct concomitant cytotoxic activites, *J. Immunol.* **120:**1415–1421.

Shih, W. W. H., Ellison, G. W., Myers, L. W., Durkos-Smith, D., and Fahey, J. L., 1982, Locus of selective depression of human natural killer cells by azathioprine, *Clin. Immunol. Immunopathol.* **23:**672–681.

Sibbitt, W. L., Jr., Likar, L., Spellman, C. W., and Bankhurst, A. D., 1983, Impaired natural killer cell activity in systemic lupus erythematosus: Relationship to interleukin-2 production, *Arthritis Rheum.* **26:**1316–1320.

Sibbitt, W. L., Jr., Mathews, P. M., and Bankhurst, A. D., 1984, Impaired release of a soluble natural killer cytotoxic factor in systemic lupus erythematosus, *Arthritis Rheum.* **27:**1095–1100.

Silver, R. M., Redelman, D., Zvaifler, N. J., and Naides, S., 1982, Studies of rheumatoid synovial fluid lymphocytes. I. Evidence for activated natural killer-(NK) like cells, *J. Immunol.* **128:**1758–1763.

Struyf, N. J., Snoeck, H. W., Bridts, C. H., De Clerck, L. S., and Stevens, W. J., 1990, Natural killer cell activity in Sjøgren's syndrome and systemic lupus erythematosus: Stimulation with interferons and interleukin-2 and correlation with immune complexes, *Ann. Rheum. Dis.* **49:**690–693.

Sørskaar, D., Førre, Ø., Albrechtsen, D., and Stavem, P., 1986, Decreased natural killer cell activity versus normal natural killer cell markers in mononuclear cells from patients with smoldering leukemia, *Scand. J. Haematol.* **37:**154–161.

Takasugi, M., Mickey, M. R., and Terasaki, P. I., 1973, Reactivity of lymphocytes from normal persons on cultured tumor cells, *Cancer Res.* **33:**2989–2902.

Takasugi, M., Koide, Y., Akira, D., and Ramseyer, A., 1977, Specificities in natural cell-mediated cytotoxicity by the cross-competition assay, *Int. J. Cancer* **19:**291–297.

Targan, S., and Dorey, F., 1980, Interferon activation of "pre-spontaneous killer" (pre-SK) cells and alteration in kinetics of lysis of both "pre-SK" and active SK cells, *J. Immunol.* **124:**2157–2161.

Taylor, H. G., Nixon, N., Sheeran, T. P., and Dawes, P. T., 1989, Rheumatoid arthritis and chronic lymphatic leukaemia, *Clin. Exp. Rheumatol.* **7:**529–532.

Thiele, D. L., and Lipsky, P. E., 1985, Modulation of human natural killer cell function by L-leucine methyl ester: Monocyte-dependent depletion from human peripheral blood mononuclear cells, *J. Immunol.* **134:**786–793.

Thoen, J., Waalen, K., and Førre, Ø., 1987, Natural killer (NK) cells at inflammatory sties in patients with rheumatoid arthritis and in IgM rheumatoid factor positive polyarticular juvenile rheumatoid arthritis, *Clin. Rheumatol.* **6:**215–225.

Thoen, J., Helgetveit, K., Førre, Ø., Haile, Y., and Kåss, E., 1988, Effects of piroxicam and D-penicillamine on T lymphocyte subpopulations, natural killer cells and rheumatoid factor production in rheumatoid arthritis, *Scand. J. Rheumatol.* **17:**91–102.

Tilden, A. B., Abo, T., and Balch, C. M., 1983, Suppressor cell function of human granular lymphocytes identified by HNK-1 (Leu-7) monoclonal antibody, *J. Immunol.* **130:**1171–1175.

Timonen, T., Ranki, A., Saksela, E., and Hayry, P., 1979, Fractionation, morphological and functional characterization of effector cells responsible for human natural killer activity against cell-line targets, *Cell. Immunol.* **48:**121–132.

Timonen, T., Ortaldo, J. R., and Herberman, R. B., 1982a, Analysis by a single cell cytotoxicity of natural killer (NK) cell frequencies among human large granular lymphocytes and of the effects of IFN on their activity, *J. Immunol.* **128:**2514–2521.

Timonen, T., Ortaldo, J. R., Stadler, B. M., Onnard, G. D., Sharrow, S. O., and Herberman, R. B., 1982b, Cultures of purified human natural killer cells: Growth in the presence of interleukin 2, *Cell. Immunol.* **72:**178–185.

Ucker, D. S., 1987, Cytotoxic T lymphocytes and glucocorticoids activate an endogenous suicide process in target cells, *Nature* **327:**62–64.

Ullberg, M., and Jondal, M., 1981, Recycling and target binding capacity of human natural killer cells, *J. Exp. Med.* **153**:615–628.

Versluis, D. J., Metselaar, H. J., Bijma, A. M., Vaessen, L. M. B., Wenting, G. J., and Weimar, W., 1988, The effect of long-term cyclosporine therapy on natural killer cell activity, *Transplant. Proc.* (Suppl. 2) **20**:179–185.

Whiteside, T. L., and Herberman, R. B., 1989, The role of natural killer cells in human disease, *Clin. Immunol. Immunpathol.* **53:** 1–23.

Yocum, D. E., Wilder, R. L., Dougherty, S., Klippel, J. H., Pillemer, S., and Wahl, S., 1990, Immunologic parameters of response in patients with rheumatoid arthritis treated with cyclosporine A, *Arthritis Rheum.* **9**:1310–1316.

Ytterberg, S. R., and Schnitzer, T. J., 1982, Serum interferon levels in patients with systemic lupus erythematosus, *Arthritis Rheum.* **25**:401–406.

Zarling, J. M., Clouse, K. A., Biddison, W. E., and Kung, P. C., 1981, Phenotypes of human natural killer cell populations detected with monoclonal antibodies, *J. Immunol.* **127**:2575–2580.

Chapter 6

INTERLEUKINS

Molecular and Biological Properties

Sudhir Gupta

1. INTRODUCTION

Interleukins are a family of communication molecules that play a critical role in the differentiation and maturation of effector immune responses. Several of these molecules are pleiotropic with regard to cells of origin and targets for their effects. To date, eight interleukins (IL-1 through IL-8) have been identified and I believe many more will be discovered. Most of the interleukins have been purified to homogeneity, sequenced, gene cloned, and their cDNA expressed in *Escherichia coli*. Furthermore, their receptors have been purified and sequenced and their genes have been cloned. Because of these developments, their biological properties are better defined. It is almost impossible to review the properties of each of the interleukins, therefore I will review only IL-1, IL-2, and IL-6 because of their possible role in autoimmune diseases. Not to say that other interleukins play no role in autoimmune diseases, but they have not been extensively studied in relation to autoimmune diseases. Some of these interleukins have been recently reviewed (Gupta, 1985, 1988; Oppenheim *et al.*, 1986; Dinarello, 1988; Zvaifler and Firestein, 1988; Kishimoto, 1989).

2. INTERLEUKIN-1

Interleukin-1 is a polypeptide with pleiotropic effects on three major networks in the body, namely, nervous system, endocrine system, and immune system networks. This polypeptide hormone appears to play an important role in protective inflammatory and immunological responses to invading organisms and cancer and in tissue injury associated with disease process (e.g., type I diabetes mellitus). Interleukin-1 is comprised of two species whose genes have been cloned and cDNA expressed in *E. coli*. Interleukin 1 exerts its biological activity via IL-1 receptor (IL-1R). Recently IL-1 has been crystallized (Priestle *et al.*, 1988). The molecular and biological characteristics of IL-1 and its receptors will be discussed in subsequent sections.

Sudhir Gupta • Division of Basic and Clinical Immunology, University of California, Irvine, Irvine, California 92717.

Immunopharmacology in Autoimmune Diseases and Transplantation, edited by Hans Erik Rugstad *et al.* Plenum Press, New York, 1992.

2.1. Molecular Characteristics of IL-1

Two structurally related but biologically distinct IL-1 molecules were cloned in 1984. One was murine IL-1 (Lomedico *et al.*, 1984) and the other was human IL-1 (Auron *et al.*, 1984). The murine IL-1 (pI 5.0) cDNA coded for a 270-amino acid polypeptide precursor with a molecular weight of 31 kDa and lacked a signal peptide. Human IL-1 cDNA clone blood monocyte, which codes for a 269-amino acid precursor, also lacks a signal peptide. The murine IL-1 precursor includes the 152 amino acids contained in the 17-kDa extracellular form of IL-1 (pI 7.0). The human IL-1 is cleaved to produce a product with most biological activities assigned to IL-1. A 20% homology at the peptide level and 45% at the nucleotide level was observed between murine IL-1 (pI 5.0) and human IL-1 (pI 7.0). The discovery of second human IL-1 was made by the isolation of two distinct but distantly related cDNA clones encoding proteins sharing biological activities of IL-1 (March *et al.*, 1985). These molecules were referred to as IL-1 alpha and IL-2 beta and showed considerable homology to murine and human cDNA isolated by Lomedico *et al.* (1984) and Auron *et al.* (1984). The pI 7.0 IL-1 cDNA sequence reported by March *et al.* (1985) was almost identical to IL-1 cDNA reported by Auron *et al.* (1984). A 26% homology in amino acid sequences and 45% homology in nucleotide sequences was observed between human pI 5.0 and pI 7.0 IL-1 cDNAs. Furthermore, there is 62% homology between nucleotide sequences of human and murine pI 5.0 IL-1. Each IL-1 is encoded by separated genes that are located on chromosome 2, and each gene contains seven exons. The regulation of IL-1 production is predominantly controlled at the level of transcription. March *et al.* (1985) also demonstrated that biological activities of IL-1 alpha and IL-1 beta are conveyed by 159 and 153 amino acids from their C-terminal, respectively. The mRNA for IL-1 beta but not IL-1 alpha mRNA is present in unstimulated human monocytes. However, using more sensitive dot blot analysis, observed mRNA for both IL-1 alpha and IL-1 beta is detected in monocyte populations. The mRNA for IL-1 alpha in unstimulated monocytes is present in lesser amounts than mRNA for IL-1 beta. Following lipopolysaccharide (LPS) stimulation, mRNA of IL-1 alpha increases to two- to fourfold whereas IL-1 beta mRNA increases to 40-fold over unstimulated level. It is well established that both IL-1 species are produced by a population of macrophages but it would be of interest to know if one single macrophage could produce both molecules. It would also be of interest to determine whether both IL-1 alpha and IL-1 beta are independently regulated. Recently, Fenton *et al.* (1988) have demonstrated that human pro-IL-1 beta gene expression in monocyte cells is regulated by two distinct pathways. They demonstrated that stimulation of THP-1 (a human monocytic leukemia cell line) with LPS and phorbol myristate acetate (PMA) resulted in differential expression of both pro-IL-1 beta mRNA and protein. PMA-induced transcription, unlike that for LPS, was not affected by cyclohexamide, suggesting a lack of requirement for *de novo* protein synthesis. In addition to being transcriptionally regulated, pro-IL-1 beta expression is also controlled at posttranscriptional level. PMA and LPS regulate the expression of IL-1 beta gene by distinct pathways at both the transcription and posttranscription level.

2.2. Synthesis and Secretion of IL-1

2.2.1. Cell Source of IL-1

Although monocyte–macrophage lineage cells are the predominant source of IL-1, several cell types produce IL-1. Table I lists the cell sources for IL-1. The biochemical properties of the IL-1 activities have been defined in a few cell types. The monocyte-derived

TABLE I. Cellular Sources of IL-1 Activities

Cell type	Stimulants[a]
Monocytes and macrophages	LPS, particles, immune complexes, PMA, ionophores, gamma interferon, colony-stimulating factor
Synovial fibroblasts	MDP
Keratinocytes and Langerhans cells	LPS
Mesangial cells of the kidney	Cell cycle-dependent
Dendritic cells	LPS
Large granular lymphocytes	LPS
B cells and B cell lines	LPS, anti-IgM or spontaneously produced
Astrocytes and microglial cells	LPS
Vascular endothelial cells	LPS
Thymic epithelial cells	PMA
Neutrophils	Aluminum hydroxide
Adult T cell leukemia cell line	Spontaneously produced

Abbreviations: LPS, lipopolysaccharide; PMA, phorbol myristate acetate; MDP, muramyldipeptide.

cDNA for IL-1 beta hybridizes with a keratinocyte-derived mRNA. This would suggest that two cell types produce closely related forms of IL-1. Because most nonmacrophage cells produce IL-1 with the same molecular weight and major pI as monocyte-derived IL-1, it would suggest that most of these cells produce IL-1 alpha and IL-1 beta. IL-1-like factor produced by B cell lines may differ from both IL-1 alpha and IL-1 beta (Matsushima *et al.*, 1987). IL-1 produced by Epstein-Barr virus (EBV)-transformed B cell line has a molecular weight of approximately 25 kDa with a pI of 5.5. In contrast, normal human B cell-derived IL-1 has a molecular weight of 20 kDa with pIs of 5.0, 6.0, and 7.0, and therefore resembles monocyte-derived IL-1.

2.2.2. Production and Secretion of IL-1

A majority of cells and cell lines produce IL-1 upon activation with a variety of stimuli, although some cell line spontaneously produce IL-1. The most common stimuli, both *in vivo* and *in vitro*, are bacterial products, phagocytosis, and immunological agents, including complement components, gamma interferon, leukotriene B4, and colony-stimulating factors (Dinarello, 1988; Dinarello *et al.*, 1989). Following stimulation with LPS, intracellular IL-1 activity appears within 30 min and secreted IL-1 can be detected within 1 hr with maximum levels found within 6 hr. This increase is blocked by cycloheximide and actinomycin D, indicating RNA and protein synthesis. Following stimulation, there is a short period of transcription; however, stimulants have a major effect on translation and processing of the IL-1 precursor. The period of transcription can be increased by suppressing the synthesis of a repressor protein (Fenton *et al.*, 1988). Because of the lack of a cleavage sequence, a significant amount of IL-1 remains cell-associated, either intracellularly (Lepe-Zuniga and Gery, 1984) or as part of a cell membrane. The 31-kDa and 22-kDa forms are cell-associated and could form membrane-bound IL-1 (Lepe-Zuniga and Gery, 1984; Matsushima *et al.*, 1987). Membrane-bound IL-1 is biologically active (Kurt-Jones *et al.*, 1985) and may be responsible for most of the immunostimulatory property of IL-1 in local tissues, including skeletal joints and skin. A majority of membrane-bound IL-1 is in alpha form; the beta form is secreted into extracellular fluid. The membrane-bound IL-1 is also important in antigen presentation.

IL-1 production can be affected at several levels. Corticosteroids reduce IL-1 production by acting at the level of transcription and translation of IL-1 beta (Kern *et al.*, 1988). Prostaglandins and prostacyclins induce cAMP, which in turn reduces IL-1 production at a posttranscription level (Dinarello *et al.*, 1984). Gamma interferon reduces IL-1-induced IL-1 production but up-regulates endotoxin-induced IL-1 production (Ghezzi and Dinarello, 1988). Arend *et al.* (1985) reported that the regulation of IL-1 beta in cultured human monocytes is regulated at multiple levels. There is evidence to suggest that CD8$^+$ T cells suppress IL-1 production from large granular lymphocytes (Scala *et al.*, 1984).

2.3. IL-1 Receptors

The diverse biological activities of IL-1 are mediated by binding to its receptors. Both forms of IL-1 bind to the same receptors. An 80-kDa IL-1 specific binding protein has been recognized on a variety of cell lines (Lowenthal and MacDonald, 1986). Lowenthal and MacDonald (1986) described the presence of high- and low-affinity IL-1R on EL4 T cells. The majority of IL-1R bind IL-1 with a dissociation constant (Kd) of 200–500 pM (low-affinity IL-1 receptors), whereas high-affinity IL-1R, making up 1–2% of the total, bind to IL-1 with a Kd of 3–8 pM. High-affinity IL-1R can internalize IL-1, whereas low-affinity IL-1R cannot do so. The biological activities of IL-1 are mediated exclusively via interaction with the minor class of high-affinity IL-1R. All IL-1R$^+$ T cells express both high- and low-affinity classes of IL-1R. Normal T cells express very low numbers of high-affinity IL-1R (-10/cell). In the lymph node cells, only L3T4$^+$ T cells express IL-1R. So far, no function has been assigned to low-affinity IL-1R, but it is possible that they represent an external pool of nonfunctioning receptors that can be recruited into the high-affinity functional IL-1R. IL-1 regulates its own receptors (Dinarello *et al.*, 1989). In human synovial cells, IL-1 beta binds with a Kd of 6.6×10^{-11}M (Chin *et al.*, 1988).

It has recently been demonstrated that IL-1 transduces a signal via the mechanism of phospholipid hydrolysis (Rosoff *et al.*, 1988). In Jurkat T cells, IL-1 increases the liberation of diacylglycerol (DAG), which takes place in the absence of phosphatidyl inositol turnover. There is no increase in cytosolic free Ca^{2+} (Abraham *et al.*, 1987). Jurkat cells release phosphoryl choline from phosphatidyl choline within seconds of exposure to IL-1. In pre-B cells, IL-1, following binding to IL-1R, induces fluxes of Na^{2+}/K$^+$ and Ca^{2+} across the plasma membrane (Mizel *et al.*, 1988).

2.4. Biological Activities of IL-1

IL-1 exerts many biological effects on neurological and endocrinological systems and on various metabolic processes. These biological activities recently have been reviewed (Oppenheim *et al.*, 1986; Dinarello, 1988). Using *in vivo* administration of synthetic peptide and a monoclonal antibody-recognizing nonapeptide of IL-1 beta, Boraschi *et al.*, (1989) showed that a nonapeptide, position 163–173, of IL-1 beta possesses immunostimulatory activity but lacks pyrogenic and inflammatory activity. In this section I will detail the immunological effects of IL-1 and briefly review some of the biological effects of IL-1 on bone and cartilage metabolism because of their relevance to autoimmune connective tissue diseases. It is interesting to note that IL-1 shares many immunological effects with tumor necrosis factors (reviewed by Lee and Vilcek, 1987; Gupta, 1988) as summarized in Table II.

2.4.1. Effects on T-Cell-Mediated Immune Responses

IL-1 plays a crucial role in T-cell activation and proliferation. The production of IL-2, expression of IL-2 receptors (IL-2R) and binding of IL-2 to IL-2R are important and absolute ingredients for the progression of resting T cells to undergo proliferation and clonal

TABLE II. Biological Properties of IL-1 and TNF[a]

Functions	Tumor necrosis factor	IL-1
T-cell activation	+	+
B-cell activation	+	+
Induction of c-myc and c-fos in T cells	?	+
Induction of c-fos and c-myc in fibroblasts	+	+
Inhibition of c-myc in tumor cells	+	?
Expression of MHC class I antigens	+	+
Expression of MHC class II antigen	+	?
Expression of ICAM 1 on astrocytes	+	+
Expression of ICAM 1 on keratinocytes	+	+
Induction of IL-1 synthesis	+	+
Induction of TNF synthesis	+	+
Induction of GM-CSF synthesis	+	+
Induction of IL-2 synthesis	?	+
Induction of IL-4 synthesis	?	+
Induction of IL-6	+	+
Induction of EGF receptors	+	?
Induction of IL-2 receptors	+	+
Increased PGE_2 and collagenase synthesis	+	+
Activation of neutrophils	+	+
Endothelial cells		
Induction of procoagulant activity	+	+
Induction of surface antigens (CDw18)	+	+
Mitogenic action on fibroblasts	+	+
Osteoclast activation	+	+
Cartilage reabsorption		
Proteoglycan degradation	+	+
Inhibition of synthesis	+	+
Antiviral activity	+	+
Cytotoxic/cytostatic action on tumor cells	+	±
Inhibition of lipoprotein lipase	+	+
Pyrogenic action	+	+
Induction of acute-phase proteins	+	+
Cytotoxicity for pancreatic beta cells	+	+

[a]Modified from Gupta (1988).

expansion. IL-1 does not activate resting T cells (G0-Gla), but acts as a costimulant with antigen or mitogen (Bettens et al., 1982; Kristensen et al., 1982). Cells in a Gla phase will respond to IL-1 by progressing to S phase (Kristensen et al., 1982). IL-1 induces transcription, synthesis, and secretion of IL-2, as well as expression of IL-2R. During an antigen-specific immune response, the initial signal is provided by an antigen in the context of major histocompatibility (MHC) class II antigen, and the second signal is provided by IL-1. DeLuca and Mizel (1985) showed that IL-1 may be required for generating medullary T cells in the thymus and may also up-regulate MHC class II antigen expression or amplify Ia-dependent induction of self-recognizing thymocytes. Falk et al. (1989) showed that IL-1 induces high-affinity IL-2R expression on double-negative CD4–CD8-thymocytes. IL-1 induces an acute phase protein, SAP, that has been shown to augment IL-1-induced T-cell proliferation (Sarto and Mortensen, 1985). In contrast, IL-1 induces PGE_2 production, which inhibits T-cell proliferation. Kovacs et al. (1986) showed that IL-1 alpha induces c-fos and c-myc expression in T cells. In addition to IL-2 production, IL-1 also induces production of other cytokines, namely gamma interferon, colony-stimulating factors, IL-5, and IL-6 (Dinarello, 1988). IL-1 is also chemotactic for human T cells.

2.4.2. Effects of IL-1 on B-Cell-Mediated Immune Response

IL-1 appears to act on both pre-B and mature B cells. In pre-B cells, IL-1 induces maturation as evidenced by kappa chain synthesis followed by membrane expression of assembled Ig molecules (Giri et al., 1984). The precise role of IL-1 in B-cell proliferation and differentiation is unclear and controversial. Some investigators have shown that IL-1 promotes the clonal expansion of B cells following antigenic stimulation (Wood et al., 1976; Hoffmann, 1980). Howard and Paul (1983), however, found no requirement of IL-1 in B-cell proliferation. They showed that IL-1 works with B-cell stimulatory factor-1 (BSF-1) for anti-immunoglobulin-induced DNA synthesis in murine B cells. IL-1 also has been shown to work with IL-5. Gordon et al. (1986) demonstrated that IL-1 will induce DNA synthesis in EBV-transformed B lymphocytes (when cultured at a density below which there is no autostimulation of B cells) but not in lymphocytes stimulated by anti-μ antibody. Therefore, it is possible that IL-1 plays an autocrine role in the growth of EBV-transformed cells that produce their own IL-1, but has no role in the activation or DNA synthesis of antigen-primed B cells; perhaps their role in B-cell DNA synthesis is obligatory. The effects of IL-1, then, appear to be indirect and occur via stimulation of production of a cascade of cytokines that influence B-cell activation, proliferation, and differentiation.

2.4.3. Effects of IL-1 on Monocyte Functions

IL-1 induces synthesis of PGE_2 that could result in indirect inhibitory effects of IL-1 on T-cell proliferation and on Ia expression on monocytes. IL-1 is known to induce its own synthesis in macrophages, increase macrophage migration, induce synthesis of TNF alpha and colony-stimulating factors, and increase monocyte cytotoxic activity. Philip and Epstein (1986) suggested that IL-1-mediated enhanced monocyte tumoricidal activity appears to be a result of the induction of TNF alpha synthesis. Lachman et al. (1986) showed that IL-1 beta itself, independent of TNF alpha, is capable of killing human melanoma cells.

2.4.4. Effects of IL-1 on Natural Killer Cells

IL-1 works with IL-2 and interferons for tumor lysis by natural killer (NK) cells, increases conjugation between effector NK cells and target cells, and induces cytokine production by NK cells (review by Dinarello, 1988).

2.4.5. Effects of IL-1 on Hematopoietic Cells

IL-1 has no direct effect on bone marrow cells. IL-1 stimulates the synthesis of granulocyte macrophage-colony stimulating factor (GM-CSF) in cultured lung fibroblasts and induces B-cell tumor cell line to synthesize CSF (Zucali et al., 1986). IL-1 acts synergistically with bone marrow growth factors in reconstituting hematopoioiesis.

2.4.6. Effects of IL-1 on Bone and Cartilage Metabolism

Originally, osteoclast-activating factor was detected in the supernatants of peripheral blood leukocytes. Dewhirst et al. (1985) purified human osteoclast-activating factor to homogeneity and found it to be identical to IL-1 beta. This factor stimulates bone resorption. IL-1 also induces cartilage resorption. IL-1 causes cartilage to degrade its proteoglycan and inhibits the synthesis of new proteoglycan (Tyler, 1985). Loss of proteoglycan, which occurs in rheumatoid arthritis and other joint diseases, results in severe impairment of cartilage function. Therefore, IL-1 appears to have a role in normal bone remodeling and plays a role in the bone and cartilage pathology observed in rheumatoid and other arthritides.

2.5. IL-1 Inhibitors

Theoretically, functions of IL-1 can be blocked at multiple levels: molecules that directly interact with IL-1, receptor antagonist, or by interfering with intracellular pathways activated by IL-1. It should be stressed that the use of bioassay to demonstrate inhibitory activity against IL-1 might be due to an inhibition of other cytokines that act as costimulators. Several investigators have demonstrated IL-1 inhibitors that act by direct IL-1 receptor blockade. There are several sources of native IL-1 inhibitors. These include urine-derived inhibitors; monocyte–macrophage-derived inhibitors; inhibitors derived from neutrophils, keratinocytes, submandibular glands, and B lymphoblastoid lines; and transmembrane envelop protein (P15E) from type C avian and murine retroviruses (reviewed by Larrick, 1989). The best-characterized urine-derived inhibitor is a 15- to 25-kDa molecular weight protein found in the urine of patients with acute monocytic leukemia (Seckinger et al., 1987a,b). This inhibitor blocks both IL-1 alpha- and beta-induced PGE_2 and collagenase production by human synovial cells and fibroblasts. This factor is a specific competitive inhibitor of IL-1 binding to target cells. Liao et al. (1985) described a 30- to 35-kDa protein from the urine of febrile patients that appears to act at a site distinct from IL-1 or the IL-1 receptors. Uromodulin is a glycoprotein present in the urine of pregnant women. It appears to bind to PHA and to IL-1.

Barak et al. (1986) described an IL-1 inhibitor with a molecular weight of 50 kDa from a myelomonocytic leukemic cell line (M20). This cell line also produces IL-1. It appears likely that the IL-1 inhibitor in the urine and serum of patients with juvenile rheumatoid arthritis is related to this inhibitor (Prieur et al., 1987). The inhibitor produced by immune complex-stimulated human monocytes is a 22-kDa protein. Roberts et al. (1986) showed that IL-1 and IL-1 inhibitor with a molecular weight of 95 kDa are released by influenza virus and respiratory syncytial virus-infected macrophages. Berman et al. (1986) described spontaneous production of a low-molecular-weight (8 kDa with a pI of 4.5) IL-1 inhibitor by human immunodeficiency virus (HIV)-infected macrophages, which inhibits soluble antigen-specific responses by T cells but does not inhibit mitogen-induced responses. It also inhibits T-cell-dependent antibody response by murine and human B cells. It is likely that IL-1 inhibitors might play a role in immune dysfunctions in patients infected with viruses, including HIV, in tumor-bearing patients and in uncontrolled inflammatory disorders.

3. INTERLEUKIN-2

Interleukin-2 is one of the best-characterized cytokines, and has a pivotal role in the antigen-specific clonal proliferation of T lymphocytes. In addition, IL-2 has been shown to act on B lymphocytes, macrophages, natural killer cells (NK), and lymphokine-activated killer cells (LAK). Interleukin-2 was discovered as a T-cell growth factor by Morgan et al. (1976). They showed that normal human T cells could be cultured for extended periods in media that had been conditioned by growth of PHA-stimulated peripheral blood mononuclear cells (MNC). Interleukin-2 is a single polypeptide that is released from antigen or mitogen-stimulated T cells within hours of activation. IL-2 functions to switch T cells from G1 to S, G2, and M phases of cell cycle.

3.1. Production of IL-2

Freshly isolated lymphocytes do not contain intracellular IL-2 or release IL-2 spontaneously; however, they produce IL-2 upon stimulation with mitogens or antigens. The factors that are considered crucial or important for optimum IL-2 production include binding of lectin–antigen to the cell surface receptor, interaction with Ir gene products (Ia, DR), and IL-1 produced by monocytes–macrophages (Smith et al., 1979). Neefe et al. (1981) demonstrated that adherent cells are absolute requirements for PHA-induced IL-2 production. Interleukin-2 is probably produced in the G1 phase of the cell cycle (Stadler et al., 1981). Phorbol esters increase the levels of IL-2 mRNA in mitogen-stimulated T cells (Hirano et al., 1984). Recently, Mills et al. (1989) have shown that physiological activation of protein kinase C (PKC) limits IL-2 secretion, whereas prolonged activation of PKC augments IL-2 production. Mills et al. (1985) also demonstrated that an increase in intracellular calcium was necessary for IL-2 production but not for the expression of IL-2R. Corticosteroids inhibit T-cell proliferation by inhibiting IL-2 production. Cyclosporine A and vitamin D_3 also inhibit IL-2 production, and synergistically inhibit IL-2 production (Gupta et al., 1989). IL-2 is produced by mature T cells. Although the report of large granular lymphocyte (LGL) clones producing IL-2 have been published, the phenotype of this clone had T-cell marker (OKT11). It is likely, then, that IL-2 is the only cytokine that is produced exclusively by T cells. IL-2 is produced by both CD4$^+$ and CD8$^+$ T cells, depending on the nature of stimulus; however, CD4$^+$ T cells appear to be the predominant cell type. Salmon et al. (1988) investigated the production of IL-2 in subsets of CD4$^+$ T cells using monoclonal antibodies 2H4 and 4B4. They observed that CD4$^+$CD45R$^-$4B4$^+$ cells produced IL-2 and proliferated in response to lectin stimulation. In contrast, CD4$^+$CD45R$^+$4B4$^-$ cells produced no IL-2 and proliferated poorly to lectin stimulation but expressed IL-2 receptors. Furthermore, this latter population responded to exogenous IL-2. These observations would suggest that two subsets of CD4$^+$ cells are not independent, or counteracting, but rather that the generation of T-cell help is likely to involve cooperative interactions between two subsets. Recently it has been shown that CD4$^+$CD45R$^+$ and CD4$^+$CD45R$^-$ cells are not functionally distinct subsets, but rather represent naive and memory stages of same cell type (Sanders et al., 1988). In the murine system, it was found that when stimulator–responder MHC antigens differed at only the I region, Lyt 1$^+$ T cells and not Lyt 2$^+$ T cells produced IL-2. In contrast, when the mixed lymphocyte reaction (MLR) combination differed singularly at the K/D region of MHC, the Lyt 2$^+$ and not Lyt 1$^+$ T cells produced IL-2 (Okada et al., 1979; Okada and Henney, 1980). At the clonal level, the average of IL-2 activity produced by Lyt 2$^+$ T cells is about eightfold less than that produced by Lyt 2$^-$ cells. It was also observed that the capacity to produce IL-2 and the cytotoxic activity were mutually exclusive.

3.2. Molecular Characteristics of IL-2

Biochemical analyses show that all the activity could be ascribed to a glycoprotein with a molecular weight of 15.5 kDa and a pI of 8.2 (Robb and Smith, 1981). Definitive evidence that IL-2 activity resides in a single molecule came following the development of anti-IL-2 antibodies. A number of structural and functional properties suggest that IL-2 from human, rat, murine, and ape lymphocytes are analogous to one another. Murine IL-2 behaves on gel filtration as a noncovalent dimer of a 15,000 to 17,000 molecular weight subunit.

In the short five-year period since the development of bioassay, the molecular properties of IL-2 have been defined (Robb and Smith, 1981), monoclonal antibodies against IL-2 developed, and IL-2 purified to homogeneity, and cDNA (Taniguchi, 1983) as well as genomic DNA clones isolated and sequenced (Fujita et al., 1983). Several investigators have isolated mRNA from human and gibbon IL-2-producing cells and transfected *Xenopus laevis* to produce biologically active IL-2 (Lin et al., 1982). mRNA from human tonsil lymphocytes is around 10 S. A minor species of mRNA (13 to 13.5 S) has been detected in human cells that can be translated to produce biologically active IL-2. The overall genomic organization of IL-2 is encoded by four exons separated by one short and two long introns (Fujita et al., 1983). Human IL-2 consists of a 133-amino acid single polypeptide containing a single intramolecular disulfide bridge between two cysteins in position 58 and 105. This bond plays an important role in maintaining active conformation of the molecule. The truncated segment of an IL-2 sequence cannot promote T-cell growth (Ciardelli et al., 1987) and the reduction of a disulfide bond between residues 58 and 105 destroys biological activity of IL-2 (Yamada et al., 1987). This would indicate that the tertiary, folded structure of IL-2 is obligatory for stimulating growth. The nucleotide sequence derived from transformed and nontransformed T cells reveal that the cDNA codes for a molecule of 153 amino acid containing an amino terminal signal sequence of 20 amino acids (Devos et al., 1983; Taniguchi et al., 1983), that is removed prior to secretion of IL-2 (Robb and Smith, 1981). Because there is a single copy of the gene for IL-2, apart from allelic differences, all heterogeneity of human IL-2 appears to be due to posttranslational modifications (Robb et al., 1983). IL-2 production is controlled at the mRNA transcription level. Recently, IL-2 has been crystallized. It shows that the core structure is made up of antiparallel alpha helices and contains no segments of beta secondary structure (Brandhuber et al., 1987). The gene for IL-2 is located on human chromosome 4q (Seigal et al., 1984).

IL-2 mRNA is not synthesized constitutively in resting T cells but only after stimulation with T-cell activators. Induced transcription in human and murine T cell lines and in human T cell blasts is blocked by cyclosporine A. Shaw et al. (1988) examined the mechanism regulating the levels of IL-2 mRNA in T lymphocytes. IL-2 mRNA has a half-life of 1–2 hr in T cell lines and in activated human peripheral blood lymphocytes. Jurkat T cells show a rapid increase of mRNA on induction of IL-2 synthesis, followed by an equally rapid decline 4–6 hr later. The decline occurs despite a high rate of synthesis and appears to be due to an enhanced rate of mRNA degradation. The degradation of IL-2 mRNA is sensitive to cycloheximide and actinomycin D. June et al. (1989) showed evidence for the involvement of three signals in the induction of IL-2 gene expression in human T lymphocytes. The induction of maximum IL-2 gene expression required three signals provided by CD28, phorbol ester, and calcium ionophore. The three-signal requirement did not reflect differential regulation of IL-2 gene expression between the CD4 and CD8 subsets. IL-2 mRNA is induced by the stimulation of T cells with optimal concentration of phorbol ester and calcium ionophore and is completely suppressed by cyclosporine A. Addition of anti-CD28 monoclonal antibody to PMA and calcium ionophore causes significant induction of IL-2 gene expression that is resistant to cyclosporine A. The expression of IL-2 is restricted to T cells and its induction is dependent on an increased rate of transcription (Fujita et al., 1986).

3.3. IL-2 Receptor

Although it is well known that T cells produce and respond to IL-2, the information on the molecular mechanisms underlying the IL-2-mediated signal transduction is limited. However, it is now evident that intracellular signaling produced by IL-2 are mediated by high-affinity IL-2 receptors (Smith and Cantrell, 1985; Depper et al., 1985). The IL-2 receptor (IL-2R) is present in three forms: high-, intermediate-, and low-affinity forms with respect to binding ability to IL-2, and respective dissociation constants (Kd) of 10^{-11} M, 10^{-9} M, and 10^{-8} M (Robb et al., 1984; Tsudo et al., 1986; Teshigawara et al., 1987). Uchiama et al. (1981) developed a monoclonal antibody (anti-Tac) that was found to compete for radiolabeled IL-2 binding. After the IL-2R (Tac antigen, p55) was characterized (Leonard et al., 1984; Nikaido et al., 1984), it became evident that IL-2Rp55 constitutes the low-affinity form and is not functional in IL-2 internalization and signal transduction unless it is associated with the specific membrane component of lymphoid cells (Kondo et al., 1986; Robb, 1986). The intermediate-affinity IL-2R, a protein of 75 kDa, has been detected by cross-linking with ^{125}I-labeled IL-2 (Sharon et al., 1986; Tsudo et al., 1986; Teshigawara et al., 1987; Robb et al., 1987; Dukovich et al., 1987). There is evidence that IL-2-induced signal transduction is mediated by IL-2Rp75. IL-2 induces intracellular signaling in cells expressing IL-2Rp75 and not in cells expressing IL-2Rp55 alone (Siegel et al., 1987; Bich-Thuy et al., 1987; Smith, 1988a). Furthermore, internalization of IL-2 is mediated by the high-affinity IL-2R or IL-2Rp75 but not by IL-2Rp55 (Robb and Green, 1987; Tanaka et al., 1988). Takeshita et al. (1989) have recently developed a monoclonal antibody (TU27) that defines IL-2Rp75. This antibody blocks the T-cell proliferation of a T cell line, MT-2C41, conforming the role of IL-2Rp75 in intracellular signalling effect of IL-2. The high-affinity IL-2R consists of intermediate-affinity IL-2R (IL-2Rp75) and low-affinity IL-2R (Tac, IL-2Rp55) (Tsudo et al., 1986; Teshigawara et al., 1987). It is interesting to note that IL-2Rp75 and IL-2Rp55 are not connected via a covalent disulfide bond; instead, two proteins interact via noncovalent forces to form a heterodimeric high-affinity IL-2R. The IL-2 binding sites on IL-2Rp75 are distinct from the IL-2 binding sites on IL-2Rp55. When both chains are expressed together on the same cell, then only high affinity IL-2R (Kd 10 M) are detected (Teshigawara et al., 1987). When expressed individually, each IL-2Rp75 and IL-2Rp55 interacts with IL-2 with different kinetics and equilibrium-binding constants (Smith, 1988a). IL-2 binds to and dissociates from IL-2Rp75 much more slowly than its binding to and dissociation from IL-2Rp55. For the high-affinity IL-2R, the association rate of the heterodimer is contributed by IL-2Rp55 (fast) and the dissociation rate is derived from IL-2Rp75 (slow). IL-2Rp55 has been shown to be expressed by activated T cells, a subset of B cells, natural killer cells, and thymocytes. IL-2Rp75 has recently been defined and antibodies against this protein have just been developed. Therefore, cellular distribution of this receptor is not fully known. IL-2Rp75 is expressed on activated T cells and natural killer cells (Tsudo et al., 1987; Siegel et al., 1987). De la Hera et al. (1985) showed that IL-2 promotes the growth and cytolytic activity of human (CD3+ CD4- CD8-) thymocytes. More recently, Toribio et al. (1988) have shown a role for IL-2 in the gene rearrangement and expression of both alpha/beta and gamma/delta T-cell receptor (TCR) genes in human prothymocytes and immature thymocytes. Therefore, it is highly likely that IL-2Rp75 is expressed on prothymocytes (CD3-,CD4-,CD8-,CD2-,CD7+CD45+) and immature thymocytes.

3.4. Regulation of IL-2R Expression

Resting T cells do not express functional IL-2R until they are stimulated by lectin or specific antigens. Following activation of T cells, there is a coordinated transcription of IL-2 gene and IL-2R genes. Because 5' flanking regions of IL-2 gene differ from those of IL-2Rp55 gene, it appears that different promoter–enhancer mechanisms might be responsible for activating each of these genes (Fujita et al., 1986). Following TCR activation, high-affinity

IL-2R are expressed on the surface of T cells in modest numbers. When IL-2 binds to high-affinity IL-2R, the following changes occurs: within the first hour, the density of high-affinity IL-2R decreases by 40–50%. Subsequently, over the next 24 hr, isolated IL-2Rp55 accumulates on the cell surface outnumbering high-affinity IL-2R. The accumulation of IL-2Rp55 on the cell surface is associated with transcriptional activation and accumulation of its mRNA. In the absence of IL-2, the high-affinity IL-2R returns to its original density within 1–2 hr, whereas the excess of IL-2Rp55 persists for many hours before gradually decreasing. IL-2 bound to IL-2Rp55 and high-affinity IL-2R heterodimer (IL2Rp55–IL-2Rp75) is internalized with a half-life of 15 min. The IL-2 binding to its receptor forms a hormone receptor complex, which, upon internalization, leads to down-regulation of homologous receptors. IL-2R disappears ten times faster in the presence of IL-2 than in the absence of IL-2. IL-2-mediated regulation of IL-2Rp75 occurs at the cell surface, whereas the regulation of IL-2Rp55 occurs at the genetic level (Smith, 1988b).

Because of only recent delineation of IL-2Rp75, various factors regulating its expression are not fully known. However, a number of factors are known to regulate the expression of IL-2Rp55. Malek and Shevach (1984) have shown that IL-2Rp55 expression on murine T cells is accessory cell-dependent. Kaye et al. (1984) showed the requirement of IL-1 for IL-2Rp55 induction in murine T-cell clones. Several investigators have claimed that IL-1 can replace the requirement of accessory cells in the induction of IL-2R (IL-2Rp55) in human T cells. In contrast, we have observed that freshly isolated peripheral blood T cells rigorously depleted of accessory cells do not express IL-Rp55 upon activation with soluble anti-CD3 or WT31 monoclonal antibody (that defines alpha/beta TCR) in the presence of recombinant IL-1 (Gupta et al., 1991). However, IL-2R expression is observed when 5% adherent cells are added to T cells. IL-2 has also been shown to up-regulate its own receptor (IL-2Rp55) on T cells (Welte et al., 1984) and B cells (Waldmann et al., 1984). The expression of IL-2Rp55 is inhibited by actinomycin D and cycloheximide but not by mitomycin or irradiation (Depper et al., 1984; Waldmann et al., 1984), demonstrating the requirement of de novo protein and RNA synthesis but not of DNA synthesis. Activation of protein kinase C (PKC) induces IL-2Rp55 expression. Farrar and Ruscetti (1986) showed that anti-CD3 and phorbol esters could increase IL-2Rp55 expression on day 5 and 12 activated T cells that were at G0/G1 stage of cell cycle. IL-2Rp55 mRNA was detected within 2 hr of activation. In contrast, IL-2 could only enhance IL-2Rp55 expression on day 5 and not on day 12 activated T cells. IL-2 acts synergistically with phorbol ester and anti-CD3 for IL-2Rp55 expression. It appears that PKC activation is necessary for IL-2Rp55 expression. In contrast, another "second messenger," influx of calcium (intracellular calcium) was necessary for IL-2 production but not for IL-2Rp55 expression (Mills et al., 1985). The effect of cyclosporine A on IL-2Rp55 are controversial. Miyawaki et al. (1983) showed that cyclosporine A does not inhibit IL-2Rp55 on lectin-stimulated T cells. We have recently shown that cyclosporine A inhibits IL-2Rp55 expression on lectin-activated T cells and vitamin D_3 appears to potentiate the effect of cyclosporine A on IL-2Rp55 expression (Gupta et al., 1989a). Vitamin D_3 inhibits IL-2 production but not the expression of IL-2Rp55 (Gupta et al., 1989a). We found similar results with ion channel blockers that inhibited IL-2 production but had little or no effect on IL-2R expression (Gupta et al., 1985, 1989b), further supporting the view that the genes for IL-2 and IL-2R are independently regulated.

3.5. Biological Effects of IL-2

Most circulating lymphocytes are quiescent and the specific clones of T cells proliferate and differentiate into effector cells capable of mediating cytolysis, help, or antibody production only upon introduction of antigen. IL-2 plays a critical role in the differentiation and proliferation of T cells. The concentration of IL-2 produced, expression of IL-2R, and the period during which IL-2 is available to interact with IL-2R become primary determinants of the magnitude and extent of IL-2-mediated T-cell proliferation.

3.5.1. Effect of IL-2 on Helper T Cells

Schreier et al. (1980) developed antigen-specific helper T-cell clones in the presence of IL-2. These clones will support an antibody response to the antigen by splenic B cells. Restimulation with antigen and accessory cells is not a prerequisite for the maintenance of specific helper function. It has been shown that T-cell clones specific for influenza virus, which provide B cell help, do not produce IL-2 (Lamb et al., 1983). Salmon et al. (1988) showed that CD4+CD45R+ T cells do not produce IL-2, but such cells express IL-2Rp55 upon lectin stimulation and do indeed proliferate in the presence of exogenous IL-2.

3.5.2. Effect of IL-2 on Suppressor T Cells

IL2- is known to support the generation and maintenance of suppressor T cells in mice, primates, and humans. A number of suppressor T-cell lines and clones have been generated in the presence of IL-2 (Fresno et al., 1981; Cantor 1981). Ting et al. (1984) reported generation of suppressor T cells with IL-2. In nu/nu mice spleen cells, low concentrations of IL-2 generate alloreactive cytotoxic T lymphocytes (CTL), whereas higher concentrations of IL-2 support the T-cell growth. It has also been shown that high concentrations of IL-2 suppress the generation of alloreactive CTL in mixed lymphocyte culture (MLC) reaction but generates antigen nonspecific suppressor T cells in normal splenic cell cultures and augments the antigen-specific suppressor T cells in MLC.

3.5.3. Effect of IL-2 on Cytotoxic T Cells

After interaction with specific antigen, precursors of cytotoxic T lymphocytes (pCTL) express receptors for IL-2; the binding of IL-2 to its receptors leads to differentiation and proliferation of pCTL into effector CTL (Teh and Teh, 1980). It is likely that more than one factor is required for optimal CTL generation (Wagner et al., 1982; Sharma and Gupta, 1986). However, a number of CTL cell lines have been established in the presence of IL-2. Although both CTL and helper T-cell clones have absolute requirements of IL-2 for their growth, only helper and not CTL clones interact with accessory cells to release IL-2 in cultures (Schreier et al., 1980).

3.5.4. Effect of IL-2 on Natural Killer Cells

Human NK cells have been shown to express high-affinity IL-2Rp75 (Tsudo et al., 1987) and have been propogated in the presence of IL-2. IL-2-mediated enhancement of NK activity has been reported in human and murine cells (Henney et al., 1981; Trinchiari et al., 1984). The stimulation of NK by IL-2 is more pronounced than that of interferon and is synergistic to the stimulatory effect of interferon (Ortaldo et al., 1984).

3.5.5. Role of IL-2 in the Generation of Lymphokine-Activated Killer Cells

Peripheral blood mononuclear cells incubated in vitro with IL-2 for 4–14 days acquire non-MHC-restricted cytotoxicity against NK-sensitive and NK-resistant targets. These cells have been termed lymphokine-activated killer cells (LAK). The antitumor effect in nonimmunogenic tumors is mediated by LAK cells and in weakly immunogenic tumors by T cells as well as LAK cells (Lotze and Rosenberg, 1988). LAK cells differ from NK cells in that they are CD3$^+$ and IL-2-dependent. Gamma interferon appears to enhance IL-2-induced LAK activity. The physiological significance of LAK cells is presently unclear.

3.5.6. Effect of IL-2 in the Production of Other Cytokines

Interleukin-2 is known to induce secretion of gamma interferon, tumor necrosis factor, and B-cell growth factor I (BCGF-I) (Howard et al., 1983; Lotze, et al., 1985; Ernstoff et al., 1987). BCGF-I induces proliferation of anti-Ig-stimulated B cells. Recently it has been shown that IL-2 is synergistic with IL-6 in the differentiation of peripheral blood B cells to immunoglobulin-producing cells. Therefore, some of the biological effects of IL-2 could be secondary to the induction of other cytokines.

4. INTERLEUKIN-6

Originally IL-6 was described as a factor produced by T cells that induces immunoglobulin production in activated human B lymphocytes and lymphoblastoid cell lines (Hirano et al., 1985). Subsequently, it became apparent that IL-6, like IL-1 and tumor necrosis factor, is a pleiotropic cytokine with a multiple cell source of its production and many immune and nonimmune cells as targets of its effect. In 1986, IL-6 was cloned (Hirano et al., 1986). Molecular cloning and biological activity of several other factors demonstrated molecular identity of IL-6 to interferon beta 2, 26-kDa protein, myeloma–plasmacytoma growth factor, hepatocyte-stimulating factor, macrophage–granulocyte-inducing factor 2, and cytotoxic T-cell differentiation factor (reviewed by Kishimoto, 1989).

4.1. Molecular Structure of IL-6

The cDNA of IL-6 has been cloned, expressed in E. coli, and the recombinant IL-6 has been purified. IL-6 consists of 212 amino acids including a hydrophobic signal sequence of 28 amino acids. The secreted IL-6, therefore, consists of 184 amino acids with two potential N-glycosylation sites and four cysteine residues (Hirano et al., 1986). The cDNA sequence of human IL-6 shows 65% homology at the DNA level and 42% at the protein level with murine IL-6. The position of four cysteine residues and nine amino acid residues (56 to 65) between two cysteine residues (50 and 75) are identical between human and murine IL-6, suggesting that this region of the secreted protein may play a critical role in biological activity of IL-6 (Kishimoto, 1989). Recently, a biologically active rIL-6 gene was chemically synthesized (Jambou et al., 1988). The bioengineered and biologically active IL-6 is cysteine-free, suggesting that cysteine residues might not be required for biological activity of IL-6.

Among all other cytokines, IL-6 shows a significant homology with granulocyte-colony stimulating factor (G-CSF) (Hirano et al., 1986). The gene organization of IL-6 shows a distinct similarity with the G-CSF gene (Yashukawa et al., 1987). Both genes have the same number of introns and exons and the size of each exon is similar. This would suggest these two cytokines might be evolutionarily derived from a common ancestor gene. The position of four cysteine residues of IL-6 matches those of G-CSF. There are some similarities in their biological activities as well.

4.2. Regulation of IL-6 Expression

IL-6 is produced by a variety of normal cells, cell lines, and tumor cells. These include T cells, B cells, monocytes, fibroblasts, keratinocytes, endothelial cells, astrocytes, bone marrow stroma cells, mesangial cells, human T lymphotropic virus-I (HTLV-1) transformed T cell lines U937 and P388D1 (both monocyte lines), MG63 osteosarcoma cell line, T24 bladder carcinoma cell line, A549 lung carcinoma cell line, SK-MG-4 glioblastoma line, U373 astrocytoma line, atrial myxoma cells, myeloma cells, hypernephroma cells, pancreatic beta cells, and so on. IL-6 produced by T cells and macrophages has different kinetics, and therefore might exert distinct effects during different phases of immune response. IL-6 produced by T cells requires the presence of macrophages, whereas monocytes produce IL-6 spontaneously (Hori et al., 1988). Mitogen and antigen stimulation result in IL-6 production by T cells, while lipopolysaccharide (LPS) enhances IL-6 production by monocytes and fibroblasts (Hori et al., 1988). Cytokines that enhance IL-6 gene expression in a variety of cells include IL-1, tumor necrosis factor, platelet-derived growth factor, interferon beta, and serum poly(I)poly(C) (Kishimoto, 1989). Phorbol esters enhances IL-6 mRNA (Sehgal et al., 1987; Zhang et al., 1988). In addition, various viruses induce IL-6 production in fibroblasts and the central nervous system (Frei et al., 1988). Recently, human immunodeficiency virus I has been shown to induce IL-6 production by human macrophages (Nakajima et al., 1988). Glucocorticoids are powerful inhibitors of IL-6 gene expression in various tissues and cells (Helfgott et al., 1987).

4.3. IL-6 Receptor

cDNA for IL-6R has been cloned, using high-efficiency COS cell expression vector (Yamasaki et al., 1988). The IL-6R consists of 468 amino acids with a single transmembrane segment. The mature protein is comprised of 449 amino acids. The intracytoplasmic portion consists of 82 amino acids and does not have a tyrosine kinase domain. The sequence analysis puts IL-6 in the C2 set of the immunoglobulin supergene family. Genomic organization shows five exons. IL-6R has five possible N-glycosylation sites and the molecular weight of the mature protein is 80 kDa. The IL-6R consists of two polypeptide chains, a ligand-binding chain, and a nonligand-binding signal-transducing chain. IL-6R are expressed on activated B cells, resting T cells, EBV-transformed B cell line, Burkitt's lymphoma line, myeloma cells and myeloma cell lines, hepatoma cell lines, myeloid leukemia cell lines, and rat pheochromocytoma.

4.4. Biological Effects of IL-6

IL-6 was originally described as a B cell differentiation factor that induces final differentiation of B cells to immunoglobulin-producing cells (Muraguchi et al., 1988; Hirano et al., 1986). IL-6 is not a B cell growth factor. Beagley et al. (1989) have shown that both human and murine IL-6 induce high-rate IgA secretion in IgA-committed B lymphocytes. IL-6 induces IL-2R and IL-2 production in mitogen-stimulated T cells and thymocytes (German et al., 1987). IL-6 promotes the growth of phytohemagglutinin (PHA)-stimulated thymocytes and peripheral blood T cells (Lotz et al., 1988). IL-6 induces proliferation and differentiation of cytotoxic T lymphocytes in the presence of IL-2 from murine and human thymocytes and splenic T cells (Takai et al., 1988; Okada et al., 1988).

IL-6 acts synergistically with IL-3 in supporting the formation of multilineage blast cell colonies in murine spleen cell cultures (Ikebuchi *et al.*, 1987). IL-6 acts on multipotent progenitor cells and activates them at G0 stage to enter G1 phase (Koike *et al.*, 1988). IL-6 has also been shown to induce the differentiation of mouse myeloid cells into macrophages and induced expression of Fc and C3d receptors and enhanced phagocytosis (Miyaura *et al.*, 1988). A number of cytokines are known to induce acute-phase reaction. IL-6 also induces various acute-phase reactants, including fibrinogen, alpha-1-antichymotrypsin, alpha-1-acid glycoprotein, heptoglobin, serum amylase A, C-reactive protein, and alpha-1-antitrypsin.

IL-1 induces the expression of IL-6 mRNA in glioblastoma and astrocytoma cells. IL-6 induces differentiation of PC12 cells into neural cells (Satoh *et al.*, 1988). IL-6 was found to induce the transient expression of *c-fos* and an increase in the number of voltage-dependent Na^{2+} channels in PC12 cells.

5. INTERLEUKINS IN RHEUMATOID ARTHRITIS

A number of interleukins (both proteins and mRNA) have been examined in the peripheral blood and synovial fluid and synovial tissues of patients with rheumatoid arthritis. The significance of these interleukins and other cytokines in the pathogenesis of rheumatoid arthritis remains unclear. A number of investigators have reported production of IL-1 synovial fluid from patients with rheumatoid arthritis (reviewed by Gupta, 1985). Increased IL-1 mRNA and high levels of IL-1 alpha in rheumatoid joint cell culture supernatants have been reported by Burmester *et al.* (1983). Feldmann *et al.* (1988) also found IL-1 mRNA in synovial fluid. Waalen *et al.* (1986) reported high amounts of IL-1 produced by rheumatoid arthritis dendritic cells. Goto *et al.* (1987) have shown that a cloned adherent synovial cells with certain characteristics of dendritic cells spontaneously produce IL-1 activity. The rheumatoid synovial dendritic cells together with synovial macrophages may be responsible for the high amounts of IL-1 found in synovial effusion in rheumatoid arthritis. Hopkins *et al.* (1988) demonstrated the presence of both biologically active and immunoreactive IL-1 in synovial fluid from patients with rheumatoid as well as osteoarthritis. They also showed the presence of IL-1 inhibitors of endogenous and exogenous IL-1 in synovial fluids. Therefore, it is important to exclude the possibility of IL-1 inhibitor (if bioassays are used) where IL-1 production is negligible. About six years back, it was proposed that synovial macrophages in rheumatoid arthritis chronically produce IL-1, which perpetuates the inflammation characteristic of rheumatoid arthritis. Interleukin-1 in joint space elicits fibroblast proliferation and enhanced collagenase and prostaglandin synthesis. Miyasaka *et al.* (1988) observed potent IL-1 activity in culture supernatants from synovium from patients with rheumatoid arthritis, but not from nonrheumatoid arthritis patients. Production of IL-1 correlated with the findings of inflammation on arthroscopy, cells expressing HLA class II antigens (predominantly T cells), and joint changes detected on roentgenography. These findings would suggest a role of IL-1 in joint destruction in rheumatoid arthritis. The role of IL-1 in rheumatoid joint pathology is further supported by a fact that chloroquine, which is known to inhibit IL-1 secretion, has some beneficial effect in rheumatoid arthritis. More recently, Brennan *et al.* (1989) have shown that synovial cells from patients with rheumatoid arthritis produce significant amounts of both IL-1 and tumor necrosis factor alpha, whereas in osteoarthritis spontaneous IL-1 production is low, despite high concentrations of tumor necrosis factor alpha. Furthermore, they showed that anti-tumor necrosis factor alpha monoclonal antibodies inhibit IL-1 production by rheumatoid synovial cells but not by osteoarthritis cells. This would suggest that tumor necrosis factor alpha probably may be the main inducer of IL-1 in rheumatoid arthritis. These authors suggested that anti-tumor necrosis factor alpha agents may be useful for the treatment of rheumatoid arthritis.

There is less consensus regarding IL-2 production in rheumatoid arthritis, since low, normal, and high levels of IL-2 have been reported (reviewed Gupta, 1985). Ruschen et al. (1988) found increased IL-2 in synovial fluids and not in the peripheral blood from patients with rheumatoid arthritis. Kitas et al. (1988) observed decreased IL-2 production that correlated with disease activity. Defective IL-2 production was partially corrected by removal of monocytes, suggesting a role of macrophages in decreased IL-2 production in rheumatoid arthritis. Feldmann et al. (1988) and Førre et al. (1988) observed increased levels of mRNA for IL-2 in rheumatoid arthritis synovial T cells. Førre et al. (1988) also observed increased levels of mRNA for IL-2R in rheumatoid synovial T cells compared to nonactivated T cells. The decreased levels of IL-2 in synovial fluid could be due in part to absorption/ utilization of IL-2 by increased numbers of T cells expressing IL-2R. Waalen et al. (1987) have shown that spontaneous proliferation of rheumatoid inflammatory T cells is due in part to a continuous production and consumption of IL-2.

IL-6, because of its role in B-cell differentiation, has been examined in rheumatoid joints. Hirano et al. (1988) reported high levels of IL-6 in synovial fluids from patients with active rheumatoid arthritis. The synovial cells as well as the infiltrated T cells and B cells constitutively produced IL-6. Feldmann et al. (1988) and Førre et al. (1988) also reported increased mRNA for IL-6 in T cells from joints of rheumatoid arthritis patients. The infiltration of plasma cells into synovial tissues, autoantibody production, and elevated acute-phase proteins, including C-reactive protein and serum amyloid A, in rheumatoid joints could be explained by elevated levels of IL-6. Because IL-6 also supports the growth of EBV-transformed B lymphoblastoid cells, it would explain the presence of abnormally elevated numbers of circulating EBV-infected B cells in rheumatoid arthritis patients.

6. SUMMARY

In this chapter, I have briefly summarized the molecular and biological characteristics of IL-1, IL-2, and IL-6 because they are most extensively studied and might play a role in the pathogenesis of joint pathology in rheumatoid arthritis. It would be safe to say that these interleukins play a role in perpetuating the pathology of joint destruction in rheumatoid arthritis. Other cytokines whose mRNA and/or protein have been observed in rheumatoid arthritis include IL-4, gamma interferon, tumor necrosis factor alpha and beta, GM-CSF, G-CSF, transforming growth factor (TGF) beta, and platelet-derived growth factor (PDGF) (Zvaifler and Firestein, 1988; Feldmann et al., 1988; Førre et al., 1988). Although it has been suggested that antibodies against some of the cytokines (e.g., anti-tumor necrosis factor alpha) might be used in the treatment of rheumatoid arthritis, because of the pleiotropic nature of many of these cytokines it is likely that even intra-articular treatment would be associated with undesirable side effects. However, such approaches should be tried in experimental models.

ACKNOWLEDGMENT. The work cited was supported in part by grant USPHS AI-25456.

REFERENCES

Abraham, R. T., Ho, S. N., Barna, T. S., and McKean, D. J., 1987, Transmembrane signalling during interleukin 1-dependent T cell activation, J. Biol. Chem. 262:2719–2728.

Arend, W. P., Gordon, D. F., Wood, W. M., Janson, R. W., Joslin, F. G., and Jamed, S., 1989, 1L-1β production in cultured human monocytes is regulated at multiple levels, *J. Immunol.* **143**:118–126.

Auron, P. E., Webb, A. C., Rossenwasser, L. J., Mucci, S. F., Rich, A., Wolff, S. M., and Dinerallo, C. A., 1984, Nucleotide sequence of human monocyte interleukin 1 precursor cDNA, *Proc. Natl. Acad. Sci. USA* **81**:7907–7911.

Barak, V., Treves, A. J., Yanai, P., Helperin, M., Wasserman, D., Schoshana, B., and Braun, S., 1986, Interleukin 1 inhibitory activity secreted by a human myelomonocytic cell line (M20), *Eur. J. Immunol.* **16**:1446–1452.

Beagley, K. W., Eldridge, J. H., Lee, F., Kiyono, H., Everson, M. P., Koopman, W. J., Hirano, T., Kishimoto, T., and McGhee, J. R., 1989, Interleukins and IgA synthesis. Human and murine interleukin 6 induce high rate IgA secretion in IgA-committed B cells, *J. Exp. Med.* **169**:2133–2148.

Berman, M. A., Sandborg, C. I., Calabia, B. S., Andrew, B. S., and Friou, G. J., 1986, Studies of an interleukin 1 inhibitor. Characterization and clinical significance, *Clin. Exp. Immunol.* **64**:136–145.

Bettens, F., Kristensen, F., and deWeck, A. L., 1982, Effect of macrophages on the G0-G1 and G1-transition of thymocytes, *Immunology* **74**:140–149.

Bich-Thuy, L. T., Dukovich, M., Peffer, N. J., Fauci, A. S., Kehrl, J. H., and Greene, W. C., 1987, Direct activation of human resting T cells by IL-2: The role of an IL-2 receptor distinct from the protein, *J. Immunol.* **139**:1550–1556.

Boraschi, D., Volpini, G., Villa, L., Nencioni, L., Scapighati, G., Nucci, D., Antoni, G., Mattencci, G., Cioli, F., and Tagliabue, A., 1989, A monoclonal antibody to the IL-1 beta peptide 163-171 blocks adjuvanticity but not pyrogenicity of IL-1 beta in vivo, *J. Immunol.* **143**:131–134.

Brandhuber, B. J., Boone, T., Kenney, W. C., and McKay, D. B., 1987, Three-dimensional structure of interleukin 2, *Science* **238**:1707–1709.

Brennan, F. M., Chantry, D., Jackson, A., Maini, R. N., and Feldmann, M., 1989, Inhibitory effect of TNF alpha antibodies on synovial cell interleukin 1 production in rheumatoid arthritis, *Lancet* **2**:244–247.

Burmester, G. R., Di-Mitriu-Bona, A., Waters, S. J., and Winchester, R. J., 1983, Identification of three major synovial lining cell populations by monoclonal antibodies directed to Ia antigen and antigens associated with monocytes/macrophages and fibroblasts, *Scand. J. Immunol.* **17**:69–82.

Cantor, H., 1981, Regulation of immune response: Analysis with lymphocyte clones, *Cell* **25**:7–8.

Chin, J., Ruppe, E., Cameron, P. M., McNaul, K. L., Lotke, P. A., Tocci, M. J., and Schmidt, J. A., 1988, Identification of a high affinity receptor for interleukin 1 alpha and interleukin 1 beta on cultured human rheumatoid synovial cells, *J. Clin. Invest.* **82**:420–426.

Ciardelli, T. L., Smith, K. A., Cohen, F. E., and Kosen, P. A., 1987, Interleukin 2: A structural perspective, in: *Immune Regulation by Characterized Polypeptides* (G. Goldstein, J. F., Bach, and H. Wigzell, eds.), Liss Publication, New York, pp. 315–322.

De la Hera, A., Toribio, M. L., Marquez, C., and Martinez, A. C., 1985, Interleukin 2 promotes growth and cytolytic activity in human T3+4−8− thymocytes, *Proc. Natl. Acad. Sci. USA* **82**:6268–6272.

DeLuca, D., and Mizel, S. B., 1985, Ia positive non-lymphoid cells, interleukin 1 and T cell development in murine fetal thymus organ culture, in: *The Physiologic, Metabolic and Immunologic Action of Interleukin 1* (M. J. Kluger, J. J. Oppenheim, and M. C. Powanda, eds.), Alan R. Riss, New York, pp. 241–250.

Depper, J. M., Leonard, W. J., Kronke, M., Noguchi, P. D., Cunningham, R. E., Waldmann, T. A., and Gre, W. C., 1984, Regulation of interleukin 2 receptor expression: Effects of phorbol diester, phospholipase C, and reexposure to lectin or antigen, *J. Immunol.* **133**:3054–3061.

Depper, J. M., Leonard, W. J., Drogula, C., Kronke, M., Waldmann, T. A., and Greene, W. C., 1985, Interleukin 2 (IL-2) augments transcription of the IL-2 receptor gene, *Proc. Natl. Acad. Sci. USA* **82**:4230–4234.

Devos, R., Plaetinct, G., Cheronte, H., Simons, G., Degrave, W., Traverniere, J., Remout, E., and Fiers, W., 1983, Molecular cloning of human IL-2 cDNA and its expression in *E. coli*, *Nucleic Acid Res.* **11**:4307–4323.

Dewhirst, F. E., Stashenko, P. P., Mole, J. E., and Tsurumachi, T., 1985, Purification and partial sequence of human osteoclast-activating factor: Identity with interleukin 1 beta, *J. Immunol.* **135**:2562–2568.

Dinarello, C. A., 1988, Biology of interleukin 1, *FASEB J.* **2**:108–115.

Dinarello, C. A., Bishai, I., and Rossenwasser, L. J., 1984, The influence of lipoxygenase inhibitor on the *in vitro* production of human leukocyte pyrogen and lymphocyte activating factor (interleukin 1), *Int. J. Immunopharmacol.* **6**:43–50.

Dinarello, C. A., Clark, B. D., Puren, A. J., Savage, N., and Rosoff, P. M., 1989, The interleukin 1 receptor, *Immunol. Today* **10**:49–51.

Dukovich, M., Wano, Y., Thuy, L. B., Katz, P., Cullen, B. R., Kerhl, J. H., and Greene, W. C., 1987, A second human interleukin 2 binding protein that may be a component of high affinity interleukin 2 receptors, *Nature* **327**:518–522.

Ernstoff, M. S., Trautman, T., Davis, C. A., Rekh, S. D., Witman, P., Balser, J., Rudnick, S., and Kirkwood, J. M., 1987, A randomized phase I/II study of continuous versus intermittent intravenous interferon gamma in patients with metastatic melanoma, *J. Clin. Oncol.* **5**:1804–1810.

Falk, W., Mannel, D. N., Darjes, H., and Krammer, P. H., 1989, IL-1 induces high affinity IL-2 receptor expression of CD4-8- thymocytes, *J. Immunol.* **143**:513–517.

Farrar, W. L., and Ruscetti, F. W., 1986, Association of protein kinase C activity with IL-2 receptor expression, *J. Immunol.* **136**:1266–1273.

Feldmann, M., Kissonerghis, A. M., Buchan, G., Turner, M., Haworth, C., Barrett, K., Chantry, D., Ziegler, A., and Maini, R. N., 1988, Role of HLA class II and cytokine expression in rheumatoid arthritis, *Scand. J. Immunol.* (Suppl.) **76**:39–46.

Fenton, M. J., Vermeulen, M. W., Clark, B. D., Webb, A. C., and Auron, P. E., 1988, Human pro-IL-1 b gene expression in monocyte cells is regulated by two distinct pathways, *J. Immunol.* **140**:2267–2273.

Førre, O., Waalen, K., Natvig, J. B., and Kjeldsen-Kragh, J., 1988, Evidence of activation of rheumatoid synovial T lymphocytes. Development of rheumatoid T cell clones, *Scand. J. Rheumatol.* (Suppl.) **76**:153–160.

Frei, K., Leist, T. P., Meager, A., Gallo, P., Leppert, D., Zinkernagel, R. M., and Fontana, A., 1988, Production of B cell stimulatory factor 2 and interferon gamma in the central nervous system during viral meningitis and encephalitis, *J. Exp. Med.* **168**:448–453.

Fresno, M., Nabel, G., McVay-Bourdeau, L., Furthmeyer, H., and Cantor, H., 1981, Antigen specific T lymphocyte clones. I. Characterization of T cell clone expressing antigen-specific suppressive activity, *J. Exp. Med.* **153**:1245–1259.

Fujita, T., Shibuya, H., Ohashi, T., Yamanishi, K., and Taniguchi, T., 1986, Regulation of human interleukin 2 gene. Functional DNA sequences in the 5′ flanking region for the gene expression in activated T lymphocytes, *Cell* **46**:401–407.

Fujita, T., Takaoka, C., Matsui, H., and Tamiguchi, T., 1983, Structure of the human interleukin-2 gene, *Proc. Natl. Acad. Sci. USA* **80**:7437–7441.

German, R. D., Jacobs, K. A., Clark, S. C., and Raulet, D. H., 1987, B-cell-stimulatory factor (beta 2 interferon) functions as a second signal for interleukin 2 production by mature murine T cells, *Proc. Natl. Acad. Sci. USA* **84**:7629–7633.

Ghezzi, P., and Dinarello, C. A., 1988, IL-1 induces IL-1. III. Specific inhibition of IL-1 production by interferon gamma, *J. Immunol.* **140**:4238–4244.

Giri, J. G., Kincade, P. W., and Mizel, S. B., 1984, Interleukin 1-mediated induction of κ-light chain synthesis and surface immunoglobulin expression on pre-B cells, *J. Immunol.* **132**:223–228.

Gordon, J., Guy, G., and Walker, L., 1986, Autocrine model of B lymphocyte growth. II. Interleukin 1 supports the proliferation of transformed lymphoblasts but not the stimulation of resting B cells triggered through their receptors for antigen, *Immunology* **57**:419–423.

Goto, M., Sasano, M., Yamanaka, H., Miyasaka, N., Kamatani, N., Inoue, K., Nishiko, K., and Miyamot, T., 1987, Spontaneous production of an interleukin 1-like-factor by cloned rheumatoid synovial cells in long-term culture, *J. Clin. Invest.* **80**:786–796.

Gupta, S., 1985, Interleukins. Molecular and biological characteristics, in: *Immunology of Rheumatic Diseases* (S. Gupta and N. Talal, eds.), Plenum Press, New York, pp. 109–139.

Gupta, S., 1987, Autologous mixed lymphocyte reaction in man. XVII. *In vitro* effect of ion channel blocking agents on the autologous mixed lymphocyte reaction, *Cell Immunol.* **104**:290–295.

Gupta, S., 1988, Cytokines—molecular and biological characteristics, *Scand. J. Rheumatol.* (Suppl.) **76**:109–121.

Gupta, S., Chandy, K. G., Vayuvegula, B., Ruhlig, M., DeCoursey, T. E., and Cahalan, M. D., 1985, Role of potassium channels in interleukin 1 and interleukin 2 synthesis and interleukin 2 receptor expression, in: *Cellular and Molecular Biology of Lymphokines* (C. Sorg and A. Schimple, eds.), Academic Press, New York, pp. 39–44.

Gupta, S., Fass, D., Shimizu, M., and Vayuvegula, B., 1989a, Potentiation of immunosuppressive effect of cyclosporin A by 1,25-dihydroxyvitamin D3, *Cell. Immunol.* **121**:290–297.

Gupta, S., Shimizu, M., Batra, R., and Vayuvegula, B., 1989b, Early and late steps of T cell activation by monoclonal antibody WT31, in: *Lymphocyte Activation and Immune Regulation III* (S. Gupta and W. E. Paul, eds.), Plenum Press, New York, pp. 35–44.

Gupta, S., Shimizu, M., Ohira, K., and Vayuvegula, B., 1991, Activation of human T cells via the T cell receptor: A comparison between WT31 (defining α/β TCR)-induced and anti-CD3-induced activation of human T lymphocytes, *Cell. Immunol.* **132**:26–44.

Helfgott, D. C., May, L. T., Sthoeger, Z., Tamm, I., and Sehgal, P., 1987, Bacterial lipopolysaccharide (endotoxin) enhances expression and secretion of β₂ interferon by human fibroblasts, *J. Exp. Med.* **166**:1300–1309.

Henney, C. S., Kuribayasashi, K., Kern, D. E., and Gillis, S., 1981, Interleukin 2 augments natural killing activity, *Nature* **291**:335–338.

Hirano, T., Fujimoto, K., Teranishi, T., Nishino, N., Onoue, K., Maeda, S., and Shimada, K., 1984, Phorbol ester increases level of interleukin 2 mRNA in mitogen-stimulated human lymphocytes, *J. Immunol.* **312**:2165–2167.

Hirano, T., Taga, T., Nakano, N., Yasukawa, K., Kashiwamura, S., Shimizu, K., Nakajima, K., Pyun, K., and Kishimoto, T., 1985, Purification to homogeneity and characterization of human B cell differentiation factor (BCDF or BSFp2), *Proc. Natl. Acad. Sci. USA* **82**:5490–5492.

Hirano, T., Yasukawa, K., Harada, H., Taga, T., Watanabe, Y., Matsuda, T., Kashiwamura, S., Nakajima, K., Koyama, K., Iwamatsu, A., Tsunasawa, S., Sakiyama, F., Matsui, H., Takahara, Y., Taniguchi, T., and Kishimoto, T., 1986, Complementary DNA for a novel human interleukin (BSF-2) that induces B lymphocytes to produce immunoglobulin, *Nature* **324**:73–76.

Hirano, T., Matsuda, T., Turner, M., Miyasaka, N., Buchan, G., Tang, B., Sato, K., Shimizu, M., Maini, R., Feldman, M., and Kishimoto, T., 1988, Excessive production of interleukin 6/B cell stimulatory factor-2 in rheumatoid arthritis, *Eur. J. Immunol.* **18**:1797–1801.

Hoffmann, M. K., 1980, Macrophage and T cell control distinct phases of B cell differentiation in humoral immune response *in vitro*, *J. Immunol.* **125**:2076–2081.

Hopkins, S. J., Humphreys, M., and Jayson, M. I. V., 1988, Cytokines in synovial fluid. I. The presence of biologically active and immunoreactive IL-1, *Clin. Exp. Immunol.* **72**:422–427.

Hori, Y., Muraguchi, A., Suematsu, S., Matsuda, T., Yoshizaki, K., Hirano, T., and Kishimoto, T., 1988, Regulation of BSF-2/IL-6 production by human mononuclear cells: Macrophage-dependent synthesis of BSF-2/IL-6 by T cells, *J. Immunol.* **141**:1529–1535.

Howard, M., and Paul, W. E., 1983, Regulation of B-cell growth and differentiation by soluble factors, *Immunol. Rev.* **1**:307–333.

Howard, M., Matis, L., Malek, T. R., Shevach, E., Kell, W., Cohen, D., Nakanishi, K., and Paul, W. E., 1983, Interleukin 2 induces antigen-reactive T cell lines to secrete BCGF-1, *J. Exp. Med.* **158**:2024–2039.

Ikebuchi, K., Wong, G. G., Clark, S. C., Ihle, J. N., and Ogawa, M., 1987, Interleukin 6 enhancement of interleukin 3-dependent proliferation of unipotential hemopoietic progenitors, *Proc. Natl. Acad. Sci. USA* **84**:9035–9039.

June, C. H., Ledbetter, J. A., Lindsten, T., and Thompson, C. B., 1989, Evidence for the involvement of three distinct signals in the induction of IL-2 gene expression in human T lymphocytes, *J. Immunol.* **143**:153–161.

Kaye, J., Gillis, S., Mizel, S. B., Shevach, E. M., Malek, T. R., Dinarello, C. A., Lachman, L. B., and Janeway, C. A., 1984,

Growth of a cloned helper T cell line induced by a monoclonal antibody specific for antigen receptor: Interleukin 1 is required for the expression of receptors for IL-2, *J. Immunol.* **133**:1339–1345.

Kern, J. A., Lamb, R. J., Reed, J. C., Daniele, R. P., and Nowell, P. C., 1988, Dexamethasone inhibition of interleukin 1 beta production by human monocytes. Posttranscriptional mechanisms, *J. Clin. Invest.* **81**:237–244.

Kishimoto, T., 1989, The biology of interleukin 6, *Blood* **74**:1–10.

Kitas, G. D., Salmon, M., Farr, M., Gaston, J. S. H., and Bacon, P. A., 1988, Deficient interleukin 2 production in rheumatoid arthritis: Association with active disease and systemic complications, *Clin. Exp. Immunol.* **73**:242–249.

Koike, K., Nakahata, T., Takagi, M., Kobayashi, T., Ishiguro, A., Tsuji, K., Naganuma, K., Okano, A., Akiyama, Y., and Akabane, T., 1988, Synergism of BSF2/interleukin 6 and interleukin 3 on development of multipotential hemopoietic progenitors, *J. Exp. Med.* **168**:879–890.

Kondo, S., Shimizu, A., Saito, Y., Kinoshita, M., and Honjo, T., 1986, Molecular basis for two different affinity states of the interleukin 2 receptor: Affinity conversion model, *Proc. Natl. Acad. Sci. USA* **83**:9026–9030.

Kovacs, E. J., Oppenheim, J., and Young, H., 1986, Induction of c-fos and c-myc expression in T lymphocytes after treatment with recombinant interleukin-alpha, *J. Immunol.* **137**:3649–3651.

Kristensen, F., Walker, C., Bettens, F., Joncourt, F., and DeWeck, A. L., 1982, Assessment of interleukin 1 and interleukin 2 effects on cycling and noncycling murine thymocytes, *Cell Immunol.* **74**:140–149.

Kurt-Jones, E. A., Kiely, J. M., and Unanue, E. R., 1985, Conditions required for expression of membrane IL-1 on B cells, *J. Immunol.* **135**:1548–1550.

Lachman, L. B., Dinarello, C. A., Llansa, N. D., and Fidler, I. J., 1986, Natural and recombinant human interleukin 1-beta is cytotoxic for human melanoma cells, *J. Immunol.* **136**:3098–3102.

Lamb, J. R., Zenders, E. D., Feldman, M., Lake, P., Exkles, D. D., Woody, J. N., and Bevereley, P. C. L., 1983, The dissociation of interleukin 2 production and antigen-specific helper activity by clonal analysis, *Immunology* **50**:397–405.

Larrick, J. W., 1989, Native interleukin 1 inhibitors, *Immunol. Today* **10**:61–66.

Lee, J., and Vilcek, J., 1987, Tumor necrosis factor and interleukin 1: Cytokines with multiple overlapping biological activities, *Lab. Invest.* **56**:234–248.

Leonard, W. J., Depper, J. M., Crabtree, G. R., Rudikoff, S., Pumphrey, J., Robb, R. J., Kronke, M., Svetlik, P. B., Peffer, N. J., Waldmann, T. A., and Greene, W. C., 1984, Molecular cloning and expression of cDNAs for the human interleukin 2 receptor, *Nature* **311**:626–631.

Lepe-Zuniga, B., and Gery, I., 1984, Production of intracellular and extracellular interleukin 1 (IL-1) by human monocytes, *Clin. Immunol. Immunopathol.* **31**:222–230.

Liao, Z., Haimovitz, A., Chen, Y., Chan, J., and Rosenstriech, D. L., 1985, Characterization of a human interleukin 1 inhibitor, *J. Immunol.* **134**:3882–3886.

Lin, Y., Stadler, P. M., and Rabin, H., 1982, Synthesis of biologically active interleukin 2 by *Xenopus* oocytes in response to poly A-RNA from a gibbon T cell line, *J. Biol. Chem.* **257**:1587–1590.

Lomedico, P. T., Gubler, U., Hellman, C. P., Dukovich, M., Giri, J. G., Pan, Y. E., Collier, K., Semionow, R., Chua, A. O., and Mizel, S. B., 1984, Cloning and expression of murine interleukin 1 in *Escherichia coli*, *Nature* **312**:458–462.

Lotze, M. T., and Rosenberg, S. A., 1988, The immunologic treatment of cancer, *Cancer J. Clin.* **38**:68–94.

Lotze, M. T., Frana, L. W., Sharrow, S. O., Robb, R. J., and Rosenberg, A., 1985, *In vivo* administration of purified human interleukin 2. I. Half-life and immunologic effects of the Jurkat cell line-derived interleukin 2, *J. Immunol.* **134**:157–166.

Lotz, M., Jirik, F., Kabouridis, R., Tsoukas, C., Hirano, T., Kishimoto, T., and Carson, D. A., 1988, BSF-2/IL-6 is costimulant for human thymocytes and T lymphocytes, *J. Exp. Med.* **167**:1253–1258.

Lowenthal, J. W., and MacDonald, H. R., 1986, Binding and internalization of interleukin 1 by T cells. Direct evidence for high and low affinity classes of interleukin 1 receptor, *J. Exp. Med.* **164**:1060–1074.

Malek, T. R., and Shevach, E. M., 1984, Cellular and humoral requirements for the induction of IL-2 receptor expression on T cell subpopulations, *Leukemia Res.* **3**:257.

March, C. J., Mosley, B., Larsen, A., Serretti, D. P., Braedt, G., Price, V., Gillis, S., Henny, C. S., Kronheim, S. R., Grabstein, K., Conlon, P. J., Hopp, T. P., and Cosman, D., 1985, Cloning sequence and expression of two distinct human interleukin 1 complimentary cDNA, *Nature* **315**:641–647.

Matshushima, K., Taguchi, M., Kovacs, E. J., Young, H. A., and Oppenheim, J. J., 1987, Intracellular localization of human monocyte associated interleukin 1 (IL-1) activity and release of biologically active IL-1 from monocytes by trypsin and plasmin, *J. Immunol.* **136**:2883–2891.

Mills, G. B., Cheung, R. K., Grinstein, S., and Gelfand, E. W., 1985, Increase in cytosolic free calcium concentration is an intracellular messenger for the production of interleukin 2 but not for expression of the interleukin 2 receptor, *J. Immunol.* **134**:1640–1643.

Mills, G. B., May, C., Hill, M., Ebanks, R., Roifman, C., Mellors, A., and Gelfand, W. E., 1989, Physiologic activation of protein kinase C limits Il-2 secretion, *J. Immunol.* **142**:1995–2003.

Miyasaka, N., Sato, K., Goto, M., Sasano, M., Natsuyama, M., Inoue, K., and Nishioka, K., 1988, Augmented interleukin 1 production and HLA-DR expression in the synovium of rheumatoid arthritis patients. Possible involvement in joint destruction, *Arthritis Rheumat.* **31**:480–486.

Miyaura, C., Onozaki, K., Akiyama, Y., Taniyama, T., Hirano, T., Kishimoto, T., and Suda, T., 1988, Recombinant human interleukin 6 (B-cell stimulatory factor 2) is a potent inducer of differentiation of mouse myeloid leukemia cells (M1), *FEBS Lett.* **234**:17–21.

Miyawaki, T., Yachie, A., Ohzeki, S., Nagaoki, T., and Taniguchi, N., 1983, Cyclosporin A does not prevent expression of Tac antigen, a possible TcGF receptor molecule, on mitogen stimulated human T cells, *J. Immunol.* **130**:2727–2742.

Mizel, S. B., Shirakawa, F., and Chedid, M., 1988, cAMP and signal transduction pathway for interleukin 1, *Lymphokine Res.* **7**:262.

Morgan, D. A., Ruscetti, F. W., and Gallo, R. C., 1976, Selective in vitro growth of T lymphocytes from normal human bone marrow, Science 193:1007–1009.

Muraguchi, A., Hirano, T., Tang, B., Matsuda, T., Horii, Y., Nakajima, K., and Kishimoto, T., 1988, The essential role of B cell stimulatory factor 2 (BSF-2/IL6) for the terminal differentiation of B cells, J. Exp. Med. 167:332–344.

Nakajima, K., Martinez-Maza, O., Hirano, T., Nishanian, P., Salazar-Gonzalez, J. F., Fahey, J. L., and Kishimoto, T., 1988, Induction of interleukin 6 (BSF-2/IFN-beta 2) production by human immunodeficiency virus (HIV), J. Immunol. 142:531–538.

Neefe, J. R., Curl, R., and Woody, J. N., 1981, Absolute requirement for adherent cells in the production of human interleukin 2 (IL-2), Immunology 67:71–80.

Nikaido, T., Shimizu, A., Ishida, N., Sabe, H., Teshigwara, K., Maeda, M., Uchiama, T., Yodoi, J., and Honjo, T., 1984, Molecular cloning of cDNA encoding human interleukin 2 receptor, Nature 311:631–635.

Okada, M., and Henney, C. S., 1980, The differentiation of cytotoxic T cells in vitro. II. Amplifying factor(s) produced in primary mixed lymphocyte cultures against K/D stimuli required for the presence of Lyt2+ cells but not Lyt1+ cells, J. Immunol. 125:300–307.

Okada, M., Klimpel, G. R., Kupper, R. C., and Henney, C. S., 1979, The differentiation of cytotoxic T cells in vitro. I. Amplifying factor(s) in primary response is Lyt1+ cell dependent, J. Immunol. 122:2527–2533.

Okada, M., Kitahara, M., Kishimoto, S., Matsuda, T., Hirano, T., and Kishimoto, T., 1988, BSF-2/IL-6 functions as a killer helper factor in the in vitro induction of cytotoxic T cells, J. Immunol. 141:1543–1549.

Oppenheim, J. J., Kovacs, E. J., Matsushima, K., and Durum, S. K., 1986, There is more than one interleukin 1, Immunol. Today 7:45–56.

Ortaldo, J. R., Mason, A. T., Gerard, J. P., Henderson, L. E., Farra, W., Hopkins, R. F., III, Herberman, R. B., and Rabin, H., 1984, Effects of natural and recombinant IL-2 on regulation of interferon gamma production and natural killer activity: Lack of involvement of the Tac antigen for these immunoregulatory effects, J. Immunol. 133:779–783.

Philip, R., and Epstein, L. B., 1986, Tumor necrosis factor as immunomodulator and mediator of monocyte cytotoxicity induced by itself, gamma interferon and interleukin 1, Nature 323:86–89.

Priestle, J. P., Schaer, H. P., and Gruetter, M. G., 1988, Crystal structure of the cytokine interleukin 1, EMBO J. 7:339–343.

Prieur, A-M., Kaufman, M-T., Griscelli, C., and Dayer, J-M., 1987, Specific interleukin 1 inhibitor in serum and urine of children with systemic juvenile chronic arthritis, Lancet 2:1240–1242.

Robb, R. J., 1986, Conversion of low affinity interleukin 2 receptors to a high affinity state following fusion of membranes, Proc. Natl. Acad. Sci. USA 83:3992–3996.

Robb, R. J., and Greene, W. C., 1987, Internalization of interleukin 2 is mediated by the beta chain of the high affinity interleukin 2 receptor, J. Exp. Med. 165:1201–1206.

Robb, R. J., and Smith, K. A., 1981, Human T-cell growth factor is glycosylated, Mol. Immunol. 18:1087–1094.

Robb, R. J., Kutney, R. M., Panico, M., Morris, H., DeGrado, W. F., and Chowdlvey, V., 1983, Posttranslation modification of human T cell growth factor, Biochem. Biophys. Res. Commun. 116:1049–1055.

Robb, R. J., Greene, W. C., and Rusk, C. M., 1984, Low and high affinity cellular receptors for interleukin 2. Implications for the level of Tac antigen, J. Exp. Med. 160:1126–1146.

Robb, R. J., Rusk, C. M., Yodoi, J., and Greene, W. C., 1987, Interleukin 2 binding molecule distinct from the Tac protein: Analysis of its role in formation of high affinity receptor, Proc. Natl. Acad. Sci. USA 84:2002–2006.

Roberts, B. C., Prill, A. H., and Mann, T. N., 1986, Interleukin 1 and interleukin 1 inhibitor production by human macrophages exposed to influenza virus or respiratory syncytial virus, J. Exp. Med. 163:511–519.

Rosoff, P. M., Savage, N., and Dinerallo, C. A., 1988, Interleukin 1 stimulates diacyleglycerol production in T lymphocytes by a novel mechanism, Cell 54:73–81.

Ruschen, S., Lemm, G., and Watnatz, H., 1988, Interleukin 2 secretion by synovial fluid lymphocytes in rheumatoid arthritis, Br. J. Rheumatol. 27:350–356.

Salmon, M., Kitas, G. D., Hill-Gaston, J. S., and Bacon, P. A., 1988, Interleukin 2 production and response by helper T cell subsets in man, Immunology 65:81–85.

Sanders, M. E., Makgoba, M. W., and Shaw, S., 1988, Naive and memory T cells, Immunol. Today 9:195–199.

Sarto, K. T., and Mortensen, R. F., 1985, Enhanced interleukin 1 (IL-1) production mediated by mouse serum amyloid P component, Cell Immunol. 93:398–405.

Satoh, T, Nakamura, S., Taga, T., Matsuda, T., Hirano, T., Kishimoto, T., and Kaziro, Y., 1988, Induction of neural differentiation in PC 12 cells by B cell stimulatory factor 2/interleukin 6, Mol. Cell. Biol. 8:3546–3549.

Scala, G., Allavena, P., Djeu, J. Y., Kasahara, T., Ortaldo, J. R., Herberman, R. B., and Oppenheim, J. J., 1984, Human large granular lymphocytes are potent producers of interleukin 6, Nature 309:56–59.

Schreier, M. H., Iscove, N. N., Tees, R., Aarden, L., and VonBoehmer, H., 1980, Clones of killer and helper T cells: Growth requirements, specificity and retention of function in long-term culture, Immunol. Rev. 51:315–336.

Seckinger, P., Williamson, K., Balavaine, J-F., Mach, B., Mazzei, G., Shaw, A., and Dayer, J-M., 1987a, A urine inhibitor of interleukin 1 activity affects both interleukin 1α and 1β but not tumor, J. Immunol. 139:1541–1545.

Seckinger, P., Lowenthal, J. W., Williamson, K., Dayer, J-M., and McDonald, H. R., 1987b, A urine inhibitor of interleukin 1 activity that blocks ligand binding, J. Immunol. 139:1546–1549.

Sehgal, P. B., Walther, Z., and Tamm, I., 1987, Rapid enhancement of beta 2 interferon/B-cell differentiation factor BSF-2 gene expression in human fibroblasts by diacylglecerol and calcium ionophore A23187, Proc. Natl. Acad. Sci. USA 84:3663–3667.

Seigal, L. J., Harper, M. E., Wong-Stall, F., Gallo, R. C., Nash, W. G., and O'Brien, S. J., 1984, Gene for T cell growth factor. Location on human chromosome 4q and feline chromosome B1, Science 233:175–178.

Sharma, B., and Gupta, S., 1985, Antigen specific cytotoxic T cells in patients with AIDS and AIDS-related complex (ARC), Clin. Exp. Immunol. 62:296–303.

Sharon, M., Klausner, R. D., Cullen, B. R., Chizzomoto, R., and Leonard, W. J., 1986, Novel interleukin-2 receptor subunit detected by cross-linking under high-affinity conditions, *Science* **234**:859–863.

Shaw, J., Meerovitch, K., Bleackley, R. C., and Paetkan, V., 1988, Mechanisms regulating the levels of IL-2 mRNA in T lymphocytes, *J. Immunol.* **140**:2243–2248.

Siegel, J. P., Sharon, M., Smith, P. L., and Leonard, W. J., 1987, The IL-2 receptor beta chain (p70): Role in mediating signals for LAK, NK, and proliferative activities, *Science* **238**:75–78.

Smith, K. A., 1988a, Interleukin 2: Inception, impact, and implication, *Science* **240**:1169–1176.

Smith, K. A., 1988b, The interleukin 2 receptor, *Adv. Immunol.* **82**:864–868.

Smith, K. A., and Cantrell, D. A., 1985, Interleukin 2 regulates its own receptor, *Proc. Natl. Acad. Sci. USA* **82**:864–868.

Smith, K. A., Gillis, S., Baker, P. E., McKenzie, D., and Ruscetti, F. W., 1979, T cell growth factor mediated T cell proliferation, *Ann. NY Acad. Sci.* **332**:423–432.

Stadler, B. M., Dougherty, S. F., Farrar, J. J., Oppenheim, J. J., 1981, Relationship of cell cycle to recovery of IL-2 activity from human mononuclear cells, human and mouse T cell lines, *J. Immunol.* **127**:1936–1940.

Takai, Y., Wong, G. G., Clark, S. C., Burakoff, S. J., and Herrmann, S. H., 1988, B-cell stimulatory factor-2 is involved in the differentiation of cytotoxic T cells, *J. Immunol.* **140**:508–512.

Takeshita, T., Goto, Y., Tada, K., Nagata, K., Asao, H., and Sugamura, K., 1989, Monoclonal antibody defining a molecule possibly identical to the p75 subunit of interleukin 2 receptor, *J. Exp. Med.* **169**:1323–1332.

Tanaka, T., Saiki, O., Doi, S., Fuji, M., Sugamura, K., Hara, H., Negoro, S., and Kishimoto, S., 1988, Novel receptor-mediated internalization of interleukin 2 in B cells, *J. Immunol.* **140**:866–870.

Taniguchi, T., Matsui, H., Fujita, T., Takaoka, C., Kashima, N., Yoshimoto, R., and Hamuro, J., 1983, Structure and expression of a cloned cDNA for human interleukin 2, *Nature* **302**:305–310.

Teh, M. S., and Teh, S. J., 1980, Direct evidence for two signal mechanism of cytotoxic T cell activity, *Nature* **285**:163–165.

Teshigawara, K., Wang, H-M., Kato, K., and Smith, K. A., 1987, Interleukin 2 high affinity receptor expression requires two distinct binding proteins, *J. Exp. Med.* **165**:233–238.

Ting, C. C., Yang, S. S., Hargrove, M. E., 1984, Induction of suppressor T cells by interleukin 2, *J. Immunol.* **133**:261–266.

Toribio, M. L., de la Hera, A., Borst, J., Marcos, M. A. R., Marquez, C., Alonso, J. M., Barcena, A., and Martinez, A. C., 1988, Involvement of the interleukin 2 pathway in the rearrangement of both alpha/beta and gamma/delta T cell receptor genes in human T cell precursors, *J. Exp. Med.* **168**:2231–2249.

Trinchiari, G., Matsumoto-Kobayashi, M., Clark, S. C., Seehra, J., London, L., and Perussia, B., 1984, Response to human peripheral blood natural killer cells to interleukin 2, *J. Exp. Med.* **160**:1147–1169.

Tsudo, M., Kozak, R. W., Goldman, C. K., and Waldmann, T. A., 1986, Demonstration of a non-Tac peptide that binds interleukin 2: A potential participant in a multichain interleukin 2 receptor complex, *Proc. Natl. Acad. Sci. USA* **83**:9694–9698.

Tsudo, M., Goldman, C. K., Bongiovanni, K. F., Chan, W. C., Winton, E. F., Yagita, M., Grimm, E. A., and Waldmann, T. A., 1987, The p75 peptide is the receptor for IL-2 expression on large granular lymphocytes and is responsible for the IL-2 activation of these cells, *Proc. Natl. Acad. Sci. USA* **84**:5394–5398.

Tyler, J. A., 1985, Articular cartilage cultured with catabolin (pig interleukin 1) synthesizes a decreased number of normal proteoglycan molecules, *Biochem. J.* **227**:869–878.

Uchiama, T., Broder, S., and Waldmann, T. A., 1981, A monoclonal antibody (anti-Tac) reactive with activated and functional mature human T cells: I. Production of anti-Tac monoclonal antibody and distribution of Tac (+) cells, *J. Immunol.* **126**:1393–1397.

Waalen, K., Duff, G. W., Forre, O., Dickens, E., Kvarnes, L., and Nuki, G., 1986, Interleukin 1 activity produced by human rheumatoid and normal dendritic cells, *Scand. J. Immunol.* **23**:365–371.

Waalen, K., Førre, O., Linker-Israeli, M., and Thoen, J., 1987, Evidence of an activated T cell system with augmented turnover of interleukin 2 in rheumatoid arthritis. Stimulation of human T lymphocytes by dendritic cells as a model for rheumatoid T cell activation, *Scand. J. Immunol.* **25**:367–373.

Wagner, H. C., Hardt, C., Rouse, B. T., Rollinghoff, M., Schewrich, P., and Pfzenmaier, K., 1982, Dissection of the proliferative and differentiation signals controlling murine cytotoxic T lymphocyte response, *J. Exp. Med.* **155**:1876–1881.

Waldmann, T. A., Goldman, C., Robb, R. J., Depper, J. M., Leonard, W. J., Sharrow, S. O., Bongiovanni, K. F., Korsmeyer, K. F., and Greene, W. C., 1984, Expression of interleukin 2 receptor on activated B cells, *J. Exp. Med.* **160**:1523–1538.

Welte, K., Andreeff, M., Platzer, E., Holloway, K., Rubin, B. Y., Moore, M. A. S., and Mertelsmann, R., 1984, Interleukin 2 regulates the expression of Tac antigen on peripheral blood T lymphocytes, *J. Exp. Med.* **160**:1390–1403.

Wood, D. D., Cameron, P. M., Poe, M. T., and Morris, C. A., 1976, Resolution of a factor that enhances the antibody response of T-cell-derived murine splenocytes from several other monocyte products, *Cell. Immunol.* **21**:86–96.

Yamada, T., Fujishima, A., Kawahara, K., Kato, K., Nishimura, A., 1987, Importance of disulfide linkage for constructing the biologically active human interleukin 2, *Arch. Biochem. Biophys.* **257**:194–199.

Yamasaki, K., Taga, T., Hirata, Y., Ywata, H., Kawanishi, Y., Seed, B., Taniguchi, T., Hirano, T., and Kishimoto, T., 1988, Cloning and expression of the human interleukin 6 (BSF-2/IFN beta) receptor, *Science* **241**:825–828.

Yasukawa, K., Hirano, T., Watanabe, Y., Muratani, K., Matsuda, T., and Kishimoto, T., 1987, Structure and expression of human B cell stimulatory factor 2 (BSF-2/IL6) gene, *EMBO J.* **6**:2939–2945.

Zhang, Y., Lin, J-X., and Vilcek, J., 1988, Synthesis of interleukin 6 (interferon beta 2/B-cell stimulatory factor 2) in human fibroblasts triggered by an increase in intracellular cyclic AMP, *J. Biol. Chem.* **263**:6177–6182.

Zucali, J. R., Dinarello, C. A., Oblon, D. J., Gross, M. A., Anderson, L., and Weiner, R. S., 1986, Interleukin 1 stimulates fibroblasts to produce granulocyte-macrophage colony stimulating activity and prostaglandin E2, *J. Clin. Invest.* **77**:1857–1862.

Zvaifler, N. J., and Firestein, G. S., 1988, Cytokines in chronic inflammatory synovitis, *Scand. J. Immunol.* (Suppl.) **76**:203–210.

Chapter 7

THE IMMUNOLOGIC NETWORK

Possibilities for a New Immunopharmacology

Norman Talal

1. INTRODUCTION

Conventional therapy in autoimmune diseases and transplantation, although at times quite effective, brings with it a host of undesirable side effects ranging from severe osteoporosis and iatrogenic Cushing's syndrome (with corticosteroids) to generalized immunosuppression and increased risk for opportunistic infection (with cyclophosphamide and azathioprine). Based on new developments in our understanding of the functioning and regulation of the immunologic network, a new immunopharmacology has been quietly developed over the past decade whose goals are more precise and defined treatment rationale with specific targeting of drugs to specific molecular sites.

Autoimmunity and transplantation have much in common from an immunologic standpoint. Although the etiology of the former is unknown and the latter attributable to the introduction of foreign tissue or cells, once the immune network of regulation is perturbed, similar destructive processes ensue. Research findings in one field will contribute greatly to the other, and the development of new therapeutic approaches will benefit both types of patients. In this current era, research is dominated by cellular immunity and rapidly expanding knowledge of cytokines, which are factors released by cells that function normally to mediate the controlled processes of the immune response but also function pathologically in immune-mediated inflammation and tissue destruction. The major emphasis in the new immunopharmacology is based on restoring regulation through control of these cells and their products. This chapter presents an overview of the current status of this field and serves as an introduction to the more detailed chapters that follow. In a sense, it is a bridge between the effectors of immunity and immunopathology, which precede this chapter, and the hoped-for restorers of regulation, which follow.

Basic and clinical immunologists are defining precisely how the latest advances in molecular and cellular immunology might be transferred into medicine through the develop-

Norman Talal • Clinical Immunology Section, Audie L. Murphy Memorial Veterans Hospital, and the Department of Medicine, The University of Texas Health Science Center at San Antonio, San Antonio, Texas 78284.
Immunopharmacology in Autoimmune Diseases and Transplantation, edited by Hans Erik Rugstad *et al.* Plenum Press, New York, 1992.

ment of these new immunopharmacologic strategies. Recent conceptual as well as techno-
logical progress in research and development have moved fast enough so that clinical
immunologists are already undertaking the first therapeutic endeavors designed to restore
immunologic control in transplant and autoimmune disease patients. This specifically
targeted therapy, based as it is on precise pathophysiological mechanisms and molecular
engineering, represents a vastly different approach than conventional therapy such as
corticosteroids and generalized immunosuppression. Table I lists the cellular targets for
specific immunologic intervention. These targets are either the specific cells involved in the
immune response or the products of these cells. Since the number of defined cytokines is
expanding at a tremendously rapid rate, there will be more and more opportunities for
intervention at the level of cytokine products.

2. MONOCLONAL ANTI-Ia ANTIBODIES

The immune response starts by the appropriate presentation of antigen in association
with class II major histocompability (MHC) molecules on the surface of macrophages. The
macrophages first ingest and process the antigen before they present it on the cell surface
where the already-present class II MHC proteins act as a restriction element, thereby
conferring genetic regulation to the immune response. These activated macrophages or
antigen-presenting cells secrete tumor necrosis factor alpha (TNFα), which in turn induce
the secretion of interleukin-1, both molecules vitally important in the T-cell activation
process. Recent studies suggest that class II MHC molecules may be occupied *in vivo* by
natural peptides and displaced by exogenous digested antigen to initiate the immune
response to foreign antigens.

There is a twofold rationale behind the use of monoclonal anti-Ia antibodies in the
treatment of autoimmune disorders. One is to block the physiological presentation of
autoantigen in an effort to reduce lymphocyte activation generally. The other is to block the
aberrant expression of Ia molecules, which can be found in the salivary gland in Sjögren's
syndrome, the thyroid epithelium in autoimmune thyroiditis, and on many different cells
in the inflamed synovium of rheumatoid arthritis. Both induced diseases such as experimental allergic encephalomyelitis (EAE) as well as spontaneous autoimmune disorders such as
systemic lupus erythematosus developing in NZB/NZW mice can be suppressed with
monoclonal anti-Ia antibodies (Sriram and Steinmann, 1983; Adelman et al., 1983).
Significant therapeutic effects have been achieved in all of these experimental models. This
therapeutic strategy is based on the demonstrated ability of antibodies to class II MHC
molecules to suppress the immune response to specific antigens known to be under immune
response gene control (McDevitt et al., 1984). The precise mechanism by which these
antibodies act has not been determined, but it is thought to involve suppressor cells.

TABLE I.   Targets for Specific Immunologic Intervention

Cellular	Cytokines
Antigen-presenting cells	Interleukins (IL-1 through IL-10)
T-cell surface markers	Tumor necrosis factor
B-cell surface markers	

3. THERAPY TARGETED TO T CELLS

Most immunologic intervention is directed at the T cells themselves since they are the great orchestrators of the immune response and much is known about their physiology. T cells produce what is probably the single most important and studied cytokine discovered to date, interleukin-2 (IL-2). We know more about IL-2 and the IL-2 receptor than we do about most other molecules involved in immune regulation (Waldmann, 1986). Indeed, much of the evidence that autoimmune diseases are T-cell driven has come from the ability to suppress these diseases by specific immunologic intervention. Prior to these therapeutic studies, the evidence that autoimmune diseases are T-cell driven was largely dependent on the beneficial effect of neonatal thymectomy, the ability to induce experimental auto-immune diseases with T-cell clones to sensitized autoantigens, and the development of a generalized autoimmune syndrome with overlap features in patients receiving bone marrow transplants and undergoing chronic graft versus host disease (Table II).

Specific immunologic intervention directed at T cells is illustrated in Table III. This includes monoclonal antibodies to a variety of cell surface markers as well as for the T-cell antigen receptor, a heterodimer conjugated to the CD3 molecular complex (a pan-T-cell determinant). The heterodimer recognizes antigen presented in association with class II MHC molecules on the surface of macrophages. The CD3 molecular complex functions to transduce the activation signal into the nucleus. Clinical trials using anti-CD3 in patients demonstrate efficacy in acute renal transplant rejection, but this treatment is less successful for more chronic immunologically mediated diseases. Furthermore, many of these studies have the problem that the recipients become sensitized to the foreign immunoglobulins, thereby limiting the utility of the therapy. Administration of mouse antibodies to humans usually results in modulation of T-cell surface markers without much cytotoxicity, whereas rat antibodies given to mice induce significant cell destruction.

Eight patients with chronic multiple sclerosis (Hafler et al., 1988) were treated with anti-CD4 and anti-CD2 monoclonal antibody infusions, which demonstrated some degree of immunosuppression without alteration in T-cell populations. The authors explain their results as representing possible induction of negative signals or blocking of a modulating T-cell surface receptor for molecules that may be important in T-cell activation. Some patients developed anti-mouse immunoglobulin responses and a few developed an anti-idiotype response after infusion of anti-T-cell monoclonal antibodies. In experimental animals, a single high dose of anti-L3T4 (CD4) will induce tolerance, thereby allowing an F(ab)'2 fragment to be as effective as the intact anti-L3T4 molecule itself. There was a greater than 80% survival and no significant infiltrates found in the kidneys of NZB/NZW mice.

Experimental allergic encephalomyelitis, the animal model for multiple sclerosis, can be suppressed by anti-Ia or anti-CD4 antibodies prior to immunization with myelin basic protein. Reversal of disease was achieved in animals already paralyzed, both in rodents and in nonhuman primates.

TABLE II. Evidence That Autoimmune Diseases Are T-Cell Driven

Beneficial effect of neonatal thymectomy
Induction with T-cell clones
Human chronic graft versus host disease
Suppression by therapy targeted to T cells

TABLE III.   Therapy Directed at T Cells

Monoclonal antibodies to CD2, CD4
   Cell surface markers CD3, CD5 (L3T4)
   Antigen receptor
Block effects of IL-2
   Monoclonal antibody to IL-2 receptor (anti-Tac)
Toxin conjugation (ricin, diphtheria, *Pseudomonas*)
Vaccination with T cell lines
Cyclosporine

Recent studies show a very limited heterogeneity of the T-cell antigen receptors used by encephalitogenic T-cell clones sensitized to myelin basic protein peptide (Acha-Orbea *et al.*, 1988). Antibodies specific for this T-cell receptor were able to prevent or reverse EAE, similar to the effects achieved with anti-Ia and anti-CD4. This was attributable to the limited heterogeneity of these T-cell receptors in which all the T-cell clones used the same Vα gene element and at least 80% use the same Vβ gene element. Most of the clones utilize the same Jα element. Thus, there was a very strong selection *in vivo* for a particular T-cell receptor specificity. The authors conclude that this limited heterogeneity of T-cell receptor primary structure raises definite possibilities for immune intervention using monoclonal antibody therapy.

Several approaches, based on cytokines and receptor science, offer great promise for new directions in specific immunosuppression. The IL-2 receptor consists of a low-affinity component (p55, Tac) and an intermediate-affinity component (p75). The binding of IL-2 to the p75 component induces the production of Tac and these two molecules together constitute a high-affinity receptor. Monoclonal antibodies to the IL-2 receptor greatly extend allograft survival and can induce immunologic tolerance (Kupiec-Weglinski *et al.*, 1986). It also suppresses murine diabetic insulitis and lupus nephritis in NZB/NZW mice (Kelley *et al.*, 1988). Adult T-cell leukemia is a disease caused by the human T-cell leukemia (HTLV-I) virus in which T-cell infiltrates with 10–35,000 Tac receptors per cell infiltrate the skin. Anti-Tac antibodies conjugated to *Pseudomonas* endotoxin have been able to induce remissions in some patients with adult T-cell leukemia.

Using recombinant DNA methodology, fusion genes have been created combining IL-2 with diphtheria toxin as a means of killing IL-2 receptor positive cells (Bacha *et al.*, 1988). The diphtheria toxin conjugate requires high-affinity IL-2 receptors to work and has been used successfully to prevent delayed hypersensitivity, to induce tolerance to heart grafts, and to permit islet cell engraftment.

Toxin conjugation has also proved efficacious in the treatment of chronic graft versus host disease and may have extension into the field of autoimmune diseases. Ricin conjugated monoclonal antibodies to CD5 were used in these human trials.

Yet another approach to specific immunosuppression of EAE involves vaccination with T cell lines specifically reactive with the inductive antigen, myelin basic protein (Ben-Nun *et al.*, 1981). The cell line employed originated in rats that had developed EAE as a consequence of immunization with basic protein. The cell line was itself capable of inducing EAE after intravenous inoculation. However, attenuation of the cell line by irradiation or exposure to mitomycin c or high pressure rendered it capable of transferring resistance to EAE following immunization with myelin basic protein. Autoimmune arthritis can also be suppressed using attenuated T cell lines (Holoshitz *et al.*, 1983).

The synthesis of IL-2 can be prevented by the drug cyclosporine A. More than 40 autoimmune diseases have now been treated with cyclosporine A with some notable successes, particularly in uveitis (Kahan, 1988). In France, it has proved efficacious in clinical trials in the treatment of insulin-dependent diabetes mellitus, particularly when treatment is started early. Renal toxicity continues to be the main problem with cyclosporine A. Some patients have also developed malignant lymphomas which may regress when therapy is discontinued. The future for this agent may depend on the development of less toxic cyclosporine analogues as well as drug combinations in which cyclosporine can be used in lower doses.

4. THERAPY DIRECTED AT B CELLS

In addition to the interest in T cells, it is important to appreciate that B cells play an important role in many autoimmune disorders. Great interest has centered on the role of CD5$^+$ B cells, which are increased in patients with rheumatoid arthritis (Plater-Zyberk et al., 1985) and primary Sjögren's syndrome (Dauphinee et al., 1988). These cells correlate with disease activity although their exact clinical significance for these autoimmune diseases is still unknown. The CD5$^+$ B cell is the circulating cell in chronic lymphocytic leukemia and is capable of producing rheumatoid factor. The murine analogue of this cell is increased in autoimmune mice where it produces most of the autoantibodies to single-stranded DNA and to mouse erythrocytes. CD5 B cells are present in normal newborn mice but then decline with age. In autoimmune mice they persist into adulthood, function to produce autoantibodies, and can even become clonal in aged autoimmune mice, taking on malignant characteristics reminiscent of lymphomas that develop in Sjögren's syndrome patients. We have recently found that estrogen can induce normal murine CD5 B cells to increase production of anti-mouse erythrocyte antibodies, a finding relevant to the female predominance of many autoimmune diseases. If monoclonal antibodies to CD5 prove successful in T-cell depletion, they could theoretically also be tried to suppress CD5$^+$ B cells in autoimmune patients.

Another form of therapy potentially useful in the depletion of B cells is based on anti-idiotype specificity, although this therapy might be active against idiotype positive T cells as well. The suppression of pathogenic antibodies to DNA has been achieved by repeated inoculation of NZB/NZW mice with monoclonal anti-idiotypic antibodies directed against the major cross-reactive idiotype on anti-DNA antibodies in these mice (Hahn and Ebling, 1984). There was a transient suppression in disease manifestations but this was followed by the appearance of large quantities of anti-DNA that did not bear the major cross-reactive idiotype.

5. GENERAL BIOLOGICAL APPROACHES

Sex steroid hormones also influence normal immune mechanisms with androgens suppressing and estrogens augmenting (Ahmed et al., 1985). Androgens can suppress several autoimmune models including lupus in B/W and MRL/lpr mice, experimental allergic myesthenia gravis (EAMG), thyroiditis, and polyarthritis. The effects of sex hormones on autoimmunity probably represent physiological actions being expressed on aberrant systems of immunoregulation. The possible utilization of these effects in the treatment of human autoimmune disease is being studied in several laboratories.

Calorie restriction of NZB and B/W mice had a profound influence on the development of autoimmunity and immune dysregulation. Dietary restriction of NZB mice inhibits early thymic involution, delays the development of splenomegaly, and resulted in the prolonged maintenance of T-cell immune function (Fernandes, 1984). Restriction of total calorie intake in B/W mice more than doubled the life span and decreased immune complex deposition in the kidneys. Well-fed B/W mice showed earlier thymic involution, disorganization and dysfunction of the T-cell system, and the earlier onset of renal disease, accelerated autoimmunity, and death.

Dietary restrictions also retarded the lymphoproliferative disease and autoimmunity that occurs in MRL/*lpr* mice. Dietary restriction more than doubles the life span of these mice and inhibited the development of both lymphoproliferation and autoimmunity.

Studies on the mechanism of these effects are currently underway. Whether specific nutrients or total calorie manipulation can ultimately be employed for patients with the autoimmune disorders is uncertain at this time.

Another general biological approach that has been tried in autoimmunity is totally lymphoid irradiation (TLI). Initially developed for the treatment of Hodgkin's disease, TLI has been studied both in experimental models and in patients with systemic lupus erythematosus and rheumatoid arthritis (Kotzin and Strober, 1985).

Although the future clinical role of TLI in autoimmune diseases remains unclear, results thus far indicate that TLI is a unique immunosuppressive regimen when compared to currently used immunosuppressive drugs that are relatively nonselective and have short-lived effects. TLI is thought to produce a more selective and long-lasting reduction in the number and function of helper T cells. TLI is also associated with the appearance of antigen-nonspecific suppressor cells.

REFERENCES

Acha-Orbea, H., Mitchell, D. J., Timmermann, L., Wraith, D. C., Tausch, G. S., Waldor, M. K., Zamvil, S. S., McDevitt, H. O., and Steinman, L., 1988, Limited heterogeneity of T cell receptors from lymphocytes mediating autoimmune encephalomyelitis allows specific immune intervention, *Cell* **554**:263–273.

Adelman, N. E., Watling, D. L., and McDevitt, H. O., 1983, Treatment of (NZB × NZW)F$_1$ disease with anti-I-A monoclonal antibodies, *J. Exp. Med.* **158**:1350–1355.

Ahmed, Ansar, S., Penhale, W. J., and Talal, N., 1985, Sex hormones, immune responses and autoimmune diseases: Mechanisms of sex hormone action, *Am. J. Pathol.* **121**:531–551.

Bacha, P., Williams, D. P., Waters, C., Williams, J. M., Murphy, J. R., and Strom, T. B., 1988, Interleukin-2 receptor-targeted cytotoxicity. Interleukin-2 receptor-mediated action of a diphtheria toxin-related interleukin-2 fusion protein, *J. Exp. Med.* **167**:612–622.

Ben-Nun, A., Wekerle, H., and Cohen, I. R., 1981, Vaccination against autoimmmune encephalomyelitis using attenuated cells of a T lymphocyte line reactive against myelin basic protein, *Nature* **292**:60–61.

Dauphinee, M., Tovar, Z., and Talal, N., 1988, B cells expressing CD5 are increased in Sjogren's syndrome, *Arthritis Rheum.* **31**:642–647.

Fernandes, G., 1984, Nutritional factors: Modulating effects on immune function and aging, *Pharmacol. Rev.* **36**:123S–129S.

Hafler, D. A., Ritz, J., Slossman, S. F., and Weiner, H. L., 1988, Anti-CD4 and anti-CD2 monoclonal antibody infusions in subjects with multiple sclerosis. Immunosuppressive effects and human anti-mouse responses, *J. Immunol.* **141**:131–138.

Hahn, B. H., and Ebling, F. M., 1984, Suppression of murine lupus nephritis by administration of an anti-idiotypic antibody to anti-DNA, *J. Immunol.* **132**:187–190.

Holoshitz, J., Naparstek, Y., Ben-Nun, A., and Cohen, I., 1983, Lines of T lymphocytes induce or vaccinate against autoimmune arthritis, *Science* **219**:56–58.

Kahan, B. D., 1988, *Transplantation Proceedings*, Vol. XX, No. 3, Suppl. 4, Grune and Stratton, Philadelphia.

Kelley, V. E., Gaulton, G. N., Hattori, M., Ikegami, H., Eisenbarth, G., and Strom, T. B., 1988, Anti-interleukin-2 receptor antibody suppresses murine diabetic insulitis and lupus nephritis, *J. Immunol.* **140**:59–61.

Kotzin, B. L., and Strober, S., 1985, Total lymphoid irradiation, in: *Immunology of Rheumatic Diseases* (S. Gupta and N. Talal, eds.), Plenum Press, New York, pp. 793–809.

Kupiec-Weglinski, J. W., Diamantstein, T., Tilney, N. L., and Sron, T. B., 1986, Therapy with monoclonal antibody to interleukin-2 receptor spares suppressor T cells and prevents or reserves acute allograft rejection in rats, *Proc. Natl. Acad. Sci. USA* **83**:2624–2627.

McDevitt, H., Adelman, N., Watling, D., Steinmann, L., and Subramanian, S., 1984, The use of monoclonal anti-Ia antibodies for haplotype specific immunosuppression in animal models of autoimmune disease, in: *Immunogenetics: Its Application to Clinical Medicine* (T. Sasazuki and T. Tada, eds.), Academic Press, New York, pp. 85–94.

Plater-Zyberk, C., Maini, R. N., Lam, K., Kennedy, T. D., and Janossy, G., 1985, A rheumatoid arthritis B cell subset expresses a phenotype similar to that in chronic lymphocytic leukemia, *Arthritis Rheum.* **28:**971–976.

Sriram, S., and Steinmann, L., 1983, Anti-I-A antibody suppresses active encephalomyelitis: Treatment model for diseases linked to IR genes, *J. Exp. Med.* **158:**1362–1367.

Waldmann, T. A., 1986, The structure, function, and expression of interleukin-2 receptors on normal and malignant lymphocytes, *Science* **232:**727–732.

Part II

PHARMACOLOGY AND GENERAL THERAPEUTIC PRINCIPLES OF IMMUNOMODULATING DRUGS

Chapter 8

STEROIDS

Bruce W. Kirkham and *Gabriel S. Panayi*

1. INTRODUCTION

Glucocorticoids continue to have an important role in the treatment of many connective tissue and allergic diseases. In the 1980s, knowledge of how glucocorticoids function increased enormously, in parallel with the great growth of knowledge in immunology and molecular biology. We have concentrated on these new findings and have confined our review mainly to reports on human subjects or cells, as interspecies differences occur in some glucocorticoid activities.

The natural prototype of the glucocorticoid group is cortisol (hydrocortisone) (Figure 8.1), which is derived from cholesterol. Modifications of the basic cortisol structure have produced synthetic glucocorticoids with increased anti-inflammatory potency and reduced mineralocorticoid properties. These increases in anti-inflammatory potency result from alterations in the pharmacokinetics (Meikle and Tyler, 1977), improved ability to bind to steroid receptors (Ballard *et al.*, 1975), and perhaps from increased effectiveness at the site of action (Haynes and Murad, 1985). The relative anti-inflammatory potencies of glucocorticoids have been derived from models of inflammation and assessments of clinical responses. Metabolic effects such as hyperglycemia are also used as a guide to *in vivo* activity. Haynes and Murad (1985) provide a good review of the structure and function of the different glucocorticoids.

Some investigators have attempted to define the immunosuppressive properties of glucocorticoids separately from anti-inflammatory properties. They have used *in vitro* systems of lymphocyte stimulation by mitogen as models of cell-mediated immunity and assessed the levels of glucocorticoids required to suppress these reactions (Cantrill *et al.*, 1975; Langhoff and Ladefoged, 1983). As Table I shows, relative immunosuppressive potency as assessed by these methods does not give consistent results and shows no clear differences from the accepted anti-inflammatory potency spectrum.

Bruce W. Kirkham and *Gabriel S. Panayi* • Rheumatology Unit, United Medical and Dental Schools, Guy's Hospital, London SE1 9RT, England.

Immunopharmacology in Autoimmune Diseases and Transplantation, edited by Hans Erik Rugstad *et al.* Plenum Press, New York, 1992.

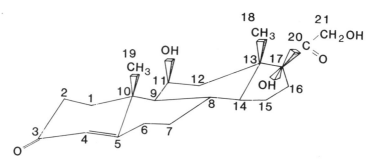

FIGURE 8.1.   Schematic three-dimensional structure of cortisol (hydrocortisone).

2. PHARMACOKINETICS

We will consider the detailed pharmacokinetics of prednisolone and prednisone since these drugs illustrate the important pharmacokinetic properties of glucocorticoids and are widely used. An excellent review of glucocorticoid pharmacokinetics by Begg and colleagues (1987) gives details of the differences within the glucocorticoid group.

2.1. Absorption

Prednisone is a pro-drug that, after oral administration, is rapidly converted to prednisolone, the active metabolite, in the liver (Meikle et al., 1975). The concentration–time profile of prednisone is very similar to that of prednisolone with almost complete availability of prednisolone from both preparations (Uribe et al., 1978; Pickup, 1979). Enteric coating delays the absorption of prednisolone and there is conflicting evidence of whether the extent of this absorption is reduced (Hulme et al., 1975; Hayes et al., 1983). Marked individual variations in peak plasma prednisolone levels occur after low- and high-dose oral prednisolone (Needs et al., 1988). At low doses of prednisolone (5–10 mg), there is no correlation between dose per kilogram body weight and the resulting plasma predniso-lone levels. In a study of 83 patients with rheumatic diseases, Hayes et al. (1983) also found no correlation between peak plasma prednisolone levels and disease-remitting effects. Other glucocorticoid preparations such as enemas and topical preparations are absorbed system-ically in appreciable amounts. Intra-articular administration of prednisolone sodium phos-

TABLE I.   Relative Anti-inflammatory and Immunosuppressive Properties of Glucocorticoids

Name	Relative immunosuppressive potency		Relative anti-inflammatory potency
	Langhoff and Ladefoged (1983)	Cantrill et al. (1975)	Haynes and Murad (1985)
Cortisol (hydrocortisone)	1	1	1
Cortisone	0.02	—	0.8
Prednisolone	0.3	2.43	4
6 methylprednisolone	9	—	5
Betamethasone	12	—	25
Dexamethasone	0.8	24.7	25

phate results in systemic absorption of about 50% of the dose, with the resulting suppression of endogenous cortisol levels (Reeback et al., 1980). Armstrong et al. (1981) found that peak serum levels of methylprednisolone occurred 2–12 hr after intra-articular injection; methylprednisolone was detectable for 3–5 days, with suppression of endogenous cortisol for approximately seven days. Intravenous prednisolone sodium phosphate is very rapidly hydrolyzed to prednisolone, with peak prednisolone levels found 5 min after injection (Bergrem et al., 1983). As shown in Figure 8.2, the pharmacokinetic profile of high-dose oral prednisolone (1 g) is very similar to that of intravenous high-dose methylprednisolone succinate, with similar clinical responses to both forms of treatment (Needs et al., 1988).

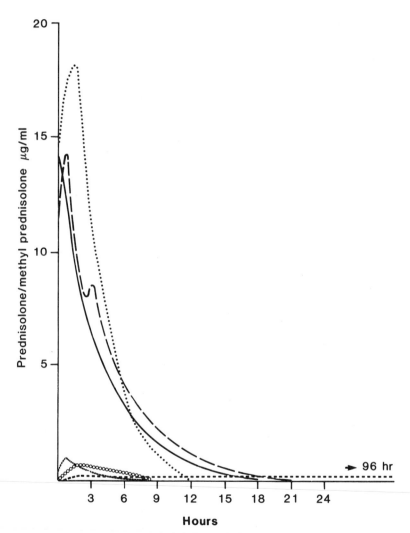

FIGURE 8.2. Glucocorticoid plasma concentration versus time for intravenous (IV), intra-articular (IA), and oral metylprednisolone or prednisolone. [. . ., Methylprednisolone hemisuccinate, 10 mg/kg IV (Derendorf et al., 1985); _____, methylprednisolone sodium succinate, 1 g IV (Needs et al., 1988); _____, prednisolone 1 g oral (Needs et al., 1988); ..., methylprednisolone hemisuccinate, 80 mg IV (Derendorf et al., 1985); ooo, methylprednisolone hemisuccinate, 80 mg oral (Derendorf et al., 1985); ___, Methylprednisolone acetate, 80 mg IA (Armstrong et al., 1981)].

2.2. Distribution

Prednisolone binds with high affinity but low capacity to a naturally occurring alpha-1-glycoprotein called transcortin and with low affinity but large capacity to albumin (Agabeyoglu *et al.*, 1979). The diurnal rhythm of endogenous cortisol results in a diurnal rhythm in prednisolone pharmacokinetics at low doses (< 7.5 mg). In the morning, competition between the elevated cortisol levels and prednisolone for binding sites increases free prednisolone, and competition for common metabolic pathways reduces prednisolone clearance (English *et al.*, 1983). This occurs at a time when the hypothalmic–pituitary–adrenal axis has an increased resistance to suppression by circulating glucocorticoids (Nichols *et al.*, 1965). These facts make a strong case for using single morning doses of prednisolone. These circadian variations in the pharmacokinetics of prednisolone are unimportant at higher doses (10–20 mg) of prednisolone and in long-term treatment where endogenous cortisol is suppressed (Meffin *et al.*, 1984a).

2.3. Elimination

Most prednisone and prednisolone are metabolically eliminated mainly in the liver by hydroxylation and conjugation. Drug half-lives are a function of volume of distribution and clearance. As these variables change in parallel with the dose of glucocorticoids, the half-life for prednisolone is approximately 3 hr (range 2.6–5 hr) (Begg *et al.*, 1987).

2.4. Drug Interactions

These are uncommon but have important clinical implications. Enzyme-inducing agents such as barbiturates, rifampicin, and phenytoin can significantly increase the clearance of prednisolone with a half-life less than 50% of the normal value (Gambertoglio *et al.*, 1980). As glucocorticoid doses are kept to the minimum effective level in clinical practice, an increase in glucocorticoid clearance may have serious consequences for disease control, particularly in organ transplant recipients. At low doses of corticosteroids, oral contraceptives can significantly decrease the clearance of glucocorticoids (Meffin *et al.*, 1984b).

3. SIDE EFFECTS

Physiological levels of cortisol have widespread homeostatic effects that involve regulation of carbohydrate, protein, and lipid metabolism. The supraphysiological levels of glucocorticoids used in therapy have equally widespread adverse effects. Most common irreversible side effects arise during long-term therapy. Daily doses of 10 mg prednisolone will eventually produce side effects in adults (Cochrane, 1983), with the elderly being adversely affected at lower doses (Thomas, 1984). In contrast, short-term glucocorticoid therapy, even at high doses (oral prednisolone 100 mg daily for up to 21 days, intra-articular glucocorticoids or intravenous "pulse" methylprednisolone), is associated with few side effects, most of which are transient and reversible when glucocorticoids are withdrawn (Seale and Compton, 1986). The side effects associated with short-term and long-term therapy are summarized in Table II.

TABLE II.   Side Effects of Glucocorticoid Therapy

I. Short-Term Therapy
   Weight gain
   Fluid retention, mild
   Insomnia
   Mood changes
     Euphoria, depression
     Psychosis
     Underreported
   Hyperglycemia
   Ketoacidosis, in diabetic patients
   Hypokalemia
   Superficial gastric mucosal ulceration
   Hypothalamic–pituitary–adrenal axis suppression; normal function usually returns within days
   Intra-articular crystalline glucocorticoids
     Transient increase in joint pain—?crystal synovitis
     Facial flushing
   Intravenous glucocorticoids
     All rare, especially now infusions given slowly (over 15–30 min)
     Anaphylactoid reactions in asthmatic patients; difficult to detect
     Hypotension
     Sudden death
   Intramuscular/subcutaneous
     Subcutaneous tissue atrophy
     Localized vitiligo
II. Long-Term Therapy
   Metabolic disturbance
     Hyperglycemia
     Hypokalemia ⎫
     Alkalosis   ⎬   not with 16 substituted compounds
                  ⎭
     Cushingoid habitus
       "moon face," central obesity
       "buffalo hump"
   Osteoporosis
     Especially post menopausal women
     Reduced bone mass
       Decreased osteoblast activity
       Decreased calcium absorption from gastrointestinal tract
       Increased renal calcium excretion
       Secondary hyperparathyroidism causing increased osteoclast activity
   Avascular necrosis of bone: usually femoral head but includes humerus
   Peptic ulceration: small increase in risk
   Hypertension: only with doses more than 10 mg daily prednisolone
   Myopathy
     Shoulder and pelvic girdles
     Slow sometimes incomplete recovery
   Pancreatitis: rare
   Occular effects
     Increased intraocular pressure: especially if preexisting myopia or diabetes
     Posterior subcapsular cataracts: increased incidence in children and rheumatoid arthritis
   Cutaneous effects
     Easy bruising, purpura
     Hirsutism
     Acne
   Reduced growth in children
     Can occur at low doses

(continued)

TABLE II.   (*Continued*)

Reduced by alternate day treatment
Monitor growth and weight during glucocorticoid treatment
Raised intracranial pressure: children and young women
    benign intracranial hypertension develops on dose reduction
Increased susceptibility to infection, including reactivation of tuberculosis
Hypothalamic–pituitary–adrenal axis suppression: may persist for up to 9 months after cessation of long-term
        daily treatment
    Reduced by
        Single morning doses
        Alternate day treatment
Corticosteroid withdrawal syndrome: fever, malaise, myalgia, arthralgia on dose reduction.

4. SUBCELLULAR MECHANISMS OF ACTION

4.1. Regulation of Gene Transcription

4.1.1. Gene Transcription

Glucocorticoids function by inducing or suppressing the transcription of a large number of genes. We will begin this section with a brief description of the processes that regulate gene transcription and protein production. Cellular differentiation and function are mediated by proteins produced by that cell. Protein production begins with transcription of the DNA coding for a protein to form nuclear RNA, which is then processed to produce messenger RNA (mRNA) (Figure 8.3). This leaves the nucleus and on reaching the cytoplasmic ribosomes translation of the mRNA produces the protein product. This product

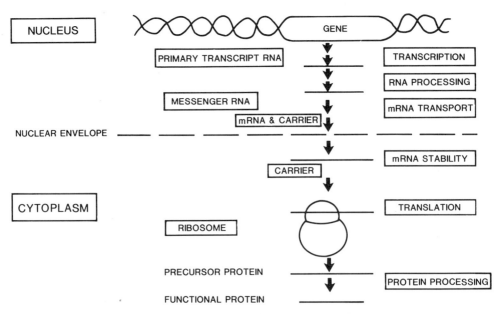

FIGURE 8.3.   Intracellular pathway of protein production.

is often in a precursor form and is processed before or after release from the cell to form the final functioning protein. Therefore, effector protein production has many potential control points.

Regulation of transcription of genes is under the control of regulatory DNA sequences. Transcription takes place when an enzyme, RNA polymerase, binds at the appropriate site and initiates RNA production. The original work on the control of bacterial genes demonstrated two main mechanisms of control called *cis* and *trans*. *Cis* describes a situation in which the regulatory DNA sequences are very close to the gene they regulate and are important sequences in the actual transcription of that DNA. These sequences are usually within 50–100 base pairs upstream (i.e., just before the site of initiation of RNA transcription) and are the sites of regulatory protein binding, which may inhibit or enhance RNA polymerase binding. The other situation is that of *trans* control, in which the regulatory sequences are distant from the regulated gene and are thought to form a gene that encodes a regulatory protein. This protein may increase or decrease the transcription of one or several genes (Darnell *et al.*, 1986).

Glucocorticoids are thought to act on transcription primarily in a *trans*-acting manner, although they probably have a less important *cis* action (Lan *et al.*, 1984). They can also regulate protein production at the level of mRNA translation and protein processing, as demonstrated by their effect on interleukin-1 production described in Section 5.6.1.

4.1.2. Glucocorticoid Receptors

Glucocorticoids are fat-soluble derivatives of cholesterol and pass freely through cell membranes into the cellular cytosol where they bind cytosolic glucocorticoid receptors (GR) (Lan *et al.*, 1984). This hormone–receptor interaction results in receptor transformation or activation. The untransformed GR is a 9S complex, consisting of a single 4S glucocorticoid-binding protein and at least one molecule of a non-glucocorticoid-binding heat-shock protein (Catelli *et al.*, 1985; Bresnick *et al.*, 1988). Binding of glucocorticoid with the GR results in dissociation of the 9S hetero-oligomer, with the release of the 4S glucocorticoid-binding protein that is capable of entering the nucleus and binding to DNA (Groyer *et al.*, 1987). In whole cell preparations the presence of glucocorticoid is mandatory for the transformed receptor to enter the nucleus. Rat, mouse, and human GR have similar structures and exceed the exclusion limit of approximately 70 kDa for passive diffusion through nuclear pores. Rat GRs have been shown to contain two nuclear localization signals, which are also found on other proteins that accumulate in the nucleus (Picard and Yamamoto, 1987) (Figure 8.4). Transformation of the GR culminates in accumulation of glucocorticoid–GR complexes in the nucleus where they associate with specific glucocorticoid response elements (Scheidereit *et al.*, 1986; Munck *et al.*, 1990).

4.1.3. Glucocorticoid Response Elements

Association of GR complexes with glucocorticoid response elements initiates transcription of the gene controlled by that element. Transcription at this site has now been shown to be induced by other classes of steroids and the term "hormonal response element" (HRE) is used for the region located -202 to -595 base pairs upstream of the transcription initiation site of the gene (Ponta *et al.*, 1985; Cato *et al.*, 1986). The transcriptional-activating properties of the HRE are similar to enhancer elements found in other viral or cellular genomes including SV40, moloney murine leukemia virus, and the immunoglobulin gene. Complex interactions govern the control of transcription. *Trans*-acting factors may specifically modify glucocorticoid initiation of transcription by interaction with the amino

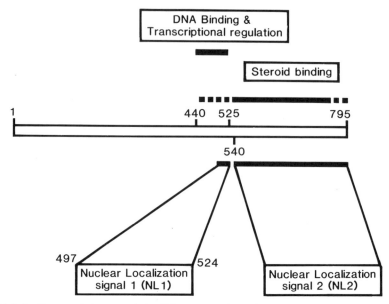

FIGURE 8.4. Functional domains of the 795 amino acid rat glucocorticoid receptor. Adapted with kind permission of Picard and Yamamoto (1987).

terminal of the DNA-bound glucocorticoid receptor (Cato *et al.*, 1988). These factors may provide cell-specific "fine-tuning" of responses to glucocorticoids and have been described in other systems (Nowock *et al.*, 1985; Miksicek *et al.*, 1987).

4.2. Glucocorticoid Anti-inflammatory Actions

4.2.1. The Acute Inflammatory Response

The acute inflammatory response is mediated by a combination of powerful pro-inflammatory mediators. Prominent among these are the lipid-derived products of which the prostaglandins, leukotrienes and platelet-activating factor (PAF) are the most important. These mediators are secreted by migrant and local cells (Oppenheim and Potter, 1984). Activation of these cells results in membrane perturbation and calcium influx, which initiates the generation of cell membrane-derived inflammatory mediators. The initial step is the enzymatic action of phospholipase A2, or a combination of phospholipase C and diglyceride lipase, on membrane phospholipids to form either free fatty acids, mainly arachidonic acid, or glycerolipids, mainly PAF (Barnes, 1990). Arachidonic acid is then metabolized either by the cyclo-oxygenase pathway to form prostaglandins or thromboxane A2 or by the lipoxygenase pathway to form leukotrienes; lyso-PAF is metabolized by acetylation to form active PAF (Oates *et al.*, 1988; Laue *et al.*, 1988; Russo-Marie, 1990).

4.2.2. Phospholipase A2 Inhibition

Unlike the aspirinlike nonsteroidal anti-inflammatory drugs, glucocorticoids do not directly inhibit cyclo-oxygenase activity. They are thought to exert many of their potent anti-inflammatory effects by inhibiting phospholipase A2. This inhibition suppresses the release of both fatty acids and glycerolipids, not only reducing prostaglandin release (as the aspirinlike drugs do), but also leukotriene and PAF release. Other mechanisms not dependent on phospholipase A2 inhibition also have been shown (Goppelt-Struebe et al., 1989). These inhibitory activities of glucocorticoids are suppressed by actinomycin D (an inhibitor of gene transcription) and cycloheximide (an inhibitor of protein synthesis), indicating that these glucocorticoid activities involve RNA and protein synthesis (Danon and Assouline, 1978; Flower and Blackwell, 1979; Raz et al., 1989) and are mediated by protein products. Glucocorticoid-induced proteins with antiphospholipase activities have been isolated by several groups and termed "lipocortins" (Hirata, 1984; Flower et al., 1984; DiRosa et al., 1984).

4.2.3. Lipocortins and Antiphospholipase A2 Proteins

Lipocortins are a group of phospholipase inhibitory glycoproteins present in many tissues and cells. They can be found in unstimulated cells and their synthesis can be induced by glucocorticoids. They were first discovered in culture media in which macrophages, neutrophils, and kidney cells were cultured with glucocorticoids. Two cDNA clones encoding lipocortins I and II have been isolated and the derived amino acid sequences give them molecular weights of 36 and 37 kDa, respectively (Wallner et al., 1986; Huang et al., 1986). They are composed of four nonidentical repeats that have an average 41% homology. The lipocortin family of proteins is identical to the placental proteins p35 and p36 and is related to a larger group of proteins with antiphospholipase activity, including calectrins.

Miele and colleagues (1988) constructed synthetic oligopeptides corresponding to a region of high amino acid sequence similarity between uteroglobin, a rabbit protein with antiphospholipase A2 activity, and lipocortin I. These peptides have potent antiphospholipase A2 activity in vitro and striking anti-inflammatory effects in vivo. The mechanism of lipocortin phospholipase A2 inhibitory activity is unclear but may involve the formation of phospholipase A2–lipocortin complexes (Hirata et al., 1987). The importance of lipocortins as glucocorticoid "second messengers" is still unclear. Variability in the six lipocortin protein preparations isolated by different groups has been proposed as a cause of the differences in anti-inflammatory effects reported to date and should be resolved by the use of recombinant proteins (Peers and Flower, 1990). One unresolved question of the actual glucocorticoid inducibility of lipocortins may reflect differing tissue responses to glucocorticoid (Isacke et al., 1989; Russo-Marie, 1990). Goulding and colleagues (1990) have shown a median increase of 225% of intracellular lipocortin I in peripheral blood monocytes from normal human volunteers after an intravenous bolus of hydrocortisone.

5. CELLULAR MECHANISMS OF ACTION

5.1. Cell Traffic

Changes in peripheral blood leukocyte numbers occur in response to the physiological diurnal rhythms of cortisol levels. Glucocorticoids induce a peripheral blood neutrophilia and lymphopenia that affects T lymphocytes more than B lymphocytes. Monocyte and eosinophil numbers also fall. These changes reach a maximum 4 hr after an intravenous bolus of glucocorticoid and return to normal levels by 24 hr (Cupps and Fauci, 1982). After a bolus of glucocorticoid, the CD4 positive T helper lymphocyte subset numbers fall more than the CD8 suppressor/cytotoxic T-lymphocyte subset (Hermanns *et al.*, 1982; Silverman *et al.*, 1984). Lymphocytes are thought to localize in lymph nodes and the bone marrow, although the mechanisms governing these changes are unknown (Bloemena *et al.*, 1990). A recent study by Smith and colleagues (1988) investigated glucocorticoid-mediated changes of the leukocyte numbers in an extravascular inflammatory site. They analyzed synovial fluid leukocyte numbers sequentially in rheumatoid arthritis patients receiving 1 g intravenous methylprednisolone bolus treatment. Their results showed a profound synovial fluid neutropenia and a modest lymphocytosis, with the CD4 T lymphocyte subset increasing by a smaller proportion than the CD8 subset. In contrast to peripheral blood changes usually lasting 24 hr, the synovial fluid neutropenia and lymphocytosis was still present two weeks after treatment. Thus the glucocorticoid effects on cellular traffic in inflammatory sites is prolonged and may contribute to the clinical improvement, often lasting several weeks after a single intravenous bolus of methylprednisolone (Richter *et al.*, 1983).

5.2. T-Lymphocyte Function

5.2.1. T-Lymphocyte Cytokines

In vivo, T lymphocytes are thought to be activated through their recognition of nominal antigen on the surface of an antigen-presenting cell in the context of major histocompatibility antigens. Following activation of T lymphocytes, the expression of various lymphokines and surface receptor genes is induced. The controlled transcription of these genes plays a crucial role in the proliferation, differentiation, and function of T lymphocytes and the immune response (Figure 8.5).

Glucocorticoids have major suppressive effects on *in vivo* cell-mediated immune responses and *in vitro* studies show they profoundly suppress T-lymphocyte proliferation to both mitogens and antigens (Cupps and Fauci, 1982; Dupont *et al.*, 1986). This suppression of proliferation can be partially or completely reversed by exogenous interleukin-2 (IL-2) (Gillis *et al.*, 1979). It has been shown that glucocorticoids such as dexamethasone suppress IL-2 gene transcription at pharmacological levels (Arya *et al.*, 1984). This suppression of lymphokine gene transcription has also been shown for interferon-gamma (Arya *et al.*, 1984), IL-3 (Culpepper and Lee, 1985), and granulocyte/ macrophage colony-stimulating factor (GM-CSF) (Kelso and Munck, 1984). The mechanism of this suppressive action is unknown. Prednisolone at pharmacological levels did not suppress the increased expression of the biologically active high-affinity receptor for IL-2 on phytohemagglutinin (PHA) stimulated lymphoblasts (Bloemena *et al.*, 1988). However, suprapharmacological levels of prednisolone (10^{-4} M) reduced the numbers of high-affinity IL-2 receptors on T lymphoblasts stimulated by PHA (Reed *et al.*, 1986). Glucocorticoids suppress lymphotoxin (tumor necrosis factor beta) production (Williams and Granger, 1969). The above data on lymphokine and receptor expression come from *in vitro* cell culture experiments. The results for IL-2 have been confirmed by an *in vivo* study that demonstrated that spontaneous IL-2 secretion and IL-2 mRNA production by bronchoalveolar lavage lymphocytes from patients with pulmonary sarcoidosis were undetectable after treatment with 1 mg/kg prednisolone daily for one month (Pinkston *et al.*, 1987).

5.2.2. T-Lymphocyte Activity

Hanson *et al.* (1986) assessed peripheral blood lymphocyte function in patients with chronic hepatitis B infection treated with daily prednisolone. At high daily doses of

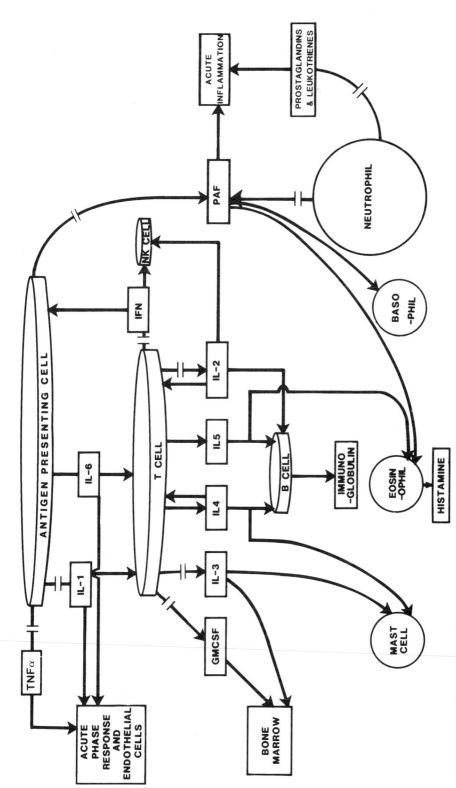

FIGURE 8.5. Glucocorticoid effects on immune and inflammatory mediator production. (⊣⊢, Glucocorticoid suppression of production.) Glucocorticoid effects on IL-4, IL-5, and IL-6 production not published to date.

prednisolone (60 mg), helper T-lymphocyte function, as measured by increases of *in vitro* immunoglobulin synthesis in the presence of lymphocytes from treated patients, was decreased. No decrease in helper function was detectable at 30 mg of prednisolone daily. In contrast, T suppressor cell function was decreased at both doses. These results correlated with the *in vivo* effects seen in these patients. A small decrease in serum immunoglobulin (predominantly decreased helper function) was seen at 60 mg/day and an increase in immunoglobulin levels occurred at the lower dose (predominantly decreased suppressor function). Paavonen (1985) has also demonstrated *in vitro* that human peripheral blood CD8 subset suppressor function is reduced by pharmacological amounts of glucocorticoids in contrast to CD4 helper function, which remained unchanged. Piccolella and colleagues (1985) demonstrated that dexamethasone at pharmacological levels prevented the development of suppressor cell function in the later stages of an antigen-induced response. This prevention of development of suppressor function could not be corrected by exogenous IL-2.

5.3. B-Lymphocyte Function

Studies of B-cell function have been difficult to perform since the commonly used measure of B-cell activation, immunoglobulin reproduction, is a terminal function of B-cell activation, influenced by both B cell, T cell, and accessory cell changes. Recently the sequential activation pathway of human B-lymphocytes has been clarified and has enabled the effects of glucocorticoids on B-cell function to be analyzed (Muraguchi *et al.*, 1983). *In vitro* T-cell activation of unstimulated B lymphocytes is suppressed by physiological levels of glucocorticoids (Cupps and Fauci, 1982). Bowen and Fauci (1984) have demonstrated that glucocorticoids prevent anti-μ antibody-induced enlargement of small tonsillar B cells, prevent expression of surface activation markers in response to anti-μ, and suppress small B-cell proliferation in response to anti-μ combined with cell growth factor (BCGF) and to *Staphylococcus aureus* Cowan. These suppressive actions occurred only if glucocorticoids were introduced within the first 24 hr of stimulation. *In vitro* or *in vivo* preactivated B cells were resistant to these suppressive activities of glucocorticoids.

Cupps and colleagues (1985) confirmed the above findings and extended the previous study to investigate glucocorticoid effects on the later steps of B-cell activation. They found that in contrast to the suppressive effects in the early stages of B-cell activation, the presence of glucocorticoid either did not change or increased the differentiation of plaque-forming (immunoglobulin-secreting) B cells in response to antigen or mitogen. They also showed that the suppressive effect of glucocorticoids on B-cell proliferation in response to *S. aureus* Cowan was much greater in the presence of monocytes, indicating the importance that glucocorticoid modification of accessory cell properties has on B-cell function. The complexity of the effects of glucocorticoids on B-cell activation is demonstrated by Akahoshi and colleagues (1988) who found that resting peripheral blood B cells express markedly elevated levels of high-affinity IL-2 receptor when cultured in the presence of pharmacological levels of glucocorticoids.

5.4. Lymphocyte Lysis

In vitro, glucocorticoids are found to cause lysis of rat and murine thymocytes, peripheral blood lymphocytes, and lymphoma cells. This cytolytic effect is not seen when human thymocytes or peripheral blood B and T lymphocytes are cultured with glucocorticoid (Claman, 1972). Galili (1983), however, has shown that certain human lymphocyte subsets are lysed *in vitro* by upper physiological (10^{-6} M) and pharmacological (10^{-5} M) concentrations of cortisol. These subsets include prothymocytes and peripheral blood lymphocytes activated in a one-way mixed lymphocyte reaction but not by the lectin phytohemagglutinin. *In vivo*-activated T lymphocytes from rheumatoid arthritis synovial fluid were also lysed. Chronic lymphocytic leukemia cells from all subjects tested and acute lymphocytic leukemia cells from half of the tested subjects showed extensive lysis after culture with 10^{-5} cortisol for 20 hr. Acute and chronic myeloid leukemic cells were all resistant to lysis. The role that differences in glucocorticoid receptor density has in these results is unresolved at present (Lowenthal and Jestrimski, 1986). The lytic process is dependent on mRNA and protein synthesis. Compton and Cidlowski (1987), using a rat model, have proposed that glucocorticoids induce a nucleolytic "lysis gene" product that is responsible for the cytolytic process characteristic of programmed cell death (apoptosis).

5.5. Natural Killer Cells and Antibody-Dependent Cellular Cytotoxicity

Onsrud and Thorsby (1981) investigated natural killer (NK) cell function after an *in vivo* bolus of hydrocortisone (300 mg). They found changes in natural killer activity (a decrease at 4 hr and an increase at 24 hr) of peripheral blood mononuclear cells (PBMNC). When corrected for changes in lymphocyte numbers, however, no medication-related change was found and they concluded that the changes seen were due to a reversible redistribution of cells affecting mainly non-NK cells and that no intrinsic glucocorticoid change in NK cell function had occurred. Nair and Schwartz (1984) investigated *in vitro* changes due to glucocorticoids. They demonstrated that NK activity of PBMNC was reduced in the presence of pharmacological levels of prednisolone (1×10^{-6} M). These suppressive effects on NK activity of prednisolone were reversed by the addition of interferon γ (IFN-γ) but not IL-2.

Parrillo and Fauci (1978) have also demonstrated significant decreases in spontaneous cellular cytotoxicity by pharmacological levels of dexamethasone with no changes in antibody-dependent cellular cytotoxicity (ADCC). In a study of ADCC of an enriched monocyte population, pharmacological levels of dexamethasone were found either not to change or to increase ADCC (Shen *et al.*, 1986). Interferon-γ-stimulated ADCC also was not suppressed and at times was augmented by dexamethasone.

5.6. Accessory Cell Function

5.6.1. Interleukin-1

IL-1 is mainly produced by cells of the monocyte/macrophage series, although epidermal, epithelial, lymphoid, and vascular tissues can also secrete IL-1. There are two biochemically distinct but structurally related forms, IL-1 alpha and IL-1 beta. These two forms share only small stretches of amino acid homology (26% in humans). Both forms are primarily translated as 31-kDa precursor molecules, and the generation of the amino terminus of the mature peptide (17.5 kDa) and smaller peptides then occurs by the action of serine proteases. Messenger RNA encoding for IL-1 beta predominates over that for IL-1 alpha, and the IL-1 beta peptide is the main extracellular IL-1 form. Receptors for IL-1 recognize both forms equally and both forms possess the same biological properties (Dinarello, 1988). Since Snyder and Unanue (1982) reported that murine macrophage IL-1 production was inhibited by glucocorticoids, the mechanisms of this inhibition have been elucidated. It seems likely that glucocorticoids control IL-1 production at both the transcriptional and posttranscriptional levels of the production process.

Knudsen and colleagues (1987) investigated the effects of dexamethasone on IL-1 production using the monocytelike tumor line, U937. Dexamethasone (10^{-8} M) completely blocked accumulation of IL-1β mRNA, indicating transcriptional control of IL-1β synthesis. Prestimulated cells when treated with 5×10^{-7} M dexamethasone had reductions of IL-1 release although IL-1β mRNA levels were unchanged, indicating the presence of posttranscriptional mechanisms. Glucocorticoid mechanisms were mediated by glucocorticoid receptors. The inhibition of release of IL-1 was accompanied by transient increases in cAMP levels, which are thought to block posttranscriptional IL-1 synthesis. Lee *et al.* (1988) found similar results for IL-1β gene transcription and also demonstrated a selective decrease in the stability of the IL-1 mRNA. Lew and colleagues (1988) demonstrated similar dexamethasone suppression of IL-1β gene transcription in human peripheral blood monocytes. However, the results of Kern *et al.* (1988) are at variance. They found that dexamethasone profoundly inhibited release of IL-1 protein from human peripheral blood monocytes without reducing IL-1β gene transcription. Glucocorticoids inhibited IL-1β release in cultures of human lung tissue (Bochner *et al.*, 1987). Glucocorticoids at pharmacological levels inhibited IL-1 release by more than 50% in contrast to nonglucocorticoid steroids. Inhibition of IL-1 production occurred after a lag period of 5–16 hr, and the relative glucocorticoid potencies agreed with established anti-inflammatory potencies (Table I).

5.6.2. Tumor Necrosis Factor

Tumor necrosis factor (TNF-α), or cachectin, is thought to be predominantly secreted by cells of the monocyte/macrophage lineage, although production by T cells has been recently documented (Cuturi *et al.*, 1987). TNF-β or lymphotoxin is a lymphoid cell product. TNF-α production is inhibited by glucocorticoids with control at both transcriptional and posttranscriptional levels in a similar manner to control of IL-1 (Beutler and Cerami, 1987).

5.6.3. Accessory Cell Activation

Human monocytes and macrophages express receptors for the Fc portion of IgG (FcγR). These receptors are thought to play an important role in immune function, particularly phagocytic functions such as endocytosis of immune complexes and antibody-dependent cell-mediated lysis (ADCC) of antibody-coated erythrocytes, parasites, and tumor cells. Glucocorticoids inhibit FcγR expression on HL60 and U937 cells *in vitro*. Decreased monocyte FcγR levels have been found after *in vivo* glucocorticoid therapy. However, Girard *et al.* (1987) have shown that *in vitro* culture of monocytes with glucocorticoid did not significantly reduce expression of an important subtype of FcγR, the high-affinity FcγR. The combination of IFN-γ and dexamethasone significantly increased expression of the high-affinity FcγR. These findings may help explain the additional increases in activity of some IFN-γ-dependent mononuclear phagocyte Fc-mediated functions such as ADCC, when both IFN-γ and glucocorticoid are present.

In vitro enhancement of human monocyte MHC class I and II expression by IFN-γ was increased in the presence of pharmacological levels of dexamethasone (2×10^{-7} M) (Shen *et al.*, 1986). These findings are supported by the findings of Gerrard and colleagues (1984) that *in vitro* hydrocortisone treatment of monocytes results in increased expression of

HLA DR antigens. However, Aberer and colleagues (1984) demonstrated a dose-dependent decrease in epidermal Ia-bearing cells in mice treated with topical or systemic glucocorticoids. This decrease in number was also accompanied by reduced *in vitro* Langerhans cell-dependent immunologic functions, such as antigen-specific syngeneic or allogeneic T-cell proliferation. Similar results have also been demonstrated by other authors (Belsito *et al.*, 1982).

Leszczynski *et al.* (1986) demonstrated that *in vivo* systemic glucocorticoids reduced unstimulated rat heart and kidney tissue dendritic cell density and abolished capillary endothelial cell MHC class II Ag expression. Glucocorticoids could also inhibit IFN-γ-induced enhancement of endothelial cell class II expression and tissue dendritic cell density. An interesting finding from this study was that only high doses of methylprednisolone (300 mg/kg) were effective if given as a single bolus, but that repeated small doses were extremely effective (1–3 mg/kg per day). These *in vivo* effects of methylprednisolone are probably an indirect effect, as IFN-γ enhancement of class II expression on *in vitro* endothelial cell cultures was not reduced by methylprednisolone. *In vitro* findings of absent glucocorticoid inhibition of IFN-γ-induced expression of MHC class II antigens on human umbilical endothelial cell cultures is reported by Manyak *et al.* (1988). This group found IFN-γ and -β were inhibitory, but dexamethasone showed a slight enhancing effect on class II expression.

5.7. Acute-Phase Response

Using cultured rat, mouse, or human liver cells it has been found that the presence of glucocorticoids is essential for the production of some acute-phase proteins (APP) and that glucocorticoids alone can stimulate the production of some APP in rat liver cells (Andus *et al.*, 1988). In a model using cultured human hepatoma cells, Baumann and colleagues (1987) found that dexamethasone did not directly stimulate production of APP, but acted additively or synergistically with combinations of IL-1 and a hepatocyte-stimulating factor that was probably IL-6. However, *in vivo* glucocorticoids reduce APP levels, presumably by suppressing production of cytokines, such as IL-1, that stimulate APP release.

5.8. Glucocorticoid Resistance

The clinical impression that some patients do not respond to glucocorticoids has been investigated *in vitro*. Walker *et al.* (1985) found a wide range of individual sensitivity to the immunosuppressive effects of prednisolone in an *in vitro* system. Approximately 30% of normal subjects and renal dialysis patients required large amounts of prednisolone to suppress lymphocyte proliferation. Langhoff *et al.* (1986) applied a similar *in vitro* assay to renal transplant candidates and found "steroid resistance" was associated with an increased one-year graft failure, particularly in those patients who did not receive cyclosporine. Dumble and colleagues (1981) reported similar findings using an antibody-dependent cell-mediated cytotoxicity assay to assess steroid sensitivity. Walker *et al.* (1987) found steroid resistant subjects had higher levels of IL-2 activity in the supernatants of both steroid- and nonsteroid-treated cultures. Some asthmatic patients do not respond clinically to glucocorticoids (Carmichael *et al.*, 1981). *In vitro* assessment of glucocorticoid suppression of PBMNC proliferation correlates with *in vivo* results. It has been suggested that monocytes are central to glucocorticoid sensitivity (Wyllie *et al.*, 1986). Wilkinson *et al.* (1989) have demonstrated that PBMNC from asthmatic patients produce a factor that increases neutrophil leukotriene B4 production. *In vitro* production of this factor was suppressed by hydrocortisone in patients clinically sensitive to glucocorticoids but persisted in those patients clinically resistant to glucocorticoids.

6. SUMMARY

Glucocorticoids are potent suppressors of inflammatory and immune responses. These suppressive activities are the result of a complex series of subcellular interactions. Many of these glucocorticoid actions are mediated by the production of specific controlling peptides, which act as regulators of gene transcription or regulate cytoplasmic enzymes. A major mechanism of glucocorticoid activity is the inhibition of production of the mediators of inflammatory and immune activity. The inability of glucocorticoids to block or antagonize the direct effect of these mediators on target cells is demonstrated *in vitro* by IL-2. *In vivo*, this inability to counteract many of the direct effects of mediators such as cytokines may account for the lack of efficacy and even detrimental effects of glucocorticoids in acute conditions such as gram-negative septicemia (Bone *et al.*, 1987), in which many of the pathological events are thought to be directly mediated by cytokines. Glucocorticoids also cause profound changes in cell traffic which can be long-lasting. The powerful anti-inflammatory and immunomodulatory activities of glucocorticoids are the culmination of activities that affect most aspects of the immune system.

ACKNOWLEDGMENTS. The authors would like to thank Professor T. H. Lee and Dr. Gabrielle Kingsley for their helpful comments. Our thanks go to Mrs. R. Lewis and Mrs. P. Powell for their expert secretarial assistance. Dr. B. Kirkham is supported by the Arthritis Foundation of New Zealand, Inc.

REFERENCES

Aberer, W., Stingl, L., Pogantsch, S., and Stingl, G., 1984, Effect of glucocorticosteroids on epidermal cell-induced immune responses. *J. Immunol.* **133**:792–797.

Agabeyoglu, I. T., Bergstrom, R. F., Gillespie, W. R., Wagner, J. G., and Kay, D. R., 1979, Plasma protein binding of prednisolone in normal volunteers and arthritic patients, *Eur. J. Clin. Pharmacol.* **16**:399–404.

Akahoshi, T., Oppenheim, J. J., and Matsushima, K., 1988, Induction of high-affinity interleukin 1 receptor on human peripheral blood lymphocytes by glucocorticoid hormones, *J. Exp. Med.* **167**:924–936.

Andus, T., Geiger, T., Hirano, T., Kishimoto, T., and Heinrich, P. C., 1988, Action of recombinant human interleukin 6, interleukin 1β and tumor necrosis factor α on the mRNA induction of acute-phase proteins, *Eur. J. Immunol.* **18**:739–746.

Armstrong, R. D., English, J., Gibson, T., Chakraborty, J., and Marks, V., 1981, Serum methylprednisolone levels following intra-articular injection of methylprednisolone acetate, *Ann. Rheum. Dis.* **40**:571–574.

Arya, S. K., Wong-Staal, F., and Gallo, R. C., 1984, Dexamethasone-mediated inhibition of human T cell growth factor and γ-interferon messenger RNA, *J. Immunol.* **133**:273–276.

Ballard, P. L., Carter, J. P., Graham, B. S., and Baxter, J. D., 1975, A radioreceptor assay for evaluation of the plasma glucocorticoid activity of natural and synthetic steroids in man, *J. Clin. Endocrinol. Metab.* **41**:290–304.

Barnes, P. J., 1990, Allergic inflammatory mediators and bronchial hyperresponsiveness, in: *Immunology and Allergy Clinics of North America* (C. W. Bierman and T. H. Lee, eds.), W.H. Saunders and Co., Philadelphia, pp. 241–246.

Baumann, H., Richards, C., and Gauldie, J., 1987, Interaction among hepatocyte-stimulating factors, interleukin 1, and glucocorticoids for regulation of acute phase plasma proteins in human hepatoma (HepG2) cells, *J. Immunol.* **139**:4122–4128.

Begg, E. J., Atkinson, H. C., and Gianarakis, N., 1987, The pharmacokinetics of corticosteroid agents, *Med. J. Aust.* **146**:37–41.

Belsito, D. V., Flotte, T. J., Lim, H. W., Baer, R. l., Thorbecke, G. J., and Gigli, I., 1982, Effect of glucocorticosteroids on epidermal Langerhans cells, *J. Exp. Med.* **155**:291–302.

Bergrem, H., Grottum, P., and Rugstad, H. E., 1983, Pharmacokinetics and protein binding of prednisolone after oral and intravenous administration, *Eur. J. Clin. Pharmacol.* **24**:415–419.

Beutler, B., and Cerami, A., 1987, Cachectin: More than a tumor necrosis factor, *N. Engl. J. Med.* **316**:379–385.

Bloemena, E., van Oers, M. H. J., Weinreich, S., and Schellekens, P. Th. A., 1988, Cyclosporin A and prednisolone do not inhibit the expression of high-affinity receptors for interleukin 2, *Clin. Exp. Immunol.* **71**:308–313.

Bloemena, E., Weinreich, S., and Schellekens, P. T. A., 1990, The influence of prednisolone on the recirculation of peripheral blood lymphocytes *in vivo*, *Clin. Exp. Immunol.* **80**:460–466.

Bochner, B. S., Rutledge, B. K., and Schleimer, R. P., 1987, Interleukin 1 production by human lung tissue. II. Inhibition by anti-inflammatory steroids, *J. Immunol.* **139:**2303–2307.

Bone, R. C., Fisher, C. J., Clemmer, T. P., Slotman, G. J., Metz, C. A., and Balk, R. A., 1987, A controlled clinical trial of high-dose methylprednisolone in the treatment of severe sepsis and septic shock, *N. Engl. J. Med.* **317:**653–658.

Bowen, D. L., and Fauci, A. S., 1984, Selective suppressive effects of glucocorticoids on the early events in the human B cell activation process, *J. Immunol.* **133:**1885–1890.

Bresnick, E. H., Sanchez, E. R., and Pratt, W. B., 1988, Relationship between glucocorticoid receptor steroid-binding capacity and association of the M$_r$ 90,000 heat shock protein with the unliganded receptor, *J. Steroid. Biochem.* **30:**267–269.

Cantrill, H. L., Waltman, S. R., Palmberg, P. F., Zink, H. A., and Becker, B., 1975, *In vitro* determination of relative corticosteroid potency, *J. Clin. Endocrinol. Metab.* **40:**1073–1077.

Carmichael, J., Paterson, I. C., Diaz, P., Crompton, G. K., Kay, A. B., and Grant, I. W. B., 1981, Corticosteroid resistance in asthma, *Br. Med. J.* **282:**1419–1422.

Catelli, M. G., Binart, N., Jung Testas, I., Renoir, J. M., Baulieu, E. E., Feramisco, J. R., and Welch, W. J., 1985, The common 90-kd protein component of non-transformed "8S" steroid receptors is a heat shock protein, *EMBO J.* **4:**3131–3135.

Cato, A. C. B., Miksicek, R., Schutz, G., Arnemann, J., and Beato, M., 1986, The hormone regulatory element of mouse mammary tumour virus mediates progesterone induction, *EMBO J.* **5:**2237–2240.

Cato, A. C. B., Skroch, P., Weinmann, J., Butkeraitis, P., and Ponta, H., 1988, DNA sequences outside the receptor-binding sites differentially modulate the responsiveness of the mouse mammary tumour virus promoter to various steroid hormones, *EMBO J.* **7:**1403–1410.

Claman, H. M., 1972, Corticosteroids and the lymphoid cells, *N. Engl. J. Med.* **287:**388–389.

Cochrane, G. M., 1983, Systemic steroids in asthma, in: *Steroids in Asthma: A Reappraisal in the Light of Inhalational Therapy* (T. J. H. Clark, ed.), Adis Press, Auckland, pp. 103–120.

Compton, M. M., and Cidlowski, J. A., 1987, Identification of a glucocorticoid-induced nuclease in thymocytes: A potential "lysis gene" product, *J. Biol. Chem.* **262:**8288–8292.

Culpepper, J. A., and Lee, F., 1985, Regulation of IL-3 expression by glucocorticoids in cloned murine T lymphocytes, *J. Immunol.* **135:**3191–3197.

Cupps, T. R., and Fauci, A. S., 1982, Corticosteroid-mediated immunoregulation in man, *Immunol. Rev.* **65:**133–155.

Cupps, T. R., Gerrard, T. L., Falkoff, R. J. M., Whalen, G., and Fauci, A. S., 1985, Effects of *in vitro* corticosteroids on B cell activation, proliferation, and differentiation, *J. Clin. Invest.* **75:**754–761.

Cuturi, M. C., Murphy, M., Costa-Giomi, M. P., Weinmann, R., Perussia, B., and Trinchieri, G., 1987, Independent regulation of tumor necrosis factor and lymphotoxin production by human peripheral blood lymphocytes, *J. Exp. Med.* **165:**1581–1594.

Danon, A., and Assouline, G., 1978, Inhibition of prostaglandin biosynthesis by corticosteroids requires RNA and protein synthesis, *Nature* **273:**552–554.

Darnell, J., Lodish, H., and Baltimore, D., 1986, *Molecular Cell Biology*, Scientific American Books, Inc., New York.

Derendorf, H., Mollman, H., Rohdewald, P., Rehder, J., and Schmidt, E. W., 1985, Kinetics of methylprednisone and its hemisuccinate ester, *Clin. Pharmacol. Ther.* **37:**502–507.

Dinarello, C. A., 1988, Biology of interleukin 1, *FASEB J.* **2:**108–115.

DiRosa, M., Flower, R. J., Hirata, F., Parente, L., and Russo-Marie, F., 1984, Anti-phospholipase proteins, nomenclature announcement, *Prostaglandins* **28:**441–442.

Dumble, L. J., MacDonald, M., Kincaid-Smith, P., and Clunie, G. J. A., 1981, Correlation between ADCC resistance to *in vitro* steroid and renal graft failure, *Transplant Proc.* **13:**1569–1571.

Dupont, E., Schandene, L., Denys, C., and Wybran, J., 1986, Differential *in vitro* actions of cyclosporin, methylprednisolone, and 6-mercaptopurine: Implications for drugs' influence on lymphocyte activation mechanisms, *Clin. Immunol. Immunopathol.* **40:**422–428.

English, J., Dunne, M., and Marks, V., 1983, Diurnal variation in prednisolone kinetics, *Clin. Pharmacol. Ther.* **33:**381–385.

Flower, R. J., and Blackwell, G. J., 1979, Anti-inflammatory steroids induce biosynthesis of a phospholipase inhibitor which inhibits prostaglandin synthesis, *Nature* **278:**456–457.

Flower, R. J., Wood, J. N., and Parente, L., 1984, Macrocortin and the mechanism of action of the glucocorticoids, *Adv. Inflammation Res.* **7:**61–70.

Galili, U., 1983, Glucocorticoid induced cytolysis of human normal and malignant lymphocytes, *J. Steroid Biochem.* **19:**483–490.

Gambertoglio, J. G., Amend, W. J., and Benet, L. Z., 1980, Pharmacokinetics and bioavailability of prednisone and prednisolone in healthy volunteers and patients: A review, *J. Pharmacokinet. Biopharm.* **8:**1–52.

Gerrard, T. L., Cupps, T. R., Jurgensen, C. H., and Fauci, A. S., 1984, Increased expression of HLA-DR antigens in hydrocortisone-treated monocytes, *Cell. Immunol.* **84:**311–316.

Gillis, S., Crabtree, G. R., and Smith, K. A., 1979, Glucocorticoid-induced inhibition of T cell growth factor production. I. The effect on mitogen-induced lymphocyte proliferation, *J. Immunol.* **123:**1624–1631.

Girard, M. T., Hjaltadottir, S., Fejes-Toth, A. N., and Guyre, P. M., 1987, Glucocorticoids enhance the γ-interferon augmentation of human monocyte immunoglobulin G Fc receptor expression, *J. Immunol.* **138:**3235–3241.

Goppelt-Struebe, M., Wolter, D., and Resch, K., 1989, Glucocorticoids inhibit prostaglandin synthesis not only at the level of phospholipase A2 but also at the level of cyclo-oxygenase/PGE isomerase, *Br. J. Pharmacol.* **98:**1287–1295.

Goulding, N. J., Godolphin, J. L., Sharland, P. R., Peers, S. H., Sampson, M., Maddison, P. J., and Flower, R. J., 1990, Anti-inflammatory lipocortin 1 production by peripheral blood leucocytes in response to hydrocortisone, *Lancet* **335:**1416–1418.

Groyer, A., Schweizer-Groyer, G., Cadepond, F., Mariller, M., and Baulieu, E.-E., 1987, Antiglucocorticosteroid effects suggest why steroid hormone is required for receptors to bind DNA *in vivo* but not *in vitro*, *Nature* **328:**624–626.

Hanson, R. G., Peters, M. G., and Hoofnagle, J. H., 1986, Effects of immunosuppressive therapy with prednisolone on B and T lymphocyte function in patients with chronic type B hepatitis, *Hepatology* **6**:173–179.

Hayes, M., Alam, A. F. M. S., Bruckner, F. E., Doherty, S. M., Myles, A., English, J., Marks, V., and Chakraborty, J., 1983, Plasma prednisolone studies in rheumatic patients, *Ann. Rheum. Dis.* **42**:151–154.

Haynes, R. C., and Murad, F., 1985, Adrenocorticotrophic hormone: Adrenocorticosteroids and their synthetic analogs: Inhibitors of adrenocortical steroid biosynthesis, in: *Goodman and Gilman's The Pharmacological Basis of Therapeutics*, 7th Ed. (A. G. Gilman, L. S. Goodman, T. W. Rall, and F. Murad, eds.), MacMillan Publishing Company, New York, pp. 1459–1490.

Hermanns, P., Verbruggen, G., Veys, E. M., Vansteenkiste, M., Delanghe, J., and Mielants, H., 1982, Influence of low dose corticosteroid administration on the lymphocytes subpopulations, *J. Rheumatol.* **9**:648–649.

Hirata, F., 1984, Roles of lipomodulin, a phospholipase inhibitory protein in immunoregulation, *Adv. Inflammation Res.* **7**:71–78.

Hirata, F., Stracke, M. L., and Schiffmann, E., 1987, Regulation of prostaglandin formation by glucocorticoids and their second messenger, lipocortins, *J. Steroid. Biochem.* **27**:1053–1056.

Huang, K-S., Wallner, B. P., Mattaliano, R. J., Tizard, R., Burne, C., Frey, A., Hession, C., McGray, P., Sinclair, L. K., Chow, E. P., Browning, J. L., Ramachandran, K. L., Tang, J., Smart, J. E., and Pepinsky, R. B., 1986, Two human 35 Kd inhibitors of phospholipase A$_2$ are related to substrates of pp60 V-src and of the epidermal growth factor receptor/kinase, *Cell* **46**:191–199.

Hulme, B., James, V. H., and Rault, R., 1975, Absorption of enteric and non-enteric coated prednisolone tablets, *Br. J. Clin. Pharmacol.* **2**:317–320.

Isacke, C. M., Lindberg, R. A., and Hunter, T., 1989, Synthesis of p36 and p35 is increased when U-937 cells differentiate in culture but expression is not inducible by glucocorticoids, *Mol. Cell Biol.* **9**:232–240.

Kelso, A., and Munck, A., 1984, Glucocorticoid inhibition of lymphokine secretion by alloreactive T lymphocyte clones, *J. Immunol.* **133**:784–791.

Kern, J. A., Lamb, R. J., Reed, J. C., Daniele, R. P., and Nowell, P. C., 1988, Dexamethasone inhibition of interleukin 1 beta production by human monocytes: Posttranscriptional mechanisms, *J. Clin. Invest.* **81**:237–244.

Knudsen, P. J., Dinarello, C. A., and Strom, T. B., 1987, Glucocorticoids inhibit transcriptional and post-transcriptional expression of interleukin 1 in U937 cells, *J. Immunol.* **139**:4129–4134.

Lan, N. C., Karin, M., Nguyen, T., Weisz, A., Birnbaum, M. J., Eberhardt, N. L., and Baxter, J. D., 1984, Mechanisms of glucocorticoid hormone action, *J. Steroid. Biochem.* **20**:77–88.

Langhoff, E., and Ladefoged, J., 1983, Relative immunosuppressive potency of various corticosteroids measured *in vitro*, *Eur. J. Clin. Pharmacol.* **25**:459–462.

Langhoff, E., Ladefoged, J., Jakobsen, B. K., Platz, P., Ryder, L. P., Svegaard, A., and Thaysen, J. H., 1986, Recipient lymphocyte sensitivity to methylprednisolone affects cadaver kidney graft survival, *Lancet* **1**:1296–1297.

Laue, L., Kawai, S., Brandon, D. D., Brightwell, D., Barnes, K., Knazek, R. A., Loriaux, D. L., and Chrousos, G. P., 1988, Receptor-mediated effects of glucocorticoids on inflammation: Enhancement of the inflammatory response with a glucocorticoid antagonist, *J. Steroid. Biochem.* **29**:591–598.

Lee, S. W., Tsou, A-P., Chan, H., Thomas, J., Petrie, K., Eugui, E. M., and Allison, A. C., 1988, Glucocorticoids selectively inhibit the transcription of the interleukin 1β gene and decrease the stability of interleukin 1β mRNA, *Proc. Natl. Acad. Sci. USA* **85**:1204–1208.

Leszczynski, D., Ferry, B., Schellekens, H., v.d. Meide, P. H., and Hayry, P., 1986, Antagonistic effects of γ interferon and steroids on tissue antigenicity, *J. Exp. Med.* **164**:1470–1477.

Lew, W., Oppenheim, J. J., and Matsushima, K., 1988, Analysis of the suppression of IL-1α and IL-1β production in human peripheral blood mononuclear adherent cells by a glucocorticoid hormone, *J. Immunol.* **140**:1895–1902.

Lowenthal, R. M., and Jestrimski, K. W., 1986, Corticosteroid drugs: Their role in oncological practice, *Med. J. Aust.* **144**:81–85.

Manyak, C. L., Tse, H., Fischer, P., Coker, L., Sigal, N. H., and Koo, G. C., 1988, Regulation of class II MHC molecules on human endothelial cells: Effects of IFN and dexamethasone, *J. Immunol.* **140**:3817–3821.

Meffin, P. J., Brooks, P. M., and Sallustio, B. C., 1984a, Alterations in prednisolone disposition as a result of time of administration, gender and dose, *Br. J. Clin. Pharmac.* **17**:395–404.

Meffin, P. J., Wing, L. M. H., Sallustio, B. C., and Brooks, P. M., 1984b, Alterations in prednisolone disposition as a result of oral contraceptive use and dose, *Br. J. Clin. Pharmac.* **17**:655–664.

Meikle, A. W., and Tyler, F. H., 1977, Potency and duration of action of glucocorticoids: Effects of hydrocortisone, prednisone and dexamethasone on human pituitary–adrenal function, *Am. J. Med.* **63**:200–207.

Meikle, A. W., Weed, J. A., and Tyler, F. H., 1975, Kinetics and interconversion of prednisolone and prednisone studied with new radioimmunoassays, *J. Clin. Endocrinol. Metab.* **41**:717–721.

Miele, L., Cordella-Meile, E., Facchiano, A., and Mukherjee, A. B., 1988, Novel anti-inflammatory peptides from the region of highest similarity between uteroglobin and lipocortin I, *Nature* **335**:726–730.

Miksicek, R., Borgmeyer, U., and Nowock, J., 1987, Interaction of the TGGCA-binding protein with upstream sequences is required for efficient transcription of mouse mammary tumor virus, *EMBO J.* **6**:1355–1360.

Munck, A., Mendel, D. B., Smith, L. I., and Orti, E., 1990, Glucocorticoid receptors and action, *Am. Rev. Respir. Dis.* **141**:S2–S10.

Muraguchi, A., Kehrl, J. H., Butler, J. L., and Fauci, A. S., 1983, Sequential requirements for cell cycle progression on resting human B cells following activation by anti-Ig, *J. Immunol.* **132**:176–180.

Nair, M. P. N., and Schwartz, S. A., 1984, Immunomodulatory effects of corticosteroids on natural killer and antibody-dependent cellular cytotoxic activities of human lymphocytes, *J. Immunol.* **132**:2876–2882.

Needs, C. J., Smith, M., Boutagy, J., Donovan, S., Cosh, D., McCredie, M., and Brooks, P. M., 1988, Comparison of methylprednisolone (1g IV) with prednisolone (1 g orally) in rheumatoid arthritis: A pharmacokinetic and clinical study, *J. Rheumatol.* **15**:224–228.

Nichols, T., Nugent, C. A., and Tyler, F. H., 1965, Diurnal variation in suppression of adrenal function by glucocorticoids, *J. Clin. Endocrinol.* **25**:343–349.

Nowock, J., Borgmeyer, U., Puschel, A. W., Rupp, R. A. W., and Sippel, A. E., 1985, The TGGCA protein binds to the MMTV–LTR, the adenovirus origin of replication, and the BK virus enhancer, *Nucleic Acids Res.* **13**:2045–2061.

Oates, J. A., FitzGerald, G. A., Branch, R. A., Jackson, E. K., Knapp, H. R., and Roberts, L. J., 1988, Clinical implications of prostaglandin and thromboxane A_2 formation, *N. Engl. J. Med.* **319**:689–698.

Onsrud, M., and Thorsby, E., 1981, Influence of *in vitro* hydrocortisone on some human blood lymphocyte subpopulations. I. Effect on natural killer cell activity, *Scand. J. Immunol.* **13**:573–579.

Oppenheim, J. J., and Potter, M., 1984, Immunity and inflammation, in: *Cellular Functions in Immunity and Inflammation* (J. J. Oppenheim, D. L. Rosenstreich, and M. Potter, eds.), Elsevier, New York, pp. 1–28.

Paavonen, T., 1985, Glucocorticoids enhance the *in vitro* Ig synthesis of pokeweed mitogen-stimulated human B cells by inhibiting the suppressive effect of T8+ T cells, *Scand. J. Immunol.* **21**:63–71.

Parrillo, J. E., and Fauci, A. S., 1978, Comparison of effector cells in human spontaneous cellular cytotoxicity and antibody-dependent cellular cytotoxicity: Differential sensitivity of effector cells to *in vivo* and *in vitro* corticosteroids, *Scand. J. Immunol.* **8**:99–107.

Peers, S. H., and Flower, R. J., 1990, The role of lipocortin in corticosteroid actions, *Am. Rev. Resp. Dis.* **141**:S18–S21.

Picard, D., and Yamamoto, K. R., 1987, Two signals mediate hormone-dependent nuclear localization of the glucocorticoid receptor, *EMBO J.* **6**:3333–3340.

Piccolella, E., Vismara, D., Lombardi, G., Guerritore, D., Piantelli, M., and Ranelletti, F. O., 1985, Effect of glucocorticoids on the development of suppressive activity in human lymphocyte response to a polysaccharide purified from *Candida albicans*, *J. Immunol.* **134**:1166–1171.

Pickup, M. E., 1979, Clinical pharmacokinetics of prednisone and prednisolone, *Clin. Pharmacokinet.* **4**:111–128.

Pinkston, P., Saltini, C., Muller-Quernheim, J., and Crystal, R. G., 1987, Corticosteroid therapy suppresses spontaneous interleukin 2 release and spontaneous proliferation of lung T lymphocytes of patients with active pulmonary sarcoidosis, *J. Immunol.* **139**:755–760.

Ponta, H., Kennedy, N., Skroch, P., Hynes, N. E., and Groner, B., 1985, Hormonal response region in the mouse mammary tumor virus long terminal repeat can be dissociated from the proviral promoter and has enhancer properties, *Proc. Natl. Acad. Sci. USA* **82**:1020–1024.

Raz, A., Wyche, A., and Needleman, P., 1989, Temporal and pharmacological division of fibroblast cyclo-oxygenase expression into transcriptional and translational phases, *Proc. Natl. Acad. Sci. USA* **86**:1657–1661.

Reeback, J. S., Chakraborty, J., English, J., Gibson, T., and Marks, V., 1980, Plasma steroid levels after intra-articular injection of prednisolone acetate in patients with rheumatoid arthritis, *Ann. Rheum. Dis.* **39**:22–24.

Reed, J. C., Abidi, A. H., Alpers, J. D., Hoover, R. G., Robb, R. J., and Nowell, P. C., 1986, Effect of cyclosporin A and dexamethasone on interleukin 2 receptor gene expression, *J. Immunol.* **137**:150–154.

Richter, M. B., Woo, P., Panayi, G. S., Trull, A., Unger, A., and Shepherd, P., 1983, The effects of intravenous pulse methylprednisolone on immunological and inflammatory processes in ankylosing spondylitis, *Clin. Exp. Immunol.* **53**:51–59.

Russo-Marie, F., 1990, Glucocorticoid control of eicosanoid synthesis, *Semin. Nephrol.* **10**:421–429.

Scheidereit, C., Krauter, P., von der Ahe, D., Janich, S., Rabenau, O., Cato, A. C. B., Suske, G., Westphal, H. M., and Beato, M., 1986, Mechanism of gene regulation by steroid hormones, *J. Steroid. Biochem.* **24**:19–24.

Seale, J. P., and Compton, M. R., 1986, Side-effects of corticosteroid agents, *Med. J. Aust.* **144**:139–142.

Shen, L., Guyre, P. M., Ball, E. D., and Fanger, M. W., 1986, Glucocorticoid enhances gamma interferon effects on human monocyte antigen expression and ADCC. *Clin. Exp. Immunol.* **65**:387–395.

Silverman, E. D., Myones, B. L., and Miller, J. J., 1984, Lymphocyte subpopulation alterations induced by intravenous megadose pulse methylprednisolone, *J. Rheumatol.* **11**:287–290.

Smith, M. D., Bertouch, J. V., Smith, A. M., Weatherall, M., Ahern, M. J., Brooks, P. M., and Roberts-Thomson, P. J., 1988, The clinical and immunological effects of pulse methylprednisolone therapy in rheumatoid arthritis. 1. Clinical effects. *J. Rheumatol.* **15**:229–232.

Snyder, D. S., and Unanue, E. R., 1982, Corticosteroids inhibit murine macrophage Ia expression and interleukin 1 production, *J. Immunol.* **129**:1803–1805.

Thomas, T. P. L., 1984, The complications of systemic corticosteroid therapy in the elderly. A retrospective study, *Gerontology* **30**:60–65.

Uribe, M., Schalm, S. W., Summerskill, W. H., and Go, V. L., 1978, Oral prednisone for chronic active liver disease: Dose responses and bioavailability studies, *Gut* **19**:1131–1135.

Walker, K. B., Potter, J. M., and House, A. K., 1985, Variable inhibition of mitogen-induced blastogenesis in human lymphocytes by prednisolone *in vitro*, *Transplant. Proc.* **17**:1676–1678.

Walker, K. B., Potter, J. M., and House, A. K., 1987, Interleukin 2 synthesis in the presence of steroids: A model of steroid resistance, *Clin. Exp. Immunol.* **68**:162–167.

Wallner, B. P., Mattaliano, R. J., Hession, C., Cate, R. L., Tizard, R., Sinclair, L. K., Foeller, C., Chow, E. P., Browning, J. L., Ramachandran, K. L., and Pepinsky, R. B., 1986, Cloning and expression of human lipocortin, a phospholipase A_2 inhibitor with potential anti-inflammatory activity, *Nature* **320**:77–80.

Wilkinson, J. R. W., Crea, A. E. G., Clark, T. J. H., and Lee, T. H., 1989, Identification and characterisation of a monocyte-derived neutrophil-activating factor in corticosteroid-resistant bronchial asthma, *J. Clin. Invest.* **84**:1930–1941.

Williams, T. W., and Granger, G. A., 1969, Lymphocyte *in vitro* cytotoxicity: Correlation of derepression with release of lymphotoxin from human lymphocytes, *J. Immunol.* **103**:170–178.

Wyllie, A. H., Poznansky, M. C., and Gordon, A. C. H., 1986, Glucocorticoid-resistant asthma: Evidence for a defect in mononuclear cells, in: *Asthma. Clinical Pharmacology and Therapeutic Progress* (A. B. Kay, ed.), Blackwell Scientific Publications, Oxford, pp. 306–314.

Chapter 9

MODE OF ACTION OF THIOPURINES

Azathioprine and 6-Mercaptopurine

Jean-François Bach

1. INTRODUCTION

The thiopurines used as immunosuppressive agents are analogues of hypoxanthine, described by Elion *et al.* (1951), manufactured by Burroughs Wellcome. (For reviews, see Elion, 1972; Bach and Strom, 1985.) They depress antibody production and delayed hypersensitivity reactions in many species, including man. They are effective in preventing rejection of transplanted organs, as described by Elion (1972). Their toxicity is moderate and consists mainly of bone marrow aplasia and hepatitis.

Azathioprine (Imuran) acts in the form of thioinosinic acid, one of its metabolites. This metabolite is formed after transformation into 6-mercaptopurine under the action of the enzyme hypoxanthine-guanine-phosphoribosyl-transferase (HGPRT). Contradictory findings have been published concerning the relative immunosuppressive effects of azathioprine and 6-mercaptopurine, both of which are apparently active at the same order of molarity. Azathioprine is broken down into thiouric acid by xanthine oxidase, hence the necessity to reduce its dosage in patients who are simultaneously receiving allopurinol for the treatment of gout.

2. BIOCHEMICAL EFFECTS OF AZATHIOPRINE

The biochemical effects of azathioprine remain ambiguous (Elion, 1972; Bach and Strom, 1985). Azathioprine inhibits the synthesis of DNA, RNA, and proteins, but the mode of action of this inhibition at the molecular level is still unclear. Many hypotheses have been proposed: interference with coenzymes, incorporation into nucleic acids, enzyme inhibition, alteration of purine interconversions, and inhibition of *de novo* synthesis of purines. These effects explain the inhibition of nucleic acid synthesis for which the drug was

Jean-François Bach • Immunology Clinic, Necker Hospital, 75743 Paris Cedex 15, France.

Immunopharmacology in Autoimmune Diseases and Transplantation, edited by Hans Erik Rugstad *et al.* Plenum Press, New York, 1992.

designed but are probably also compatible with many other subcellular actions that could be at the basis of the immunosuppressive effect of the drug. The role of the imidazole nucleus (associated with hypoxanthine) is probably not negligible. Fixation of the drug to some amino acid residues of the membrane proteins could also be involved. Finally, although it is still hypothetical and poorly defined, there may be interference with adenosine metabolism. It should be noted that two congenital immune deficiencies are due to enzyme anomalies at the key site of purine metabolism. One involves adenosine deaminase, which deaminates adenosine to transform it into inosine, and the other nucleotidylphosphorylase, which transforms hypoxanthine into inosine. These various effects could explain the inhibition of rosette formation by quiescent lymphocytes within 60 min, an observation that is difficult to explain by inhibition of DNA synthesis.

3. TARGET CELLS

The target cell also remains rather elusive. Despite two isolated reports, one of depressed monocyte production in the rat (Van Furth et al., 1975) and the other of inhibited monocyte function in delayed hypersensitivity reactions in the guinea pig (Philipps and Zweiman, 1973), macrophages and monocytes do not seem to represent a significant target. Controversy is greater, however, with regard to B and T lymphocytes. A selective effect on B cells has also been suggested (Dimitriu and Fauci, 1978). In fact, most of the experimental data obtained both in animals and in man favor a preferential effect on T lymphocytes. In the first place, T-cell-dependent responses are more affected, especially at low doses, than those of B cells alone, both in vivo and in vitro. The particularly favorable effect of azathioprine in organ transplantation explains its wide use in this field, which represents its major clinical application.

Even in the case of antibody production, it has been shown that responses directed against thymus-dependent antigens, which require the presence of T helper cells, are more sensitive to the effect of azathioprine than those directed against the thymus-independent antigens. All these arguments strongly suggest that azathioprine acts preferentially on T cells. In the normal mouse, azathioprine acts on a population of spleen cells that forms rosettes with sheep erythrocytes. Rosette formation is inhibited by azathioprine and the cells lose their sensitivity to azathioprine after adult thymectomy (Bach et al., 1971; Bach and Dardenne, 1972a). In addition, T-cell-dependent immune responses, such as delayed hypersensitivity, graft rejection, or the in vitro mixed-lymphocyte reaction, are particularly sensitive to the action of the drug. Its effect on antibody production is much less clear. At usual doses (below 3 mg/kg per day in man), antibody production is not depressed, and suppression of antibody production is attained only with doses of the order of 5 to 6 mg/kg per day in man (Swanson and Schwartz, 1967). In animals, thiopurines selectively attenuate thymus-dependent experimental autoimmune diseases such as allergic thyroiditis. In the latter model, it is in fact interesting to note that antithyroglobulin antibody production is not depressed by thiopurines, whereas delayed hypersensitivity is suppressed (Spiegelberg and Miescher, 1963). Last, azathioprine given alone preferentially favors viral infections and among bacterial infections, tuberculosis and salmonellosis, all infections in which the immune defenses consist essentially of T cells. This preferential action on T lymphocytes, observed at the moderate doses used in clinical practice, is rapidly reversible since the T cells are inactivated rather than eliminated. This explains why the profile of B- and T-cell markers is generally not modified in patients treated by azathioprine.

B cells are probably also affected in some cases (Dimitriu and Fauci, 1978; Duclos et al., 1982). In the in vitro antibody response, although only thymus-dependent responses are inhibited, it seems that azathioprine selectively affects the sensitivity of B cells to signals produced by helper T cells (Duclos et al., 1982). In addition, there are multiple subfamilies of T cells, and much remains to be done before it can be determined what category of T cells is preferentially affected in any given situation. A number of reports indicate that suppressor T cells can be inhibited in certain cases (Medzihradsky et al., 1981), which complicates the problem even more since the immunosuppressive effect is then abrogated or even inversed. In such a case, 6-mercaptopurine, given before the antigen, clearly increases antibody production.

4. MODE OF ACTION

The mode of action at the cellular level is difficult to determine. The presumed biochemical effect on nucleic acid synthesis would a priori lead one to think that aza-thioprine acts on lymphocyte proliferation and thus on lymphocyte differentiation after antigen recognition. However, as we have seen, it is doubtful that there is only one biochemical mechanism of action, and many cellular effects can result from modification of purine metabolism and inhibition of lymphocyte proliferation.

The fact that the best time for giving a single dose of azathioprine is 24 hr after antigen administration has been considered a particularly important argument in favor of an antiproliferative effect of thiopurines (Berenbaum, 1967). Nevertheless, this argument is not indubitable, and it can also be conceived that azathioprine acts on the early stages of the immune response. This suggestion is corroborated by the fact that thiopurine activity is rapidly reversible in vivo, on the one hand because it is rapidly metabolized and on the other because its cellular action is not durable. If antigen recognition occurs throughout the first two to three days after antigen administration (as suggested by the loss of immunosuppressive effect of antibodies administered passively until day 3), it can be assumed that if thiopurines act on antigen recognition, they are not active if they are given before the antigen. Their activity has disappeared while the antigen is still recognized and will induce a near-normal immune response. The fact that azathioprine inhibits in vitro the mixed-lymphocyte culture only when it is added during the first 24 hr of culture, when no DNA synthesis is yet detectable, favors this interpretation (Bach and Bach, 1972). Many experimental data are also compatible with a nondirectly antiproliferative action, such as the rapid effect of azathioprine within 60 min on the expression of some membrane differentiation antigens, before any antiproliferative effect could have taken place. Even if it is still difficult and premature to propose a precise mode of action to replace the classic antiproliferative effect, it should be stressed that these "unconventional" effects of azathioprine contribute to a large degree to the mode of action of the drug at the level of lymphocyte membranes (perhaps by altering antigen recognition), an action that is essentially reversible. This would explain why lymphocytes sampled in patients receiving azathioprine have nearly normal immune compe-tence in vitro when cultures are performed in azathioprine-free medium. Azathioprine retains its immunosuppressive effect only if lymphocytes are maintained in its presence. At the end of treatment, the immunosuppressive effect is lost. We have seen that there may be a period of several days of azathioprine-induced immune hyperreactivity due to inhibition of T suppressor cells.

5. CLINICAL USES

The clinical use of azathioprine is well-defined. Effective dosage is between 2 and 3 mg/kg per day orally. A form for intravenous use is also available. Individual metabolism of the drug can be followed by rosette inhibition (Bach and Dardenne, 1971, 1972a) or high-pressure liquid chromatography. Pharmacokinetics remain unchanged in patients with renal failure (Bach and Dardenne, 1971). Conversely, immunosuppressive activity is quite depressed in cases of major liver failure (Bach and Dardenne, 1972b). Side effects are generally moderate, especially if patients are carefully followed up. They include leukopenia (rarely evolving to bone marrow aplasia) and intracellular bacterial or viral infections (in particular, hepatitis linked to immunosuppression induced by the product rather than a direct toxic effect).

6. IMMUNOLOGICAL FOLLOW-UP

The immunological follow-up of patients receiving azathioprine remains difficult. The notions discussed above, in particular the lack of direct depletion of a lymphocyte subpopulation and the reversibility of the inhibition of lymphocyte functions, explain why usual methods (markers and functions) are not applicable. In fact, these tests generally give normal results in patients receiving azathioprine alone, even at the 3 mg/kg dose, which is known to be immunosuppressive given the fact that it allows survival of a grafted kidney.

REFERENCES

Bach, M. A., and Bach, J. F., 1972, Activities of immunosuppressive agents in vitro. II. Differing timing of azathioprine and methotrexate in inhibition and stimulation of mixed lymphocyte reaction, Clin. Exp. Immunol. 11:89.

Bach, J. F., and Dardenne, M., 1971, The metabolism of azathioprine in renal failure, Transplantation 12:253.

Bach, J. F., and Dardenne, M., 1972a, Antigen recognition by T lymphocytes. I. Thymus and bone marrow dependence of rosette-forming cells in normal and neonatally thymectomized mice, Cell Immunol. 3:1–10.

Bach, J. F., and Dardenne, M., 1972b, Serum immunosuppressive activity of azathioprine in normal subjects and patients with liver diseases, Proc. Roy. Soc. Med. 65:260.

Bach, J. F., and Strom, T. B., 1985, Thiopurines, in: The Mode of Action of Immunosuppressive Agents (J. F. Bach and T. B. Strom, eds.), Elsevier, North Holland, 105–174.

Bach, J. F., Dardenne, M., and Davies, A. J. S., 1971, Early effect of adult thymectomy, Nature New Biol. 231:110.

Berenbaum, M. C., 1967, Immunosuppressive agents and the cellular kinetics of the immune response, in: Immunity, Cancer and Chemotherapy (E. Mihic, ed.), Academic Press, New York, p. 217.

Dimitriu, A., and Fauci, A. S., 1978, Activation of human B lymphocytes. XI. Differential effect of azathioprine on B lymphocytes and lymphocyte subpopulations regulating B cell function, J. Immunol. 121:2335.

Duclos, H., Maillot, M. C., and Galanaud, P., 1982, Differential effects of azathioprine on T cells regulating murine B cell function, Immunology 46:595.

Elion, G. B., 1972, Significance of azathioprine metabolites, Proc. Roy. Soc. Med. 65:257.

Elion, G. B., Hitchings, G. H., and Vanderwerff, H., 1951, Antagonists of nucleic acid derivatives. VI. Purines, J. Biol. Chem. 192:505.

Medzihradsky, J. L., Hollowell, R. P., and Elion, G. B., 1981, Differential inhibition by azathioprine and 6-MP of specific suppressor T cell generation in mice, J. Immunopharmacol. 3:1.

Philipps, S. M., and Zweiman, B., 1973, Mechanisms in the suppression of delayed hypersensitivity in the guinea pig by 6-mercaptopurine, J. Exp. Med. 137:1494–1510.

Spiegelberg, H. L., and Miescher, P. A., 1963, The effect of 6-MP and amenopterin on experimental immune thyroiditis in guinea pigs, J. Exp. Med. 118:869.

Swanson, H. A., and Schwartz, R. S., 1967, Immunosuppressive therapy. The relation between clinical response and immunologic competence, N. Engl. J. Med. 227:163.

Van Furth, R., Gassman, A. E., and Diesselhof-Den-Dulk, M. M. C., 1975, The effect of azathioprine (Imuran) on the cell cycle of promonocytes and the production of monocytes in the bone marrow, J. Exp. Med. 141:531.

Chapter 10

PHARMACOLOGY AND GENERAL THERAPEUTIC PRINCIPLES OF METHOTREXATE

Liv Endresen

1. INTRODUCTION

Methotrexate (MTX) is one of the most potent and widely used drugs in cancer chemotherapy. Synthesized in 1949 by Seeger and co-workers, it soon proved to be strikingly effective in childhood leukemia (Farber *et al.*, 1956). The immunosuppressive potential of MTX was also recognized in the 1950s; this aspect received minimal attention, however, in the following years. During the 1970s, its primary use in nonneoplastic disease was for the treatment of psoriasis, based on the assumption that the rapidly proliferating epidermal cells in psoriatic lesions are more sensitive to the effects of MTX than normal epidermal cells.

With the growing interest in the use of immunosuppressants in rheumatoid arthritis (RA), MTX received increasing attention in the late 1970s and early 1980s as a third-line agent. At present, it has proved to be effective in low doses in various inflammatory connective tissue disorders as well as for the prevention and treatment of graft versus host disease.

During the exploitation of the use of this drug in cancer chemotherapy, doses have been escalated dramatically up to megadoses of more than 30 g/m². This approach has been possible due to reversal of toxicity by the antidote leucovorin (folinic acid, citrovorum factor). Doses for autoimmune disease, however, are usually in the range of 7–15 mg per week, given as a single dose or in two to three divided doses 12 hr apart. Regimens for prevention of graft versus host disease also consist of low-dose MTX, which may be 15 mg/m² as a starting dose, then tapered to 10 mg/m² per week and continued at this level for a period of about 2 to 14 weeks.

Even though a major part of the pharmacological studies have addressed the use of MTX

Liv Endresen • Institute of Clinical Biochemistry, The National Hospital, University of Oslo, 0027 Oslo 1, Norway.

Immunopharmacology in Autoimmune Diseases and Transplantation, edited by Hans Erik Rugstad *et al.* Plenum Press, New York, 1992.

in chemotherapy, several issues recently studied concerning its clinical and biochemical pharmacology provide insight regarding its use as an immunomodulating drug. This chapter, therefore, focuses on various pharmacological aspects concluded from studies on its use in chemotherapy as well as from its use as an immunosuppressive agent.

2. BIOCHEMICAL PHARMACOLOGY

Methotrexate (4-amino-N^{10}-methyl pteroylglutamic acid) belongs to a class of tight-binding enzyme inhibitors called antifolates. Structurally, it is similar to the naturally occurring folic acid (Fig. 1). An important feature of folate biochemistry is that the folates, to be active in enzymatic reactions, must be reduced to their tetrahydro forms. The enzyme dihydrofolate reductase (DHFR), which is responsible for this conversion, is potently inhibited by MTX.

Another important feature of the folate cofactors is the glutamyl residue. Although circulating folates have a single terminal glutamate, most intracellular folates are converted to polyglutamates, which contain two to five glutamate groups linked by gamma-peptide bonds. This chain elongation also takes place with MTX intracellularly, resulting in

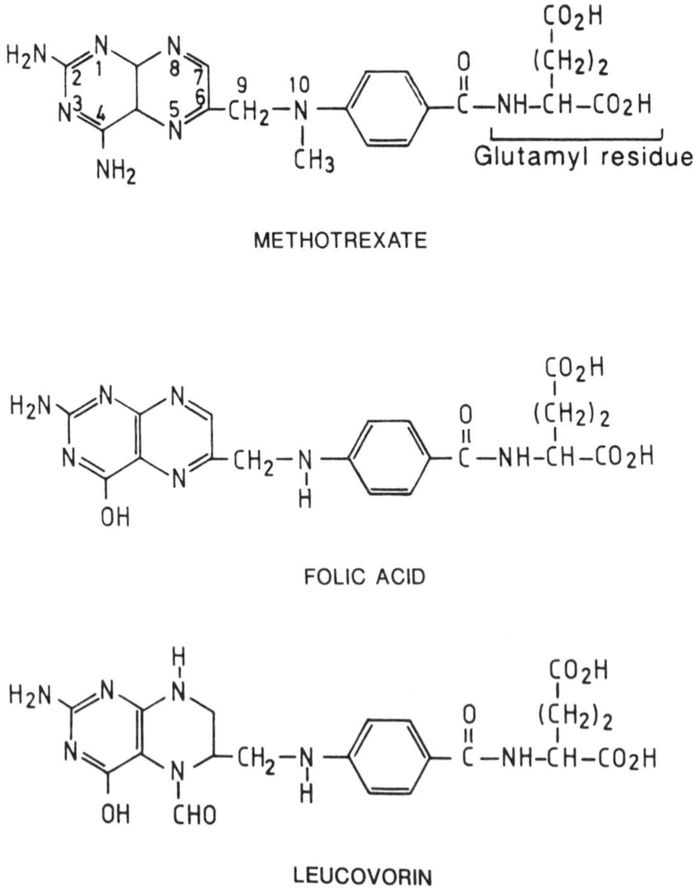

FIGURE 10.1. Structural formulas of methotrexate, folic acid, and leucovorin.

derivatives with markedly altered properties both with regard to their potency of inhibition as well as their cellular retention. Aspects of MTX biochemical pharmacology have been reviewed by several authors (Jolivet *et al.*, 1983; Chabner *et al.*, 1985; Goldman and Matherly, 1985; Evans *et al.*, 1986; Schweitzer *et al.*, 1990).

2.1. Transport across Cellular Membranes

The transport of MTX into cells and its efflux from cells is one critical element of its action. These phenomena have been extensively studied and reviewed by Goldman and associates (Goldman and Matherly, 1985).

At relatively low extracellular concentrations, transport is mediated via an active carrier system for reduced folate cofactors. It is a high-affinity, low-capacity system; thus influx is saturable. Once the carrier system is saturated, the only way additional drug can accumulate within cells is by transport via some other low-affinity process or by passive diffusion. At high plasma concentrations ($> 2 \times 10^{-5}$ M), this or these mechanisms account for the major fraction of drug that enters the cells. There is considerable evidence for distinct entry and efflux mechanisms; thus, in contrast to the influx, the efflux process seems to be nonsaturable.

2.2. Enzyme Inhibition

The reduced folate cofactors are essential in the synthesis of both purines and thymidylic acid, which in turn are essential for DNA synthesis and cell division (Fig. 2). The formation of thymidylate, which is catalyzed by the enzyme thymidylate synthetase (TS), involves both a one-carbon transfer and oxidation of reduced folate to dihydrofolate (FH_2). The actual serum concentration of MTX that is necessary for inhibition of DNA synthesis seems to be tissue-specific; thus, inhibition of DNA synthesis in mouse bone marrow was achieved with plasma concentrations above 1×10^{-8} M, whereas for intestinal epithelium the concentration necessary for a similar inhibition was 5×10^{-9} M (Chabner and Young, 1973). Pinedo and Chabner (1977) have shown that at MTX concentrations above 1×10^{-8} M, the cytotoxic effects are a function of both drug concentration and duration of exposure.

Because of the critical need for thymidylate in DNA synthesis, cells contain an excess of DHFR activity in order to ensure sufficient stores of reduced folate, even during maximal anabolic activity. During normal TS activity the cellular levels of FH_2 are therefore extremely low. Sufficient levels of MTX must be attained intracellularly for a complete DHFR inhibition. Even with approximately 95% of the enzyme inhibited, normal cellular functions will be maintained. In addition, appreciable levels of FH_2 will accumulate because of the inhibition of DHFR; consequently, this natural substrate will compete with MTX for binding sites on the enzyme (for reviews, see Jolivet *et al.*, 1983; Goldman and Matherly, 1985).

2.3. Metabolism to Polyglutamate Forms

The pharmacological implications of the conversion of MTX to polyglutamate derivatives have been reviewed by Chabner *et al.* (1985). The derivatives are formed intracellularly by the enzyme folyl polyglutamyl synthetase and up to five additional glutamate residues are added to the MTX molecule (Fig. 2). These forms are not readily transported across cellular

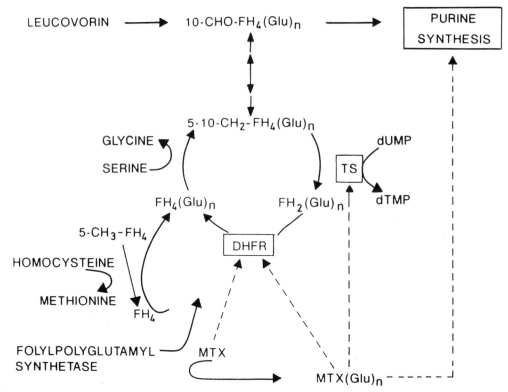

FIGURE 10.2. Major enzymatic reactions involving methotrexate and folates as cosubstrates. MTX, methotrexate; DHFR, dihydrofolate reductase; TS, thymidylate synthetase; FH_2, dihydrofolate; FH_4, tetrahydrofolate; Glu, glutamyl; dTMP, thymidylate; dUMP, dioxyuridylate. Broken lines indicate enzyme inhibition. Modified from Jolivet *et al.* (1983).

membranes. Although they bind with the same affinity as MTX to DHFR, they seem to dissociate at a significantly slower rate. Of further importance are data indicating that the higher polyglutamates possess markedly increased affinity for several other folate-dependent enzymes such as TS. During the initial high cellular levels shortly after dosing, the parent drug is the compound responsible for DHFR inhibition. The free drug that is not bound to DHFR will then be available for conversion to increasingly longer polyglutamate derivatives. Since these are substantially irreversible inhibitors of DHFR, these compounds will gradually displace the other forms of the drug from binding sites on the enzyme. Consequently, a very sustained action is achieved, even as the extracellular concentrations fall. Of particular interest for the cytotoxic effect of MTX in cancer is evidence that polyglutamation seems to be more abundant in rapidly as opposed to more slowly proliferating cells. Moreover, polyglutamation seems to occur to a greater extent in sensitive malignant cells than in normal tissues such as the bone marrow and intestinal mucosa (see Section 4).

2.4. 7-Hydroxy-Methotrexate

In addition to the conversion to polyglutamate forms, metabolic conversion to 7-OH-MTX has been reported in patients receiving high- as well as low-dose MTX. This conversion mainly takes place in the liver. The derivative has been shown to have a markedly longer half-life relative to MTX, resulting in plasma levels that by far will exceed those of MTX during the elimination phase. It will compete both with MTX and natural reduced folates for the membrane carrier and may thus affect the intracellular levels of MTX.

Due to a weak inhibitory action on DHFR *in vitro*, 7-OH-MTX was for a long time regarded to be virtually inactive *in vivo*. However, recent evidence indicates that the 7-OH-metabolite shares the same mechanisms for cellular uptake and metabolism to polygluta-mates as the parent drug, and may therefore interact with MTX at the cellular level if present in sufficient levels (Slørdal, 1987). In patients receiving low-dose MTX, significant levels of 7-OH-MTX were detected in plasma with peak levels of $0.9–1.1 \times 10^{-6}$ M compared with 1.4×10^{-6} M for MTX. Moreover, analysis of bone marrow cells obtained 24 hr after MTX showed that the majority of the drug present was the 7-OH-metabolite, with concentrations that were at least fivefold those of 7-OH-MTX and threefold those of MTX in plasma (Sonneveld *et al.*, 1986).

Because of its low aqueous solubility and thereby the possibility of renal intratubular precipitation, 7-OH-MTX has been recognized as a putative contributor to the renal toxicity seen in some patients receiving high-dose therapy. In addition, the metabolite may compete with the parent drug for active renal tubular secretion and thereby modulate MTX elimination. The extensive metabolism of MTX to the 7-OH-metabolite in the liver has been suggested to have importance for the relatively low incidence of severe hepatotoxicity with high-dose MTX therapy, because of the relatively lower cytotoxicity of the metabolite (Evans *et al.*, 1986).

2.5. Effects on Folate Stores

Certain side effects of prolonged low-dose MTX therapy may mimic symptoms of folate deficiency, including gastrointestinal intolerance and hepatic, neurologic, as well as hematological toxicity. A significant (50–80%) decrease in folate levels of hepatic and red cells (Kamen *et al.*, 1981; Kremer *et al.*, 1986) as well as of lymphocytes (Ellegaard *et al.*, 1972; Morgan *et al.*, 1987) occurs in patients following chronic low-dose treatment for several years. In rhesus monkeys treated with weekly low-dose intramuscular MTX for one year, a 90% loss of total folate in brain tissue was observed (Winick *et al.*, 1987). Whereas serum folate levels primarily reflect a recent dietary intake, folate in red cells and particularly in lymphocytes has a longer half-life.

The precise mechanisms by which MTX induces cellular folate depletion is incompletely understood, although studies of psoriatic patients gave no indication of an impaired intestinal absorption of folic acid during MTX treatment (Duhra *et al.*, 1988). Concomitant with the loss of intracellular folate, an accumulation of MTX as polyglutamates in erythrocytes and liver has been noted (Kamen *et al.*, 1981; Kremer *et al.*, 1986). This indicates that MTX and folate may compete for mechanisms of storage such as polyglutamation enzymes. Although the decrease in hepatic folate occurred in the absence of marked elevations of liver enzymes or abnormal liver histology, it is conceivable that a rapid deficiency of folate cofactors may develop during metabolic stress, when folate requirements for cellular repair or replication are increased.

Administration of daily folate supplement during 24 weeks was shown to ameliorate toxicity in RA patients during low-dose MTX therapy. Although not evaluated in long-term studies, the supplementation did not seem to affect efficacy parameters (Morgan *et al.*, 1990). Leucovorin was also evaluated in an attempt to ameliorate nausea, which is a rather common side effect in RA patients on continuous low-dose MTX (Tishler et al., 1988). Although the nausea disappeared, a significant aggravation of the disease activity occurred. Furthermore, Kremer et al. (1986) demonstrated a repletion of hepatic folate together with a decrease in hepatic levels of MTX in patients on concomitant oral leucovorin. Thus, several authors have linked the antifolate effects of MTX to its action and toxic effects (Kremer et al., 1986; Morgan et al., 1987; Tishler et al., 1988). The fact that the two antifolates, MTX and sulfasalazine, both are effective in RA has also been taken as support of this hypothesis.

Refsum and co-workers (1989) have recently shown that fasting plasma homocysteine levels are significantly and transiently raised following administration of low-dose MTX to psoriatic patients. The metabolic fate of homocysteine is closely linked to the metabolism of reduced folates (Fig. 2). Increased basal levels of plasma homocysteine and low serum folate were observed in patients with malignant disorders and psoriasis prior to therapy (Refsum, 1990). It has been suggested, therefore, that homocysteine may be a sensitive and responsive parameter of antifolate drug treatment. Also, in RA patients, high homocysteine levels prior to MTX therapy seemed to be predictive of final MTX toxicity as determined after six months of treatment. Thus, the basal levels of fasting homocysteine may be an early warning of adverse effects during long-term MTX treatment (Refsum, 1990).

3. PHARMACOKINETICS

The bioavailability of oral MTX is dose-dependent and unpredictable (Evans et al., 1986). Even at relatively low doses (< 15 mg/m^2), which previously were believed to be completely absorbed, the bioavailability is incomplete and highly variable among patients. A fractional bioavailability in the range of 0.32–0.98 has been reported in psoriatic patients (Hendel, 1985) and a mean of 0.70 in RA patients (Herman et al., 1989).

After a single oral dose of MTX, peak serum levels are reached within approximately 2 hr. The 1-hr serum levels of MTX in children with juvenile RA on long-term oral MTX were in the range from 6×10^{-8} to 1×10^{-6} M (Wallace et al., 1989). Sinnett et al. (1989) detected peak levels of $3–7 \times 10^{-7}$ M in adult RA patients following a single 7.5-mg oral dose. The ratio of synovial fluid to serum concentration has been reported to be approximately 1.0 in RA patients 4 to 24 hr after a dose of 10 mg/m^2 (Herman et al., 1989).

After conventional doses there are considerable differences in tissue accumulation of the drug, with high levels in liver, kidney, and intestines; lower concentrations in connective tissues and skin; and very low levels in the brain and spinal cord. Steady state concentrations of MTX in psoriatic patients on long-term therapy were reported to be 8×10^{-8} M in erythrocytes, 5×10^{-7} in epidermis, and 1.8×10^{-6} in liver (Hendel, 1985). Polyglutamates constituted 75% of the MTX and were significantly correlated to the steady state MTX levels in erythrocytes from children with acute lymphoblastic leukemia on weekly low-dose therapy. The polyglutamate concentrations remained constant throughout the life span of the erythrocyte; mature red blood cells did not form significant amounts, however (Schrøder and Fogh, 1988).

Following the initial distribution phase, drug disappearance from plasma has two components, the first with a half life of about 2–4 hr while the last ranges from about 8–15 hr (Evans et al., 1986). Renal excretion is the major route of elimination, constituting more than 80% of total body elimination. At low ($< 5 \times 10^{-7}$ M) concentrations, MTX clearance exceeds the glomerular filtration rate, indicating that tubular secretion is involved. There is also evidence of an active tubular reabsorption at low concentrations of the drug. In addition, MTX is to some degree excreted by the biles.

In plasma, 30–50% of the drug is protein-bound, primarily to albumin (Herman *et al.*, 1989). The 7-OH-metabolite, however, is extensively bound to albumin (> 90%). Slørdal (1987) demonstrated a significant reduction in bound fraction of 7-OH-MTX in hypo-albuminemic patients compared with healthy volunteers (82 vs. 90%). A two- to threefold increase in unbound 7-OH-MTX was also observed during coincubation of serum with MTX, at 10^{-6} M, and naproxen or ketoprofen, both at therapeutic drug concentrations. Whereas indomethacin, naproxen, and ketoprofen apparently do not significantly alter the binding of MTX to serum albumin, the possibility exists that the more extensively bound 7-OH-metabolite may be displaced from serum albumin (Slørdal, 1987).

4. THEORIES FOR A SELECTIVE ACTION ON NEOPLASTIC CELLS

Because of the rapid cellular proliferation, the two normal tissues that are the primary sites of MTX toxicity are the gastrointestinal epithelium and the bone marrow. During MTX treatment, DNA synthesis in both of these tissues is potently inhibited; however, it recovers rapidly as the extracellular concentrations of MTX fall below 10^{-8} M. Thus, it seems probable that neither of these tissues accumulates appreciable levels of polyglutamates. Indeed, it has been found that bone marrow cells and gastrointestinal cells possess markedly decreased capacity to form polyglutamates compared to susceptible tumors (Fry *et al.*, 1983; Fabre *et al.*, 1984). The capacity to accumulate sufficient levels of polyglutamates therefore seems to be a *major* determinant for cellular sensitivity to MTX. Moreover, evidence suggests that intracellular folates derived from leucovorin during rescue therapy can compete with MTX, but not MTX polyglutamates, at the level of DHFR and produce a net displacement of MTX from the enzyme (Matherly *et al.*, 1983, 1986). Thus, the differential action of MTX in cancer appears to be closely associated with the ability of various tumors to metabolize the drug to the long-acting polyglutamate forms and to the possibility of a selective rescue by leucovorin of sensitive normal tissues following high-dose MTX treatment.

5. MECHANISMS OF CELLULAR RESISTANCE. HIGH-DOSE THERAPY

Resistance to MTX is a frequent clinical phenomenon in cancer patients who are exposed repeatedly or continuously to the drug. The mechanisms behind an acquired cellular resistance against MTX have been extensively studied (for reviews, see Schimke, 1986; Jolivet, 1987). Although of obvious importance in cancer chemotherapy, the implications of these resistance mechanisms remain uncertain with respect to the decreased clinical response seen in some patients receiving long-term therapy for nonneoplastic disease. One aspect is the consensus that normal cells do not develop a significant degree of resistance.

The basic mechanisms that have been recognized in the cellular resistance to MTX are (1) decreased membrane transport, (2) alteration in affinity of MTX for DHFR, (3) decreased capacity for polyglutamation, and (4) increased cellular levels of DHFR. Defective transport of MTX was believed early on to be the most important mechanism of resistance, based on *in vitro* data from human leukemic cells in which the uptake of MTX at lower concentrations (2×10^{-7} M) was found to vary more than fivefold among different patients tested and to correlate with clinical response (Kessel *et al.*, 1968). Altered affinity of DHFR for MTX has been identified in a study on patients with acute myelogenous leukemia (Dedhar *et al.*, 1985). Recent evidence indicates that impaired intracellular polyglutamation of MTX may be one of the more prevalent clinical mechanisms of resistance (Curt *et al.*,

1985). Also, increases in DHFR activity have been identified as a clinically important resistance mechanism. Large increases of DHFR levels can be produced experimentally in tumor cells by long-term exposure to stepwise increasing concentrations of MTX. Such cells overproduce DHFR as a result of gene amplification (Schimke, 1986). Being under a constant selective pressure, the rare cells with increased copy numbers that code for DHFR will be selected, and in experimental conditions cells have been isolated that contain DHFR levels 400 times above the normal. A number of human tumors have been found to have MTX resistance related to gene-amplified DHFR levels (Curt et al., 1983; Horns et al., 1984; Trent et al., 1984; Carman et al., 1984). In tumor cells isolated from patients, the level of amplification of DHFR is of a much lower order compared with that demonstrated following resistance developed in vitro. In a study of Rodenhuis et al., (1987), RA patients who received long-term MTX therapy were shown to have markedly elevated DHFR levels in their peripheral blood mononuclear cells compared with those of a control group of RA patients receiving slow-acting drugs. The elevated DHFR levels did not result in a marked reduction of in vitro sensitivity to MTX. Considering the very low DHFR activity that is sufficient for normal folate metabolism, it is conceivable, however, that even a moderate elevation of enzyme activity may result in modified response to the drug.

To overcome resistance due to, for example, limited active transport or increased enzyme levels, increasingly higher doses of MTX have been used in cancer chemotherapy over the last years. Leucovorin or some other form of "rescue" is required for MTX dosages in excess of 100 mg/m². The rationale for high-dose treatment with leucovorin rescue within 42–48 hr is production of prolonged plasma levels of the drug in order to expose more cells during DNA synthesis, to obtain increased levels of polyglutamates, and to increase the therapeutic index through a reversal of MTX action in normal cells while creating a sustained effect in the malignant cells. Therapeutic guidelines for monitoring serum MTX have been developed to minimize risk of toxicity and optimize therapeutic efficacy of high-dose regimens in cancer therapy (Evans et al., 1986). So far, there is only limited experience with high-dose MTX therapy in autoimmune disease. Shiroky et al. (1988) reported on promising results in a preliminary study of five patients with intractable RA who were administered four courses of 500 mg/m² MTX with leucovorin rescue. Of particular interest were the clinical responses in four of the patients who had previously been treated with a low-dose regimen without success.

6. EFFECTS ON THE IMMUNE SYSTEM

Despite the extensive knowledge of the effect of MTX on cancer cells, the mode of action in autoimmune diseases and graft versus host (GvH) disease remains largely unknown.

Several authors have inferred that MTX predominantly has anti-inflammatory properties. This is based, for example, on the fact that the drug has a relatively rapid onset of action in RA, especially with regard to the improvement of synovitis and the decreased sedimentation rate, as well as a rapid exacerbation of the disease following withdrawal of the drug (Anderson et al., 1985; Weinblatt et al., 1985; Segal et al., 1990).

In active psoriatic lesions, the intraepidermal accumulation of polymorphonuclear leukocytes (PMNs) is a classical feature. In RA a similar accumulation of leukocytes in synovial fluid is believed to contribute to the destruction of synovial and joint tissues. Low-dose MTX treatment has been shown to reduce the in vitro chemotactic response of PMNs obtained from patients treated for psoriasis (Walsdorfer et al., 1983; Ternowitz and Herlin,

1985), as well as for Ra (O'Callaghan *et al.*, 1988), thus supporting the theory of an anti-inflammatory effect of MTX. The chemotactic depression was seen within the first 24 hr after MTX and persisted for a few days following the dose of MTX. The PMN has negligible amounts of DHFR. Thus, there may be a more direct enzyme inhibition on one of the other enzymes by polyglutamate derivatives of MTX. Although there have been no reports on MTX polyglutamates in mature PMNs, they have been identified in myeloid precursor cells following 24-hr incubation with the drug (Koizumi *et al.*, 1985). The mature PMN has a circulation half-life of only approximately 7 hr, whereas the inhibition of chemotaxis in psoriatic patients lasted for at least four days. Thus, there is evidence in support of an effect of MTX predominantly on PMNs resident in or newly released from the bone marrow.

There are also data available indicating that leukotriene-B_4-induced intraepidermal accumulation of PMNs in patients with psoriasis was substantially inhibited *in vivo* (Van de Kerkhof *et al.*, 1985; Lammers *et al.*, 1987). Furthermore, the inhibition correlated with the clinical efficacy of MTX (Lammers *et al.*, 1987).

A few recent studies give support to the hypothesis that MTX at low concentrations selectively inhibits the proliferation of suppressor T cells (O'Meara *et al.*, 1985; Gibbons and Lucas, 1989; Olsen and Murray, 1989). In a murine acute GvH model, MTX (in a dose comparable to the regimen used in human RA) inhibited the proliferation of donor as well as of host suppressor T cells (Lyt2$^+$Ts cells) (Gibbons and Lucas, 1989). In contrast, the helper function of donor L3T4$^+$ cells was not inhibited, indicating that MTX may be a useful modulator of pathologic suppressor cell function. The protection from the symptoms of acute GvH reaction of immunosuppression lasted for at least three weeks after withdrawal of the drug.

Studies of the immune function in patients treated with low-dose MTX have revealed marked decreases in cellular IgM-rheumatoid factor synthesis within the first 24 hr of treatment (Olsen *et al.*, 1987) and also a decrease in plasma levels. These findings may indicate that MTX affects those cells that are most activated, including those producing rheumatoid factor. In other studies, however, no correlation was observed between changes in serum rheumatoid factor and clinical improvement (Anderson *et al.*, 1985). Decreases in total IgM production have also been noted in RA patients on MTX treatment (Olsen *et al.*, 1987) as well as decreases in serum Ig levels (Anderson *et al.*, 1985; Weinblatt *et al.*, 1986). In accordance with these findings, studies using [^{3}H]deoxyuridine as a proliferation marker have demonstrated inhibition of proliferation of mononuclear cells from peripheral blood of RA patients treated with MTX (Olsen and Murray, 1989). In contrast, several previous studies, using [^{3}H]thymidine as a marker of DNA synthesis, failed to demonstrate a similar effect on mitogen-induced proliferation (Anderson *et al.*, 1985; Weinblatt *et al.*, 1985; Olsen *et al.*, 1987). There is reason to believe that [^{3}H]thymidine is not an optimal marker in such pulse-labeling studies, since the block produced by MTX on TS may make cells more avid for thymidine uptake.

Patients with RA are reported to have abnormalities in mononuclear cell subset proportions and numbers. This involves decreased total lymphocyte and T-cell counts, increased percentage of monocytes as well as increased T helper/T suppressor cell ratio (Kotzin *et al.*, 1983; Anderson *et al.*, 1985). Neither short-term (13 weeks) nor long-term (6 months) therapy of RA patients with low-dose MTX was associated with significant changes in ratios of helper to suppressor T cells (Anderson *et al.*, 1985; Duby *et al.*, 1985; Olsen *et al.*, 1987), although a modest increase in percentage of T cells and a similar decrease of monocytes were noted (Anderson *et al.*, 1985). Recently, it has been shown that MTX inhibits Il-1β activity *in vitro*. MTX competed with the binding of Il-1β to its receptor on T cells, and a "rescue" phenomenon could be observed when leucovorin was added to the cultures (for review, see Segal *et al.*, 1990). Although an inhibition of Il-1 activity may be of importance, it is at present not possible to draw definite conclusions whether the reported effects of MTX on the immune system are related to its efficacy in autoimmune disease or whether its action is predominantly immunosuppressive or inflammatory. It is likely, however, that some phenomena described are dose-dependent. At relatively high concentrations (i.e., above 10^{-7} M), the effect on the immune response is probably nonselective, that is, all lymphocyte populations are suppressed, whereas at very low concentrations, in the range of 10^{-8}–10^{-11} M, a selective effect of MTX on subpopulations may be achieved (Matheson *et al.*, 1985; O'Meara *et al.*, 1985). These concentrations are significantly lower than those previously considered to be of clinical relevance.

7. SIDE EFFECTS AND TOXICITY

Patients on long-term low-dose MTX therapy commonly experience side effects. Alarcòn *et al.* (1989) studied the prognostic factors that influence the probability of continuing MTX therapy in 152 RA patients and reported that occurrence of toxic effects was the major factor limiting long-term treatment. The probability of developing a major or minor toxic event was especially high during the first year of treatment. The overall probability of remaining on MTX was about 50% at six years. Common side effects include infections, nausea, vomiting, anorexia, diarrhea, stomatitis, and hematologic effects (leukopenia, anemia, and thrombocytopenia, all of which are usually reversible). The more rare side effects include hepatotoxicity, nephrotoxicity, and pulmonary toxicity (acute pneumonitis), which may be serious. Other side effects that have been reported are central nervous system effects, including fatigue, headache, diplopia, dysphoria, and weight loss (for review, see Tugwell *et al.*, 1989; Furst, 1990). There is an obvious need for long-term follow-up studies of long-term MTX therapy to establish more clearly the risk of developing *serious* toxic effects, as well as to assess the relative benefit of such therapy compared with other therapeutic approaches (for a recent discussion on this topic, see Furst, 1990; Willkens, 1990).

8. CONCLUSION

The increasing insights about the action of MTX at the biochemical level seem to raise several interesting questions with regard to the use of this drug as an immunomodulating agent. For example, subpopulations of immunocompetent cells may possess differential capacity of polyglutamation; this in turn may have implications for the mode and duration of action of the drug.

It seems reasonable to conclude that as long as the clinical pharmacology of MTX in immunotherapy remains elusive, the basis for its use must be empirical. However, with a broader understanding of its exact mechanisms of action in autoimmune and GvH disease, more rational approaches with regard to doses and dose schedules, as well as methods to limit toxic effects, may be developed.

REFERENCES

Alarcòn, G. S., Tracey, I. C., and Blackburn, W. D., Jr., 1989, Methotrexate in rheumatoid arthritis. Toxic effects as the major factor in limiting long-term treatment, *Arthritis Rheum.* 32:671–676.

Anderson, P. A., West, S. G., O'Dell, J. R., Via, C. S., Claypool, R. G., and Kotzin, B. L., 1985, Weekly pulse methotrexate in rheumatoid arthritis. Clinical and immunological effects in a randomized double-blind study, *Ann. Intern. Med.* **103:** 489–496.

Carman, M. D., Schornagel, J. H., Rivest, R. S., Srimatkandada, S. Portlock, C. S., Duffy, T., and Bertino, J. R., 1984, Resistance to methotrexate due to gene amplification in a patient with acute leukemia, *J. Clin. Oncol.* **2:**16–20.

Chabner, B. A., and Young, R. C., 1973, Threshold methotrexate concentration for in vivo inhibition of DNA synthesis in normal and tumorous target tissues, *J. Clin. Invest.* **52:**1804–1811.

Chabner, B. A., Allegra, C. J., Curt, G. A., Clendeninn, N. J., Baram, J., Koizumi, S., Drake, J. C., and Jolivet, J., 1985, Polyglutamation of methotrexate. Is methotrexate a prodrug? Prespectives, *J. Clin. Invest.* **76:**907–912.

Curt, G. A., Carney, D. N., Cowan, K. H., Jolivet, J., Bailey, B. D., Drake, J. C., Kao-Shan, C. S., Minna, J. D., and Chabner, B. A., 1983, Unstable methotrexate resistance in a human small-cell carcinoma associated with double minute chromosomes, *N. Engl. J. Med.* **308:**199–202.

Curt, G. A., Jolivet, J., Carney, D. N., Bailey, B. D., Drake, J. C., Clendeninn, N. J., and Chabner, B. A., 1985, Determinants of the sensitivity of human small-cell lung cancer cell lines to methotrexate, *J. Clin. Invest.* **76:**1323–1329.

Dedhar, S., Hartley, D., Fitz-Gibbons, D., Phillips, G., and Goldie, J. H., 1985, Heterogeneity in the specific activity and methotrexate sensitivity of dihydrofolate reductase from blast cells of acute myelogenous leukemia patients, *J. Clin. Oncol.* **3:**1545–1552.

Duby, S., Karsh, J., Prchal, J. F., Whitehead, V. M., and Osterland, C. K., 1985, Measurements of red blood cell methotrexate concentrations and lymphocyte subsets during therapy of rheumatoid arthritis, *Clin. Exp. Rheumatol.* **3:**5–9.

Duhra, P., Hodgson, C., Martin, J. A., and Stablefort, P. J., 1988, Intestinal folate absorption in methotrexate treated psoriatic patients, *Br. J. Dermatol.* **119:**327–332.

Ellegaard, J., Esmann, V., and Henrichson, L., 1972, Deficient folate activity during treatment of psoriasis with methotrexate diagnosed by determination of serine synthesis in lymphocytes, *Br. J. Dermatol.* **87:**248–255.

Evans, W. E., Crom, W. R., and Yalowich, J. R., 1986, Methotrexate, in: *Applied Pharmacokinetics: Principles of Therapeutic Drug Monitoring*, 2nd ed. (W. E. Evans, ed.), Vancouver, Wash., *Applied Therapeutics*, pp. 1009–1056.

Farber, S., Toch, R., Manning Sears, E., and Pinkel, D., 1956, Advances in chemotherapy of cancer in man, in: *Advances in Cancer Research* (J. P. Greenstein and A. Haddow, eds.), Academic Press, New York, pp. 2–73.

Fabre, I., Fabre, G., and Goldman, I. D., 1984, Polyglutamation, an important element in methotrexate cytotoxicity and selectivity in tumor versus murine granulocytic progenitor cells *in vitro*, *Cancer Res.* **44:**3190–3195.

Fry, D. W., Anderson, L. A., Borst, M., and Goldman, I. D., 1983, Analysis of the role of membrane transport and polyglutamation of methotrexate in gut and the Ehrlich tumor *in vivo* as factors in drug sensitivity and selectivity, *Cancer Res.* **43:**1087–1092.

Furst, D. E., 1990, Proposition: Methotrexate should not be the first second-line agent to be used in rheumatoid arthritis if NSAIDs fail, *Semin. Arthritis Rheum.* **20:**69–75.

Gibbons, J. J., Jr., and Lucas, J., 1989, Immunomodulation by low-dose methotrexate. I. Methotrexate selectively inhibits Lyt-2+ cells in murine acute graft-versus-host reactions, *J. Immunol.* **142:**1867–1873.

Goldman, I. D., and Matherly, L. H., 1985, The cellular pharmacology of methotrexate, *Pharmac. Ther.* **28:**77–102.

Hendel, J., 1985, Clinical pharmacokinetics of methotrexate in psoriasis therapy, *Dan. Med. Bull.* **32:**329–337.

Herman, R. A., Veng-Pedersen, P., Hoffman, J., Koehnke, R., and Furst, D. E., 1989, Pharmacokinetics of low-dose methotrexate in rheumatoid arthritis patients, *J. Pharm. Sci.* **78:**165–171.

Horns, R. C., Dower, W. J., and Schimke, R. T., 1984, Gene amplification in a leukemic patient treated with methotrexate, *J. Clin. Oncol.* **2:**2–7.

Jolivet, J., 1987, Biochemical and pharmacologic rationale for high-dose methotrexate, *NCI Monogr.* **5:**61–65.

Jolivet, J., Cowan, K. H., Curt, G. A., Clendeninn, J. J., and Chabner, B. A., 1983, The pharmacology and clinical use of methotrexate, *N. Engl. J. Med.* **309:**1094–1104.

Kamen, B. A., Nylen, B. M., Camitta, B. M., and Bertino, R. J., 1981, Methotrexate accumulation and folate depletion in cells as possible toxicity to the drug, *Br. J. Haematol.* **49:**355–360.

Kessel, D., Hall, T. C., and Roberts, D., 1968, Modes of uptake of methotrexate by normal and leukemic human leukocytes *in vitro* and their relation to drug response, *Cancer Res.* **28:**564–570.

Koizumi, S., Curt, G. A., Fine, R. L., Griffin, J. D., and Chabner, B. A., 1985, Formation of methotrexate polyglutamates in purified myeloid precursor cells from normal human bone marrow, *J. Clin. Invest.* **75:**1008–1014.

Kotzin, B. L., Kansas, G. S., Engleman, E. G., Hoppe, R. T., Kaplan, H. S., and Strober, S., 1983, Changes in T-cell subsets in patients with rheumatoid arthritis treated with total lymphoid irradiation, *Clin. Immunol. Immunopathol.* **27:**250–260.

Kremer, J. M., Galivan, J., Streckfuss, A., and Kamen, B., 1986, Methotrexate metabolism analysis in blood and liver of rheumatoid arthritis patients: Association with hepatic folate deficiency and formation of polyglutamates, *Arthritis Rheum.* **29:**832–835.

Lammers, A. M., Van de Kerkhof, P. C. M., and Mier, P. D., 1987, Reduction of leukotriene B4-induced intraepidermal accumulation of polymorphonuclear leukocytes by methotrexate in psoriasis, *Br. J. Dermatol.* **116:**667–671.

Matherly, L. H., Fry, D. W., and Goldman, I. D., 1983, Role of methotrexate polyglutamation and cellular energy metabolism in inhibition of methotrexate binding to dihydrofolate reductase by 5-formyl-tetrahydrofolate in Ehrlich ascites tumor cells *in vitro*, *Cancer Res.* **43:**2694–2699.

Matherly, L. H., Barlowe, C. K., and Goldman, I. D., 1986, Antifolate polyglutamation and competitive drug displacement at dihydrofolate reductase as important elements in leucovorin rescue in L1210 cells, *Cancer Res.* **46:**588–593.

Matheson, D. S., Green, B. J., Hoar, D. I., Friedman, S. J., and Inoue, M., 1985, Agents which decrease intracellular thymidine pools cause an augmentation in human natural killer activity *in vitro*, *Basic Life Sci.* **31:**461–464.

Morgan, S. L., Baggott, J. E., and Altz-Smith, M., 1987, Folate status of rheumatoid arthritis patients receiving long-term, low-dose methotrexate therapy, *Arthritis Rheum.* **30:**1348–1356.

Morgan, S. L., Baggott, J. E., Vaughn, W. H., Young, P. K., Ausin, J. V., Krumdieck, C. L., and Alarcon, G. C., 1990, The effect of folic acid supplementation on the toxicity of low-dose methotrexate in patients with rheumatoid arthritis, *Arthritis Rheum.* **33**:9–18.

O'Callaghan, J. W., Forrest, M. J., and Brooks, P. M., 1988, Inhibition of neutrophil chemotaxis in methotrexate-treated rheumatoid arthritis patients, *Rheumatol. Int.* **8**:41–45.

Olsen, N. J., and Murray, L. M., 1989, Antiproliferative effects of methotrexate on peripheral blood mononuclear cells, *Arthritis Rheum.* **32**:378–385.

Olsen, N. J., Callahan, L. F., and Pincus, T., 1987, Immunologic studies of rheumatoid arthritis patients treated with methotrexate, *Arthritis Rheum.* **30**:481–488.

O'Meara, A., Headon, B., and Reen, D. J., 1985, Effect of methotrexate on the immune response in children with acute lymphatic leukaemia, *Immunopharmacology* **9**:33–38.

Pinedo, H. M., and Chabner, B. A., 1977, Role of drug concentration, duration of exposure and endogenous metabolites in determining methotrexate cytotoxicity, *Cancer Treat. Rep.* **61**:709–715.

Refsum, H., 1990, Extracellular homocysteine as an indicator of methotrexate pharmacodynamics. Analytical methods, *in vitro* experiments, and clinical studies, thesis, Department of Pharmacology and Toxicology, University of Bergen, Norway.

Refsum, H., Helland, S., and Ueland, P. M., 1989, Fasting plasma homocysteine as a sensitive parameter of antifolate effect: A study of psoriasis patients receiving low-dose methotrexate treatment, *Clin. Pharmacol. Ther.* **46**:510–520.

Rodenhuis, S., Kremer, J. M., and Bertino, J. R., 1987, Increase of dihydrofolate reductase in peripheral blood lymphocytes of rheumatoid arthritis patients treated with low-dose oral methotrexate, *Arthritis Rheum.* **30**:369–374.

Schimke, R. T., 1986, Methotrexate resistance and gene amplification, *Cancer* **57**:1912–1917.

Schrøder, H., and Fogh, K., 1988, Methotrexate and its polyglutamate derivatives in erythrocytes during and after weekly low-dose oral methotrexate therapy of children with acute lymphoblastic leukemia, *Cancer Chemother. Pharmacol.* **21**:145–149.

Schweitzer, B. I., Dicker, A. P., and Bertino, F. R., 1990, Dihydrofolate reductase as a therapeutic target, *FASEB J.* **4**:2441–2452.

Segal, R., Yaron, M., and Tartakovsky, B., 1990, Methotrexate: Mechanism of action in rheumatoid arthritis, *Semin. Arthritis. Rheum.* **20**:190–200.

Shiroky, J., Allegra, C., Inghirami, G., Chabner, B.., Yarboro, C., and Klippel, J. H., 1988, High dose intravenous methotrexate with leucovorin rescue in rheumatoid arthritis, *J. Rheumatol.* **15**:251–255.

Sinnett, M. J., Groff, G. D., Raddatz, D. A., Franck, W. A., and Bertino, J. S., Jr., 1989, Methotrexate pharmacokinetics in patients with rheumatoid arthritis, *J. Rheumatol.* **16**:745–748.

Slørdal, L., 1987, Pharmacokinetics of methotrexate and its major extracellular metabolite 7-hydroxy-methotrexate, thesis, Institute of Medical Biology, University of Tromsø, Norway.

Sonneveld, P., Schultz, F. W., Nooter, K., and Hählen, K., 1986, Pharmacokinetics of methotrexate and 7-hydroxy-methotrexate in plasma and bone marrow of children receiving low-dose oral methotrexate, *Cancer Chemother. Pharmacol.* **18**:111–116.

Ternowitz, T., and Herlin, T., 1985, Neutrophil and monocyte chemotaxis in methotrexate-treated psoriatic patients, *Acta Derm. Venereol.* (Suppl.) (Stockh.) **120**:23–26.

Tishler, M., Caspi, D., Fishel, B., and Yaron, M., 1988, The effects of leucovorin (folinic acid) on methotrexate therapy in rheumatoid arthritis patients, *Arthritis Rheum.* **31**:906–908.

Trent, J. M., Buick, R. N., Olson, S., Horns, R. C., Jr., and Schimke, R. T., 1984, Cytologic evidence for gene amplification in methotrexate-resistant cells obtained from a patient with ovarian adenocarcinoma, *J. Clin. Oncol.* **2**:8–15.

Tugwell, P., Bennett, K., Bell, M., and Gent, M., 1989, Methotrexate in rheumatoid arthritis. Feedback on American College of Physicians Guidelines, *Ann. Int. Med.* **110**:581–583.

Van de Kerkhof, P. C. M., Bauer, F. W., and Maassen-de Grood, R. M., 1985, Methotrexate inhibits leukotriene B$_4$ induced intraepidermal accumulation of polymorphonuclear leukocytes, *Br. J. Dermatol.* **113**:251a–255a.

Wallace, C. A., Bleyer, W. A., Sherry, D. D., Salomonson, D. L., and Wedgewood, R. J., 1989, Toxicity and serum levels of methotrexate in children with juvenile rheumatoid arthritis, *Arthritis Rheum.* **32**:677–681.

Walsdorfer, V., Christophers, E., and Schroeder, J-M., 1983, Methotrexate inhibits polymorphonuclear leukocyte chemotaxis in psoriasis, *J. Dermatol.* **108**:451–456.

Weinblatt, M. E., Coblyn, J. S., Fox, D. A., Fraser, P. A., Holdsworth, D. E., Glass, D. N., and Trentham, D. E., 1985, Efficacy of low-dose methotrexate in rheumatoid arthritis, *N. Engl. J. Med.* **312**:818–822.

Weinblatt, M. E., Coblyn, J. S., Fraser, P. A., Holdsworth, D. E., Falchuk, K. R., and Trentham, D. E., 1986, Long-term prospective study of methotrexate in rheumatoid arthritis (abstract), *Arthritis Rheum.* (Suppl.) **29**:76.

Willkens, R. F., 1990, Resolve: Methotrexate is the drug of choice after NSAIDs in rheumatoid arthritis, *Semin. Arthritis Rheum.* **20**:76–80.

Winick, N. J., Kamen, B. A., Balis, F. M., Holchenberg, J., Lester, C. M., and Poplack, D. G., 1987, Folate and methotrexate polyglutamate tissue levels in rhesus monkeys following chronic low-dose methotrexate, *Cancer Drug Deliv.* **4**:25–31.

Chapter 11

ALKYLATING AGENTS

A. M. Denman, D. J. Denman, and *R. G. Palmer*

1. INTRODUCTION

Since the 1960s, alkylating agents have been used to treat immune disorders. These agents have also been commonly used in bone marrow transplantation in order to condition the graft recipient, thereby reducing the risk of graft rejection. Cyclophosphamide has been included less frequently in immunosuppressive protocols for other transplant procedures, including renal transplantation. Their most controversial role, however, is in the treatment of autoimmune and chronic inflammatory diseases, particularly those resistant to conventional treatment. This chapter considers the place of alkylating agents in the management of immune disorders. Their contribution to transplantation is described in the appropriate literature. Only chlorambucil and cyclophosphamide are considered in detail because, for practical purposes, these are the only alkylating agents regularly used to treat immune disorders.

2. PHARMACOLOGY OF ALKYLATING AGENTS

Alkylating agents are compounds that attach their alkyl groups covalently to other molecules, including phosphate, amino, sulfhydryl, carboxyl, and imidazole groups. In terms of their application to clinical immunosuppression, binding to purine bases in DNA is probably their most important effect, since this interferes with DNA replication in lymphocytes as well as other proliferating cell populations. The 7-nitrogen atom of guanine is particularly susceptible to covalent bonding with alkylating agents and may be the most important target for these drugs (Calabresi and Parks, 1980). The DNA strand is weakened, resulting in damage and breakage. This commonly affects mitosis, meaning that these drugs are ultimately lethal for target cells. In addition, the oxazaphosphorine cyclophosphamide is bifunctional (i.e., it has two active groups), so that it cross-links DNA covalently, thereby preventing strand separation during mitosis. The formulae of chlorambucil and cyclophosphamide are given in Fig. 1.

A. M. Denman, D. J. Denman, and *R. G. Palmer* • Division of Immunological Medicine, Clinical Research Centre, Northwick Park Hospital, Harrow, Middlesex HA1 3UJ, England. *Present address R. G. P.:* Solihull Hospital, Solihull, West Midlands, B91 2JL, England.

Immunopharmacology in Autoimmune Diseases and Transplantation, edited by Hans Erik Rugstad *et al.* Plenum Press, New York, 1992.

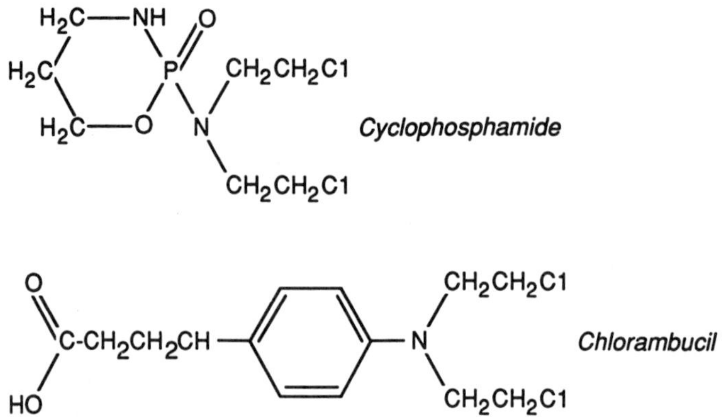

FIGURE 11.1.   Chemical formulae of cyclophosphamide and nlorambucil.

Cyclophosphamide itself has no alkylating activity and is not cytotoxic, but many of its metabolites do have these properties (Hilgard, 1987; Moore *et al.*, 1988) (Fig. 2). It is activated initially by hydroxylation at the 4-carbon atom of the oxazaphosphorine ring by liver microsomes and to some extent in mitochondria. The initial oxidation product is 4-hydroxycyclophosphamide, which is highly cytotoxic but also chemically unstable. The primary metabolite is rapidly deactivated by reversible interaction with endogenous thiols and by enzymatic conversion with aldehyde dehydrogenase to 4-ketocyclophosphamide and carboxyphosphamide. By an alternative metabolic pathway, the oxazaphosphorine ring of 4-hydroxycyclophosphamide opens spontaneously to form aldophosphamide, which, after the release of the 3-carbon unit acrolein, in turn forms phosphoramide mustard. While the latter is the final molecule produced by this pathway, 4-hydroxycyclophosphamide is more cytotoxic than its metabolites, suggesting that it serves as a carrier molecule for transporting phosphoramide mustard across the cell membrane.

3. PHARMACOKINETICS

There is considerable knowledge concerning the distribution and clearance of alkylating agents in other species, but similar information in man is necessarily more limited and has mainly been obtained in cancer patients after the intravenous injection of labeled cyclophosphamide. The value of earlier data was also limited by technical difficulties in measuring the concentration of cyclophosphamide and its metabolites. The situation has been improved by the introduction of better assays, utilizing high-performance liquid chromatography. This method makes use of an isocratic, paired-ion, reversed-phase technique for rapid analysis of these compounds in biological materials (Workman *et al.*, 1987; Moore *et al.*, 1988). Cyclophosphamide is rapidly though incompletely absorbed from the gut, but shows great individual variability (Powis *et al.*, 1987). Maximum serum concentrations of 1–2 g/ml are reached some 2 hr after an oral dose of 2–3 mg/kg. After larger intravenous injections, that is some 25 mg/kg, plasma concentrations may reach 40–50 g/ml.

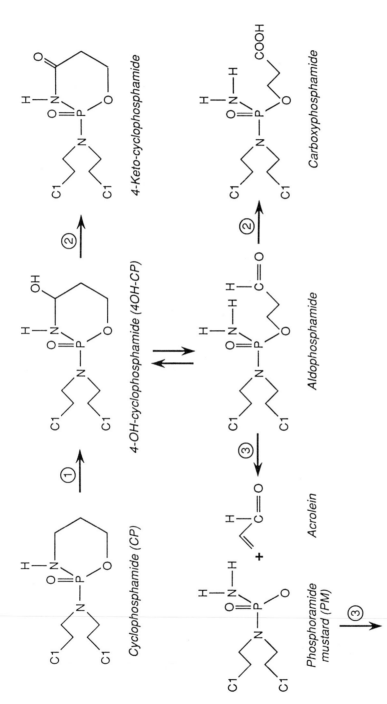

FIGURE 11.2. Metabolism of cyclophosphamide. (1) P-450 microsomal oxidation; (2) aldehyde dehydrogenase; (3) spontaneous degradation.

The mean plasma half-life after intravenous injection is some 5 hr (Moore *et al.*, 1988), but with wide variation reported between 108 and 960 min (Powis *et al.*, 1987). The half-life is probably shorter after oral administration. The plasma half-life of cyclophosphamide's metabolites is considerably shorter. Following the intravenous injection of radiolabeled cyclophosphamide, less than 20% is excreted unchanged in the urine. Urinary excretion of carboxyphosphamide accounts for some 50% and 4-ketocyclophosphamide for a further 15% of the initial compound (Kovarsky, 1983). These excretory rates are slowed some threefold in uremia. The average half-life of intravenously injected cyclophosphamide is some 6–7 hr and that of its metabolites is considerably shorter. It is probable that these values are similar after oral administration. In rhesus monkeys, these metabolites reach the cerebrospinal fluid in concentrations cytotoxic *in vitro* for tumor cells (Arndt *et al.*, 1988).

Of importance to the design of clinical dose regimens, it seems likely that the intravenous administration of cyclophosphamide in high dose induces activating enzymes. This results in a doubling of the speed of clearance of cyclophosphamide itself, but a two- to threefold increase in the plasma concentration of non-protein-bound cytotoxic metabolites (Schuler *et al.*, 1987; Moore *et al.*, 1988). However, clearance may decrease after repeated bolus infusions (Erlichman *et al.*, 1988). As a result of liver enzyme induction, the clearance of simultaneously administered dexamethasone is also accelerated. These observations have implications for clinicians devising dose schedules, particularly those schedules involving a combination of cyclophosphamide and corticosteroids. Moreover, the plasma half-life of cyclophosphamide is itself affected by concomitant treatment with enzyme-inducing drugs. This factor, combined with inaccurate assay techniques, may account for the controversial results reported in clinical pharmacology (Kovarsky, 1983). Physical factors probably alter the pharmacokinetics of the drug; thus, there is a significant decrease in body weight (Powis *et al.*, 1987). It is also possible that cyclophosphamide activation is genetically determined by a genotype controlling the aldehyde dehydrogenase concerned in carboxylation (Hadidi *et al.*, 1988).

Some direct evidence about chlorambucil distribution in cells has been obtained with the newer, high-performance liquid chromatography methods (Bank *et al.*, 1989). The drug accumulated in chronic lymphocytic leukemia cells by simple diffusion and drug-binding to DNA was temperature sensitive, increasing in relation to the period of incubation. Drug–DNA adducts could be directly detected, most of the binding being to purines; both phenyl groups and ethyl chains were found in the adducts.

4. IMMUNOSUPPRESSIVE EFFECTS

4.1. General

The immunosuppressive effects of alkylating agents have been analyzed in great detail because of their clinical applications (Table I). The interpretation of the results is complicated partly by species differences and partly by the great differences in experimental outcome with different experimental conditions. In particular, the timing of drug treatment relative to antigen challenge and the amount of antigen administered influence the nature of the immune response. In general terms, alkylating agents affect immune responses mainly through their antiproliferative effects on lymphocytes and accessory cells, but these drugs also have toxic effects on mature lymphocytes. In humans, primary antibody responses are relatively sensitive to the effects of alkylating agents, whereas established antibody responses are relatively resistant; this point has been amply demonstrated in studies employing novel or recall antigens (Rees and Lockwood, 1982). Conventional, secondary antibody responses are

TABLE I. Principal Immunosuppressive Effects of Alkylating Agents

Population	Effect	Comments
T cells	Numbers reduced	
	Suppressor cells selectively ablated	Dose dependent
	Tolerance induction aided	Dose dependent
B cells	Numbers reduced	Especially sensitive in man
	Primary antibody responses suppressed	
	Secondary antibody responses resistant	
	Autoantibody production suppressed	
Interleukin production	Inhibited in high dose	More information needed
Nonspecific	Monocyte–macrophages inhibited	Dose dependent
	Natural killer function inhibited	Dose dependent

not affected by low-dose cyclophosphamide (0.5–1 mg/kg per day), and are only slightly suppressed by higher doses (2–3 mg/kg per day, either by mouth or by pulse intravenous high doses).

4.2. Suppressor Mechanisms

An intriguing feature of cyclophosphamide's effects in experimental animals is the apparently selective ablation of suppressor cell populations. As in other experimental systems, achieving this effect in a defined immune response depends on the timing of drug administration with respect to antigen challenge and also on antigen dose (Sy *et al.*, 1977). Thus contact sensitivity reactions in mice are increased if drug administration coincides with suppressor cell proliferation in response to supraoptimal doses of contact-sensitizing agents, thereby ablating this lymphocyte population (Turk, 1987).

Paradoxically, high-dose cyclophosphamide induces the production of suppressor cells in the bone marrow (Nikcevich *et al.*, 1987), emphasizing the importance of taking dose-dependent effects into account. Since cytokine production clearly influences the magnitude and duration of immune responses, there is an obvious possibility that cyclophosphamide might act through selective effects on interleukin production. However, it has proved difficult to correlate augmented delayed-type hypersensitivity responses with changes of this kind (Sewell *et al.*, 1987). There are claims that immune responses can be augmented in man by ablating T suppressor cells with cyclophosphamide (Berd and Mastrangelo, 1987, 1988), but the difficulties in characterizing this population in man makes this interpretation of the results very speculative. Nevertheless, these experimental observations may be relevant to clinical situations in which it is desirable to augment immune responses to defined target cells.

4.3. Tolerance

Another experimental effect of possible clinical importance is cyclophosphamide's ability to induce tolerance to defined antigens in appropriate experimental conditions (Aisenberg and Davis, 1968). There are many clinical situations in which it would be desirable to induce tolerance, for example, to drugs or proteins administered to hypersensitive patients or to autoantigens in organ-specific autoimmune diseases. Theoretically, one would wish to try restoring tolerance to autoantigens associated with autoimmune disease by administering such antigens at the time of cyclophosphamide treatment. However, there is little evidence that this ideal can be readily achieved.

4.4. Nonspecific Immunity

The effects of cyclophosphamide on nonspecific immunity are also complicated by the varying and often paradoxical effects observed with different doses. Whereas higher doses inhibit interleukin production (McBride *et al.*, 1987), lower doses may, for example, stimulate the proliferation of natural killer cell precursors (Shen *et al.*, 1988).

4.5. Immunoenhancement

Cytotoxic drugs were first given to patients with severe autoimmune diseases in the expectation that they would be immunosuppressive. However, many studies showed no correlation between responses to standard *in vitro* or *in vivo* immune stimuli and clinical response. Indeed, azathioprine is commonly immunoenhancing. Similarly, in the NZB/NZW murine model of lupus nephritis, cyclophosphamide arrests disease progression and corrects associated abnormalities in the relative numbers of circulating lymphocyte populations (Girard *et al.*, 1990). This concept needs further exploration in clinical practice.

5. IMMUNOSUPPRESSIVE EFFECTS IN CLINICAL USE

It is difficult to assess the immunosuppressive effects of alkylating agents in clinical practice, mainly because of the near impossibility of dissociating changes directly attributable to the drug from those resulting from altered disease activity. Lymphopenia is common and can to some extent be correlated with daily and cumulative dosage. With most oral schedules not exceeding 3 mg/kg per day cyclophosphamide or 0.7 mg/kg per day chlorambucil, primary antibody responses are usually but not invariably suppressed, but secondary antibody responses are little affected. Delayed hypersensitivity-type skin reactions are also little impaired. The effects on *in vitro* lymphocyte transformation responses to standard mitogens and antigens are hard to quantitate because of the need to take challenge doses and cultured cell concentrations into account. While some degree of suppression is common, this is not an invariable finding. There is relatively little information about the effects of high-dose, intravenous pulse injections.

In vitro observations suggested that B cells are more sensitive than T lymphocytes to alkylating agents (Stevenson and Fauci, 1980), but *in vivo* this selectivity does not appear to operate (Clements and Levy, 1977). Judged by phenotypic criteria, T helper cells are especially sensitive (Brinkman *et al.*, 1984), although their numbers recover within 6–12 months of stopping treatment (Feehally *et al.*, 1984). The relevance of these observations to the therapeutic efficacy of immunosuppression in man is uncertain; the pattern of immune responses observed in patients taking azathioprine or chlorambucil is very varied in terms of skin test reactions, antibody titers, and *in vitro* lymphocyte transformation, there being little correlation with clinical response (Swanson and Schwartz, 1967; Denman *et al.*, 1970).

6. CLINICAL INDICATIONS

Several human autoimmune and chronic inflammatory diseases have been treated with chlorambucil or cyclophosphamide (Table II).

TABLE II.   Principal Immunological Disorders Treated with Alkylating Agents

Rheumatoid arthritis	Systemic lupus erythematosus
Vasculitis	Glomerulonephritis
Rheumatoid vasculitis	Nephrotic syndrome
Polyarteritis	Other forms of nephritis
Wegener's granulomatosis	Renal amyloidosis
Behçet's syndrome	Pemphigus
Takayasu's disease	Multiple sclerosis

6.1. Rheumatoid Arthritis

Several groups of patients with rheumatoid arthritis have been treated with cyclo-phosphamide with undoubted benefit. Improvement has been confirmed in controlled trials (American Rheumatism Association, 1970; Williams *et al.*, 1980). The efficacy of low-dose oral cyclophosphamide has also been shown (Currey *et al.*, 1974). Chlorambucil has also been used to treat patients with rheumatoid arthritis (for example, Amor and Mery, 1983; Cannon *et al.*, 1985) with an efficacy comparable to that of cyclophosphamide. There is also an increasing reliance on combined drug regimens in patients with intractable rheumatoid arthritis (Paulus, 1990). In most trials, clinical and laboratory improvement occurs in 40–60% of patients and prolonged remissions of up to 1 year have been observed. More recently, concern over the side effects of alkylating agents has reduced enthusiasm for this class of immunosuppressive drugs, and they have been used more sparingly.

6.2. Vasculitis

Following the first reports by Fauci and colleagues (1979), cyclophosphamide has been used with undoubted success to treat rheumatoid vasculitis (Scott and Bacon, 1984; Fort and Abruzzo, 1988) and polyarteritis (Scott *et al.*, 1982, Gudbjornsson and Hallgren, 1990). It is often used in combination with pulse intravenous methylprednisolone (Euler *et al.*, 1990). However, controlled comparisons with other immunosuppressive regimens are lacking.

6.3. Wegener's Granulomatosis

Wegener's granulomatosis also responds to cyclophosphamide, and it has been claimed that cyclophosphamide treatment for this disease is essential (Fauci *et al.*, 1983). Neverthe-less, some disease features may respond better to intravenous corticosteroids than to cyclophosphamide (Kroneman and Pevzner, 1986). There is suggestive but incompletely controlled evidence that cyclophosphamide prevents disease relapses, particularly if disease activity is monitored by measuring antineutrophil cytoplasmic antibody (ANCA) titers (Cohen-Tervaert *et al.*, 1990).

Not all disease manifestations can be prevented by cyclophosphamide, as shown, for example, in a patient with Wegener's granulomatosis who developed severe subglottic stenosis while receiving this drug (Strange *et al.*, 1990).

6.4. Behçet's Syndrome

Behçet's syndrome, a disorder with a vasculitic basis, is commonly treated with chlorambucil or cyclophosphamide, especially if it is associated with progressive retinal vascular disease, neuro-Behçet's (O'Duffy *et al.*, 1984), or renal disease (Tietjen and Moore, 1990). However, these trials are mainly uncontrolled, and while vigorous immunosuppression has improved the chances of retaining vision in this disorder (Tessler and Jennings, 1990), it is not clear that alkylating agents are indispensable.

6.5. Systemic Lupus Erythematosus

Several uncontrolled studies indicate that relatively steroid-resistant systemic lupus erythematosus (SLE) responds to regular intravenous cyclophosphamide (see, for example, Sessoms and Kovarsky, 1984). There are few reports of controlled trials of cyclophosphamide in comparison with other immunosuppressive drugs; but an impressive study of different therapeutic regimens in lupus nephritis showed that intravenous cyclophosphamide combined with low-dose oral prednisone was superior to other treatment regimens in preventing renal failure (Austin *et al.*, 1986). There is also a preliminary, uncontrolled report that monthly intravenous injections of cyclophosphamide in high dosage induce sustained remissions of steroid-resistant SLE affecting multiple systems and that this improvement is associated with sustained reduction of several circulating T-cell subsets (McCune *et al.*, 1988). Similar success has been reported in seven patients with autoimmune thrombocytopenia complicating SLE who were resistant to conventional corticosteroid treatment (Boumpas *et al.*, 1990).

6.6. Renal Disease

Alkylating agents and other cytotoxic drugs have been used to treat several forms of renal disease with a presumed immunopathological basis; they are most commonly used in patients with renal diseases that have proved resistant to corticosteroids. In children, steroid-resistant nephrotic syndrome often responds to alkylating agents; cyclophosphamide and chlorambucil appear equally beneficial.

In other forms of glomerulonephritis, particularly in adults, alkylating agents have been used from the beginning (Brahm *et al.*, 1988). Chlorambucil has also been reported to arrest the deterioration of idiopathic membranous nephropathy resistant to steroids in adults (Mathieson *et al.*, 1988). Controlled trials proving the efficacy of alkylating agents are especially valuable (Ponticelli *et al.*, 1989).

According to uncontrolled trials, renal amyloidosis responds well to chlorambucil, and the hitherto poor prognosis leaves little choice but to resort to this drug in such patients (Berglund *et al.*, 1987).

6.7. Pemphigus

The severe immune disorder pemphigus responds well to combined treatment with dexamethasone and cyclophosphamide (Pasricha *et al.*, 1988), and four patients with pemphigus resistant to azathioprine treatment also responded to cyclophosphamide (Ahmed and Hombal, 1987).

6.8. Other Immune Disorders

Alkylating agents have been used in other, uncommon immune disorders, with isolated reports of success. Cases include hypoprothrombinemia in a patient with lupus anticoagulant (Simel *et al.*, 1987), colonic pneumatosis intestinalis associated with SLE (Laing, 1988), pure red cell aplasia (Firkin and Maher, 1988), and antibody-mediated polyneuropathy (Pestronk *et al.*, 1988). However, it is difficult to validate their value in rare disorders.

6.9. Multiple Sclerosis

There are several reports of controlled trials claiming that cyclophosphamide reduces the frequency and duration of relapses in multiple sclerosis (Killian *et al.*, 1988; Carter *et al.*, 1988a,b). Furthermore, combined cyclophosphamide and steroid treatment has been reported to reduce the concentrations of basic myelin protein and immunoglobulin G in the cerebrospinal fluid of treated patients (Lamers *et al.*, 1988). This remains a contentious issue, however, and many neurologists maintain that equally good results can be obtained with accepted steroid regimens (Likosky, 1988).

7. MECHANISMS OF ACTION

It is tacitly accepted that the therapeutic benefits of alkylating agents are attributable to their immunosuppressive effects. This is a reasonable conclusion in those diseases where successful treatment is associated with the complete or partial disappearance of autoantibodies likely to account for the immunopathological features. However, there are many inflammatory disorders in which the etiology is less clear; in these situations, immunosuppression may be a secondary and indeed an undesirable consequence of treatment with alkylating agents. The benefits of treatment may be more correctly attributable to the inactivation of rapidly proliferating cell populations that contribute to the inflammation in an immunologically nonspecific manner. There is also the possibility that successful treatment may be dependent on selective immunoenhancement. Even in experimental models of autoimmune disease, it is difficult to discern which immunosuppressive effects are therapeutically decisive. For example, cyclophosphamide prevents the onset of autoimmune phenomena in MRL/1 mice (Shiraki *et al.*, 1984; Jonsson *et al.*, 1988), but suppresses both polyclonal B-cell activation and T helper cell function (Shiraki *et al.*, 1984). In this same murine model, cyclophosphamide also modulates the transcription of the proto-oncogene *c-myb* (Mountz *et al.*, 1985). The possibility that alkylating agents affect immunoproliferation through their selective actions on abnormally expressed growth-regulating genes has scarcely been explored.

8. DOSE SCHEDULE

There are obvious differences in opinion about the manner in which alkylating agents should be administered; contentious points include dose schedules, duration of treatment, and route of administration. In theory, the guiding principles are cumulative experience in specific diseases, the extent of the resulting immunosuppression and the clinical response in individual patients.

There are relatively few immunological diseases in which sufficiently many controlled data have accrued to allow rational decisions based on clinical experience. Rheumatoid arthritis is a possible exception in that it can be adequately treated with cyclophosphamide in an oral dose of 0.75–2 mg/kg per day. In contrast, while lupus nephritis often responds satisfactorily to pulse, high-dose cyclophosphamide, there is little to suggest that treatment schedules employing conventional oral doses of the same drug are unacceptable.

Laboratory tests are of limited value in treating immunological disorders with alkylating agents. Routine hematological and biochemical tests are, of course, essential for reducing the risk of toxicity. Similarly, established immunological methods help to monitor the response of autoimmune disorders to treatment. It is also important to avoid prolonged drug-induced hypogammaglobulinemia. However, assays of immunological function are of little value because the results correlate so poorly with clinical responses. Indeed, total lymphocyte counts provide as good a working guide to the effects of alkylating agents as counts of specific lymphocyte subpopulations or assays of specific immune function. However, even in this context, there is no virtue in achieving lymphopenia for its own sake. The main difficulty is the lack of assays for titrating the effects of immunosuppressive agents on the relevant immunopathological processes, and this situation will continue until these have been better elucidated.

At present, the only reliable guide to the management of these disorders with alkylating agents is the clinical response judged by conventional criteria.

9. SIDE EFFECTS

The alopecia, stomatitis, and gastrointestinal symptoms induced by high, cumulative doses of cyclophosphamide are rarely problems in the low oral (< 2 mg/kg per day) or intravenous (< 15 mg/kg per month) doses used to treat most immune disorders (Table III). Similarly, the cumulative dose of cyclophosphamide in most courses does not exceed 15 g/70 kg. Bladder toxicity, usually presenting as hematuria, is also uncommon with these dose schedules. While it is important to encourage a reasonable fluid intake in the 24 hr following pulse cyclophosphamide (usually < 15 mg/kg per infusion per month), there is no point in using Mesna (sodium 2-mercaptoethanesulfonate) as a routine precaution. Nevertheless, Mesna has virtually eradicated this hazard of high-dose cyclophosphamide treatment (Shaw, 1987; Stillwell and Benson, 1988); however, occasional routine urinalysis for microscopic hematuia is a reasonable precaution.

TABLE III.   Side Effects of Alkylating Agents

Antiproliferative
Alopecia
Bone marrow depression
Gastrointestinal symptoms
Sterility
Toxic
Cystitis
Other
Infections
Mutagenic
Neoplasia
Teratogenesis

9.1. Hematology

Hematological monitoring is routine, and it is advisable to withhold further doses if the blood granulocyte count falls below 2.0×10^6/liter or the platelet count below 80×10^6/liter. Hemoglobin concentrations are more difficult to interpret because of the often concomitant anemia of disease but may be the first indicator of bone marrow depression. It is possible that the bone marrow of patients with connective tissue diseases is abnormally sensitive to cytotoxic drugs. It is noteworthy, too, that granulocyte colony formation is inhibited for prolonged periods after cyclophosphamide treatment (Thomas et al., 1983). Thus while it is usually possible to resume treatment in reduced dosage, the possibility of sudden bone marrow suppression must be kept constantly in mind. It is also important to note that macrocytosis is common in patients on these drugs but is not an indication of either serious bone marrow toxicity or vitamin B_{12} or folic acid deficiency.

9.2. Infections

Intercurrent infections are a cause of concern in these patients, in the form of either unusually severe infections by commonly encountered organisms or opportunistic infections by unusual agents. In a recent study (Bradley et al., 1989), 17 episodes of infection were observed in 201 patient months of cyclophosphamide treatment in Wegener's granulomatosis, and two patients died of pneumonia. The most commonly encountered organisms were Enterobacter, Pseudomonas, and Staphylococcus. However, interpretation is complicated by the age of the patients, since infection was usually encountered in men over 60 years of age, and by concomitant steroid treatment. In rheumatoid arthritis, herpesvirus and fungal infections are the main problem. In our experience at this center, using intensive immunosuppression with various treatment regimens often incorporating cyclophosphamide, intercurrent infection has not been a problem in multiple sclerosis (Mertin et al., 1982), in severe connective tissue diseases (Hollingworth et al., 1982), or in 160 patients with Behçet's syndrome followed over a mean period of ten years. The immunosuppression associated with immunoproliferative diseases itself predisposes to intercurrent infections. Appropriate "immunosuppressive" treatment commonly restores a more normal pattern of immune responses, thereby increasing resistance to infections (Denman, 1982).

9.3. Sterility

Sterility in males is almost inevitable after relatively low doses of chlorambucil or cyclophosphamide. Amenorrhea and sterility in females are less predictable, but may still affect as many as 30% of those at risk (Schilsky et al., 1980). In female patients, serum gonadotropin levels rise significantly after two months of treatment with alkylating agents. Accurate long-term data are less readily available, and the long-term risks in children may be greater than in adults. Experimental studies in animals suggest possible means of protecting the gonads by hormonal manipulation. In mice, ovarian function was protected by concomitant treatment with the synthetic androgen danazol, a drug that limits the development of susceptible ovarian follicles (Budel et al., 1988). In contrast, attempts to protect spermatogenesis in dogs by analogous maneuvers were unsuccessful (Goodpasture et al., 1988). More experimental work of this kind is needed before such techniques can be introduced into clinical practice.

9.4. Neoplasia

The mutagenic effects of alkylating agents impose oncogenic hazards. Isolated instances of malignancy probably induced by these drugs have been commonly reported; for example, diffuse histiocytic lymphoma (Ambrus and Fauci, 1984), Hodgkin's lymphoma (Colburn *et al.*, 1985), acute myeloblastic leukemia (Ohyashiki *et al.*, 1986), and Kaposi's sarcoma (Erban and Sokas, 1988) have all been reported in patients with Wegener's granulomatosis treated with cyclophosphamide. Some of the cancers recorded in patients receiving alkylating agents have been so unusual that there is little doubt that the drugs were responsible. For example, leiomyosarcoma of the bladder has been reported in two patients receiving cyclophosphamide for lupus nephritis (Thrasher *et al.*, 1990).

The chances of developing neoplasms in given age groups and any underlying diseases also have to be taken into account in calculating the oncogenic risks of therapy, however. These risks can only be properly assessed in large numbers of patients followed long-term. Cyclophosphamide carries a small but definite risk of inducing cancer in nontransplanted patients, particularly of the lymphoid system and skin (Kinlen, 1985). Patients with rheumatoid arthritis have been particularly well studied, where the risk of hematological and lymphoreticular malignancies is increased fourfold (Baltus *et al.*, 1983). Interestingly, the risks of inducing tumors are comparable in patients treated with alkylating agents and azathioprine, and similar kinds of cancer are induced (Table IV) (Csuka *et al.*, 1986; Baker *et al.*, 1987; Pitt *et al.*, 1987; Wessel *et al.*, 1988; Silman *et al.*, 1988). However, in comparison with other cytotoxic drugs, cyclophosphamide may have the additional hazard of inducing carcinoma of the bladder, although these data have accrued from studies of patients with other forms of malignant disease (Pedersen-Bjergaard *et al.*, 1988). However, Mesna may

TABLE IV. Principal Recent Reports of Neoplasia Developing in Patients with Connective Tissue Diseases Treated with Cytostatic Drugs

Drug	Diagnosis	(No. treated)	Neoplasms No.	Neoplasms Type	Comparative risk (where control series)	References
CYC	RA	(81)	2	Lymphomas	4.1	Baltus *et al.* (1983)
AZA/CYC	CTD	(1634) (inc. 643 RA)	13	Carcinomas (mainly)	10.9 variable	Kinlen (1985)
			6	Lymphomas		
			59	Carcinomas (mainly)		
CYC	RA	(119)	4	Lymphoma/leukemia	2.3 overall	Baker *et al.* (1987)
			6	Bladder carcinoma		
			27	Other		
AZA	RA	(41)	3	Lymphomas	—	Pitt *et al.* (1987)
AZA	RA	(36)	2	Carcinomas	—	Wessel *et al.* (1988)
	SLE	(36)	0			
CL	RA	(39)	8	Skin cancer	—	Patapanian *et al.* (1988)
			3	Leukemia		
AZA	RA	(30)	1	Skin		
AZA	RA	(202)	4	Lymphomas	RA × 5	Silman *et al.* (1988)
			31	Carcinomas	RA + AZA × 10 compared controls	

Abbreviations: RA, rheumatoid arthritis; SLE, systemic lupus erythematosus; CTD, connective tissue diseases; AZA, azathioprine; CL, chlorambucil; CYC, cyclophosphamide.

have some protective value against the mutagenic effects that presumably operate in the induction of this tumor (Pool et al., 1988).

The mechanisms of tumor induction by alkylating agents remain speculative. Lymphocytes are susceptible to chromosome damage by chlorambucil and by mutagenic metabolites of cyclophosphamide activated in the liver or by lymphocytes themselves (Sargent et al., 1987). In vitro, both 4-hydroxycyclophosphamide and phosphoramide mustard are potent inducers of sister chromatid exchanges (Bryant et al., 1989). In the rat, the major DNA adduct of cyclophosphamide has been identified as N-(2-hydroxyethyl)-N-[2-(7-guaninyl)-ethyl]amine (Benson et al., 1988), which means that more refined studies of excision and repair proficiency should be possible.

This damage is reflected in an increased frequency of sister chromatid exchanges in the lymphocytes of patients with connective tissue diseases treated with chlorambucil; the increase is dose-dependent and cumulative (Palmer et al., 1984). A similar increase is noted in children with juvenile chronic arthritis treated with this drug (Palmer et al., 1985). Judged by this criterion, cyclophosphamide is more potent than chlorambucil in inducing chromosome damage (Palmer et al., 1986). Moreover, these abnormalities persist for many years after treatment. In addition, a high incidence of T cells resistant to thioguanine has been detected in patients with connective tissue diseases (Palmer et al., 1988) and with multiple sclerosis (Ammenheuser et al., 1988) treated with cyclophosphamide. These findings are evidence for mutation specifically at the hypoxanthine-guanine phosphoribosyl transferase (HGPRT) locus.

These studies indicate that lymphocytes with chromosome damage and specific mutations survive for prolonged periods after treatment with alkylating agents. Nevertheless, despite the cumulative genotoxic damage, malignancy is a relatively uncommon event, indicating that other factors must be involved. One possibility is that other genotoxic agents, including drugs, may have a synergistic effect (Ford and Warnick, 1988). Conversely, cyclophosphamide may increase the risks imposed by other mutagenic agents; for example, it enhances the incidence of radiation-induced mutations, possibly by interfering with repair mechanisms (Ehling and Neuhauser-Klaus, 1988). There is also some evidence that patients with connective tissue disease may be particularly susceptible to malignancies induced by chlorambucil compared with other patient groups (Palmer and Denman, 1984). There is nothing to suggest that lymphocytes from such patients are abnormally sensitive to these drugs on the basis of a putative DNA repair defect (Palmer et al., 1987). However, there is some evidence that the lymphocytes of patients with connective tissue diseases may be relatively deficient in repairing the powerful, promutagenic, directly miscoding base lesion O6-methylguanine bases, compared with normal controls and patients with other diseases (Lawley et al., 1988). The propensity of alkylating agents to induce lymphoreticular malignancies also raises the possibility that impaired antiviral immune responses may be a cofactor (Kinlen, 1982).

The mutagenic effects of alkylating agents demand that hospital and industrial workers exposed to these be fully protected and properly monitored (Thompson, 1990). Evidence of chromosome damage can be obtained in such personnel when safety precautions are inadequate. Equally, abnormalities are not detectable when the handling of these drugs is properly regulated (Sorsa et al., 1988; Yager et al., 1988).

9.5. Teratogenesis

Since there is a strong suspicion that alkylating agents are teratogenic to human fetuses (Kirshon et al., 1988), it is obviously advisable to avoid prescribing this drug in early pregnancy. Cyclophosphamide directly inhibits cell division during morphogenesis (Padmanabhan, 1988; Lahdetie, 1988) and inflicts other potentially heritable defects (Backer *et al.*, 1988). The teratogenicity induced in cultured rat embryos is probably attributable to phosphoramide mustard and to acrolein (Slott and Hales, 1988), suggesting a possible link between cyclophosphamide's mutagenic and teratogenic actions.

9.6. Other Side Effects

The reactivity of alkylating agents with molecules other than purines may account for some of the more unusual side effects that they have occasionally been reported to induce, notably hemolytic anemia (Doll and Weiss, 1985), lung toxicity (Lauta *et al.*, 1987; Giles *et al.*, 1990), abnormalities of the central nervous system (Ciobanu *et al.*, 1987; Vandenberg *et al.*, 1988), and liver damage (Shaunak *et al.*, 1988; Honjo *et al.*, 1988). Reports of this kind, however, such as transitory increases in liver enzyme concentrations in the blood, are hard to interpret because of concomitant treatment with complex drug regimens. Florid hypersensitivity skin reactions to chlorambucil occurs (Hitchins *et al.*, 1987), albeit rarely, with cross-reactivity to cyclophosphamide (Kritharides *et al.*, 1987).

10. ANALOGUES OF ALKYLATING AGENTS

Unlike other classical alkylating agents, cyclophosphamide inhibits *de novo* DNA synthesis. It also inhibits several metabolic pathways and interacts biochemically with cell membrane constituents (Hilgard, 1987). There is interest in developing analogues of the parent molecule or identifying metabolites, which do not need bioactivation *in vivo* and which have more selective biological effects. In particular, immunomodulating analogues that lack cyclophosphamide's toxic and mutagenic effects would have obvious clinical advantages. Some compounds of this nature have now been tested. For example, 4-hydroxyperoxycyclophosphamide has immunomodulatory features resembling those of cyclophosphamide, including the ability to suppress the generation of T-cell subsets *in vitro* (Smith *et al.*, 1987).

Mafosfamide is a cyclophosphamide derivative that does not need *in vivo* enzymatic activation. There is some evidence that a given dose is less toxic and a more selective regulator of T-cell activity than cyclophosphamide itself (Pohl *et al.*, 1987). There are also preliminary hints from experimental models and clinical studies that mafosfamide enhances macrophage and natural killer cell function (Klein *et al.*, 1987).

To date, no analogues have been developed that warrant serious comparison with the alkylating agents and other immunosuppressive agents used to treat immunological disorders.

11. FUTURE PROSPECTS

Several lines of current research suggest that the efficacy and safety of alkylating agents, particularly oxazaphosphorine cytostatics, can be improved (Table V). There has been considerable progress in developing analogues of cyclophosphamide with a higher therapeutic ratio (Brock, 1989), even though their clinical application has so far been very limited. In addition, some entertainingly simple suggestions have been made for protecting patients from some of the side effects of this class of drugs. Thus dietary carrot may have an

TABLE V.   Future Prospects for Treatment with Alkylating Agents

Analogues
Potentiation by other agents
Selective action on immunological effector cells by administering growth
    factors for other proliferating precursor cells
Tolerance induction to autoantigens
Local administration
Targeting using monoclonal antibodies as carriers

antimutagenic effect (Darroudi et al., 1988), and some Indian medicinal plants have been reported to block cyclophosphamide-induced neutropenia (Thatte et al., 1987). In similar vein, a rice-rich diet is reported to increase the immunoenhancing effects of cyclophosphamide in mice (Kodama and Kodama, 1988). The therapeutic activity of cyclophosphamide may also be improved by other drugs: potentiation of its therapeutic activity has been reported in mice given the adjuvant N-acyldehydroalanine (Allemon et al., 1987).

Concomitant immunomanipulation, of the kind used to improve the antitumor effects of cyclophosphamide in experimental and clinical studies, has scarcely been explored in the treatment of immune disorders. A clear possibility is the simultaneous administration of recombinant cytokines such as interleukin-2 (Hosokawa et al., 1988; Kolitz et al., 1988).

There are also reports that cyclophosphamide can be used to promote tolerance for therapeutic purposes; thus, immune tolerance to factor VIII has been induced in this way in hemophiliac patients with antibody to factor VIII (Nilsson et al., 1988). The same theme has been pursued in animals with experimentally induced demyelinating disease associated with autoimmunity to myelin basic protein (Eidinoff, 1988). The disease process can be ameliorated if this protein is administered in conjunction with cyclophosphamide in order to restore tolerance to autologous myelin basic protein. The theoretical relevance of these observations to the management of multiple sclerosis is self-evident.

By extrapolating from experimental antitumor therapy (Scheper et al., 1987), local injection of active metabolites might prove beneficial in patients with chronic inflammatory lesions such as rheumatoid arthritis. Finally, it is reasonable to consider the targeting of alkylating agents combined with monoclonal antibodies to defined immunoproliferative populations (Smyth et al., 1987).

12. CONCLUSIONS

The inevitable side effects and long-term risks of alkylating agents limit their routine use in immunological disorders. Nevertheless, the morbidity and often mortality attendant upon these disorders make it reasonable to consider using these drugs in patients who have failed to respond to less toxic drugs or in whom the prognosis is unequivocally bad. The main difficulty in choosing between alkylating agents and other immunosuppressive measures is the scarcity of comparative trials with adequate periods of follow-up. While clinicians faced with acute problems cannot always afford the luxury of academic reflection and decision, there are few situations in which there is not at least a priori evidence that other immunosuppressive regimens might be equally effective. For example, severe rheumatoid arthritis responds to cyclophosphamide, but it has also been successfully treated with a combination of high-dose prednisolone, azathioprine, and antilymphocyte globulin (Binder et al., 1986). The recent resurgence of interest in treating rheumatoid arthritis with methotrexate (Mason and Furst, 1989) also prompts serious comparison between this drug and alkylating agents. Similarly, severe inflammatory connective tissue diseases respond to some combinations excluding alkylating agents (Hollingworth *et al.*, 1982), and there are still legitimate doubts that cyclophosphamide is necessarily superior to azathioprine in treating lupus nephritis. There are also diseases that have been treated with alkylating agents for speculative reasons in which subsequent controlled trials proves that these drugs are entirely ineffective; scleroderma is a recent example (Furst *et al.*, 1989).

Indeed, there are scarcely any immune disorders whose management would not benefit from properly planned and documented trials, often necessitating multicenter cooperation when the diseases are uncommon. This need is made more urgent by the advent of more sophisticated and selective immunological manipulation. Moreover, only proper documentation will ensure that long-term natural history, clinical correlations, and drug toxicity are properly recorded for analysis. Unfortunately, in most countries only financial institutions seem to collect long-term data with the required assiduousness. For the moment, one must conclude that alkylating agents are an often effective but undesirably toxic means of treating severe immunological disorders in an era of nonspecific, pragmatic immunosuppression that all clinicians hope is drawing to its close.

REFERENCES

Ahmed, A. R., and Hombal, S., 1987, Use of cyclophosphamide in azathioprine failures in pemphigus, *J. Am. Acad. Dermatol.* **17**:437–442.

Aisenberg, A. C., and Davis, C., 1968, The thymus and recovery from cyclophosphamide induced tolerance to sheep erythrocytes, *J. Exp. Med.* **128**:35–46.

Allemon, A. M., Buc Calderon, P., and Roberfroid, M., 1987, Potentiation of the therapeutic activity of cyclophosphamide by an original N-acyldehydroalanine, *Drugs. Exp. Clin. Res.* **13**:359–365.

Ambrus, J. L., and Fauci, A. S., 1984, Diffuse histiocytic lymphoma in a patient treated with cyclophosphamide for Wegener's granulomatosis, *Am. J. Med.* **76**:745–747.

American Rheumatism Association, 1970, A controlled trial of cyclophosphamide in rheumatoid arthritis, *N. Engl. J. Med.* **283**:883–889.

Ammenheuser, M. M., Ward, J. B., Jr., Whorton, E. B., Jr., Killian, J. M., and Legator, M. S., 1988, Elevated frequencies of 6-thioguanine-resistant lymphocytes in multiple sclerosis patients treated with cyclophosphamide: A prospective study, *Mutat. Res.* **204**:509–520.

Amor, B., and Mery, C., 1983, Chlorambucil in rheumatoid arthritis, in: *Anti-rheumatic Drugs* (I. Huskisson, ed.), Praeger, New York, pp. 605–622.

Arndt, C. A. S., Balis, F. M., McCully, C. L., Colvin, O. M., and Poplack, D. G., 1988, Cerebrospinal fluid penetration of active metabolites of cyclophosphamide and ifosfamide in rhesus monkeys, *Cancer Res.* **48**:2113–2115.

Austin, H. A., III, Klippel, J. H., Balow, J. E., Le Riche, N. G. H., Steinberg, A. D., Plotz, P. H., and Decker, J. L., 1986, Therapy of lupus nephritis: Controlled trial of prednisone and cytotoxic drugs, *N. Engl. J. Med.* **314**:614–619.

Backer, L. C., Gibson, J. B., Moses, M. J., and Allen, J. W., 1988, Synaptonemal complex damage in relation to meiotic chromosome aberrations after exposure of male mice to cyclophosphamide, *Mutat. Res.* **203**:317–330.

Baker, G. L., Kahl, L. E., Zee, B. C., Stolzer, B. L., Agarwal, A. K., and Medsger, T. A., Jr., 1987, Malignancy following treatment of rheumatoid arthritis with cyclophosphamide, *Am. J. Med.* **83**:1–9.

Baltus, J. A. M. Boersma, J. W., Hartman, A. P., and Vandenbroucke, J. P., 1983, The occurrence of malignancies in patients with rheumatoid arthritis treated with cyclophosphamide: A controlled retrospective follow-up, *Ann. Rheum. Dis.* **42**:368–373.

Bank, B. B., Kanganis, D., Liebes, L. F., and Silber, R., 1989, Chlorambucil pharmacokinetics and DNA binding in chronic lymphocytic leukemia lymphocytes, *Cancer Res.* **49**:554–559.

Benson, A. J., Martin, C. N., and Gardner, R. C., 1988, N-(2-nydroxytheyl)-N-[2-(7-guaninyl)ethyl]amine, the putative major DNA adduct of cyclophosphamide *in vitro* and *in vivo* in the rat, *Biochem. Pharmacol.* **37**:2979–2985.

Berd, D., and Mastrangelo, M. J., 1987, Elimination of immune suppressor mechanisms in humans by oxazaphosphorines, *Methods Find. Exp. Clin. Pharmacol.* **9**:569–577.

Berd, D., and Mastrangelo, M. J., 1988, Effect of low dose cyclophosphamide on the immune system of cancer patients: Depletion of CD4+, 2H4+ suppressor-inducer T-cells, *Cancer Res.* **48**:1671–1675.

Berglund, K., Keller, C., and Thysell, H., 1987, Alkylating cytostatic treatment in renal amyloidosis secondary to rheumatic disease, *Ann. Rheum. Dis.* **46**:757–762.

Binder, A. I., So, A., Ansell, B. M., and Denman, A. M., 1986, Intensive immunosuppression in intractable rheumatoid arthritis, *Br. J. Rheumatol.* **25**:380–383.

Boumpas, D. T., Barez, S., Klippel, J. H., and Balow, J. E., 1990, Intermittent cyclophosphamide for the treatment of autoimmune thrombocytopenia in systemic lupus erythematosus, *Ann. Intern. Med.* **112**:674–677.

Bradley, J. D., Brandt, K. D., and Katz, B. P., 1989, Infectious complications of cyclophosphamide treatment for vasculitis, *Arthritis Rheum.* **32**:45–53.

Brahm, M., Balslov, J. T., Brammer, M., Brun, C., Gerstoft, J., Jorgensen, H. E., Kamper, A., Larsen, S., Lorenzen, I., and Thomsen, A. C., 1988, Cytostatic treatment of glomerular diseases. V. Treatment of glomerulonephritis with cyclophosphamide plus prednisone, azathioprine plus prednisone and cyclophosphamide as monotherapy. A comparative study. A report from a Copenhagen study group of renal diseases, *Acta Med. Scand.* **224**:605–610.

Brinkman, C. J. J., Nillesen, W. M., and Hommes, O. R., 1984, The effect of cyclophosphamide on T lymphocytes and T lymphocyte subsets in patients with chronic progressive multiple sclerosis, *Acta Neurol. Scand.* **69**:90–96.

Brock, N., 1989, Oxazaphosphorine cytostatics: Past–present–future. Seventh Cain Memorial Award Lecture, *Cancer Res.* **49**:1–7.

Bryant, M. F., Erexson, G. L., and Kligerman, A. D., 1989, A comparison of sister-chromatid exchange in mouse peripheral blood lymphocytes exposed *in vitro* and *in vivo* to phosphoramide mustard and 4-hydroxycyclophosphamide, *Mutat. Res.* **222**: 271–277.

Budel, V., Kiss, R., de Launoit, Y., Danguy, A., Atassi, G., Pasteels, J. L., and Paridaens, R., 1988, Prevention of ovarian damage induced by cyclophosphamide in adult female mice by hormonal manipulations, *J. Reprod. Fert.* **84**:625–633.

Calabresi, P., and Parks, R. E., 1980, Antiproliferative agents and drugs used for immunosuppression, in: *The Pharmacological Basis of Therapeutics*, VIth ed. (A. G. Gilman *et al.*, eds.), Macmillan, New York, p. 1256.

Cannon, G. W., Jackson, C. G., Samuelson, C. O., Jr., Ward, J. R., Williams, H. J., and Clegg, D. O., 1985, Chlorambucil therapy in rheumatoid arthritis: Clinical experience in 28 patients and literature review, *Semin. Arthritis Rheum.* **15**:106–118.

Carter, J. L., Dawson, D. M., Hafler, D. A., Fallis, R. J., Stazzone, L., Orav, J., and Weiner, H. L., 1988a, Cumulative experience with high-dose intravenous cyclophosphamide and ACTH therapy in chronic progressive multiple sclerosis, *Ann. NY Acad. Sci.* **540**:535–536.

Carter, J. L., Hafler, D. A., Dawson, D. M., Orav, J., and Weiner, H. L., 1988b, Immunosuppression with high-dose IV cyclophosphamide and ACTH in progressive multiple sclerosis: Cumulative 6-year experience in 164 patients, *Neurology* **38**:9–14.

Ciobanu, N., Runowicz, C., Gucalp, R., Frank, M., Charuvanki, V., Kaufman, D., and Wiernik, P. H., 1987, Reversible central nervous system toxicity associated with high-dose chlorambucil in autologous bone marrow transplantation for ovarian carcinoma, *Cancer Treat. Rep.* **71**:1324–1325.

Clements, P. J., and Levy, J., 1977, Relative cell sizes of lymphocyte populations: The effect of immunosuppressive therapy, *Clin. Immunol. Immunopathol.* **7**:69–76.

Cohen-Tervaert, J. W., Hultema, M. G., Hene, R. J., Sluiter, W. J., The, T. H., van der Hem, G. K., and Kallenberg, C. G., 1990, Prevention of relapses in Wegener's granulomatosis by treatment based on antineutrophil cytoplasmic antibody titre, *Lancet* **336**:709–711.

Colburn, K. K., Cao, J. D., Krick, E. H., Mortensen, S. E., and Wong, L. G., 1985, Hodgkin's lymphoma in a patient treated for Wegener's granulomatosis with cyclophosphamide and azathioprine, *J. Rheumatol.* **12**:599–602.

Csuka, M. E., Carrera, G. F., and McCarty, J., 1986, Treatment of intractable rheumatoid arthritis with combined cyclophosphamide, azathioprine, and hydroxychloroquine: A follow-up study, *J. Am. Med. Assoc.* **255**:2315–2319.

Currey, H. L. F., Harris, J., Mason, R. M., Woodland, J., Beveridge, T., Roberts, C. J., Vere, D. W., Dixon, A. St. J., Davies, J., and Owen-Smith, B., 1974, Comparison of azathioprine, cyclophosphamide and gold in treatment of rheumatoid arthritis, *Br. Med. J.* **3**:763–766.

Darroudi, F., Targa, H., and Natarajan, A. T., 1988, Influence of dietary carrot on cytostatic drug activity of cyclophosphamide and its main directly acting metabolite: Induction of sister-chromatid exchanges in normal human lymphocytes, Chinese hamster ovary cells, and their DNA repair-deficient call lines, *Mutat. Res.* **198**:327–335.

Denman, A. M., 1982, Immunosuppression and the rheumatic diseases, *Ann. Rheum. Dis.* **41**:S3–8.

Denman, E. J., Denman, A. M., Greenwood, B. M., Gall, D., and Heath, R. B., 1970, Failure of cytotoxic drugs to suppress immune responses of patients with rheumatoid arthritis, *Ann. Rheum. Dis.* **29**:220–231.

Doll, D. C., and Weiss, R. B., 1985, Hemolytic anemia associated with antineoplastic agents, *Cancer Treat. Rep.* **69**:777–782.

Ehling, U. H., and Neuhauser-Klaus, A., 1988, Induction of specific-locus and dominant-lethal mutations by cyclophosphamide and combined cyclophosphamide-radiation treatment in male mice, *Mutat. Res.* **199**:21–30.

Eidinoff, H., 1988, Suppression of the immune reaction in multiple sclerosis might be achieved by intravenous injections of myelin basic protein, concomitant with the administration of an immunosuppressant and a corticosteroid, *Med. Hypotheses* **26**: 103–106.

Erban, S. R., and Sokas, R. K., 1988, Kaposi's sarcoma in an elderly man with Wegener's granulomatosis treated with cyclophosphamide and corticosteroids, *Arch. Intern. Med.* **148**:1201–1203.

Erlichman, C., Soldin, S. J., Hardy, R. W., Thiessen, J. J., Sturgeon, J. F. G., Fine, S., and Baskerville, T., 1988, Disposition of cyclophosphamide on two consecutive cycles of treatment in patients with ovarian carcinoma, *Arzneimittelforsch.* **38**:839–842.

Euler, H. H., Gutschmidt, H. J., Schmuecking, M., Schroeder, J. O., and Loffler, H., 1990, Induction of remission in severe SLE after plasma exchange synchronized with subsequent pulse cyclophosphamide, *Prog. Clin. Biol. Res.* **337**:319–320.

Fauci, A. S., Katz, P., Haynes, B. F., and Wolff, S. M., 1979, Cyclophosphamide therapy of severe systemic necrotizing vasculitis, *N. Engl. J. Med.* **301**:235–238.

Fauci, A. S., Haynes, B. F., Katz, P., and Wolff, S. M., 1983, Wegener's granulomatosis: Prospective clinical and therapeutic experience with 85 patients for 21 years, *Ann. Intern. Med.* **98**:76–85.

Feehally, J., Beattie, T. J., Brenchley, P. E., Coupes, B. M., Houston, I. B., Mallick, N. P., and Postelthwaite, R. J., 1984, Modulation of cellular immune function by cyclophosphamide in children with minimal-change nephropathy, *N. Engl. J. Med.* **310**:415–420.

Firkin, F. C., and Maher, D., 1988, Cytotoxic immunosuppressive drug treatment strategy in pure red cell aplasia, *Eur. J. Haematol.* **41**:212–217.

Ford, C. D., and Warnick, C. T., 1988, DNA damage and repair in patients receiving high-dose cyclophosphamide and radiation, *NCI Monogr.* **6**:41–44.

Fort, J. G., and Abruzzo, J. L., 1988, Reversal of progressive necrotizing vasculitis with intravenous pulse cyclophosphamide and methylprednisolone, *Arthritis Rheum.* **31**:1194–1198.

Furst, D. E., Clements, P. J., Hillis, S., Lachenbruch, P. A., Miller, B. L., Sterz, M. G., and Paulus, H. E., 1989, Immunosuppression with chlorambucil, versus placebo, for scleroderma, *Arthritis Rheum.* **32**:584–593.

Giles, F. J., Smith, M. P., and Goldstone, A. H., 1990, Chlorambucil lung toxicity, *Acta Haematol. Basel* **83**:156–158.

Girard, D., Aloisi, R. M., Bliven, M. L., Cunningham, A. C., and Otterness, I. G., 1990, Cyclophosphamide and 15(S)-15 methyl PGE1 correct the T/B lymphocyte ratios of NZB/NZW mice, *Agents Actions* **29**:333–341.

Goodpasture, J. C., Bergstrom, K., and Vickery, B. H., 1988, Potentiation of the gonadotoxicity of cytoxan in the dog by adjuvant treatment with a luteinizing hormone-releasing hormone agonist, *Cancer Res.* **48**:2174–2178.

Gudbjornsson, B., and Hallgren, R., 1990, Cutaneous polyarteritis nodosa associated with Crohn's disease. Report and review of the literature, *J. Rheumatol.* **17**:386–390.

Hadidi, A. H., Coulter, C. E., and Idle, J. R., 1988, Phenotypically deficient urinary elimination of carboxyphosphamide after cyclophosphamide administration to cancer patients, *Cancer Res.* **48**:5167–5171.

Hilgard, P., 1987, The metabolism of oxazaphosphorines—An introduction, *Methods Find. Exp. Clin. Pharmacol.* **9**:551–553.

Hitchins, R. N., Hocker, G. A., and Thomson, D. B., 1987, Chlorambucil allergy—A series of three cases, *Aust. NZ J. Med.* **17**:600–602.

Hollingworth, P., de Vere Tyndall, A., Ansell, B. M., Platts-Mills, T., Gumpel, J. M., Mertin, J., Smith, D. S., and Denman, A. M., 1982, Intensive immunosuppression versus prednisolone in the treatment of connective tissue diseases, *Ann. Rheum. Dis.* **41**:557–562.

Honjo, I., Suou, T., and Hirayama, C., 1988, Hepatotoxicity of cyclophosphamide in man: Pharmacokinetic analysis, *Res. Comm. Chem. Pathol. Pharmacol.* **61**:149–165.

Hosokawa, M., Sawamura, Y., Morikage, T., Okada, F., Xu, Z. Y., Morikawa, K., Itoh, K., and Kobayashi, H., 1988, Improved therapeutic effects of interleukin-2 after the accumulation of lymphokine-activated killer cells in tumor tissue of mice previously treated with cyclophosphamide, *Cancer Immunol. Immunother.* **26**:250–256.

Jonsson, R., Tarkowski, A., and Backman, K., 1988, Effects of immunomodulating treatment on autoimmune sialadenitis in MRL/Mp-1pr/1pr mice, *Agents Actions* **25**:368–374.

Killian, J. M., Bressler, R. B., Armstrong, R. M., and Huston, D. P., 1988, Controlled pilot trial of monthly intravenous cyclophosphamide in multiple sclerosis, *Arch. Neurol.* **45**:27–30.

Kinlen, L. J., 1982, Immunosuppressive therapy and cancer, *Cancer Surv.* **1**:565–583.

Kinlen, L. J., 1985, Incidence of cancer in rheumatoid arthritis and other disorders after immunosuppressive treatment, *Am. J. Med.* **78**:44–49.

Kirshon, B., Wasserstrum, N., Willis, R., Herman, G. E., and McCabe, E. R. B., 1988, Teratogenic effects of first-trimester cyclophosphamide therapy, *Obstet. Gynecol.* **72**:462–464.

Klein, H. O., Kreysch, H. G., Coerper, C., Voigt, P., and Ruff, I., 1987, Preclinical and early clinical trial with mafosfamide as immune modulator, *Methods Find. Exp. Clin. Pharmacol.* **9**:627–640.

Kodama, M., and Kodama, T., 1988, Effect of a rice-rich diet on the therapeutic efficacy of cyclophosphamide with special reference to the enhancement of transplantation immunity, *Jpn J. Cancer Res.* **79**:608–617.

Kolitz, J. E., Wong, G. Y., Welte, K., Merluzzi, V. J., Egbert, A., Bialas, T., Polivka, A., Bradley, E. C., Konrad, M., Gnecco, C., Oettgen, H. F., and Mertelsmann, R., 1988, Phase I trial of recombinant interleukin-2 and cyclophosphamide: Augmentation of cellular immunity and T cell mitogenic response with long-term administration of rIL-2, *J. Biol. Response Mod.* **7**:457–472.

Kovarsky, J., 1983, Clinical pharmacology and toxicology of cyclophosphamide: Emphasis on use in rheumatic diseases, *Sem. Arthritis Rheum.* **12**:359–372.

Kritharides, L., Lawrie, K., and Varigos, G. A., 1987, Cyclophosphamide hypersensitivity and cross-reactivity with chlorambucil, *Cancer Treat. Rep.* **71**:1323–1324.

Kroneman, O. C., III, and Pevzner, M., 1986, Failure of cyclophosphamide to prevent cerebritis in Wegener's granulomatosis, *Am. J. Med.* **80**:526–527.

Lahdetie, J., 1988, Induction and survival of micronuclei in rat spermatids. Comparison of two meiotic micronucleus techniques using cyclophosphamide, *Mutat. Res.* **203**:47–53.

Laing, T. J., 1988, Gastrointestinal vasculitis and pneumatosis intestinalis due to systemic lupus erythematosus: Successful treatment with pulse intravenous cyclophosphamide, *Am. J. Med.* **85**:555–558.

Lamers, K., Uitdehaag, B. M. J., Hommes, O. R., Doesberg, W., Wevers, R., van Geel, W. J. A., 1988, The short-term effect of an immunosuppressive treatment on CSF myelin basic protein in chronic progressive multiple sclerosis, *J. Neurol. Neurosurg. Psychiatry* **51**:1334–1337.

Lauta, V. M., Valerio, G., Greco, A., and Minutolo, M. C., 1987, Early-onset diagnosis of lung toxicity caused by cyclophosphamide, melphalan and procarbazine therapy, *Tumori* **73**:351–358.

Lawley, P. D., Topper, R., Denman, A. M., Hylton, W., Hill, I. D., and Harris, G., 1988, Increased sensitivity of lymphocytes from patients with systemic autoimmune diseases to DNA alkylation by the methylating carcinogen N-methyl-N-nitrosourea, *Ann. Rheum. Dis.* **47**:445–451.

Likosky, W. H., 1988, Experience with cyclophosphamide in multiple sclerosis—The cons, *Neurology* **38**:14–18.

Mason, D. H., Jr., and Furst, D. E., 1989, Methotrexate in rheumatoid arthritis and related diseases, *Curr. Opinion Rheumatol.* **1**:44–51.

Mathieson, P. W., Turner, A. N., Maidment, C. G. H., Evans, D. J., and Rees, A. J., 1988, Prednisolone and chlorambucil treatment in idiopathic membranous nephropathy with deteriorating renal function, *Lancet* **2**:869–872.

McBride, W. H., Hoon, D. B, Jung, T., Naungayan, J., Nizze, A., and Morton, D. L., 1987, Cyclophosphamide-induced alterations in human monocyte functions, *J. Leukocyte Biol.* **42**:659–666.

McCune, W. J., Golbus, J., Zeldes, W., Bohlke, P., Dunne, R., and Fox, D. A., 1988, Clinical and immunologic effects of monthly administration of intravenous cyclophosphamide in severe systemic lupus erythematosus, *N. Engl. J. Med.* **318**:1423–1431.

Mertin, J., Rudge, P., Kremer, M., Healey, M. J. R., Knight, S. C., Compston, A., Batchelor, J. R., Thompson, E. J., Halliday, A. M., Denman, A. M., and Medawar, P. B., 1982, Double-blind controlled trial of immunosuppression in the treatment of multiple sclerosis: Final report, *Lancet* **2**:351–354.

Moore, M. J., Hardy, R. W., Thiessen, J. J., Soldin, S. J., and Erlichman, C., 1988, Rapid development of enhanced clearance after high-dose cyclophosphamide, *Clin. Pharmacol. Ther.* **44**:622–628.

Mountz, J. D., Mushinski, J. F., Smith, H. R., Kilman, D. M., and Steinberg, A. D., 1985, Modulation of c-myb transcription in autoimmune disease by cyclophosphamide, *J. Immunol.* **135**:2417–2422.

Nikcevich, D. A., Duffie, G. P., Young, M. R., Ellis, N. K., Kaufman, G. E., and Wepsic, H. T., 1987, Simulation of suppressor cells in the bone marrow and spleens of high-dose cyclophosphamide-treated C57Bl/6 mice, *Cell Immunol.* **109**:349–359.

Nilsson, I. M., Berntorp, E., and Zettervali, O., 1988, Induction of immune tolerance in patients with hemophilia and antibodies to factor VIII by combined treatment with intravenous IgG, cyclophosphamide, and factor VIII, *N. Engl. J. Med.* **318**:947–950.

O'Duffy, J. D., Robertson, D. M., and Goldstein, N. P., 1984, Chlorambucil in the treatment of uveitis and meningoencephalitis of Behçet's disease, *Am. J. Med.* **76**:75–84.

Ohyashiki, K., Kocova, M., Ryan, D. H., Rowe, J. M., and Sandberg, A. A., 1986, Secondary acute myeloblastic leukemia with a Ph translocation in a treated Wegener's granulomatosis, *Cancer Genet. Cytogenet.* **19**:331–333.

Padmanabhan, R., 1988, Light microscopic studies on the pathogenesis of exencephaly and cranioschisis induced in the rat after neural tube closure, *Teratology* **37**:29–36.

Palmer, R. G., and Denman, A. M., 1984, Malignancies induced by chlorambucil, *Cancer Treat. Rev.* **11**:121–129.

Palmer, R. G., Dore, C. J., and Denman, A. M., 1984, Chlorambucil-induced chromosome damage to human lymphocytes is dose-dependent and cumulative, *Lancet* **1**:246–249.

Palmer, R. G., Varonos, S., Dore, C. J., Denman, A. M., and Ansell, B. M., 1985, Chlorambucil induced chromosome damage in juvenile chronic arthritis, *Arch. Dis. Child.* **60**:1008–1013.

Palmer, R. G., Dore, C. J., and Denman, A. M., 1986, Cyclophosphamide induces more chromosome damage than chlorambucil in patients with connective tissue diseases, *Q. J. Med.* **228**:395–400.

Palmer, R. G., Smith-Burchnell, C. A., Dore, C. J., and Denman, A. M., 1987, Sensitivity of lymphocytes from patients with systemic lupus erythematosus to the induction of sister chromatid exchanges by alkylating agents and bromodeoxyuridine, *Ann. Rheum. Dis.* **46**:110–113.

Palmer, R. G., Smith-Burchnell, C. A., Pelton, B. K., Hylton, W., and Denman, A. M., 1988, Use of T cell cloning to detect *in vivo* mutations induced by cyclophosphamide, *Arthritis Rheum.* **31**:757–761.

Pasricha, J. S., Thanzama, J., and Khan, U. K., 1988, Intermittent high-dose dexamethasone–cyclophosphamide therapy for pemphigus, *Br. J. Dermatol.* **119**:73–77.

Patapanian, H., Graham, S., Sambrook, P. N., Browne, C. D., Champion, G. D., Cohen, M. L., and Day, R. O., 1988, The oncogenicity of chlorambucil in rheumatoid arthritis, *Br. J. Rheumatol.* **27**:44–47.

Paulus, H. E., 1990, The use of combinations of disease-modifying antirheumatic agents in rheumatoid arthritis, *Arthritis Rheum.* **33**:113–120.

Pedersen-Bjergaard, J., Ersboll, J., Hansen, V. L., Sorensen, B. L., Christoffersen, K., Hou-Jensen, K., Nissen, N. I., Knudsen, J. B., and Hansen, M. M., 1988, Carcinoma of the urinary bladder after treatment with cyclophosphamide for non-Hodgkin's lymphoma, *N. Engl. J. Med.* **318**:1028–1032.

Pestronk, A., Cornblath, D. R., Ilyas, A. A., Baba, H., Quarles, R. H., Griffin, J. W., Anderson, K., and Adams, R. N., 1988, A treatable multifocal motor neuropathy with antibodies to GM1 ganglioside, *Ann. Neurol.* **24**:73–78.

Pitt, P. I., Sultan, A. H., Malone, M., Andrews, V., and Hamilton, E. B. D., 1987, Association between azathioprine therapy and lymphoma in rheumatoid disease, *J. R. Soc. Med.* **80**:428–429.

Pohl, J., Reissmann, T., and Voegeli, R., 1987, Oxazaphosphorine effects in L 5222 rat leukemia, *Methods Find. Exp. Clin. Pharmacol.* **9**:589–594.

Ponticelli, C., Zucchelli, P., Passerini, P., Cagnoli, L., Cesana, B., Pozzi, C., Pasquali, S., Imbasciati, E., Grassi, C., Redaelli, B., Sasdelli, M., and Locatelli, F., 1989, A randomized trial of methylprednisolone and chlorambucil in idiopathic membranous nephropathy, *N. Engl. J. Med.* **320**:8–13.

Pool, B. L., Bos, R. P., Niemeyer, U., Theuws, J. L. G., and Schmahl, D. 1988, *In vitro/in vivo* effects of Mesna on the genotoxicity and toxicity of cyclophosphamide—A study aimed at clarifying the mechanism of Mesna's anticarcinogenic activity, *Toxicol. Lett.* **41**:49–56.

Powis, G., Reece, P., Ahmann, D. L., and Ingle, J. N., 1987, Effect of body weight on the pharmacokinetics of cyclophosphamide in breast cancer patients, *Cancer Chemother. Pharmacol.* **20**:219–222.

Rees, A. J., and Lockwood, C. M., 1982, Immunosuppressive drugs in clinical practice, in: *Clinical Aspects of Immunology,* IVth ed. (P. J. Lachmann and D. K. Peters, eds.), Blackwells, Oxford, pp. 507–564.

Sargent, L. M., Roloff, B., and Meisner, L. F., 1987, Mechanisms in cyclophosphamide induction of cytogenetic damage in human lymphocyte cultures, *Cancer Genet. Cytogenet.* **29**:239–243.

Scheper, R. J., Limpens, J., Tan, B. T. G., Valster, H., Claessen, A. M. E., and Claessen, M. E., 1987, Immunotherapeutic effects of local chemotherapy with an active metabolite of cyclophosphamide, *Methods Find. Exp. Clin. Pharmacol.* **9**:611–615.

Schilsky, R. L., Lewis, B. J., Sherins, R. J., and Young, R. C., 1980, Gonadal dysfunction in patients receiving chemotherapy for cancer, *Ann. Intern. Med.* **93:**109–114.

Schuler, U., Ehninger, G., and Wagner, T., 1987, Repeated high-dose cyclophosphamide administration in bone marrow transplantation: Exposure to activated metabolites, *Cancer Chemother. Pharmacol.* **20:**248–252.

Scott, D. G. I., and Bacon, P. A., 1984, Intravenous cyclophosphamide plus methylprednisolone in treatment of systemic rheumatoid vasculitis, *Am. J. Med.* **76:**377–384.

Scott, D. G. I., Bacon, P. A., Elliott, P. J., Tribe, C. R., and Wallington, T. B., 1982, Systemic vasculitis in a district general hospital 1972–1980: Clinical and laboratory features, classification and prognosis of 80 cases, *Q. J. Med.* **51:**292–311.

Sessoms, S. L., and Kovarsky, J., 1984, Monthly intravenous cyclophosphamide in the treatment of severe systemic lupus erythematosus, *Clin. Exp. Rheumatol.* **2:**247–251.

Sewell, W. A., de Moerloose, P. A., Hamilton, J. A., Schrader, J. W., Mackay, I. R., and Vadas, M. A., 1987, Potentiation of delayed-type hypersensitivity by pertussigen or cyclophosphamide with release of different lymphokines, *Immunology* **61;** 483–488.

Shaunak, S., Munro, J. M., Weinbren, K., Walport, M. J., and Cox, T. M., 1988, Cyclophosphamide-induced liver necrosis: A possible interaction with azathioprine, *Q. J. Med.* **67:**309–317.

Shaw, I. C., 1987, Mesna and oxazaphosphorine cancer chemotherapy, *Cancer Treat. Rev.* **14:**359–364.

Shen, R. N., Hornback, N. B., Shidnia, H., Lu, L., Broxmeyer, H. E., and Brahmi, Z., 1988, Effect of whole-body hyperthermia and cyclophosphamide on natural killer cell activity in murine erythroleukemia, *Cancer Res.* **48:**4561–4563.

Shiraki, M., Fujiwara, M., and Tomura, S., 1984, Long-term administration of cyclophosphamide in MRL/1 mice. I. The effects on the development of immunological abnormalities and lupus nephritis, *Clin. Exp. Immunol.* **55:**333–339.

Silman, A. J., Petrie, J., Hazleman, B., and Evans, S. J. W., 1988, Lymphoproliferative cancer and other malignancy in patients with rheumatoid arthritis treated with azathioprine: A 20 year follow-up study, *Ann. Rheum. Dis.* **47:**988–992.

Simel, D. L., St. Clair, E. W., Adams, J., and Greenberg, C. S., 1987, Correction of hypoprothrombinemia by immunosuppressive treatment of the lupus anticoagulant-hypoprothrombinemia syndrome, *Am. J. Med.* **83:**563–566.

Slott, V. L., and Hales, B. F., 1988, Role of the 4-hydroxy intermediate in the *in vitro* embryotoxicity of cyclophosphamide and dechlorocyclophosphamide, *Toxicol. Appl. Pharmacol.* **92:**170–178.

Smith, J. J., Mihich, E., and Ozer, H., 1987, *In vitro* effects of 4-hydroxyperoxycyclophosphamide on human immunoregulatory T subset function, *Methods Find. Exp. Clin. Pharmacol.* **9:**555–568.

Smyth, M. J., Pietersz, G. A., and McKenzie, I. F. C., 1987, The cellular uptake and cytotoxicity of chlorambucil–monoclonal antibody conjugates, *Immunol. Cell. Biol.* **65:**315–321.

Sorsa, M., Pyy, L., Salomaa, S., Nylund, L., and Yager, J. W., 1988, Biological and environmental monitoring of occupational exposure to cyclophosphamide in industry and hospitals, *Mutat. Res.* **204:**465–479.

Stevenson, H. C., and Fauci, A. S., 1980, Activation of human B lymphocytes. XII. Differential effects of *in vitro* cyclophosphamide on human lymphocyte subpopulations involved in B cell activation, *Immunology* **39:**391–397.

Stillwell, T. J., and Benson, R. C., 1988, Cyclophosphamide-induced hemorrhagic cystitis, *Cancer* **61:**451–457.

Strange, C., Halstead, L., Baumann, M., and Sahn, S. A., 1990, Subglottic stenosis in Wegener's granulomatosis: Development during cyclophosphamide treatment with response to carbon dioxide laser therapy, *Thorax* **45:**300–301.

Swanson, M. A., and Schwartz, R. S., 1967, Immunosuppressive therapy: The relation between clinical response and immunologic competence, *N. Engl. J. Med.* **277:**163–170.

Sy, M. S., and Miller, S. D., and Claman, H. N., 1977, Immune suppression with supraoptimal doses of antigen in contact sensitivity, *J. Immunol.* **119:**240–244.

Tessler, H. H., and Jennings, T., 1990, High-dose short-term chlorambucil for intractable sympathetic ophthalmia and Behçet's disease, *Br. J. Ophthalmol.* **74:**353–357.

Thatte, U. M., Chhabria, S. N., Karandikar, S. M., and Dahanukar, S. A., 1987, Protective effects of Indian medical plants against cyclophosphamide neutropenia, *J. Postgrad. Med.* **33:**185–188.

Thomas, M. R., Robinson, W. A., Boyle, D. J., Day, J. F., Entringer, M. A., and Steigerwald, J. F., 1983, Long-term effects of cyclophosphamide on granulocyte colony formation in patients with rheumatoid arthritis, *J. Rheumatol.* **10:**778–783.

Thompson, C. A., 1990, Safe handling of cyclophosphamide, *Am. J. Hosp. Pharm.* **47:**75–76.

Thrasher, J. B., Miller, G. J., and Wettlaufer, J. N., 1990, Bladder leiomyosarcoma following cyclophosphamide therapy for lupus nephritis, *J. Urol.* **143:**119–121.

Tietjen, D. P., and Moore, W. J., 1990, Treatment of rapidly progressive glomerulonephritis due to Behçet's syndrome with intravenous cyclophosphamide, *Nephron* **55:**69–73.

Turk, J. L., 1987, Enhancement of the delayed-type hypersensitivity reaction by oxazaphosphorines, *Methods Find. Exp. Clin. Pharmacol.* **9:**605–610.

Vandenberg, S. A., Kulig, K., Spoerke, D. G., Hall, A. H., Bailie, V. J., and Rumack, B. H., 1988, Chlorambucil overdose: Accidental ingestion of an antineoplastic drug, *J. Emerg. Med.* **6:**495–498.

Wessel, G., Abendroth, K., and Wisheit, M., 1988, Malignant transformation during immunosuppressive therapy (azathioprine) of rheumatoid arthritis and systemic lupus erythematosus. A retrospective study, *Scand. J. Rheum.* **67:**73–75.

Williams, H. J., Reading, J. C., Ward, J. R., and O'Brien, W. M., 1980, Comparison of high and low dose cyclophosphamide therapy in rheumatoid arthritis, *Arthritis Rheum.* **23:**521–527.

Workman, P., Oppitz, M., Donaldson, J., and Lee, F. Y. F., 1987, High-performance liquid chromatography of chlorambucil analogues, *J. Chromatogr.* **422:**315–321.

Yager, J. W., Sorsa, M., and Selvin, S., 1988, Micronuclei in cytokinesis-blocked lymphocytes as an index of occupational exposure to alkylating cytostatic drugs, *IARC Sci. Publ.* **89:**213–216.

Chapter 12

CYCLOSPORIN A

Pharmacology and Therapeutic Use in Autoimmune Diseases

Gilles Feutren and *Beat von Graffenried*

1. INTRODUCTION

Cyclosporin A (CyA, Sandimmun®, Sandoz) is a potent immunosuppressive agent. First trials in human transplantation started in 1978, and since that time very wide experience has been gained in its use (Beveridge, 1986). It is now considered a reference treatment, especially for liver and heart transplantation.

On theoretical grounds, the mechanism of action of CyA in human autoimmune diseases is not as easy to understand as in organ transplantation (Di Padova, 1989). Whereas in transplantation CyA is given at the time of antigenic challenge, before the immune system is sensitized against the antigen, in autoimmune diseases CyA can only be administered while the abnormal immune reaction is already fully ongoing. However, despite the fact that CyA poorly inhibits differentiated T or B lymphocytes, the drug has proven to be effective as preventive or curative therapy in animal models, as well as in several autoimmune diseases in man. For this reason, not only may the efficacy of CyA contribute to improving the methods used against selected diseases but it may also provide new insights into their pathogenesis.

2. PHARMACOLOGICAL BASIS

2.1. Biochemistry and Pharmacology

Cyclosporin A is a cyclic, neutral, and hydrophobic polypeptide containing 11 amino acids. Its pharmacokinetic characteristics have been extensively studied (Kahan, 1985; Lemaire *et al.*, 1986). After a single oral dose, the peak blood concentration is achieved

Gilles Feutren and *Beat von Graffenried* • Clinical Research/Immunology, Sandoz Pharma Ltd., CH-4002 Basle, Switzerland.

Immunopharmacology in Autoimmune Diseases and Transplantation, edited by Hans Erik Rugstad *et al.* Plenum Press, New York, 1992.

after 2 to 6 hr. The bioavailability of the oral form is approximately 30%. The mechanisms of intestinal absorption remain unknown. Within the body, the drug accumulates in most of the tissues, mainly in the liver, kidneys, skin, and adipose tissue (Niederberger *et al.*, 1983). In the blood, 80% of CyA is associated with red cells. The remaining plasmatic fraction is mainly bound (90%) to proteins and lipoproteins.

The drug is eliminated in a biphasic manner with half-lives of 4–6 and 27 hr, respectively. Ninety-nine percent of CyA is metabolized by the liver, and metabolites are excreted in the bile. Less than 1% of the parent compound is excreted in the urine. At least ten metabolites have been identified in the blood. Some of them have a weak immunosuppressive activity, which is, however, clearly less potent than that of unchanged CyA (Ryffel *et al.*, 1988). CyA is extensively metabolized through the liver microsomal oxidative system involving the P 450 cytochromes. Drugs that interfere with this system may induce major changes in CyA pharmacokinetics by increasing the blood concentration (Table I), for example, ketoconazole, or decreasing the levels, for example, phenytoin or rifampicin (Cockburn and Krupp, 1989a).

2.2. Pharmacological Monitoring

Systematic measurement of CyA concentration in blood or plasma has been the rule since the first clinical trials in transplantation (Kahan, 1985). The method now recommended is the measurement of the trough (predose) concentration in whole blood by a method specific for the parent compound (HPLC or RIA, using a specific monoclonal antibody) (Critical issues in cyclosporine monitoring, 1987).

The aim of the pharmacological monitoring was initially to tailor the dosage for each patient in order to attain a therapeutic window in all cases. In autoimmune diseases, the therapeutic range is estimated between 100 to 200 ng/ml with respect to the whole blood trough level of the parent compound (specific measurement). But the level that may be necessary for achieving efficacy obviously differs according to many parameters, in particular the disease itself (e.g., very low dose, and therefore low levels are active in psoriasis), and combination or not with other immunosuppressants, especially steroids. Hence, no clear usefulness of CyA level monitoring has been shown in autoimmune disease, at variance with what is the rule in transplantation. Blood level monitoring remains, however, of interest in

TABLE I.   Pharmacokinetic Interactions with Cyclosporin A

Drugs decreasing SIM blood levels	Drugs increasing SIM blood levels	
Isoniazid	Acetazolamide	Methyltestosterone
Nafcillin	Amikacin	Metoclopramide
Octreotide	Danazol	Metronidazole
Phenobarbitone	Desogestrel-ethinylestradiol	Nicardipine
Phenytoin	Diltiazem	Norethisterone
Rifampicin	Erythromycin	Norfloxacin
Sulphadimidine	Imipenem	Pristinamycin
	Itraconazole	Sulindac
	Josamycin	Ticarcillin
	Ketoconazole	Tobramycin
	Levonorgestrel-ethinylestradiol	Verapamil

difficult cases, for example, to determine patient compliance to the treatment or to detect drug interactions.

2.3. Mechanism of Action

2.3.1. Immunosuppressive Properties

The main targets of CyA are the helper T lymphocytes, which are reversibly and quite selectively inhibited (Hess and Colombani, 1986). In contrast with other immunosuppressants such as azathioprine or cyclophosphamide, CyA is not cytotoxic at therapeutic doses and does not interfere with DNA metabolism. Consequently, it is not endowed with bone marrow toxicity or mutagenicity and does not induce lymphopenia.

The central point of impact of CyA seems to be the inhibition of lymphokine production, especially interleukin-2 (IL-2) but also other T-cell lymphokines such as gamma-interferon or B-cell growth factors (Fig. 12.1). This inhibition occurs at the nuclear level, where CyA prevents the IL-2 promoter-binding activity of transcription factors NF-AT and NF-kappaB. In all probability, CyA prevents the cytosolic component of these factors from translocating to the nucleus, hence preventing their binding to the DNA, which in turn inhibits IL-2 gene transcription (Emmel et al., 1989). This inhibition can be reversed by the addition of exogenous IL-2) (Fig. 12.1). The inhibition of helper T lymphocytes results in the complete abolishment of both cellular and humoral immune responses when the drug is given at the time of the first antigenic challenge. Conversely, when an immune activation preexists to the CyA administration, cytotoxic T lymphocytes that are already differentiated are not modified. However, the inhibition of lymphokine production may result in the disappearance of the inflammation. Through inhibition of gamma-interferon production,

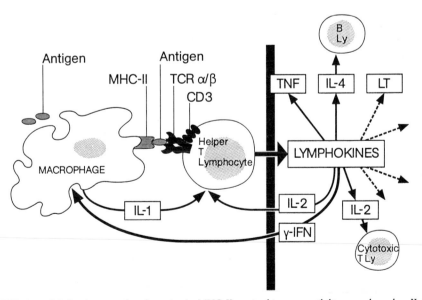

FIGURE 12.1. Mode of action of cyclosporin A. MHC-II, major histocompatibility complex, class II; TCR, T-cell receptor; IL, interleukin; γ-IFN, gamma interferon; TNF, tumor necrosis factor; LT, lymphotoxin; Ly, lymphocyte. The black bar represents the inhibitory action of CyA.

the expression of major histocompatibility antigens will also be diminished, thereby inhibiting both inducer and effector mechanisms (Autenried and Halloran, 1985).

In some conditions, CyA may inhibit B lymphocytes, mainly at an early stage of maturation. Furthermore, it inhibits the T/B cooperation required in the presence of T-dependent antigen. But, in most cases, CyA does not decrease a preestablished antibody production (Kunkl and Klaus, 1980).

In contrast to corticosteroids, CyA does not directly paralyze the functions of neutrophils or of macrophages (Janco and English, 1983). However, activation of macrophages is reduced, especially IL-1 secretion, mainly as a result of inhibition of macrophage-stimulating lymphokines at the T helper cell level (Thomson et al., 1983).

It is now established that CyA binds potently to a ubiquitous cytosolic protein, cyclophilin (Handschumacher et al., 1984), which is a folding enzyme (Fischer et al., 1989). In turn, the CyA–cyclophilin complex binds directly to calcineurin and potently inhibits its Ca^{2+} and calmodulin-stimulated serine–threonine phosphatase activity (McKeon, 1991). There is indirect evidence that the inhibition of the calcineurin phosphorylase activity may play a key role in the immunosuppressive properties of CyA.

2.3.2. Nonimmunosuppressive Properties

Nonimmunological effects of CyA on skin components such as increased B adrenergic adenylate cyclase activity in pig epidermis have been observed (Kato et al., 1988). CyA was also reported to have a direct inhibitory effect on animal or human keratinocyte proliferation *in vitro* and *in vivo*. This effect has been detected at concentrations similar to those found in the skin after oral administration of CyA in psoriatic patients (Nickoloff et al., 1988; Furue and Katz, 1988; Urabe et al., 1989).

3. ANIMAL MODELS OF AUTOIMMUNE DISEASES

The results of CyA treatment in animal models of autoimmunity correlate well with our knowledge of the mechanism of action of the drug (reviewed in Borel and Gunn, 1986) because it is more effective on T-cell-mediated than on B-cell-mediated diseases.

3.1. Preventive Treatment

Experimental autoimmune diseases induced by the injection of purified autoantigen were in most cases completely prevented by the administration of CyA given at the time of antigen injection. This is the case for T-cell-mediated diseases such as rat arthritis induced by Freund's adjuvant (Borel et al., 1976) or type II collagen sensitization, rat uveitis following the injection of retinal S antigen (Nussenblatt et al., 1981), or experimental allergic encephalomyelitis following immunization against the encephalitogenic basic protein (Bolton et al., 1982). Cyclosporine also prevented the appearance of autoantibodies and the related diseases such as experimental myasthenia gravis (Drachman et al., 1985), Heyman's nephritis, acute serum sickness of the rabbit, and autoimmune hemolytic anemia of the mouse. In some cases, short-term CyA treatment resulted in the long-term prevention of the disease, and in the uveitis model it was possible to demonstrate the existence of antigen-specific suppressor T cells.

Similar features were found in spontaneous models of autoimmune diseases. The continuous administration of CyA before the age of onset of the disease resulted in the prevention of insulin-dependent diabetes mellitus (IDDM) in the BB rat (Laupacis *et al.*, 1983) or NOD mouse (Mori *et al.*, 1986) and of systemic lupus in (NZB × W) F1 (Israel-Biet *et al.*, 1983) or MLR 1pr/1pr mice (Mountz *et al.*, 1987). On the other hand, no effect was detected in spontaneous thyroiditis of the obese chicken (Wick *et al.*, 1982), which is a purely B-lymphocyte-mediated disease since it is prevented by bursectomy and not by thymectomy.

3.2. Curative Treatment

The effect of CyA given as a curative treatment in cases of established autoimmune diseases is less clear-cut. Even when it is effective, as in the cases of T-lymphocyte-mediated diseases, the effect is sometimes difficult to demonstrate if the active immunological aggression results in irreversible lesions that do not have any chance to improve, even when the immunological process is stopped by CyA. This was obviously the case for IDDM in the BB rat or NOD mouse.

In most diseases directly mediated by autoantibodies, once they are established CyA has no effect either on autoantibody levels or on the symptoms or the lesions, as shown in myasthenia gravis. The case is more complicated in MLR 1pr/1pr lupus mice (Mountz *et al.*, 1987). CyA administration resulted in histologically proven improvement of joints, kidneys, and lymph nodes, although humoral abnormalities (anti-DNA antibodies, immune complexes, rheumatoid factor, immunoglobulin levels) remained unchanged. This suggests that in some diseases known to be antibody-mediated, CyA-sensitive cellular immune effectors may be involved and lead to clinical improvement.

4. CLINICAL TRIALS IN AUTOIMMUNE DISEASES

After the superiority of CyA immunosuppression had been demonstrated over conventional therapy in organ transplantation, it appeared logical to start clinical trials in autoimmune diseases. Clinical indications were selected on the basis of the experimental results in animal models of autoimmunity and on the medical need, as therapy was still unsatisfactory in some indications.

At the present time, the efficacy and the clinical benefit have been demonstrated for severely affected patients in four diseases: rheumatoid arthritis, autoimmune uveitis, idiopathic nephrotic syndrome, and psoriasis (Table II).

4.1. Rheumatoid Arthritis

The first attempt for treating arthritic patients with CyA was in 1978 (Herrmann and Müller, 1979), when appreciable improvement was obtained in five of six patients treated with CyA for up to ten months.

In uncontrolled studies with a CyA dose of 5 to 10 mg/kg per day, dose-dependent improvements were reported in pain and morning stiffness by between 43–87% of patients, joint tenderness (Ritchie or ARA joint index) by 38–67%, and grip strength by 15–98%, with an average "responder rate" by 70% (Weinblatt *et al.*, 1987; Førre *et al.*, 1987; Dougados *et al.*, 1987). The reduction of concomitant steroid dosage reported in some studies suggests the possible use of the drug in a "steroid-sparing" capacity. Cessation of treatment in

TABLE II. Autoimmune Diseases in Which the Efficacy of Cyclosporin A Has Been Proved

Proven efficacy		Uncertain efficacy	Under study
Proven benefit	Questionable benefit		
Rheumatoid arthritis	Myasthenia gravis	Endocrine ophthalmopathy	Primary biliary cirrhosis
Severe psoriasis	Insulin-dependent diabetes	Sjögren syndrome	Severe aplastic anemia
Idiopathic nephrotic	mellitus		Multiple sclerosis
syndrome	Crohn's disease		
Autoimmune uveitis	Atopic dermatitis		
	Primary biliary cirrhosis		
	Severe aplastic anemia		

responsive patients was followed by recurrence of symptoms within two to ten weeks in most of them.

This positive effect of CyA was confirmed in three double-blind studies (van Rijthoven *et al.*, 1986; Dougados *et al.*, 1988; Tugwell *et al.*, 1990). On 5 mg/kg per day CyA, the overall responder rate was 54% on CyA and 7% on placebo. Interestingly, this clinical effect was observed despite the absence of change in ESR, rheumatoid factor, or immunoglobulin concentration. However, even if CyA is efficacious in the treatment of active rheumatoid arthritis, its place in the hierarchy of drug treatment in RA still remains to be determined.

4.2. Autoimmune Uveitis

The most frequently studied subgroups of endogenous uveitis were Behçet's disease, involving the posterior segment of the eye, "idiopathic" uveitis, pars planitis, retinal vasculitis, Vogt–Koyanagi–Harada uveitis, birdshot chorioretinopathy, and sarcoid uveitis. Patients included in trials with CyA were suffering from severe sight-threatening uveitis (Nussenblatt *et al.*, 1983; Ben Ezra *et al.*, 1988; Le Hoang *et al.*, 1988). CyA was given at an initial loading dose of 5 to 10 mg/kg per day followed by a dose reduction according to ocular inflammatory activity and tolerability. Improvement of intraocular inflammation and visual acuity was observed in over 60% of patients within the first two to four weeks. However, in many cases relapses of the inflammatory processes have been observed when rapid discontinuation of CyA has been attempted.

In Behçet's disease with ocular involvement, CyA had a remarkable therapeutic effect on the intraocular inflammatory process, prolonging the periods of remission and therapy arresting the inevitable gradual loss of vision (Ben Ezra, 1986). This effect was confirmed by a double-masked trial of 4-month duration where 48% of the patients responded well to CyA compared to 13% of responders in the control group who received colchicine (Masuda *et al.*, 1989). The beneficial effects on the systemic manifestations of the disease, however, were less obvious and may require combining CyA with low-dose steroids. Detailed treatment guidelines have been published (Ben Ezra, 1988).

4.3. Idiopathic Nephrotic Syndrome

Idiopathic nephrotic syndrome (NS) (hypoalbuminemia due to massive proteinuria with edema) includes minimal-change nephropathy (MCN) and focal-segmental glomerulosclerosis (FSGS). The empirical treatment of this heterogeneous patient group consists primarily of corticosteroids, which are very effective, especially in MCN. Steroid-resistant patients and steroid-sensitive patients with frequent relapses and/or those who relapse during tapering off of steroids (steroid-dependent) are subgroups in need of alternate therapy. Immunosuppression with alkylating agents is used in such problem patients with relatively good results in children and steroid-dependent NS, the majority of which is MCN. However, much poorer results are obtained in FSGS.

Clinical studies with CyA in idiopathic NS (reviewed by Meyrier, 1989) have been performed almost exclusively in either steroid-resistant (mostly FSGS) or steroid-dependent patients (mostly MCN), in adults (Meyrier et al., 1986; van Hooff et al., 1988), and in children (Tejani et al., 1988; Niaudet et al., 1988; Brodehl et al., 1988). Many of these patients were also resistant to alkylating agents. In steroid-dependent idiopathic NS, the starting dose of CyA averaged 6 mg/kg per day in children and 5 mg/kg per day in adults. Treatment duration ranged from 3 to 24 months. Complete remission was reported in over 80% of patients after a median duration of treatment of two months. In the majority of these patients, steroid-induced remissions could be maintained by CyA despite the withdrawal of steroids. In steroid-resistant idiopathic NS, complete remissions were achieved in 27% and partial remissions in an additional 27% of cases. CyA-induced remissions were usually achieved within the first three to six months, that is, clearly less rapidly than in steroid-dependent NS. After CyA was discontinued, most of the patients relapsed in a few weeks. The lowest, still effective dose seems to be quite individually variable.

The side effect profile of CyA in NS is similar to that in other autoimmune diseases. However, several patients with FSGS, especially if renal function was abnormal at the start of CyA therapy, showed marked deterioration of renal function, which in some cases did not improve on discontinuation of CyA. It is difficult to assess whether this was due to CyA or to the natural course of the disease.

Renal biopsies have been performed in 42 patients after 2–18 months of continuous CyA therapy. In one series (Niaudet et al., 1988), slight to moderate changes suggestive of CyA nephrotoxicity were reported in 5 of 22 biopsies in children, whereas no relevant changes were reported in other series. In some biopsies, progression of FSGS was recorded despite CyA therapy.

Many questions relating to the optimal use of CyA in NS remain open. Despite this, it appears that CyA can provide benefit for steroid-sensitive patients with steroid toxicity and that therapeutic testing of CyA can be considered in steroid-resistant NS.

4.4. Psoriasis

It is unclear whether the hyperproliferative epidermis, which is the hallmark of psoriasis, represents a primary defect in keratinocyte growth regulation or is of immunological origin. The clinical effect of CyA in psoriasis, which was detected by pure chance (Müller and Herrmann, 1979) in patients treated with CyA in a trial in psoriatic arthropathy, gives ground to the latter hypothesis.

Studies have been conducted in patients with severe, generalized chronic plaque-form psoriasis. Most of them had long-standing disease and had been treated previously with either PUVA, methotrexate, or/and retinoids. In placebo-controlled studies, a remission ($\geq$ 75% improvement) was observed in 55% of the patients after only four weeks' CyA treatment at a dose of 5 mg/kg per day versus 3% only on placebo (van Joost et al., 1988; Ellis et al., 1991). In dose-finding studies, a clear dose–response remission rate was observed.

After three months of treatment, remission rate was 25–30% on 1.25 mg/kg per day CyA, 50% on 2.5 mg/kg per day, and 90–95% on 5 mg/kg per day (Timonen et al., 1990). The efficacy of low doses is especially interesting, since renal tolerance is clearly better. Unfortunately, most patients brought into remission have relapsed within two to ten weeks after therapy is withdrawn (Higgins et al., 1989). Four months after stopping therapy, approximately 25% of the patients are still in remission. This indicates that most patients need continued therapy of psoriasis with doses of CyA as low as possible. However, in a small cohort of patients, discontinuous therapy may be an option and each patient should be evaluated individually in this respect.

4.5. Other Autoimmune Diseases

4.5.1. Insulin-Dependent Diabetes Mellitus

The hypothesis that autoimmune mechanisms are involved in the destruction of pancreatic beta cells in insulin-dependent diabetes mellitis (IDDM) (Eisenbarth, 1986; Bach, 1988) and the observation that immune intervention with CyA is capable of modifying the natural course of the disease in animal models have led to an exciting new era in clinical research on IDDM. The problem of immune intervention in IDDM is that extensive beta cell destruction has already occurred at the time of clinical diagnosis. The aim is to prevent the autoimmune destruction of the few remaining beta cells.

Two double-blind randomized studies (Feutren et al., 1986; Canadian-European Randomized Control Group Trial, 1988) have confirmed the initial pilot study data in adults (Stiller et al., 1984; Assan et al., 1985): with CyA doses of 7.5–10 mg/kg per day significantly more patients attained complete remission (defined as good metabolic control without exogenous insulin) at 12 months than patients treated with placebo—17–32% on CyA versus 0–10% on placebo. Clinical remission in CyA-treated patients was associated with a sustained increase in the endogenous secretion of insulin as assessed by C-peptide measurements.

The major problem in all patient series was that clinical remissions were progressively lost even on continuous CyA therapy. It is obviously very difficult to assess the risk benefit ratio of CyA in IDDM, and therefore such therapy must still be regarded as experimental procedure only justified within a limited number of controlled clinical trials (Rubenstein and Pyke, 1987).

4.5.2. Gastroenterology, Hepatology

Results of several pilot studies in Crohn's disease suggested that oral doses of CyA ranging from 5 to 15 mg/kg per day are effective in most, but not all, patients with chronic active disease, but a rapid relapse was seen after stopping therapy. The efficacy of CyA in chronic active Crohn's disease was confirmed by a placebo-controlled study where 6 mg/kg per day CyA was associated with a success rate of 59% versus 32% on placebo after three months of treatment (Brynskov et al., 1989).

Positive results have been published in a small number of patients with ulcerative colitis (Lichtiger et al., 1990).

Considerably more clinical research is ongoing in primary biliary cirrhosis. As early as 1980, an improved liver function has been reported in six patients receiving 5 to 10 mg/kg per day of CyA, but substantial toxicity occurred (Routhier et al., 1980). A placebo-controlled study in 29 patients has confirmed the improvement of clinical symptoms and the decrease of laboratory liver abnormalities after one year of treatment (Wiesner *et al.*, 1990). A large placebo-controlled, long-term study (more than 300 patients followed for two to five years) is ongoing with the aim of evaluating whether disease progression can be influenced.

4.5.3. Neurology

Three double-blind, randomized studies have been completed in multiple sclerosis. Two trials compared CyA to placebo (Rudge *et al.*, 1989; The Multiple Sclerosis Study Group, 1990) and the other CyA to azathioprine (Kappos *et al.*, 1988). Treatment duration was two years. No relevant difference between both groups was detected in the incidence of relapses or in the rate of progression of the disease in either study.

A placebo-controlled study in patients with progressively worsening generalized myasthenia gravis (MG), who had not yet been treated with thymectomy, steroids, or other immunosuppressants, showed that patients on CyA (6 mg/kg per day) had significantly more improvement in strength after six months of therapy than patients on placebo (Tindall *et al.*, 1987). More studies are needed to define more clearly the potential of CyA in MG and to define its place in relation to corticosteroids and azathioprine. It is of interest that in most responders the titers of antiacetylcholine receptor antibodies did not fall.

4.5.4. Hematology

In several very limited series of patients with severe aplastic anemia treated with CyA the response rate on CyA seemed to be similar to that reported with antilymphocyte globulins (ALG). It is interesting that some nonresponders to ALG went into remission on CyA. Full efficacy was mostly obtained within the first three months. Relapses occurred frequently within three months of stopping CyA. A further randomized study was comparing the combination of CyA and ALG alone (Frickhofen *et al.*, 1991). After three months, 7 of 15 patients (47%) responded to ALG and 15 of 20 patients (75%) to CyA plus ALG. Too-limited numbers of patients have been treated with CyA in other hematological autoimmune diseases to allow a definitive conclusion concerning efficacy.

4.5.5. Varia

Improvement or steroid-sparing effect was reported in three open studies with CyA in systemic lupus erythematosus (SLE). In two of them, which included a total of 54 patients, CyA dose was 5 mg/kg per day (Feutren *et al.*, 1987; Miescher *et al.*, 1988). No relevant changes were found in anti-DNA titers. Hypertension and reversible renal dysfunction were the most serious side effects. The available experience with CyA in SLE is still quite limited. However, it seems that steroid sparing could be an important benefit of CyA therapy in this disease. In Sjögren's disease, 5 mg/kg per day CyA did not exert relevant clinical effects in a placebo-controlled study (Drosos *et al.*, 1986). Several investigators have studied CyA in severe, mostly therapy-resistant cases of Graves' ophthalmopathy. The results were quite varied, with some publications reporting excellent subjective and objective improvements (Weetmann *et al.*, 1983) and some without apparent effect (Brabant *et al.*, 1984). Case reports have been published on Wegener's granulomatosis, pulmonary sarcoidosis due to immune hepatitis, male autoimmune infertility, relapsing polychondritis, giant cell arteritis, and myocarditis.

In addition to psoriasis (mentioned above), CyA has been administered in further dermatological autoimmune diseases: dermatomyositis (Heckmatt *et al.*, 1989), bullous pemphigoid, pemphigus, pyoderma gangrenosum, and alopecia areata. The results are more convincing in severe atopic dermatitis (Van Joost *et al.*, 1987; Sowden *et al.*, 1991). Finally, despite some positive results CyA should be contraindicated in scleroderma because of the risk of unpredictable severe acute renal failure.

5. ADVERSE EVENTS

The side effect profile of CyA in autoimmune diseases is similar to the one extensively reported in transplant patients (von Graffenried and Krupp, 1986).

5.1. Infections

Infections have been surprisingly infrequent and followed an uncomplicated course. In long-term controlled studies in diabetes and multiple sclerosis, the frequency of urinary, skin, and respiratory tract infections was not significantly higher in CyA-treated patients than in those on placebo (Feutren *et al.*, 1986; Canadian–European Randomized Control Trial Group, 1988).

5.2. Lymphoproliferative Disorders

As of December 1991, malignant non-Hodgkin's lymphomas had developed in 3 out of about 3,700 patients treated for autoimmune diseases (data on file, Sandoz): two B-cell lymphomas and one T-cell lymphoma. The mechanism of induction of B lymphomas is well known. They are not specific of CyA therapy since the drug is not mutagenic, but they are associated with immunosuppression and the Epstein-Barr virus (EBV). Pronounced immunosuppression blocks anti-EBV cytotoxic T-lymphocyte response and subsequently facilitates the uncontrolled overproliferation of EBV-infected B lymphocytes. After a period of polyclonal B-lymphocyte proliferation, reversible if immunosuppression is stopped, a malignant clone may subsequently arise, resulting in irreversible widespreading monoclonal malignant B lymphoma.

The Sandoz Postmarketing Surveillance Study has shown in over 4,000 prospectively followed transplant patients on CyA that the incidence of lymphomas developing is the same as that in patients with other forms of immunosuppression (Cockburn and Krupp, 1989b).

5.3. Renal Dysfunction

The side effects that most limit the therapeutic potential of CyA are renal dysfunctional and structural changes in the kidney. It is useful to separate functional alteration from chronic histological alteration. Impairment of renal dysfunction is characterized by a reduction in the renal plasma flow and subsequently in the glomerular filtration rate. The main laboratory abnormalities are increases in serum creatinine and urea. Increase in potassium and uric acid, as well as decrease in serum magnesium, may also occur in relation with an impairment of tubular function. Often, however, the changes remain within the "normal" range.

Renal dysfunction has been analyzed in large numbers of autoimmune patients (Dieterle *et al.*, 1988). In this study, a dose-dependent drop in renal function started within the first two weeks of CyA therapy and it reached a nadir around month 6. At this time, the mean decrease of calculated creatinine clearance was 17% from baseline. There was no significant further decline, indicating that the functional disturbance is not progressive for up to two years of continuous therapy. Renal dysfunction is worsened by concomitant medication with nephrotoxic compounds, including nonsteroidal anti-inflammatory drugs (Ludwin *et al.*, 1988). Renal dysfunction is reversible. It is the general experience that serum creatinine drops within one to two weeks after dose reduction or termination of therapy. In most patients complete recovery is attained within 12 weeks after termination of CyA therapy, but in a minority baseline values are not reached completely. The more pronounced the impairment of renal function was, the more probable the incomplete return to baseline renal function.

5.4. Cyclosporin Nephropathy

More relevant than functional and reversible renal dysfunction are the histological lesions that have been found in renal biopsies of CyA-treated autoimmune patients. CyA nephropathy has been described as a combination of arteriolopathy, acellular interstitial fibrosis (striped form), and tubular atrophy within areas of fibrosis (Mihatsch, 1985). Results of over 200 renal biopsies are available in IDDM, SLE, rheumatoid arthritis, uveitis, nephrotic syndrome, and various other diseases. More than "minimal" or "slight" lesions (which cannot be attributed with certainty to CyA) were found in 47 of 210 (22%) patients, with reported frequencies ranging from 0 to 100% (Palestine *et al.*, 1986; Miescher *et al.*, 1987; Feutren, 1988). This large variation is most likely due to the quite different treatment dosages used. In a group of 192 biopsied patients (Feutren and Mihatsch, 1992), maximal creatinine increase was 101% $\pm$ 77 (mean $\pm$ SD) in the subset of patients with relevant histological lesions, whereas it was 50% $\pm$ 33 in the group with normal biopsies or with minor changes only ($p < 0.01$). In patients on CyA in whom the maximal serum creatinine level was double the baseline value, lesions were found in 15 of 26 (59%) compared to only 3 of 42 (7%) patients in whom creatinine was never increased by more than 30% above baseline. Based on these data, it appeared that the risk of developing relevant histological lesions in the kidney was low when the dose of CyA was not greater than 5 mg/kg per day and when the dose was adjusted in such a way as to avoid increases of serum creatinine greater than 30% over patients' own baseline. The safety of this approach was confirmed by a series of 43 patients with SLE and rheumatoid arthritis and in 14 patients with psoriasis (Miescher *et al.*, 1987; International Kidney Biopsy Registry, 1990) treated with low doses (3–5 mg/kg per day) in whom only very discrete impairment of renal function and no CyA-induced renal pathological lesions were found.

5.5. Other Adverse Events

The cause of the frequently observed hypertrichosis is unknown; there is no clinical or laboratory evidence for an endocrine origin. Gingival hyperplasia, due to fibrous hyperplasia, is rarely seen on low-dose CyA. It has been suggested that CyA-induced hypomagnesemia, a quite frequent finding, is responsible for some of the neurological side effects (Thompson *et al.*, 1984). However, tremor and paresthesia (often expressed as a feeling of heat), which are frequent during the first weeks of treatment, very often disappear thereafter without change of dose despite persistent hypomagnesemia. The same is true for slight increases in serum bilirubin. Only rarely did this side effect require discontinuation of treatment. A mild normochromic normocytic anemia with a reduction in hemoglobin of about 1 g/dl has been observed in several studies. This effect may be due to the inhibition of lymphokines regulating erythropoiesis. In most patients the intensity of these side effects was only slight or moderate. Of 938 patients included in various studies, the withdrawal rates because of side effects were 4% in diabetes, 6% in multiple sclerosis, 12% in uveitis, and 22% in rheumatoid arthritis. By far the most frequent reason for withdrawal was gastrointestinal symptoms. Renal dysfunction was the reason for drug withdrawal in only 27 of 938 patients (3%) (Table III).

In 11% of 321 treated patients, mild to moderate hypertension developed within the first six months of CyA therapy (Dieterle et al., 1988). If therapy was required, conventional treatment of various kinds was successful. In the light of experimental data, calcium channel inhibitors not interfering with CyA pharmacokinetics, such as isradipidine or nifedipine, should be tried first. There was a significant association between the extent of renal dysfunction and hypertension.

6. CONCLUSIONS

This chapter illustrates that cyclosporin A is efficacious in many autoimmune diseases, both for the induction and the maintenance of remission. Efficacy has been established in randomized controlled studies in rheumatoid arthritis, uveitis, psoriasis and atopic dermatitis, nephrotic syndrome, Crohn's disease, insulin-dependent diabetes mellitus, primary biliary cirrhosis, severe aplastic anemia, and myasthenia gravis. Convincing evidence of efficacy was demonstrated in uncontrolled trials in systemic lupus erythematosus and various hematological and dermatological autoimmune diseases.

Common features of the clinical effects of CyA are the relatively quick onset of effect (2–12 weeks, dependent on dose) and the occurrence of relapses when treatment is stopped. These facts are presumably linked to the rapid onset and reversibility of the inhibitory effect of CyA on lymphokine secretion. The autoimmune reaction is temporarily "frozen" without abrogation of the intrinsic autoimmune defect.

Guidelines have now been established to administer CyA in such a way as to minimize

TABLE III.   Adverse Drug Reactions of CyA
(Dose ≤6 mg/kg per day) in Autoimmune Diseases

	Psoriasis (n = 631)	Nephrotic syndrome (n = 661)	Rheumatoid arthritis (n = 378)
Discontinuation because of			
Renal dysfunction	1.9%	3.7%	6.1%
Hypertension	1.0%	0.6%	2.9%
Other	4.5%	3.1%	20.6%
Hypertension[a]	12.0%	14.0%	15.0%
CyA nephropathy	risk < 5.0%	risk < 5.0%	risk < 5.0%
Malignancies			
Lymphoma	risk ≤ 0.1%	risk ≤ 0.1%	risk ≤ 0.1%
Squamous cell carcinoma	1.0%	0%	0%
Kaposi sarcoma	0%	0%	0%

[a]WHO/ISH definition of mild hypertension.

the risk of irreversible functional or structural renal damage. Initial doses of CyA should not exceed 5 mg/kg per day (except in life-threatening emergency situations). The dose should be reduced whenever serum creatinine increases by more than 30–50% over baseline. If such "conservative" dosages do not lead to an optimal therapeutic result, it might be better to consider combining CyA with other immunosuppressive agents, for example, steroids, rather than increasing the dose.

ACKNOWLEDGMENTS. The authors thank Drs. D. Friend, W. Schiess, N. Shand, and P. Timonen for their kind collaboration, and Mrs. P. Isenring for her expert secretarial help.

REFERENCES

Assan, R., Feutren, G., Debray-Sachs, M., Quiniou-Debrie, M. C., Laborie, C.,. Thomas, G., Chatenoud, M., and Bach, J. F., 1985, Metabolic and immunological effects of cyclosporin in recently diagnosed type 1 diabetes mellitus, *Lancet* 1:67–71.

Autenried, P., and Halloran, P. F., 1985, Cyclosporine blocks the induction of Class I and Class II MHC products in mouse kidney by Graft-VS-Host disease, *J. Immunol.* 135:3922–3928.

Bach, J. F., 1988, Mechanisms of autoimmunity in insulin-dependent diabetes mellitus, *Clin. Exp. Immunol.* 72:1–8.

Ben Ezra, D., 1986, Cyclosporin A in Behçet's disease—An overview, in: *Recent Advances in Behçet's Disease* (T. Lehner and C. G. Barnes, eds.), Royal Society of Medical Service, London, pp. 319–325.

Ben Ezra, D., Cohen, E., Rakotomalala, M., de Courten, C., Harris, W., Chajek, T., Friedman, G., and Matamoros, N., 1988a, Treatment of endogenous uveitis with cyclosporin A, *Transplant. Proc.* 20(Suppl. 4):122–127.

Ben Ezra, D., Nussenblatt, R. B., and Timonen, P. (eds.), 1988b, Optimal use of Sandimmun® in endogenous uveitis, Springer-Verlag, Berlin.

Beveridge, T., 1986, Clinical transplantation—Overview, *Prog. Allergy* 38:269–292.

Bolton, C., Borel, J. F., Cuzner, M. L., Davison, A. N., and Turner, A. M., 1982, Immunosuppression by cyclosporin A of experimental allergic encephalomyelitis, *J. Neurol. Sci.* 56:147–153.

Borel, J. F., and Gunn, H., 1986, Cyclosporine as a new approach to therapy, *Ann. NY Acad. Sci.* 475:307–319.

Borel, J. F., Feurer, C., Gubler, H. U., and Stähelin, H., 1976, Biological effects of cyclosporin A: A new antilymphocyte agent, *Agents Actions* 6:468–475.

Brabant, G., Peter, H., Becker, H., Schwarzrock, R., Wonigeit, K., and Hesch, R. D., 1984, Cyclosporine in infiltrative eye disease, *Lancet* 1:515–516.

Brodehl, J., Hoyer, P. F., Oemar, B. S., Helmchen, U., and Wonigeit, K., 1988, Cyclosporin treatment of nephrotic syndrome in children, *Transplant. Proc.* 20(Suppl. 4):269–274.

Brynskov, J., Freund, L., Rasmussen, S. N., Lauritsen, K., Schaffalitsky de Muckadell, O., Williams, N., MacDonald, A. S., Tanton, R., Molina, F., Campanini, M. C., Bianchi, P., Ranzi, T., Quarto di Palo, F., Malchow-Moller, A., Thomsen, O. O., Tage-Jensen, U., Binder, V., and Riis, P., 1989, A placebo-controlled, double-blind randomized trial of cyclosporine therapy in active chronic Crohn's disease, *N. Engl. J. Med.* 321:845–850.

Canadian–European Randomized Control Trial Group, 1988, Induction of remission of type 1 diabetes mellitus by cyclosporin is dependent on early intervention and associated with maintained enhancement of insulin secretion through one year of treatment, *Diabetes* 37:1574–1582.

Cockburn, I., and Krupp, P., 1989a, An appraisal of drug interactions with Sandimmun®, *Transplant Proc.* 21:3845–3850.

Cockburn, I. T. R., and Krupp, P., 1989b, The risk of neoplasms in patients treated with cyclosporine, *J. Autoimmunity* 2:723–731.

Critical issues in cyclosporin monitoring: Report on the task force on cyclosporin monitoring, 1987, *Clin. Chem.* 33:1269–1288.

Dieterle, A., Abeywickrama, K., and von Graffenried, B., 1988, Nephrotoxicity and hypertension in patients with autoimmune diseases treated with cyclosporine, *Transplant Proc.* 20(Suppl. 4):349–355.

DiPadova, F., 1989, Pharmacology of cyclosporine (Sandimmune). Pharmacological effect on immune function: *In vitro* studies, *Pharmacol. Rev.* 41:373–405.

Dougados, M., Amor, B., 1987, Cyclosporin A in rheumatoid arthritis: Preliminary clinical results of an open trial, *Arthritis Rheum.* 30:83–87.

Dougados, M., Awada, H., and Amor, B., 1988, Cyclosporin in rheumatoid arthritis: A double-blind controlled study in 52 patients, *Ann. Rheum. Dis.* 47:127–133.

Drachman, D. B., Adams, R. N., McKintosh, K., Pestrank, A., 1985, Treatment of experimental myasthenia gravis with cyclosporin A, *Clin. Immunol. Immunopathol.* 34:174–188.

Drosos, A. A., Skopouli, F. N., Costopoulos, J. S., Papadimitriou, C. S., and Moutsopoulos, M. H., 1986, Cyclosporin A in primary Sjögren's syndrome: A double-blind study, *Ann. Rheum. Dis.* 45:731–735.

Eisenbarth, G. S., 1986, Type 1 diabetes mellitus. A chronic autoimmune disease, *N. Engl. J. Med.* 314:1360–1368.

Ellis, C. N., Fradin, M. S., Messana, J. M., Brown, M. D., Siegel, M. T., Hartley, A. H., Rocher, L. L., Wheeler, S., Hamilton, T. A., Parish, T. G., Ellis-Madu, M., Duell, E., Annesley, T. M., Cooper, K. D., and Voorhees, J. J., 1991, Cyclosporine for plaque-type psoriasis: Results of a multidose, double-blind trial, *N. Engl. J. Med.* 324:277–284.

Emmel, E. A., Verweij, C. L., Durand, D. B., Higgins, K. M., Lacy, E., and Crabtree, G. R., 1989, Cyclosporine A specifically inhibits function of nuclear proteins involved in T cell activation, *Science* 246:1617–1620.

Feutren, G., 1988, Functional consequences and risk factors of chronic cyclosporin nephrotoxicity in type 1 diabetes trials, *Transplant. Proc.* **20**(Suppl. 4):356–366.

Feutren, G., and Mihatsch, M. J., 1992, Risk factors for cyclosporine-induced nephropathy in patients with autoimmune diseases, *N. Engl. J. Med.* **326**:1654–1660.

Feutren, G., Papoz, L., Assan, R., Vialettes, B., Karsenty, G., Vexiau, P., Du Rostu, H., Rodier, M., Sirmai, J., Lallemand, A., and Bach, J. F., 1986, Cyclosporine increases the rate and length of remissions in insulin-dependent diabetes of recent onset, *Lancet* **2**:119–124.

Feutren, G., Querin, S., Noel, L. H., Chatenoud, L., Beaurain, G., Tron, F., Lesavre, P., and Bach, J. F., 1987, Effects of cyclosporine in severe systemic lupus erythematosus, *J. Pediatr.* **111**:1063–1068.

Fischer, G., Wittmann-Liebold, B., Lang, K., Kiefhaber, T., and Schmid, F. X., 1989, Cyclophilin and peptidyl-prolyl *cis-trans* isomerase are probably identical proteins, *Nature* **337**:476–478.

Førre, O., Bjerkjoel, F., Salversen, G. F., Berg, K. J., Rugstad, H. E., Saelid, G., Mellbye, O. J., and Käss, E., 1987, An open, controlled, randomized comparison of cyclosporine and azathioprine in the treatment of rheumatoid arthritis: A preliminary report, *Arthritis Rheum.* **30**:88–92.

Frickhofen, N., Kaltwasser, J. P., Schrezenmeier, H., *et al.*, 1991, Treatment of aplastic anemia with antilymphocyte globulin and methylprednisolone with or without cyclosporine, *N. Engl. J. Med.* **324**:1297–1304.

Furue, M., and Katz, S. I., 1988, The effect of cyclosporine on epidermal cells. I. Cyclosporine inhibits accessory cell function of epidermal Langerhans cells *in vitro*, *J. Immunol.* **140**:4139–4143.

Heckmatt, J., Hasson, N., Saunders, C., Thompson, N., Peters, A. M., Cambridge, G., Rose, M., Hyde, S. A., and Dubowitz, V., 1989, Cyclosporin in juvenile dermatomyositis, *Lancet* **1**:1063–1066.

Handschumacher, R. E., Harding, M. W., Rice, J., and Drugge, R. J., 1984, Cyclophilin: A specific cytosolic binding protein for cyclosporin A, *Science* **226**:544–547.

Herrmann, B., and Müller, W., 1979, Die Therapie der chronischen Polyarthritis mit Cyclosporin A, einem neuen Immunosuppressivum, *Akt. Rheumatol.* **4**:173–186.

Hess, A. D., and Colombani, P. M., 1986, Mechanism of action of cyclosporin: *In vitro* studies, *Prog. Allergy* **38**:198–221.

Higgins, E., Munro, C., Marks, J., Friedmann, P. S., and Shuster, S., 1989, Relapse rates in moderately severe chronic psoriasis treated with cyclosporin A, *Br. J. Dermatol.* **121**:71–74.

International Kidney Biopsy Registry of Cyclosporine A (Sandimmun®) in Autoimmune Diseases, 1990, Kidney biopsies in control or cyclosporin A-treated psoriatic patients, *Br. J. Dermatol.* **122**(Suppl. 36):95–100.

Israel-Biet, D., Noel, L. H., Bach, M. A., Dardenne, M., and Bach, J. F., 1983, Marked reduction of DNA antibody production and glomerulopathy in thymulin (FTS-Zn) or cyclosporin A treated NZB × NZW) F1 mice, *Clin. Exp. Immunol.* **54**:359–563.

Janco, R. L., and English, D., 1983, Cyclosporin and human neutrophil function, *Transplantation* **35**:501–503.

Kahan, B. D., 1985, Individualization of cyclosporine therapy using pharmacokinetic and pharmacodynamic parameters, *Transplantation* **40**:457–476.

Kappos, L., Patzold, U., Dommasch, D., Poser, S., Haas, J., Krauseneck, P., Malin, J. P., Fierz, W., von Graffenried, B., and Gugerli, U. S., 1988, Cyclosporin vs. azathioprine in the long-term treatment of multiple sclerosis—results of the German multicenter study, *Ann. Neurol.* **23**:56–63.

Kato, N., Halprin, K. M., Taylor, J. R., Ohkawara, A., 1988, Cyclosporin A induced augmentation of the beta-adrenergic adenylate cyclase response of pig epidermis, *Arch. Dermatol. Res.*, **280**:89–92.

Kunkl, A., and Klaus, G. G. B., 1980, Selective effects of cyclosporin A on functional cell subsets in the mouse, *J. Immunol.* **125**:2526–2531.

Laupacis, A., Stiller, C. R., Gardell, C., Keown, P., Dupré, J., Wallace, A. C., and Thibert, P., 1983, Cyclosporin prevents diabetes in BB Wistar rats, *Lancet* **1**:10–12.

Le Hoang, P., Girard, B., Deray, G., Le Minh, H., de Kozak, Y., Thillaye, B., Faure, J. P., and Rousselie, F., 1988, Cyclosporine in the treatment of birdshot retinochoroidopathy, *Transplant. Proc.* **20**(Suppl. 4):128–130.

Lemaire, M., Maurer, G., and Wood, A. J., 1986, Pharmacokinetics and metabolism, *Prog. Allergy* **38**:93–107.

Lichtiger, S., and Present, D. H. 1990, Preliminary report: Cyclosporin in treatment of severe active ulcerative colitis, *Lancet* **336**:16–19.

Ludwin, D., Bennett, K. J., Grau, E. M., Buchanan, W. W., Bensen, W., Bombardier, C., and Tugwell, P. X., 1988, Nephrotoxicity in patients with rheumatoid arthritis treated with cyclosporine, *Transplant Proc.* **20**(Suppl. 4):367–370.

Masuda, K., Nakajima, A., Urayama, A., Nakae, K., Kogure, M., and Inaba, G., 1989, Double-masked trial of cyclosporin versus colchicine and long-term open study of cyclosporin in Behçet's disease, *Lancet* **1**:1093–1096.

McKeon, F., 1991, When worlds collide: Immunosuppressants meet protein phophatases, *Cell* **66**:823–826.

Meyrier, A., 1989, Treatment of glomerular disease with cyclosporin A, *Nephrol. Dial. Transplant.* **4**:923–931.

Meyrier, A., Simon, P., Perret, G., Condamin-Meyrier, M. C., 1986, Remission of idiopathic nephrotic syndrome after treatment with cyclosporin A, *Brit. Med. J.* **292**:789–792.

Miescher, P. A., Favre, H.,. Chatelanat, F., Mihatsch, M. J., 1987, Combined steroid-cyclosporin treatment of chronic autoimmune diseases, *Klin. Wochenschr.* **65**:727–736.

Miescher, P. A., Favre, H., Mihatsch, M. J., Chatelenat, F., Huang, Y. P., and Zubler, R., 1988, The place of cyclosporin A in the treatment of connective tissue diseases, *Transplant. Proc.* **20**(Suppl. 4):224–237.

Mihatsch, M. J., 1985, International workshop in cyclosporine nephropathy, *Clin. Nephrol.* **24**:107–119.

Mihatsch, M. J., Bach, J. F., Coovadia, H. M., Forre, O., Mootsopoulos, H. M., Drosos, A. A., Siamopoulos, K. C., Noel, I. H., Ramsaroop, R., Hallgren, R., Svenson, K., and Bohman, S. O., 1988, Cyclosporin-associated nephropathy in patients with autoimmune diseases, *Klin. Wochenschr.* **66**:43–47.

Mori, Y., Suko, M., Okudaira, H., Matsuba, I., Tsuruoka, A., Sasaki, A., Yokoyama, H., Tanase, T., Shida, A., Nishimura, M., Terada, E., and Ikeda, Y., 1986, Preventive effect of cyclosporin in diabetes in NOD mice, *Diabetologia* **29**:244–247.

Mountz, J. D., Smith, H. R., Wilder, R. L., Reeves, J. P., and Steinberg, A. D., 1987, CS-A Therapy in MRL-1pr/1pr mice: Amelioration of immunopathology despite autoantibody production, *J. Immunol.* **138**:157–163.

Müller, W., and Herrmann, B., 1979, Cyclosporin A for psoriasis, *N. Engl. J. Med.* **301**:555.

The Multiple Sclerosis Study Group, 1990, Efficacy and toxicity of Sandimmun in multiple sclerosis: A double-blind placebo-controlled study, *Ann. Neurol.* **27**:591–605.

Niaudet, P., Tete, M. J., Broyer, M., and Habib, R., 1988, Cyclosporin and childhood idiopathic nephrosis, *Transplant. Proc.* **20**(Suppl. 4):265–268.

Nickoloff, B. J., Fischer, G. J., Mitra, R. S., and Voorhees, J. J., 1988, Additive and synergistic antiproliferative effects of cyclosporin A and gamma interferon on cultured human keratinocytes, *Am. J. Pathol.* **131**:12–18.

Niederberger, W., Lemaire, M., Maurer, G., Nussbaumer, K., and Wagner, O., 1983, Distribution and binding of cyclosporine in blood and tissues, *Transplant Proc.* **15**(Suppl. 1):2419–2421.

Nussenblatt, R. B., Rodrigues, M. M., and Wacker, W. B., 1981, Cyclosporin A-inhibition of experimental auto-immune uveitis in Lewis rats, *J. Clin. Invest.* **67**:1228–1231.

Nussenblatt, R. B., Rook, A. H., Wacker, W. B., Palestine, A. G., Scher, I., and Gery, I., 1983, Treatment of intraocular inflammatory disease with cyclosporin A, *Lancet* **2**:235.

Palestine, A. G., Austin, H. A., Balow, J. E., Antonovych, T. T., Sabnis, S. G., Preuss, H. G., and Nussenblatt, R. B., 1986, Renal histopathologic alterations in patients treated with cyclosporin for uveitis, *N. Engl. J. Med.* **314**:1293–1298.

Routhier, G., Epstein, O., Janossy, G., Thomas, A. C., and Sherlock, S., 1980, Effects of cyclosporin A on suppressor and inducer T-lymphocytes in primary biliary cirrhosis, *Lancet* **2**:1223–1225.

Rubenstein, A. H., and Pyke, D., 1987, Immunosuppression in the treatment of insulin-dependent (type 1) diabetes, *Lancet* **1**:436–437.

Rudge, P., Koetsier, J. C., Mertin, J., Mispelblom-Beyer, J. O., van Walbeek, H. K., Clifford-Janes, R., Harrison, J., Robinson, K., Mellein, B., Poole, T., Stovkis, J. C. J. M., and Timonen, P., 1989, Randomized double-blind controlled trial of cyclosporin in multiple sclerosis, *J. Neurol. Neurosurg. Psychiatr.* **52**:559–565.

Ryffel, B., Foxwell, B. M. J., Mihatsch, M. J., Donatsch, P., and Maurer, G., 1988, Biological significance of cyclosporine metabolites, *Transplant Proc.* **20**(Suppl. 2):575–584.

Sowden, J. M., Berth-Jones, J., Ross, J. S., Motley, R. J., Marks, R., Finlay, A. T., Salek, M. S., Graham-Brown, R. A. C., Allen, B. R., and Camp, R. D. R., 1991, Double-blind, controlled, crossover study of cyclosporin in adults with severe refractory atopic dermatitis, *Lancet* **388**: 137–140.

Stiller, R., Dupré, J., Gent, M., Jenner, M. R., Keown, P. A., Laupacis, A., Martell, R., Rodger, R., von Graffenried, B., and Wolfe, B. M. J., 1984, Effects of cyclosporin immunosuppression in insulin-dependent diabetes mellitus of recent onset, *Science* **223**:1362–1367.

Tejani, A., Butt, K., and Trachtman, H., 1988, Cyclosporin A induced remission of relapsing nephrotic syndrome in children, *Kidney Int.* **33**:729–734.

Thomson, A. W., Moon, D. K., Geczly, C. L., and Nelson, D. C., 1983, Cyclosporin A inhibits lymphokine production but not the responses of macrophages to lymphokines, *Immunology* **48**:291–299.

Thompson, C. B., June, C. H., Sullivan, E. M., and Thomas, E. D., 1984, Association between cyclosporine neurotoxicity and hypomagnesemia, *Lancet* **2**:1116–1120.

Timonen, P., Friend, D., Abeywickrama, K., Laburte, C., von Graffenried, B., and Feutren, G., 1990, Efficacy of low-dose cyclosporin A in psoriasis: Results of dose-finding studies, *Br. J. Dermatol.* **122**(Suppl. 36):33–39.

Tindall, R. S. A., Rollins, J. A., Phillips, J. T., Greenlee, R. G., Wells, L., and Belendiuk, G., 1987, Preliminary results of a double-blind, randomized, placebo-controlled trial of cyclosporin in myathenia gravis, *N. Engl. J. Med.* **316**:719–724.

Tugwell, P., Bombardier, C., Gent, M., Bennett, K. J., Bensen, W. G., Carette, S., Chalmers, A., Esdaile, J. M., Klinkhoff, A. V., Kraag, G. R., Ludwin, D., and Roberts, R. S., 1990, Low-dose cyclosporin versus placebo in patients with rheumatoid arthritis, *Lancet* **355**:1051–1055.

Urabe, A., Kanitakis, J., Viac, J., and Thivolet, J., 1989, Cyclosporin A inhibits directly *in vivo* keratinocyte proliferation of living human skin, *J. Invest. Dermatol.* **92**:755–757.

Van Hooff, J. P., Leunissen, K. M. L., Havenith, M. G., and Bosman, F. T., 1988, Cyclosporin and other therapy resistant nephrotic syndrome, *Transplant. Proc.* **20**(Suppl. 4):293–296.

Van Joost, T., Stolz, E., and Heule, F., 1987, Efficacy of low-dose cyclosporin in severe atopic skin disease, *Arch. Dermatol.* **123**: 166–167.

Van Joost, T. H., Bos, J. D., Heule, F., and Meinardi, M. M. H. M., 1988, Low-dose cyclosporin A in severe psoriasis. A double-blind study, *Br. J. Dermatol.* **118**:183–190.

Van Rijthoven, A. W. A. M., Dijkmans, B. A. C., Goeithe, H. S., Hermans, J., Montnor-Beckers, Y. L. M. B., Jacobs, P. C. J., and Cats, A., 1986, Cyclosporin treatment for rheumatoid arthritis: A placebo controlled, double blind, multicentre study, *Ann. Rheum. Dis.* **45**:726–731.

Von Graffenried, B., and Krupp, P., 1986, Side effects of cyclosporine (Sandimmun) in renal transplant recipients and in patients with autoimmune diseases, *Transplant Proc.* **18**:876–883.

Weetman, A. P., McGregor, A. M., Ludgate, M., Beck, L., Mills, P. V., Lazarus, J. H., and Hall, R., 1983, Cyclosporin improves Graves' ophthalmopathy, *Lancet* **2**:486–489.

Weinblatt, M., Coblyn, J. S., Fraser, P. A., Anderson, R. J., Spragg, J., Trentham, D. E., and Austen, K. F., 1987, Cyclosporin A treatment of refractory rheumatoid arthritis, *Arthritis Rheum.* **30**:11–17.

Wick, G., Müller, P. U., and Schwary, S., 1982, Effect of cyclosporin A on spontaneous auto-immune thyroiditis of obese strain (os) chickens, *Eur. J. Immunol.* **12**:877–881.

Wiesner, H., Ludwig, J., Lindor, D., Jorgensen, A., Baldus, P., Homburger, A., and Dickson, E., 1990, A controlled trial of cyclosporine in the treatment of primary biliary cirrhosis, *N. Engl. J. Med.* **322**:1419–1424.

Chapter 13

NONSTEROIDAL AND OTHER ANTI-INFLAMMATORY DRUGS

Yejun Zhao and *Marie L. Foegh*

1. INTRODUCTION

Organ transplant rejection involves an inflammatory cell infiltration of the allograft which may be a model of an inflammatory process involving the delayed cell-mediated immune response. Thus the observations and findings in transplant patients and in experimental transplant animal models may be transferred to other inflammatory diseases.

The immunosuppressants currently used in organ transplant patients are cyclosporin A (CsA) or azathioprine combined with prednisone. All three drugs possess serious side effects; CsA induces nephrotoxicity, azathioprine causes bone marrow suppression, and corticosteroids promote aseptic bone necrosis, cataracts, and diabetes. The side effects are generally dose related. New treatment modalities that will reduce the dose of CsA or azathioprine or will replace corticosteroids are of considerable clinical interest. The eicosanoids, consisting of prostaglandins (PG), thromboxane (TX), and leukotrienes (LT), are immune modulators, some of which are also considered to play a role as anti-inflammatory drugs.

The first implication of eicosanoids as modulators of the immune system was in 1971 when Franks *et al.* (1971) showed that prostaglandin E (PGE), which was known to increase cyclic adenosine monophosphate (cAMP) in most cells, also increased cAMP in thymic lymphocytes and thereby inhibited lymphocyte proliferation. The immunomodulatory effects of the eicosanoids are due not only to direct actions on cells but also indirect actions through release of other cytokines like platelet-activating factor (PAF), interleukin-1 (IL-1), interleukin-2 (IL-2), interferon-gamma (INF-γ), and other substances. Eicosanoids can be formed by all nucleated cells with the exception of lymphocytes; they are cyclo-oxygenase and lipoxygenase products of arachidonic acid and depending on the product may exert either immunostimulatory or immunoinhibitory activities (Fig. 1).

Yejun Zhao and *Marie L. Foegh* • Department of Surgery, Georgetown University Medical Center, Washington, D.C. 20007.

Immunopharmacology in Autoimmune Diseases and Transplantation, edited by Hans Erik Rugstad *et al.* Plenum Press, New York, 1992.

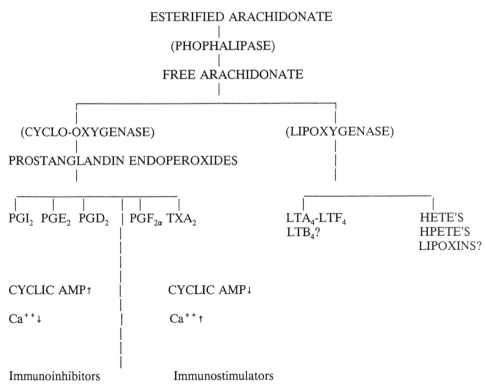

ESTERIFIED ARACHIDONATE
|
(PHOPHALIPASE)
|
FREE ARACHIDONATE
|

(CYCLO-OXYGENASE)   (LIPOXYGENASE)
|
PROSTANGLANDIN ENDOPEROXIDES
|

PGI$_2$ PGE$_2$ PGD$_2$ | PGF$_{2\alpha}$ TXA$_2$ LTA$_4$-LTF$_4$ HETE'S
                                          LTB$_4$?   HPETE'S
                                                               LIPOXINS?

CYCLIC AMP↑   CYCLIC AMP↓

Ca^{++}↓   Ca^{++}↑

Immunoinhibitors   Immunostimulators

FIGURE 13.1. The biologically active products arising from arachidonic acid oxidation. The metabolites are divided into putative pro- and antirejection products. Possible mechanisms of action are indicated.

2. ARACHIDONIC ACID METABOLITES

Arachidonic acid is released from membrane phospholipids by phospholipases during cell activation, which for example is seen in monocytes/macrophages upon both specific and nonspecific stimulations. The released arachidonate is metabolized into leukotrienes and hydroxyeicosatetraenoic acids (HETEs) by the lipoxygenase pathway and prostaglandins and thromboxane by the cyclo-oxygenase pathway. The 5-lipoxygenase, unlike cyclo-oxygenase, requires activation by calcium (Tripp *et al.*, 1985) before arachidonic acid can be utilized as a substrate. Once arachidonic acid is released from phospholipids, it is available for conversion by both enzymatic pathways. Glucocorticoids inhibit this stage. The inhibition is thought to be true induction of a protein, lipocortin (Hirata, 1986), which is a phospholipase inhibitor that blocks both enzymatic pathways by preventing arachidonate deesterification from phospholipids. Lipocortin can also inhibit a step in mitogenesis by inhibiting phospholipases. It has similar activities with respect to inhibition of arachidonate released from many cells and tissues, and exerts anti-inflammatory activity. It is observed that antiphospholipase proteins are released from neutrophils, and possibly act as modulators of inflammation.

The arachidonate metabolites might be divided into two major immunomodulatory groups according to their roles: the first group, the "antirejection" or immunoinhibitory products, namely PGE$_2$, PGI$_2$, and PGD$_2$, may act by increasing intracellular cAMP and preventing an increase in intracellular calcium (Foegh *et al.*, 1984a, 1986b, 1987a). The other group, the "prorejection" or immunostimulatory products, includes TXA$_2$, LTs, and possibly different HETEs and HPETEs. These products may exert their effects through promoting calcium influx and preventing an increase in cAMP. The metabolism of arachidonic acid can be manipulated by selective enzyme inhibitors, as illustrated in Fig. 1. Several of those inhibitors are clinically available and are listed in Table I.

3. CELLULAR SOURCES OF EICOSANOIDS

Different types of cells synthesize different eicosanoids with one notable and controversial exception, the lymphocyte. A list of eicosanoid products from different cell types involved in inflammation is given in Table II. The macrophages synthesize all eicosanoids, but there are quantitative differences. Thromboxane A_2 (TXA_2) is a major cyclo-oxygenase product of human macrophages (Foegh et al., 1983; Tripp et al., 1986a; Tripp and Needleman, 1987). The monocytes/macrophages also synthesize substantial amounts of several other products, namely, PGE_2, LTB_4, LTC_4, and LTD_4. These same cells also form, through the lipoxygenase pathways, a series of HETEs.

Some investigators have identified eicosanoids from lymphocyte cell populations, but these cell populations were impure and contained either platelets or monocytes (Goldyne, 1986), which both produce large amounts of eicosanoids. In lymphocyte cell lines the measurable eicosanoids are most likely from the serum of the cell culture medium.

The major products of polymorphonucleocytes (PMN) are the leukotrienes (Foegh, 1988b; Koller and Konig, 1990) while prostaglandins and thromboxane are very minor products (Foegh, 1988a). In contrast, another granulocyte, namely eosinophil, also synthesizes major amounts of TXA_2 and PGE_2 as well as leukotrienes (Foegh, 1988a). Eosinophil is the only circulating cell that contains substantial amounts of the enzyme 15-lipoxygenase. This feature makes it a likely major source of 15-hydroperoxyeicosatetraenoic acid (15-HPETE), which is required for synthesis of the more recently discovered lipoxins (Jorg et al., 1982; Rand et al., 1983; Turk et al., 1983; Weller et al., 1983; Payan et al., 1984; Serhan et al., 1984).

Another biologically active eicosanoid derived from platelets is 12-hydroxyeicosatetraenoic acid (12-HETE). Thus it appears that the inflammatory cells have the eicosanoid formation mainly tilted toward proinflammatory and prorejection compounds. In addition, platelets may also participate in the inflammatory response, although platelets are not generally accepted as being a part of these events.

TABLE I. Enzyme Inhibitors of Eicosanoid Synthesis

Phospholipase inhibitors
  Corticosteroids
Cyclo-oxygenase inhibitor
  Indomethacin
Lipoxygenase inhibitors
  EP 10045 (Lim et al., 1988b)
  EP 10161 (Lim et al., 1988b)
  SC 33576 (Foegh et al., 1987b)
  L 651,392 (Guindon et al., 1987)
  Dipyridamole (Foegh et al., 1987b)
Thromboxane synthase inhibitors
  OKY 1581 (Foegh et al., 1987b)
  CGS 13080 (Foegh et al., 1988)

TABLE II. Different Inflammatory Cell Types and
Platelets and Their Formation of Eicosanoids and PAF

Macrophages	LT, TXA_2, PGE_2, PAF, HETE's
Lymphocytes	Arachidonic acid
Eosinophils	PGE_2, TXA_2, 15-HPETE, LT, PAF
PMN	LT
Platelets	TXA_2, 12-HETE

4. CELL–CELL INTERACTION

The importance of lymphocytes for eicosanoid formation relates to the high content of arachidonic acid in their cell membrane; on stimulation, the lymphocytes release arachidonic acid that can be metabolized by monocytes, resulting in eicosanoid formation. There is evidence that in addition to arachidonic acid and 15-HPETE, other eicosanoids can be metabolized by adjacent cells. The best demonstrated example is the provision of prostaglandin endoperoxides by platelets to endothelial cells for metabolism to prostacyclin (PGI_2). Endothelial cells synthesize several eicosanoids in addition to PGI_2, including 13-hydroperoxyoctadecadienoic acid (13-HPOTE). The 12-HETE is derived from platelets. It may modulate cellular responses during rejection (Table II).

5. *IN VITRO* AND *IN VIVO* EFFECTS OF EICOSANOIDS AND PLATELET-ACTIVATING FACTOR ON THE CELL-MEDIATED IMMUNE RESPONSE

5.1. General

The involvement of eicosanoids has been reviewed previously (Foegh *et al.*, 1984a) and the current knowledge is illustrated in Fig. 2. The lymphocyte proliferation that takes place as a part of the cell-mediated rejection process entails an increase in the number of CD_4 (helper) and CD_8 (cytotoxic) lymphocytes. Two signals are required for initiation of T-cell proliferation. First, IL-1 is released from monocytes/macrophages and then foreign antigen is presented to the lymphocyte by these cells. In addition, the lymphocyte needs to recognize the macrophage DR antigen. The lymphokines IL-2 and INF-γ are involved; the former promotes lymphocyte proliferation and the latter promotes DR expression. The macrophages release all eicosanoids. PGE_2, PGI_2, and possibly PGD_2 decrease IL-1 release and inhibit DR antigen expression; therefore, prostaglandins inhibit lymphocyte proliferation. But TXA_2 and products of the 5-lipoxygenase pathway promote antigen expression. Corticosteroids also inhibit IL-1 and IL-2 synthesis and block both cyclo-oxygenase and lipoxygenase by preventing arachidonate deesterification from phospholipids. The important therapeutic effect of corticosteroids is more likely related to lipoxygenase product synthesis since the cyclo-oxygenase route is specifically blocked by indomethacin, which unlike corticosteroids does not improve graft survival (Foegh *et al.*, 1987b).

5.2. Prostaglandins

PGE_2 and to a lesser extent PGI_2, which is highly unstable, have been shown to inhibit antigen- and mitogen-induced lymphocyte proliferation (Leung and Mihic, 1981; Tripp

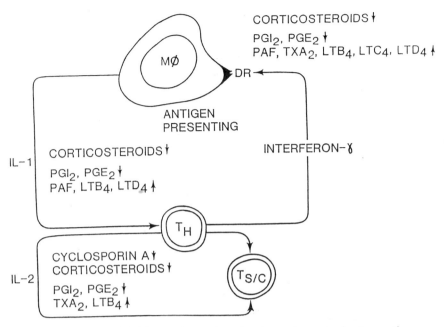

FIGURE 13.2. Modulation of macrophage–lymphocyte interaction by eicosanoids.

et al., 1986b). This inhibitory effect on proliferation is associated with inhibition of both IL-1 and IL-2 release (Farrar and Humes, 1985; Chouaib *et al.*, 1985), as well as induction of suppressor cell function. The mechanisms may be through activation of adenylate cyclase and increase of cAMP, which would reduce cytosolic calcium concentration. IL-2 also controls the effect of PGE_2 by mitigating the ability of PGE_2 to increase cAMP (Farrar and Beckner, 1986). More recently it has been shown that PGE_2 independently of cAMP prevents intracellular calcium increase in lymphocytes. Both PGE_2 and PGI_2 inhibit DR antigen expression by macrophages (Snyder *et al.*, 1982) and probably also by other cells. These prostaglandins prolong graft survival (skin, kidney, and heart) in animal models. These studies (Anderson *et al.*, 1977; Kort *et al.*, 1982; Strom and Carpenter, 1983; Rowles *et al.*, 1986) also showed that the mechanism might be inhibition of lymphocyte proliferation by PGE_2. Other mechanisms for antirejection/anti-inflammatory activity of PGE_2, PGD_2, and PGI_2 may be by preventing increase in intracellular calcium as demonstrated in TXA_2-induced increase in intracellular calcium in platelets (Foegh, 1988b). PGE_2, PGD_2, and PGI_2 are also potent vasodilators and, in addition, stabilize platelets and leukocytes. These prostaglandins have been referred to as "cytoprotective." The 6-keto-$PGF_{1\alpha}$ is the stable product of PGI_2, and is used as a measurement for production of the unstable PGI_2.

5.3. Thromboxane

TXA_2 is a platelet- and leukocyte-aggregating substance. In addition, it is a potent vasoconstrictor. TXA_2 also promotes lymphocyte proliferation. The *in vitro* effect of TXA_2 is unknown because of its relative unavailability and short half-life (20 sec). TXA_2 is rapidly hydrolyzed to TXB_2. From inhibition of TXA_2 synthase, it is inferred that TXA_2 increases T-lymphocyte clonal expansion and DR antigen expression. However, the effect on lymphocyte proliferation could also be due to shunting of endoperoxides into PGE_2 and PGI_2. The role for TXA_2 in immune stimulation was strengthened by the finding that a TXA_2 analogue promoted mitogen-induced lymphocyte proliferation. It was also found that the TXA_2 analogue reversed the inhibition of lymphocyte proliferation obtained with a TXA_2 synthase inhibitor (Ceuppens et al., 1985).

In vivo studies also support an immunostimulatory role for TXA_2. In rats, both a TXA_2 synthase inhibitor and a TXA_2 antagonist act synergistically with both azathioprine and cyclosporine to prolong cardiac allograft survival (Foegh et al., 1985b, 1986a, 1987b). During organ rejection in humans and animals, urine has been found to contain increased concentrations of immunoreactive TXB_2, which is the stable breakdown product of TXA_2 (Foegh et al., 1981, 1985a, 1987c; Khirabadi et al., 1985). The rejecting cardiac allograft from rats showed a 30-fold increase in immunoreactive TXB_2 (i-TBX_2) formation when compared with the native heart (Lim et al., 1988a).

A recent study in kidney transplant patients showed that a more than tenfold increase in the dose of the TXA_2 synthase inhibitor, which inhibited platelet TXA_2 formation, was needed for suppressing TXA_2 urinary excretion compared with the nonrejecting state (Foegh et al., 1981). This indicates that either the capacity for TXA_2 formation during rejection is increased or the TXA_2 synthase is different or less accessible in the kidney when compared with that in platelets.

5.4. Leukotrienes

Leukotrienes B_4, C_4, and D_4 (LTB_4, LTC_4, LTD_4) are the arachidonic acid metabolites of the 5-lipoxygenase pathway. Leukotriene A_4 (LTA_4) is a short-lived intermediate product that forms either LTB_4 or LTC_4. The latter is more stable and is further metabolized to LTD_4 and then to leukotriene E_4 (LTE_4). LTC_4, LTD_4, and LTE_4 increase vascular permeability; LTC_4 is the most potent. Thus, LT may contribute to the edema seen during rejection. LT may also accentuate the rejection process through effects on the immune response. An early event in lymphocyte proliferation is an influx of calcium. Some of the effects of LTB_4 may be explained by promoting calcium influx. Lymphocyte accumulation in the graft is an early stage in rejection. This accumulation may be enhanced by LTB_4, which is a chemoattractant for lymphocytes and powerful chemotactic agent rivaling complement 5a. LTB_4 may act as a calcium ionophore (Naccache et al., 1981) and it is also a potent chemoattractant for PMNs, as well as an aggregator of both PMNs and platelets (Ford-Hutchinson et al., 1980). A further amplification of the rejection process may take place because of the stimulation of LTB_4 and IL-1 and IL-2 release from macrophages and lymphocytes, respectively.

These products have numerous effects on the immune response. All LTs enhance INF-γ production and may even have the same effect as INF-γ on macrophage Ia expression, namely, an increase in the density of Ia expression. The biologic effects of LTs are summarized in (Table III). The in vitro effects of the LTs on lymphocyte proliferation may not necessarily reflect the in vivo situation where additional immunomodulating products are released. These are reflected in some of the in vitro effects of LTs, which may only be expressed if PG formation is inhibited by adding indomethacin to the lymphocyte culture. For example, LTB_4 promotes lymphocyte proliferation, but this effect is expressed only in the presence of indomethacin, which prevents the formation of PGE_2. Thus, in vivo experiments are important for elucidating the role of these products. In an animal model of cell-

TABLE III. Effects of Eicosanoids Related to Cell-Mediated Immune Response

Antirejection	Prorejection		
PGI$_2$ PGE$_2$ PGD$_2$	TXA$_2$	LTB$_4$	LTC$_4$ LTD$_4$
Vasodilation	Vasoconstriction	Vascular permeability	Vascular permeability ↑
Cytoprotection	Platelet aggregation ↑	CA^{2+} flux ↑	INF-τ ↑
Platelet aggregation ↓	Lymphocyte prolifera-	T-cell proliferation	
Leukocyte aggregation ↓	tion ↑	Leukocyte aggregation ↑	
cAMP ↑		IL1 and IL2 ↑	
IL1 and IL2 ↓		NK cell	
T-cell proliferation ↓		Cytotoxicity	
Lymphocyte migration ↓		INF-τ ↑	
DR-antigen expression ↓			

mediated rejection, lipoxygenase inhibitors act synergistically with cyclosporine in increasing graft survival (Lim et al., 1988b), suggesting that the leukotrienes are immunostimulators in vivo.

LTB$_4$ inhibits peripheral blood lymphocyte proliferation in response to mitogens and induces suppressor cells that can derive from both CD$_4$ and CD$_8$ populations but that are phenotypically CD$_8$ when exerting their suppressor activity. There is no information concerning effects of LTB$_4$ on CD$_8$ cytotoxic cells. This induction of suppressor activity by LTB$_4$ points to anti-inflammatory properties.

Natural killer (NK) cell function is enhanced by LTB$_4$. This effect is exerted both at the binding of effector to target cell and at the rate of killing (Rola-Pleszczynski and Gagnon, 1986).

5.5. Lipoxins and Hydroxyeicosatetraenoic Acids

In addition to the 5-lipoxygenase that yields leukotrienes from arachidonic acid, there are also 8-, 12- and 15-lipoxygenases. These enzymes give rise to the different hydroxyeicosatetraenoic acids and hydroperoxyeicosatetraenoic acids. Their effect on the immune system is largely unexplored; they may exert some indirect effects on enzymes like cyclooxygenase and prostacyclin synthase. Lipoxins A and B are formed from 15-HPETE. Lipoxins possess several biologic properties (Rokach and Fitzsimmon, 1986; Rowley et al., 1990). For instance, lipoxin A stimulates leukocyte chemotaxis but without provoking aggregation. Lipoxin A also causes the contraction of parenchymal strips and stimulates microvascular changes as well as activates protein phosphorylation (Dahlen et al., 1987a,b). The few studies currently available indicate that lipoxins at low doses (10^{-14} M) stimulate NK cell activity and at higher doses (10^{-8} M) inhibit NK cell activity (Rola-Pleszczynski and Gagnon, 1986). 15-HETE has been shown also to inhibit murine lymphocyte transformation (Bailey et al., 1982) and human T-cell migration, whereas 5-HETE in contrast enhances the migration of human T lymphocytes in vitro (Payan and Goetzl, 1981). The 12-HETE may modulate cellular responses during rejection and stimulates mast cell and neutrophil degranulation. Other cells, like basophils, mast cells, and endothelial cells, have been shown to contain the enzyme, but whether it plays a role in the endogenous lipoxin formation remains to be shown.

5.6. Platelet-Activating Factor

Platelet-activating factor (PAF), although not an eicosanoid, affects eicosanoid formation by stimulating arachidonic acid release. PAF is implicated as a mediator of inflammatory and acute allergic responses (Benveniste, 1985) and as contributing to the pathogenesis of antibody and complement-mediated hyperacute allograft rejection (Ito et al., 1984). PAF is released from platelets, PMNs, basophils, macrophages, lymphocytes, and endothelial cells (Chignard et al., 1979; Camussi et al., 1981, 1983, Bussolino et al., 1984; Riches et al., 1990). PAF causes peripheral vasodilation and increased vascular permeability (Inarrea et al., 1985). A possible role for PAF in acute graft rejection has been suggested by the synergistic effect of PAF antagonists and cyclosporin A in experimental cardiac allograft survival (John and Foegh, 1986). The mechanisms need to be explored and several possible mechanisms exist. Through increased vascular permeability, PAF may be implicated in the early events of cell recruitment to the allograft. PAF may also play a role in the cell-to-cell interaction within the graft. Furthermore, an enhancement of the immune response may occur through both a direct effect of PAF and a still not well understood relationship with arachidonic acid, through 2-arachidonyl PAF. The in vitro effect of PAF was first found to be the inhibition of lymphocyte proliferation and IL-1 formation; this inhibition is reversed by a PAF antagonist (Foegh et al., 1987a). In contrast, the in vivo effect of PAF is stimulation; continuous infusion of PAF in rats causes increased release of IL-1 and IL-2 from spleen cells (Pignol et al., 1988). Thus, more in vivo experiments are needed for elucidating the role of PAF.

5.7. Monitoring of Immunoreactive TXB_2 in Organ Rejection—A Cell-Mediated Immune Response

According to experiments and clinical investigations, TXA_2 increases significantly when rejection occurs. An increase in i-TXB_2 occurs before the clinical diagnosis of kidney and heart rejection (Foegh et al., 1984b,c; Khirabadi et al., 1985; Steinhauer et al., 1986) and urinary i-TXB_2 was shown to be an early indicator of rejection in renal and cardiac transplant patients. An increase in urine i-TXB_2 excretion was found to occur in rat heart transplant recipients prior to rejection. Thus, i-TXB_2 may be an indicator of an activated immune response; this remains to be shown.

6. TREATMENT WITH PROSTAGLANDINS AND INHIBITORS OF THROMBOXANE AND LEUKOTRIENE SYNTHESIS

6.1. Experimental

6.1.1. Prostaglandins

Numerous experiments have confirmed the inhibition of cell-mediated responses by PG. The protective effect of PGE_1 in skin allograft survival was demonstrated a decade ago. The first to demonstrate improved allograft survival in organ transplantation were Strom et al. (1977) who found a PGE analogue to prolong kidney allograft survival in rats. The idea that PGE compounds improve allograft survival was supported by numerous studies showing inhibition of lymphocyte proliferation by PGE. This inhibition is, as mentioned earlier, probably exerted through an increase in cAMP by activation of adenylate cyclase.

This immunosuppressant activity was confirmed by subsequent studies where PGE analogues clearly improved both cardiac (Kort *et al.*, 1982) and kidney (Strom and Carpenter, 1983) allograft survival. The other cyclo-oxygenase product, prostacyclin (PGI_2), and its analogue, iloprost, were reported to improve allograft survival in rat cardiac transplantation (John and Shaw, 1983; Rowles *et al.*, 1986). An interesting approach for studying the *in vivo* effect of PGE_2 has been the use of anti-PGE antibodies, which enhanced the *in vivo* development of cell-mediated immunity. The properties of the "antirejection" cyclo-oxygenase products PGI_2, PGE_2, and PGD_2 make them extremely suitable for use in organ preservation.

6.1.2. Thromboxane A_2 Synthase Inhibitors and Antagonists

TXA_2 may be a lymphocyte mitogen. Both a TXA_2 synthase inhibitor and a TXA_2 receptor antagonist have the same synergistic effect with CsA as prednisone in prolonging cardiac allograft survival.

6.1.3. Leukotriene–5-Lipoxygenase Inhibitors

The *in vitro* data suggest a stimulation of the cell-mediated rejection. This was found in the rat cardiac transplant model. But again the immunoinhibitory effect was only seen as a synergism with CsA and azathioprine.

These experimental data provide a conceptual basis for considering the use of TXA_2 synthase inhibitors, TXA_2 antagonists, PGE analogues, PGI_2 analogues, and 5-lipoxygenase inhibitors as agents adjunctive to decreased doses of CsA or azathioprine and may in some circumstances replace corticosteroids in immunosuppressive therapy. Tables IV and V list some drugs that may or may not prolong rat allograft survival in combination with either low-dose CsA or azathioprine.

6.2. Clinical

Lethner and co-workers treated successfully kidney transplant patients undergoing acute or chronic rejection with prostacyclin (Lethner *et al.*, 1983). Prostacyclin represents a group of drugs that could increase the therapeutic possibilities for treating graft rejection.

TABLE IV. Drugs Inhibiting Cell-Mediated Immune Events *in Vivo*

Acyl hydrolase inhibitor
  Prednisolone
Thromboxane receptor antagonists
  L640,035 (Foegh *et al.*, 1987b)
  AH 23848 (Foegh *et al.*, 1987b)
5-Lipoxygenase inhibitors
  EP 10045
  SC 33576
  Dipyridamole
  L 651,392
Prostacyclin analogue
  Iloprost (Foegh *et al.*, 1987b)

TABLE V. Drugs Which Do Not Prolong Rat Allograft Survival
in Combination with Either Low-Dose CsA or Azathioprine

Cyclooxygenase inhibitor
Indomethacin
Leukotriene D$_4$ antagonist
SC 39070 (Foegh et al., 1987b)

Misoprostol, a PGE analogue, has been used in transplant patients for protection against CsA nephrotoxicity. There was no report on effects in the immune system (Alijani et al., 1989).

7. TRANSPLANT ATHEROSCLEROSIS—CHRONIC REJECTION

Atherosclerosis is important in the pathogenesis of chronic rejection of transplanted organs (Foegh, 1990). In cardiac transplant patients accelerated coronary atherosclerosis has become the limitation for successful long-term graft survival. Transplant atherosclerosis is a rapid intimal hyperplasia (Foegh et al., 1989a). The pathophysiology is unknown. Hess et al. (1983) demonstrated a correlation between accelerated atherosclerosis and B-cell cytotoxic antibodies in their population of transplant patients. Libby et al. (1989) emphasize the response of endothelial cells and the likely participation of cytokines derived from vascular cells as well as from infiltrating leukocytes in amplification and propagation of this localized chronic immune reaction. This mechanism, which involves helper T cells interacting with class II HLA, may distinguish transplantation-associated arteriosclerosis from typical acute rejection, which may involve primarily cytolytic T cells interacting with class I HLA.

Foegh and co-workers (1989a) have suggested that stimulatory peptides mitogenic for smooth muscle cells are released following reperfusion and during activation of the immune system. The same investigators (Foegh et al., 1989b) have shown that both iloprost and angiopeptin, a somatostatin analogue, inhibit myointimal proliferation in the coronary arteries of the allograft in rabbits, and suggested that the vascular smooth muscle cell proliferation is due to lack of a putative inhibitor or presence of mitogenic peptides of smooth muscle cell growth. It is of interest to speculate that the cell proliferation in the vasculature of the transplanted organ may show similarities with the cell proliferation seen in the synovia of joints in patients with rheumatoid arthritis.

8. SUMMARY

Eicosanoids, that is, PGs, TX, and LTs, are immune modulators. Some of them also play a role as anti-inflammatory drugs. The immunomodulatory effects of eicosanoids are due to both direct actions on cells and indirect actions through release of other cytokines like PAF, IL-1, IL-2, and INF-γ. Eicosanoids can be formed by all nucleated cells with the exception of lymphocytes. They are metabolic products of arachidonic acid by the cyclooxygenase pathway or the lipoxygenase pathway, and depending on the products may exert either immunostimulatory or immunoinhibitory activities. The metabolism of arachidonic acid can be manipulated by selective enzyme inhibitors. Different types of cells and different stimulations give rise to synthesis of different eicosanoids. Macrophages synthesize all eicosanoids while PMNs only synthesize LT.

The early stage of inflammatory cell infiltration in cell-mediated rejection is lymphocyte proliferation. Eicosanoids modulate the immune response. The eicosanoids can be divided into two groups according to their immunomodulatory effects: immunoinhibitors, which have antirejection properties, and immunostimulators, which have prorejection properties.

PGs that increase intracellular cAMP and decrease influx of calcium are considered immunoinhibitory; they inhibit DR antigen expression and IL-1 and IL-2 release, and thus lymphocyte proliferation. They prolong graft survival in animal models. PGI_2 has already been applied clinically for treatment of kidney transplant patients undergoing either acute or chronic rejection. Some of their analogues can protect against CsA nephrotoxicity in transplant patients.

TX and LTs have opposite actions of PGs, and are considered immunostimulatory. They promote lymphocyte proliferation and may play a prorejection role in organ transplantation. In both experimental work and in clinical studies, TXA_2 increases significantly with rejection. Immunoreactive TXB_2 has been used to monitor organ rejection. It is observed that TXA_2 synthase inhibitors or TXA_2 receptor antagonists can prolong allograft survival in combination with CsA and azathioprine. LTs can increase vascular permeability and contribute to the edema.

PGs analogues, TXA_2 synthase inhibitors, and TXA_2 receptor antagonists may reduce the immunosuppressive dose of CsA or azathioprine and may be corticosteroid sparing.

Atherosclerosis is important in the pathogenesis of the long-term loss of transplanted organs. In cardiac transplant patients the accelerated coronary arteriosclerosis has become the limitation for successful long-term graft survival. It has been observed that this is due to myointimal proliferation in the vasculature of the transplanted organ and that the process may be inhibited by angiopeptin, a small peptide.

REFERENCES

Alijani, M. R., Benjamin, S. B., Collen, M. J., and Foegh, M. L., 1989, Misoprostol: A prostaglandin E_1 analogue versus antacid in the prevention of stress ulcers in kidney transplant patients, *Transplant. Proc.* **21**:2145.

Anderson, C. B., Jaffe, B. M., and Graff, R. J., 1977, Prolongation of murine skin allografts by prostaglandin E_1, *Transplantation* **23**:444.

Bailey, J. M., Brayant, R. W., Low, C. E., Pupillo, L. M., and Vanderhoek, J. Y., 1982, Regulation of T-lymphocyte mitogenesis by the leukocyte product 15-hydroxyeicosatetraenoic (15-HETE), *Cell. Immunol.* **67**:112.

Benveniste, J., 1985, Paf-acether (Platelet-Activating Factor), *Adv. Prostaglandin Thromboxane Leukotriene Res.* **13**:11.

Bussolino, F., Foa, R., Malauasi, F., Ferrando, M. L., and Camussi, G., 1984, Release of platelet-activating factor (PAF)-like material from human lymphoid cell lines, *Exp. Hematol.* **12**:688.

Camussi, G., Aglietta, M., Coda, R., Bussolino, F., Piacibello, W., and Tetta, C., 1981, Release of platelet-activating factor (PAF) and histamine. II. The neutrophils and basophils, *Immunology* **42**:191.

Camussi, G., Aglietta, M., Malavasi, F., Tetta, C., Piacibello, W., Sanavio, F., and Bussolino, F., 1983, The release of platelet-activating factor from human endothelial cells in culture, *J. Immunol.* **131**:2397.

Ceuppens, J. L., Vertessen, S., Deckmyn, H., and Vermylen, J., 1985, Effects of thromboxane A_2 on lymphocyte proliferation, *Cell. Immunol.* **90**:458.

Chignard, M., LeConedic, J. P., Tence, M., Vargaftig, B. B., and Benveniste, J., 1979, The role of platelet-activating factor in platelet aggregation, *Nature* **279**:799.

Chouaib, S., Welte, K., Mertelsmann, K., and Dupont, B., 1985, Prostaglandin E_2 acts at two distinct pathway of T lymphocyte activation: Inhibition of interleukin 2 production and down-regulation of transferrin receptor expression, *J. Immunol.* **135**:1172.

Dahlen, S. E.,. Raud, J.,. Serhan, C. N., Bhork, J., and Samuelsson, B., 1987a, Biological activities of lipoxin a include lung strip contraction and dilation of arterioles *in vivo*, *Acta Physiol. Scand.* **130**:643.

Dahlen, S. E., Raud, J., Serhan, C. N., Bjork, J., and Samuelsson, B., 1987b, Leukotrienes and lipoxins: Structures, biosynthesis, and biological effects, *Science* **237**:1171.

Farrar, W. L., and Beckner, S. K., 1986, Biochemical convergence of prostaglandins and interleukin 2 on the adenylate cyclase system, *Transplant. Proc.* (Suppl. 4)**18**:25.

Farrar, W. L., and Humes, J. L., 1985, The role of arachidonic acid metabolism in the activities of interleukin 1 and 2, *J. Immunol.* **135:**1153.

Foegh, M. L., 1988a, Immune regulation by eicosanoids, *Transplant. Proc.* **20**(6):1158.

Foegh, M. L., 1988b, Eicosanoids and platelet activating factor mechanisms in organ rejection, *Transplant. Proc.* **20**(6):1260.

Foegh, M. L., 1990, Chronic rejection-graft arteriosclerosis, *Transplant. Proc.* **22**(1):119.

Foegh, M. L., Zmudka, M., Cooley, C., Winchester, J. F., Helfrich, G. B., Ramwell, P. W., and Schreiner, G. E., 1981, Urine i-TXB$_2$ in renal allograft rejection, *Lancet* **2:**431.

Foegh, M. L., Maddox, Y. T., Winchester, J., Rakowski, T., Schreiner, G., and Ramwell, P. W., 1983, Prostacyclin and thromboxane release from human peritoneal macrophages, *Adv. Prostaglandin and Leukotriene Res.* **12:**45.

Foegh, M. L., Alijani, M. R., Helfrich, G. B., and Ramwell, P. W., 1984a, Eicosanoids and organ transplantation, *Ann. Clin. Res.* **16:**318.

Foegh, M. L., Alijani, M., Helfrich, G. B., Schreiner, G. H., and Ramwell, P. W., 1984b, Urine thromboxane as an immunologic monitor in kidney transplant patients, *Transplant. Proc.* **16:**1603.

Foegh, M. L., Alijani, M., Khirabadi, B. S., Shapiro, R., Goldman, M. H., Lower, R. R., and Ramwell, P. W., 1984c, Monitoring of rat heart allograft rejection by urinary thromboxane, *Transplant. Proc.* **16:**1606.

Foegh, M. L., Alijani, M. R., Helfrich, G. B., Khirabadi, B. S., Goldman, M. H., Lower, R. R., and Ramwell, P. W., 1985a, Thromboxane and leukotrienes in clinical and experimental transplant rejection, *Adv. Prostaglandin Thromboxane Leukotriene Res.* **13:**209.

Foegh, M. L., Khirabadi, B. S., and Ramwell, P. W., 1985b, Prolongation of experimental cardiac allograft survival with thromboxane-related drugs, *Transplantation* **40:**124.

Foegh, M. L., Alijani, M. R., Helfrich, G. B., Khirabadi, B. S., Kim, K., and Ramwell, P. W., 1986a, Lipid mediators in organ transplantation, *Transplant. Proc.* **18**(Suppl. 4):20.

Foegh, M. L., Alijani, M. R., Helfrich, G. B., Khirabadi, B. S., and Ramwell, P. W., 1986b, Fatty acids and eicosanoids in organ transplantation, *Prog. Lipid. Res.* **25:**567.

Foegh, M. L., Hartmann, D-P., Rowles, J. R., Khirabadi, B. S., Alijani, M. R., Helfrich, G. B., and Ramwell, P. W., 1987a, Leukotrienes, thromboxane, and platelet activating factor in organ transplantation, *Adv. Prostaglandin Thromboxane Leukotriene Res.* **17:**140.

Foegh, M. L., Khirabadi, B. S., and Ramwell, P. W., 1987b, Drugs presumably affecting macrophage and/or arachinodic acid metabolism, *Transplant. Proc.* **19:**1297.

Foegh, M. L., Lim, K-L., Alijani, M. R., Helfrich, G. B., and Ramwell, P. W., 1987c, Thromboxane and inflammatory cell infiltration of the allograft of renal transplant patients, *Transplant. Proc.* **19:**3633.

Foegh, M. L., Lim, K., Douglas, F., Turk, J., Helfrich, G. B., Taher, S. A., and Alijani, M. R., 1988, Differential effect of CGS 13080, a thromboxane synthase inhibitor, in suppressing serum and urine immunoreactive thromboxane B$_2$ in kidney transplant patients, *Transplant. Proc.* **20**(Suppl. 1):424.

Foegh, M. L., Khirabadi, B., Chambers, E., Amamoo, S., and Ramwell, P. W., 1989a, Peptide inhibition of accelerated transplant atherosclerosis, *Transplant. Proc.* **21:**3674.

Foegh, M. L., Khirabadi, B. S., Chambers, E., Amamoo, S., and Ramwell, P. W., 1989b, Inhibition of coronary artery transplant atherosclerosis in rabbits with angiopeptin, an octapeptide, *Atherosclerosis* **78:**229.

Ford-Hutchinson, A., Bray, M., Doig, M., Shipley, M,. and Smith, M., 1980, Leukotriene B, a potent chemokinetic and aggregating substance released from polymorphonuclear leukocytes, *Nature* **286:**264.

Franks, D. J., MacManus, J. P., and Whitfield, J. F., 1971, The effect of prostaglandins on cyclic AMP production and cell proliferation in thymic lymphocytes, *Biochem. Biophys. Res. Commun.* **44:**1177.

Goldyne, M. E., 1986, Lymphocyte and monocyte/macrophage interactions involving arachidonic acid metabolism, *Transplant. Proc.* **18**(Suppl. 4):37.

Guindon, Y., Girard, Y., Maycock, A., Ford-Hutchinson, A. W., Atkinson, J. G., Belanger, P. C., Dallob, A., DeSoousa, D., Dougherty, H., Egan, R., et al., 1987, L-651,392: A novel potent and selective 5-lipoxygenase inhibitor, *Adv. Prostaglandin Thromboxane Leukotriene Res.* **17A:**554.

Hess, M. L., Hastillo, A., Mohanakumar, T., Cowley, M. J., Vetrovac, G., Szentpetezy, S., Wolfgang, T. C., and Lower, R. R., 1983, Accelerated atherosclerosis in cardiac transplantation: Role of cytotoxic B-cell antibodies and hyperlipidemia, *Circulation* **68**(Suppl. II):94.

Hirata, F., 1986, Role of lipocortin as a mediator of glucocorticoids in the rejection of allografts, *Transplant. Proc.* **18**(Suppl. 4):29.

Inarrea, P., Gomez-Cambronero, J., Pascual, J., Ponte, M. C., Hermando, L., and Sanchez-Crespo, M., 1985, Synthesis of PAF-acether and blood volume changes in gram-negative sepsis, *Immunopharmacology* **9:**45.

Ito, S., Camussi, G., Tetta, C., Milgrom, F., and Andres, G., 1984, Hyperacute renal allograft rejection in the rabbit. The role of platelet-activating factor and of cationic proteins derived from polymorphonuclear leukocytes and from platelets, *Lab. Invest.* **51:**148.

John, H., and Foegh, M. L., 1986, The synergistic effect of cyclosporine and iloprost on survival of rat cardiac allografts, *Transplantation* **42:**94.

John, H., and Shaw, F. L., 1983, Prolongation of rat cardiac allograft survival by treatment with prostacyclin or aspirin during acute rejection, *Transplantation* **35:**526.

Jorg, A., Hederson, W. R., Murphy, R. C., and Klebanoff, S. J., 1982, Leukotriene generation by eosinophils, *J. Exp. Med.* **155:**390.

Khirabadi, B. S., Foegh, M. L., and Ramwell, P. W., 1985, Urine immunoreactive thromboxane B$_2$ in rat cardiac allograft rejection, *Transplantation* **39:**6.

Koller, M., and Konig, W., 1990, Arachidonic acid metabolism in heat-shock treated human leukocytes, *Immunology* **70:**458.

Kort, W. J., Bonta, I. L., Adolfs, M. J. P., and Westerbroek, D. L., 1982, Synergism of (15 s)-15-methyl-prostaglandin E₁ with either azathioprine or prednisone on the survival of heart allografts in rats, *Prostaglandins Leukotrienes Med.* **8:**661.

Lethner, C., Sinzinger, H., Schwarz, M., and Pohanka, E., 1983, Radiolabelled platelets and prostacyclin in diagnosis and treatment of transplant rejection, *Proc. Eur. Dial Transplant. Assoc.* **19:**529.

Leung, K. H., and Mihic, E., 1981, Prostaglandin modulation of development of cell-mediated immunity in culture, *Nature* **288:**597.

Libby, P., Salomon, R. N., Payne, D. D., Schoen, F. J., and Pober, J. S., 1989, Functions of vascular wall cells related to development of transplantation-associated coronary arteriosclerosis, *Transplant. Proc.* **21:**3677.

Lim, K-L., Alijani, M. R., Helfrich, G. B., and Foegh, M. L., 1988a, Correlation of renal inflammatory cell infiltrate with thromboxane, *Transplant. Proc.* **20:**256.

Lim, K-L., Khirabadi, B. S., Braquet, P., Ramwell, P. W., and Foegh, M. L., 1988b, Effect of the 5-lipoxygenase inhibitors EP 10045 and EP 10161 on cardiac graft cellular infiltrate and thromboxane formation, *Transplant. Proc.* **20**(2)**:**254.

Naccache, P. H., Sha'afi, R. I., Borgeat, P., and Goetzl, E. J., 1981, Mono- and dihydroxyeicosatetraenoic acids alter calcium homeostasis in rabbit neutrophils, *J. Clin. Invest.* **67:**1584.

Payan, D. G., and Goetzl, E. J., 1981, The dependence of human T-lymphocyte migration on the 5-lipoxygenation of endogenous arachidonic acid, *J. Clin. Immunol.* **1:**266.

Payan, D. G., Goldman, D. W., and Coetzl, E. J., 1984, Biochemical and cellular characteristics of the regulation of human leukocyte function by lipoxygenase products of arachidonic acid, in L. W. Chakrin and D. M. Bailey (Eds.), *The leukotrienes*, Academic Press, New York, p. 231.

Pignol, B., Henane, S., Sorlin, B., Rola-Pleszczynski, M., Mencia-Huerta, J-M., and Braquet, P., 1988, Effect of long-term *in vivo* treatment with platelet-activating factor on interleukin-1 and interleukin-2 production by rat splenocytes, in P. Braquet (Ed.), *New trends in lipid mediators research*, Vol. 1, Karger, Basel, p. 38.

Rand, T. H., Clanton, J. A., and Colley, D. G, 1983, Arachidonic acid metabolism in murine eosinophil stimulation promoter (ESP) on oxidative and degranulation responses of murine eosinophils, *J. Immunol.* **130:**1356.

Riches, D. W., Young, S. K., Seccomber, J. F., Henson, J. E., Clay, K. L., and Henson, P. M., 1990, The subcellular distribution of platelet-activating factor in stimulated human neutrophils, *J. Immunol.* **145**(9)**:**3062.

Rokach, J., and Fitzsimmon, B., 1986, Lipoxins—Do they have a biological role? *Transplant. Proc.* **18:**7.

Rola-Pleszczynski, M., and Gagnon, L., 1986, Natural killer cell function modulated by leukotriene B4: Mechanisms of action, *Transplant. Proc.* **18**(Suppl. 4)**:**44.

Rowles, J. R., Foegh, M. L., and Khirabadi, B. S., 1986, The synergistic effect of cyclosporine and iloprost on survival of rat cardiac allografts, *Transplantation* **42:**94.

Rowley, A. F., Pettitt, T. R., Secombes, C. J., Sharp, G. J. E., Barrow, S. E., and Mallett, A. I., 1990, Generation and biological activities of lipoxins in the rainbow trout-an overview, *Adv. Prostaglandin Thromboxane Leukotriene Res.* **21:**557.

Serhan, C. N., Hamberg, M., and Samuelsson, B., 1984, Trihydroxytetraenes: A novel series of compounds formed from arachidonic acid in human leukocytes, *Biochem. Biophys. Res. Commun.* **118:**943.

Snyder, D. S., Beller, D. I., and Unanue, E. R., 1982, Prostaglandins modulate macrophage Ia expression, *Nature* **299:**163.

Steinhauer, H. B., Wilms, H., Ruther, M., and Schollmeyer, P., 1986, Clinical experience with urine TXB₂ in acute renal allograft rejection, *Transplant. Proc.* **18:**98.

Strom, T. B., and Carpenter, C. B., 1983, Prostaglandin as an effective antirejection therapy in rat renal allograft recipients, *Transplantation* **35:**279.

Strom, T. B., Carpenter, C. B., Crago, E. J., Norris, S., Devlin, R., and Perper, R. J., 1977, Suppression of *in vivo* and *in vitro* alloimmunity by prostaglandins, *Transplant. Proc.* **9:**1075.

Tripp, C. S., and Needleman, P., 1987, Regulation of macrophage arachidonic acid metabolism during the immune response, *Adv. Prostaglandin Thromboxane and Leukotriene Res.* **17:**1085.

Tripp, C. S., Mahoney, M., and Needleman, P., 1985, Calcium ionophore enables soluble agonists to stimulate macrophage 5-lipoxygenase, *J. Biol. Chemistry* **260:**5895.

Tripp, C. S., Unanue, E. R., and Needleman, P., 1986a, Monocyte migration explains the changes in macrophage arachidonate metabolism during the immune response, *Proc. Natl. Acad. Sci. USA* **83:**9655.

Tripp, C. S., Wyche, A., Unanue, E. R, and Needleman, P., 1986b, The function significance of the regulation of macrophage Ia expression by endogenous arachidonate metabolites *in vitro*, *J. Immunol.* **137:**3915.

Turk, K., Rand, T. H., Mass, R. L., Lawson, J. A., Brash, A. R., Roberts, L. J., Cilley, D. G, and Oates, J. A., 1983, Identification of lipoxygenase products from arachidonic acid metabolism in stimulated murine eosinophils, *Biochem. Biophys. Acta* **750:**78.

Weller, P. F., Lee, C. W., Foster, D. W., Corey, E. J., Austin, K. F., and Lewis, R. A., 1983, Generation and metabolism of 5-lipoxygenase pathway leukotrienes by human eosinophils: Predominant production of leukotriene C₄, *Proc. Natl. Acad. Sci. USA* **80:**7626.

Immune Response Modifiers of Biological Origin

Chapter 14

ANTI-T-CELL MONOCLONAL ANTIBODIES AS IMMUNOSUPPRESSIVE AGENTS

Lucienne Chatenoud and *Jean-François Bach*

Anti-T-cell monoclonal antibodies represent invaluable tools for *in vivo* human serotherapy. Large panels of anti-T-cell monoclonal antibodies have been produced, which express different specificities and target efficiently functionally distinct T-cell subsets.

This chapter focuses on the various anti-T-cell monoclonals most widely used, both in experimental and clinical settings, and describes the major insights gained over the past few years into the mode of action and side effects of these important immunomodulating agents. Special attention is given to the clinical situations in which the vast array of highly sophisticated anti-T-cell monoclonal antibodies available have already been or will be applied in the near future.

1. INTRODUCTION

Less than five years since their original description in early 1980, murine monoclonal antibodies (mAbs) have progressively become invaluable tools both as biological probes and immunomodulating agents. Thus, they progressively replaced conventional serotherapy with horse or rabbit antisera in a wide variety of clinical situations, particularly in the field of immunosuppression. The use of antilymphocyte sera in organ graft recipients to prevent or treat rejection has frequently been hampered by several pitfalls, namely: (1) low titer of specific antibodies contained in the preparations, requiring the administration of large amounts of sera; (2) variabilities in antisera production and collection; (3) absence of good standardization of the antibody responsible for the therapeutic effect due to contamination by irrelevant immunoglobulins; and (4) risk of xenosensitization, provoking harmful hypersensitivity reactions. The possibility of producing indefinite amounts of highly purified

Lucienne Chatenoud and *Jean-François Bach* • Immunology Clinic, Necker Hospital, 75743 Paris Cedex 15, France.

Immunopharmacology in Autoimmune Diseases and Transplantation, edited by Hans Erik Rugstad *et al.* Plenum Press, New York, 1992.

specific mAbs has obviated most of these problems, thus offering new and broader perspectives to their therapeutic use.

This chapter essentially will focus on murine anti-T-cell mAbs administered as immunosuppressive agents since this is at present the clinical indication that has been the most widely and successfully developed. However, it is important to emphasize that all results collected from clinical studies as well as from experimental models indicate that most of the conclusions drawn by studying immunosuppressive mAbs may apply to the *in vivo* use of mAbs in other clinical settings, that is, antitumor or antivenom, or antimicrobial antibodies.

1.1. Basic Characteristics of Monoclonal Antibodies Compared to Polyclonal Antisera

Monoclonal antibodies produced by hybridomas are basically identical to antibodies present in polyclonal hyperimmune sera (Milstein, 1982). However, from a practical standpoint, the homogeneity of mAbs that are multiple copies of a single and same molecule is linked to important characteristics that distinguish them from polyclonal antibodies. Each mAb is derived from a single clone and thus possesses the unique physicochemical and specificity properties. For example, if the mAb is an IgG, it is usually an agglutinator; if it is an IgE or an IgA, it does not fix complement. Monoclonal antibodies used in clinical practice present variable isotypes, thus showing different behaviors with respect to their *in vivo* complement-fixing capacity, a property that will influence not only their therapeutic effectiveness but also the side effects.

A given mAb reacts with a single epitope, that is, a single antigenic determinant expressed by the target molecule. This essential property is of major importance since it ensures the strict specificity of the desired effect. It may also in some cases explain a paradoxical inefficacy of the antibody when the molecule recognized by the mAb is present in low amounts on target cells. Another important parameter that must be analyzed when selecting a mAb for *in vivo* clinical use is its affinity for the target molecule. When possible, one should select mAbs exhibiting the highest affinity.

The production of therapeutic mAbs does not pose problems that greatly differ from those met and now completely resolved for the production of mAbs used as *in vitro* reagents. The main point is that of quantity. Whereas limited amounts of mAb are needed for *in vitro* experiments, much higher doses, ranging from 1 to 50 mg, are usually administered per patient. Monoclonal antibodies for clinical use must, of course, be as pure as possible, particularly avoiding contamination with oncogenic viruses.

The choice of the antibody-providing species is so far limited to the mouse and the rat. A striking publication in 1980 raised the hope of producing human mAb by fusing human lymphocytes (collected from patients immunized against a given antigen) with human myelomatous B cells (Kaplan *et al.*, 1982). However, it has been nearly impossible, except in some specific settings such as cancer patients (Sikora *et al.*, 1982), to obtain stable human–human hybridomas. Alternative solutions, which gave interesting results, consisted of producing human–mouse hybrids, more difficult to obtain but stable once they have been cloned (Garchon *et al.*, 1983); deriving human B cell lines following infection by the Epstein-Barr virus; or using heteromyelomas as fusion partners (P. Lake, personal communication). Actually, this latter approach seems very interesting since it is capable of producing greater amounts of human IgG-producing hybrids. This is at variance with all the other described technologies that usually only give rise to IgM mAbs exhibiting low affinity. It must be stressed, however, that the risk of oncogenic virus transmission (often species-specific) could in theory be increased by using human mAbs.

Finally, recent reports show that by molecular engineering it is possible to replace the constant portions of the rat or murine mAb molecules by the equivalent human structures (Riechmann *et al.*, 1988). This procedure offers several advantages. First, any rat or mouse mAb can be humanized, thus compared to mAbs obtained by human–human hybridization a wider panel of specificities can be expected. Second, the procedure allows large-scale production of the chimeric immunoglobulins. Finally, one major hope is that humanized mAb will avoid patients' sensitization, although one cannot exclude that the anti-idiotypic component of the response (which is the more important one) would still occur (Chatenoud *et al.*, 1986a; Chatenoud, 1989).

All these considerations strongly suggest that it is probably not by modifying the already excellent existing production methods that further progress will be made in the clinical use of mAbs.

1.2. The Array of T-Cell Antigens

T cells express on their membrane a wide variety of antigens shown to represent reliable differentiation, function, and activation markers (Reinherz and Schlossman, 1980; Uchiyama *et al.*, 1981). Several panels of mAbs have been produced against these T-cell antigens that all represent potential immunomodulating agents. It is important to underline that some of these membrane antigens are in fact T-cell receptors that will trigger cell activation following binding a specific ligand (Reinherz *et al.*, 1982; Borst *et al.*, 1984; Kurrle *et al.*, 1986).

A major collaborative effort has been conducted by several laboratories to exchange the different series of anti-T-cell mAbs produced in order to reliably define and compare in various experimental conditions their biological capacities. The results of such extensive work have been presented in detail in annual international workshops that classified the mAb-defined molecules in an ever-growing number of differentiation clusters (i.e, CD) (Shaw, 1987). Table I summarizes the main characteristics of the CD molecules recognized by mAbs that have been used as *in vivo* immunomodulators.

TABLE I. T-Cell Antigens Characterized by Murine Monoclonal Antibodies
Used as *in Vivo* Immunomodulators

Target molecule	T3	T4	T8	T11	Tac
Differentiation cluster	CD3	CD4	CD8	CD2	CD25
Functional relevance	T3 is a molecular complex tightly linked to the T-cell receptor for antigen recognition; triggering of T3 with specific mAbs induces T-cell activation	T4 expression favors recognition of class II MHC molecules on antigen-presenting cells	T8 expression favors recognition of class I MHC molecules on antigen-presenting cells	T11 is the receptor for sheep erythrocytes (E rosette receptor); triggering of T11 epitopes with specific mAbs induces T-cell activation	Tac is the IL-2 receptor expressed on activated T cells

These mAbs may be grouped under three separate headings depending on the intrinsic properties of the target molecule:

1. Monoclonal antibodies directed against functionally relevant membrane receptors directly implicated in cell triggering. This is typically the case for mAbs directed against T3 (anti-CD3), a molecular complex that includes different polypeptide chains, tightly linked to the T-cell receptor for antigen recognition (i.e., the Ti molecule) (Reinherz et al., 1982; Borst et al., 1984; Kurrle et al., 1986). Note that mAbs that specifically recognize monomorphic epitopes on the T-cell receptor dimer itself have been characterized and recently introduced in clinical practice (Lanier and Weiss, 1986). In this category one also finds mAbs directed to the interleukin-2 (IL-2) receptor (anti-CD25); [IL-2 is a T-cell-derived soluble growth factor playing a key role in T-cell proliferation and differentiation (Uchiyama et al., 1981)]. Finally, one may mention mAbs targeting particular epitopes of the E rosette receptor (anti-CD2), which promote T-cell activation by triggering a pathway alternative to that implicated in T3-Ti activation (Reinherz, 1985).

2. Monoclonal antibodies directed against membrane molecules only expressed on distinct cell subsets, namely anti-CD4 and anti-CD8 antibodies. On a general basis, studies are concordant in showing that CD4$^+$ and CD8$^+$ T cells exhibit, respectively, helper–inducer and cytotoxic–suppressor functions (Reinherz and Schlossman, 1980). Moreover, detailed analysis of T-cell clones indicated that expression of CD4 and CD8 proteins play a fundamental role in major histocompatibility (MHC) restricted antigen recognition. Thus CD4$^+$ cells are MHC class II restricted, whereas CD8$^+$ cells are MHC class I restricted (Swain, 1983; Greenstein et al., 1984; Swain et al., 1984). Some anti-CD4 mAbs both in mice and humans have been shown to inhibit the proliferative response of CD4$^+$ lymphocytes, thus suggesting that the CD4 molecule may act as a receptor able to transduce negative signals (Bank and Chess, 1985; Tite et al., 1986). Given their active participation in physical cell-to-cell contact, that is, the formation of effector lymphocyte–target cell conjugates, the CD4 and CD8 molecules are also included in the large family of the so-called adhesion molecules (Springer et al., 1987). Under this heading one finds different molecules, not only expressed on lymphoid cells, playing a major role in cell-to-cell interactions. Main adhesion molecules present at the membrane of lymphoid cells are CD2, CD4, CD8, and LFA1. Other adhesion molecules include LFA3, MHC class II, MHC class I, and ICAM 1, which are, respectively, the natural ligands of the former, expressed by various cell types including fibroblasts, parenchymal, and endothelial cells (Springer et al., 1987).

3. Monoclonal antibodies recognizing membrane antigens such as CD6 (defined by the anti-T12 mAb) whose functional relevance is ill-defined (Kirkman et al., 1983).

1.3. Mode of Action of Therapeutic Monoclonal Antibodies

Therapeutic mAbs exert their immunosuppressive effect by means of two distinct although not mutually exclusive mechanisms: cell destruction and/or inactivation (by receptor blockade or more often by antigenic modulation, that is, the redistribution and disappearance of the target molecule from the cell membrane). As far as cell destruction is concerned, one major parameter to consider is the precise distribution of the target molecule recognized by the mAb: Is it present on all T cells or exclusively on a given T-cell subset? Conversely, in the case of cell inactivation, the functional relevance of the target molecule either physically blocked or eliminated from the cell membrane by means of antigenic modulation following mAb binding represents the main parameter to focus on (Chatenoud and Bach, 1984).

The physicochemical characteristics of the mAb itself (isotype, binding affinity, use of the entire Ig molecule or of F(ab')2 or Fab fragments, etc.) also greatly influence the therapeutic behavior. These factors correlate with the capacity of a given mAb to properly opsonize the target, thus promoting macrophage phagocytosis, complement fixation, and/or antigenic modulation. Kelley and co-workers (1987) illustrated well the role of complement activation in the *in vivo* immunosuppressive effect of mAbs. These authors investigated the *in vivo* therapeutic activity of an anti-IL-2 receptor mAb injected either into normal BALB/c mice or a C5 deficient strain. The therapeutic effect was observed only in normal mice (Kelley *et al.*, 1987).

Since, as previously mentioned, antigenic modulation represents a major mode of action of some immunosuppressive mAbs, it seems important at this stage to briefly recall the basis of the phenomenon. Antigenic modulation is the active reversible loss of membrane antigen and/or receptor expression induced by its binding to specific ligands, like a mAb (Chatenoud and Bach, 1984). The first and most simple hypothesis proposed to explain the phenomenon equates antigenic modulation with capping and/or shedding of cell surface components. Thus following mAb binding, antigen–antibody complexes move laterally to form microprecipitates (i.e., patches) that secondarily group into a cap that is either internalized or shed from the cell. *In vitro* incubation of antigenically modulated cells in the absence of the mAb induces the reappearance of the surface antigen. Due to its characteristics, antigenic modulation represents a serious adverse effect of therapeutic mAb use when total cell depletion is the major aim, namely for tumor therapy. In fact, once the antigen recognized by the injected mAb has been modulated, the target cell becomes insensitive to further coating and subsequent lysis (Dillman and Royston, 1985). In contrast, in the case of immunosuppression, the disappearance from the cell surface, by means of antigenic modulation, of functionally relevant receptors can mediate therapeutic effectiveness even in the absence of target cell depletion. As a typical example, antigenic modulation is one major mode of action of anti-CD3 antibodies that do not induce long-lasting T-cell depletion (Chatenoud *et al.*, 1982; Chatenoud and Bach, 1990).

2. EXPERIMENTAL DATA

2.1. Murine Models

In mice, rat mAbs directed to the murine equivalents of the various T-cell antigens described above have been produced and tested for their *in vivo* immunosuppressive capacity. We shall focus our attention exclusively on the mAbs that showed efficient and reproducible *in vivo* immunosuppressive activity.

The first mAb that gave impressively good results was an anti-L3T4 antibody developed by Dialynas *et al.* (1983a,b). L3T4 is the murine cell surface glycoprotein homologue of the human CD4 molecule; it identifies a functionally distinct subset of T cells called helper–inducer because it includes most T cells known to promote the differentiation or activation of

B cells as well as of suppressor or cytotoxic T cells (Cantor and Boyse, 1975; Ledbetter et al., 1980; Dialynas et al., 1983a,b). Moreover, like CD4$^+$ human T cells, L3T4$^+$ cells recognize class II MHC antigens on antigen-presenting cells (Swain, 1983; Dialynas et al., 1983b; Wilde et al., 1983; Greenstein et al., 1984; Swain et al., 1984). In vivo injection of anti-L3T4 mAbs resulted in powerful suppression of both humoral and cellular immune responses of treated mice.

One single injection of 1 mg intraperitoneally of anti-L3T4 induced a selective depletion of > 90% L3T4$^+$ cells from the blood, spleen, and lymph nodes (Wofsy et al., 1985b). Treated mice exhibited complete inhibition of humoral responses to foreign antigens. Thus, no IgG antibodies were produced following immunization with either bovine serum albumin or chicken egg ovalbumin administered in complete Freund's adjuvant (Wofsy et al., 1985b).

In vivo studies with anti-L3T4 were also extended to several murine models of autoimmune diseases. Depletion of L3T4$^+$ cells was shown to block the development of experimental allergic encephalomyelitis, a model for multiple sclerosis (Waldor et al., 1985), as well as of collagen-induced arthritis, a model for rheumatoid arthritis (Wofsy, 1985). In autoimmune (NZB × NZW)F$_1$ mice, which present a spontaneous lupuslike syndrome, weekly injection of anti-L3T4 for up to 8 months, beginning at the fourth month of age (i.e., prior to the onset of overt autoimmunity), significantly improved the disease's natural history by reducing autoantibody production, delaying the onset of proteinuria, and prolonging the actuarial survival of treated mice compared to control animals (Wofsy and Seaman, 1985). Moreover, starting the treatment at 7 months of age, when mice already exhibited an overt autoimmune pathology, significantly improved the survival (75% in treated mice compared with 17% in controls) (Wofsy and Seaman, 1987). Anti-L3T4 treatment was also effective in preventing the disease in nonobese diabetic (NOD) female mice, which spontaneously develop an autoimmune insulin-dependent type I diabetes (Shizuru et al., 1988).

Several authors could also show that anti-L3T4 treatment was effective in significantly prolonging skin allograft survival (i.e., from 9 to 18 days) (Cobbold et al., 1984; Woodcock et al., 1986). Complete tolerance, however, was not achieved in these experimental models since, although it was delayed, rejection of the skin allograft was finally observed (Woodcock et al., 1986).

Very promising results have also been obtained by injecting mice with anti-IL-2 receptor monoclonal antibodies selected according to their capacity to competitively block IL-2 binding to its receptor. This treatment can suppress delayed-type hypersensitivity reactions to foreign and syngeneic antigens (Kelley et al., 1986). Moreover, Kirkman et al. (1985) reported that an identical treatment efficiently prolonged cardiac allograft survival in mice. These data were confirmed and extended to rat recipients of cardiac allograft (Kupiec-Weglinski et al., 1986). In this experimental setting, therapy with anti-IL-2 receptor mAb was able not only to prevent but also to reverse acute allograft rejection. Additionally, spleen cells from treated rats efficiently transferred the tolerance status to syngeneic transplanted host (i.e., not receiving any mAb treatment) (Kupiec-Weglinski et al., 1986). From these results the authors concluded that, at least in rats, in vivo treatment with anti-IL-2 receptor mAb spares a subset of T cells with suppressor activity, an effect that could explain the long-lasting immunosuppressive activity of the mAb (Kupiec-Weglinski et al., 1986).

Anti-pan T-cell mAbs have also been tested in mice. The results obtained were highly variable depending on the target antigen analyzed. Thus in vivo use of anti-Lyt-1 mAb (i.e., the Lyt-1 antigen is expressed both by L3T4$^+$ and Lyt2$^+$ mouse T cells that are, respectively, the equivalent of human CD4$^+$ and CD8$^+$ lymphocytes) significantly prolonged skin allograft survival (Michaelidis *et al.*, 1981). In contrast, controversial results were obtained by using anti-Thy-1 mAbs, which also recognize all mouse T cells; clear-cut immunosuppressive effects were limited to very precise pathological conditions (mainly autoimmune diseases) in well-defined mouse strains (Wofsy *et al.*, 1985a). Striking results have recently been obtained by using a hamster mAb directed to the murine T3 molecule (Hirsch *et al.*, 1988, 1989, 1990; Hayward and Schreiber, 1989). Preliminary data confirmed the analogy existing between this mAb and OKT3, which recognizes the same molecule on human T lymphocytes. Thus *in vivo* administration of the 141 2C11 mAb induced profound immunosuppression with most of the biological effects previously described following OKT3 treatment (Hirsch *et al.*, 1988, 1989, 1990).

2.2. Monkey Models

From a chronological point of view the first extensive experimental studies on the *in vivo* immunosuppressive capacity of xenogeneic human anti-T-cell mAbs have been performed in cynomolgus and rhesus monkeys. This was made possible by the fact that most of the murine anti-human T-cell mAbs bind with good affinity to these monkey's T cells. These experiments afforded important insights into the biological effects and the potential clinical usefulness of anti-T-cell mAbs. An important exception to this approach was OKT3, since aside from human T cells it exclusively recognizes chimpanzee lymphocytes but not lymphoid cells from the experimentally more accessible rhesus monkeys.

Disappointing results were obtained when monkeys were injected with anti-pan T-cell mAbs, namely OKT11A and WT1, which binds to the CD2 molecule (i.e., the E rosette receptor) (Giorgi *et al.*, 1983; Jonker *et al.*, 1983a). OKT11A induced only a modest and nonsignificant prolongation of skin allograft survival and showed no effect at all on renal allograft survival (Giorgi *et al.*, 1983; Jonker *et al.*, 1983a). Peripheral T cells were not eliminated but underwent antigenic modulation of the CD2 antigen. The WT1 mAb showed a better immunosuppressive effect but here again without long-term T-cell depletion (Giorgi *et al.*, 1983; Jonker *et al.*, 1983a). However, all of these studies were performed by using the first-generation of anti-CD2 mAbs. It would be interesting to reconsider these results by taking advantage of recent data showing that triggering of the CD2 molecule mediates an alternative pathway of human T-cell activation distinct from that triggered by the T3-Ti complex (Reinherz, 1985). One should also evaluate the various mAbs recently characterized that are directed to different epitopes of the CD2 molecule that, at least *in vitro*, have been shown to express distinct functional capacities (Reinherz, 1985).

Contrasting results have been obtained when using in monkeys mAbs directed against the two major T-cell subsets, namely CD4$^+$ and CD8$^+$ lymphocytes. Most anti-CD4 mAbs used were immunosuppressive in monkeys receiving either skin or renal transplantation (Jonker *et al.*, 1983a, 1985). Their immunosuppressive activity was not correlated to their capacity to induce either T-cell depletion or antigenic modulation. Thus, for example, when administered alone, OKT4 exclusively bound to peripheral T cells without provoking either depletion of antibody-coated CD4$^+$ cells or modulation of the CD4 antigen. Nevertheless, OKT4 exerted a clear-cut immunosuppressive effect. Interestingly, antigenic modulation of the CD4 molecule occurred when OKT4 was injected in association to OKT4A, which recognizes a distinct epitope on the CD4 molecule (Jonker *et al.*, 1983a, 1985).

At variance with anti-CD4 mAbs, the vast majority of the anti-CD8 mAbs tested showed little or no immunosuppressive effect (Jonker *et al.*, 1983a,b). This was the case for OKT8, OKT8A (Jonker *et al.*, 1983a) and B9.8 (Jonker *et al.*, 1983b).

The only described exceptions are Leu-2a, shown by Cosimi (1983) to be immunosuppressive in unprimed monkeys receiving a mismatched kidney allograft and OKT8F shown by Jonker *et al.* (1986) to prolong skin allograft survival and to prevent early kidney allograft rejection in transfused animals. There is also experimental evidence showing that in few cases injection of a pool of anti-CD8 mAbs (B9 pool) produced by Mawas and colleagues results in prolongation of skin allograft survival (M. Jonker, unpublished data).

Encouraging results were presented in the first reports, using an anti-CD25 mAb recognizing the IL-2 receptor in monkey recipients of a renal allograft (Shapiro *et al.*, 1987). The use of such antibodies was prompted by the observation of high proportions of circulating "activated" T cells expressing the IL-2 receptor in untreated transplanted monkeys at the time of rejection. Moreover, it is well known that T cells infiltrating rejecting allografts do express high levels of functional IL-2 receptor. Since then, other reports that used different anti-CD25 mAbs recognizing distinct epitopes on the molecule have given controversial results. Very recent data obtained in cynomolgus monkeys show that anti-ICAM1 mAbs seem to be highly effective both for the prevention and treatment of rejection episodes (D. Conti and B. Cosimi, personal communication).

All these results support the conclusion that the *in vivo* immunosuppressive effectiveness of mAbs implies the recognition not only of the correct T-cell membrane antigen and/or receptor but also of the appropriate epitope within the chosen molecule.

3. CLINICAL ACTIVITY OF ANTI-T-CELL MONOCLONAL ANTIBODIES

3.1. OKT3

As mentioned, OKT3 is at present the mAb that has been the most widely used in the clinics. Confirming the initial open trial reported in 1981 by Cosimi *et al.* (1981), a multicenter randomized trial has shown that association of OKT3 to low doses of conventional immunosuppressive agents could reverse acute rejection episodes in renal allograft recipients more efficiently than corticoids (Ortho Multicenter Transplant Study Group, 1985). Similar results have been obtained in liver and cardiac transplantation (Starzl and Fung, 1986; Colonna *et al.*, 1987; Kremer *et al.*, 1987; Gordon *et al.*, 1988). OKT3 has also been used prophylactically, that is, to prevent rejection in renal allograft recipients: OKT3 administration was started at the time of transplantation and was prolonged from 14 to 30 consecutive days (Kreis *et al.*, 1985; Chatenoud *et al.*, 1986a). In all cases, as long as therapeutic serum OKT3 levels could be maintained, there was an initial total depletion of peripheral CD3$^+$ cells followed by a reappearance of antigenically modulated T3$^-$T4$^+$ or T3$^-$T8$^+$ cells (Chatenoud *et al.*, 1982, 1986a). No clinical or biological signs of allograft rejection (Kreis *et al.*, 1985) were observed as long as no T3$^+$ cells were detected in peripheral blood. OKT3 administration was generally well tolerated with the only exception of a transient, spontaneously reversible systemic reaction that followed the first injection. This reaction includes with variable intensity fever, chills, diarrhea, vomiting, and headache, and although spontaneously reversible and not life-threatening in the vast majority of cases, is highly disabling to the patient. This clinical syndrome is related to transient OKT3 induced *in vivo* monocyte/macrophage-dependent T-cell activation that provokes massive release in the circulation of some cytokines, namely, TNF, IFN-γ, and in some cases IL-2 (Chatenoud *et al.*, 1988, 1989). Peak values are recorded at 1 hr after the first OKT3 injection for TNF and at 4 hr postinjection for IFN-γ and IL-2 (Chatenoud *et al.*, 1988, 1989). Importantly, both the amount of each circulating cytokine and the intensity and duration of the clinical syndrome may be significantly reduced by administering a single high-dose corticosteroid bolus (400–500 mg of solumedrol) prior to the first mAb injection (Chatenoud *et al.*, 1991). Preliminary data we obtained in the murine model using the 145-2C11 mAb indicate that more specific means of preventing this important side effect are available, such as the administration of specific anticytokine antibodies (Ferran *et al.*, 1990, 1991).

The only important side effect that occurred with prolonged OKT3 treatment was the anti-mAb xenosensitization (see Section 4). This immunization was highly deleterious since human anti-OKT3 antibodies could totally abrogate the therapeutic effectiveness of the injected OKT3 (Chatenoud *et al.*, 1982, 1983, 1986a; Chatenoud and Bach, 1990).

3.2. Other Anti-Pan T-Cell Monoclonal Antibodies

3.2.1. Anti-CD6

An IgM mAb directed to the 120-kDa T12 molecule was selected from a series of antibodies characterized by Reinherz and co-workers (Kirkman, 1983). This mAb was selected for clinical trial because T12 expression is limited to mature T cells and, at variance with OKT3 (that is, an IgG2a), anti-T12 is not mitogenic *in vitro*. A first open clinical trial was set up to treat renal allograft recipients undergoing acute rejection within three months of transplantation. Although the clinical results of this first trial were promising (7 of the 19 patients included showed reversal of the rejection episode within the ten-day treatment period), they could not be confirmed by treating larger numbers of patients. Interestingly, at variance with OKT3, anti-T12 did not include a febrile systemic reaction. Although anti-T12 did not induce *in vitro* modulation of the T12 antigen, antigenic modulation did occur *in vivo* (Kirkman *et al.*, 1983).

3.2.2. BMA031, an Anti-T-Cell Receptor Monoclonal Antibody

BMA031 is a murine IgG2b mAb that recognizes an epitope located within the framework of the human T-cell receptor molecule (Ti) (Kurrle *et al.*, 1986). *In vitro* assays have shown that, in contrast to most anti-CD3 mAbs, BMA031 is not mitogenic for T cells and does not trigger Ca^{2+} influx although it effectively suppresses *in vitro* T-cell-dependent antibody production as well as T-cell-mediated cytotoxicity. Moreover, compared to most anti-CD3 antibodies, at least *in vitro*, BMA031 does not induce the release of significant amounts of cytokines (i.e., IFN-γ, IL-2, GM-CSF) by T cells. Preliminary trials have been performed using the BMA031 antibody to treat acute rejection in liver, heart, and kidney allograft recipients. In fewer cases the mAb has also been administered prophylactically. BMA031 was also used in the prevention of acute graft versus host disease in bone marrow transplantation. The protocols employed usually include several administrations (3 to 10) of doses ranging from 10 to 50 mg/day of BMA031. At present, nearly 80 patients receiving organ transplants have been treated. The antibody is well tolerated (only mild fever may be observed), at variance with OKT3, and no acute systemic reaction is observed. BMA031 induces both peripheral T-cell depletion and antigenic modulation of the CD3-Ti molecular complex. Interestingly, BMA031 seems to be a very potent immunogen compared to other anti-T-cell mAbs tested. Very significant titers of anti-BMA human antibodies rapidly appear even after one single injection. This precludes using the mAb for more than five to six consecutive days. Preliminary clinical data suggest that BMA031 is effective in treating acute rejection episodes. In this setting, the antibody could thus represent in the future a good alternative to OKT3. More patients are needed to judge the effectiveness of BMA031 as a prophylactic (i.e., to prevent rejection) immunosuppressive regimen.

3.3. Anti-IL-2 Receptor Monoclonal Antibody

Based on the experimental models described above showing prevention and reversal of allograft rejection subsequent to anti-IL-2 receptor mAb injection, similar therapeutic protocols were applied to human renal allograft recipients. In a pilot study reported by Soulillou et al. (1987), encouraging data subsequently were confirmed in a controlled randomized trial (J. P. Soulillou et al., personal communication). The IgG2a rat mAb 33B3.1, which interferes with IL-2 binding to its receptor, was administered prophylactically starting on the day of transplantation and then for 15 consecutive days. At a dose of 10 mg/day in association with cyclosporine, corticosteroids, and azathioprine, this antibody is well tolerated and according to this report may prevent allograft rejection as effectively as polyclonal antilymphocyte serum.

4. ANTIMONOCLONAL SENSITIZATION

As with traditional serotherapy, one of the major drawbacks of mAbs administration is linked to their xenogeneic protein nature. It is worth mentioning, however, that in contrast to the response observed with polyclonal antisera, so far, anti-mAb humoral response has never led to harmful hypersensitivity reaction. Thus the major problem left is the abrogation of the therapeutic effectiveness by neutralization and subsequently by accelerated clearance of the mAb. When mAbs are injected alone (i.e., in the absence of associated conventional immunosuppressants), rapid and intense sensitization has been observed not only in humans but also in rodents and monkeys (Chatenoud et al., 1986a; Benjamin et al., 1986; Villemain et al., 1986). The only exception to this general rule is the anti-L3T4 mAb, which was shown to be tolerogenic (Benjamin and Waldmann, 1986; Gutstein et al., 1986).

The characteristics of the anti-xenogeneic mAb response, namely isotypic diversity and fine specificity, have been well researched in OKT3-treated patients (Baudrihaye et al., 1984; Chatenoud et al., 1986a; Jaffers et al., 1986).

Several methods allow the detection of anti-mAb sensitization. Immunochemical (ELISA) or immunofluorescence assays may directly show the presence of specific anti-OKT3 antibodies (Chatenoud et al., 1986a). One may also evaluate the accelerated clearance of the mAb by measuring (by means of ELISA) OKT3 levels in the serum. Another very useful, although it may seem indirect, method to detect sensitization is monitor circulating OKT3$^+$ cells. In fact, the number of circulating T cells is dramatically reduced within 10–20 min after the first intravenous OKT3 injection. Subsequently, within the second to the fifth day posttreatment, significant although low levels of peripheral $CD3^-$ $CD4^+$ and $CD3^-CD8^+$ cells reappear that reflect the antigenic modulation provoked by OKT3 (Chatenoud et al., 1982, 1986a). As soon as serum OKT3 declines, either due to cessation of treatment or onset of neutralizing anti-OKT3 immunization, an in vivo "demodulation" is observed that is paralleled by the rapid reappearance (within 24 hr) of fully labeled $OKT3^+$ cells. One must be particularly cautious in detecting dimly labeled $OKT3^+$ cells, that is, T cells expressing decreased amounts of surface CD3 antigen that may be frequently observed in patients presenting low levels of anti-OKT3 antibodies (particularly of the IgM isotype) (Chatenoud et al., 1986a).

Anti-OKT3 antibodies present an isotype heterogeneity; both IgM and IgG are produced. Only IgG anti-OKT3 antibodies exert a clear-cut neutralizing effect on the immunosuppressive capacity of OKT3. This is probably related to the lower affinity of IgM anti-OKT3 antibodies compared to the IgG ones. Concerning their fine specificity, essentially two types of anti-OKT3 antibodies are detected and purified. The first one includes antibodies that react with all mouse IgG2 (OKT3 is an IgG2a), do not react with mouse IgG1, IgG3, or IgM, do not react with OKT3 $F(ab')_2$ fragments, and do not block OKT3 binding to T cells. These antibodies are directed to OKT3 isotypic determinants (i.e., anti-isotypic antibodies). The second type of anti-OKT3 antibodies show an anti-idiotypic specificity: they react with determinants exclusively present on the variable region of the OKT3 molecule (Fab or F(ab')2 fragments) and missing on other murine IgG2 immunoglobulins. Moreover, these anti-idiotypic antibodies have been shown to be of major clinical importance since only they can block the binding of OKT3 to T cells and their appearance in OKT3-treated patients is tightly correlated with reappearance of circulating $OKT3^+$ cells [a correlation not observed for anti-isotypic antibodies (Baudrihaye et al., 1984)].

Spectrotype analysis of anti-OKT3 antibodies by isoelectrofocusing and subsequent western blotting revealed that the anti-idiotypic response was oligoclonal [i.e., it involved a limited number of B-cell clones (Chatenoud et al., 1986b)].

As mentioned above the peculiar immunogenicity displayed by OKT3 is not unique to this mAb since the same type of restricted immune response was shown with other mAbs. Particularly detailed data have been obtained in monkeys treated with different anti-CD4 and anti-CD8 antibodies (Villemain et al., 1986) as well as in mice treated with a panel of rat mAbs presenting various specificities (Benjamin et al., 1986).

Different strategies have been developed to circumvent the deleterious anti-mAb sensitization. The association of conventional immunosuppressants is the first approach that has been explored by several groups (Ortho Multicenter Transplant Study Group, 1985; Kreis et al., 1985; Chatenoud et al., 1986a). Our experience, based at present on more than 500 renal allograft recipients who received prophylactic OKT3 treatment for 14 to 30 consecutive days, has shown that the addition of low-dose steroids in association with full-dose azathioprine is indeed effective in preventing the onset of neutralizing IgG sensitization. It must be emphasized that to be effective azathioprine must be used at full dosage of 3 mg/kg per day since strong immunization was observed in centers that used only 0.5 mg/kg per day of azathioprine (Ortho Multicenter Transplant Study Group, 1985; Chatenoud et al., 1986a; 80% of the immunized patients in the Ortho multicenter trial compared to 30% in ours). Combining cyclosporine with OKT3 is also highly effective in preventing sensitization (personal unpublished data).

Another strategy is based on the observation that the major component of the anti-mAb response is anti-idiotypic and oligoclonal (Chatenoud et al., 1986a,b). It consists in using sequentially different mAbs with the same specificity but different idiotypes. Indeed, Jonker and Den Brok (1987) succeeded in demonstrating the experimental validity of this hypothesis by consecutively injecting various anti-CD4 antibodies presenting different idiotypes into rhesus monkeys.

Humanized antibodies (Riechmann et al., 1988), of course, represent a very interesting alternative. Encouraging preliminary results have been obtained using the humanized reshaped form of the rat CAMPATH 1 mAb (Riechmann et al., 1988). Immunotoxins may also become an approach for the future, but unfortunately at present several practical problems persist that still hamper the clinical use of these products.

Major hopes were also invested in the induction of tolerance, but recent data from Benjamin et al. (1986) clearly show that it is difficult to attain full tolerance to xenogeneic mAb, at least when they bind to host cells. In fact, when mice tolerized to rat immunoglobulins are challenged with a cell-binding rat mAb, they exhibit high titers of anti-idiotypic antibodies that contrast with the absence of response to constant region determinants (i.e., anti-isotypic antibodies). From a theoretical viewpoint these results suggest that when it binds to a cell surface structure a xenogenic mAb is recognized as two distinct antigenic entities— one associated with the variable region and the other with the constant region—that undergo different pathways of processing and presentation. In this context one may speculate on the putative key role of antigenic modulation in favoring a particularly immunogenic presentation of the mAb idiotypic determinants.

CONCLUSIONS

Anti-T-cell monoclonal antibodies have now been proved to represent effective immunosuppressive agents in renal allograft recipients. One may foresee the extension of their use in transplantation involving other organs as well as possibly in other clinical settings, notably autoimmune diseases. It seems reasonable to assume that mAb will substitute for polyclonal antilymphocyte sera, thus improving the conditions of clinical serotherapy. One has to realize, however, that two limitations may still persist in some cases:

1. The sensitization problem that can be at least partly circumvented by the various approaches described. The final solution may probably come from the production of larger panels of mAbs presenting distinct idiotypes that could be used consecutively (as detailed above) when sensitization occurs.
2. The systemic reaction observed with some mAbs like OKT3.

As soon as these difficulties are solved, monoclonal anti-T-cell antibodies will surely play a major role in immunosuppression as useful complements and/or alternatives to conventional drugs, notably cyclosporine A, steroids, and azathioprine.

REFERENCES

Bank, I., and Chess, L., 1985, Perturbations of the T4 molecule transmits a negative signal to T cells, J. Exp. Med. 162:1294–1303.

Baudrihaye, M. F., Chatenoud, L., Kreis, H., Goldstein, G., and Bach, J. F., 1984, Unusually restricted anti-isotype human immune response to OKT3 monoclonal antibody, Eur. J. Immunol. 14:686–691.

Benjamin, R. J., and Waldmann, H., 1986, Induction of tolerance by monoclonal antibody therapy, Nature 320:449–451.

Benjamin, R. J., Cobbold, S. P., Clark, M. R., and Waldmann, H., 1986, Tolerance to rat monoclonal antibodies, J. Exp. Med. 163:1539–1552.

Billing, R., and Chatterjee, S., 1983, Prolongation of skin allograft survival in monkeys treated with anti-Ia and anti-blast/monocyte antibodies, *Transplant. Proc.* **15**:649–650.

Borst, J., Coligan, J. E., Oettgen, H., Pessano, S., Malin, R., and Terhorst, C., 1984, The δ and ε-chains of the human T3/T-cell receptor complex are distinct polypeptides, *Nature* **312**:455–458.

Cantor, H., and Boyse, E. A., 1975, Functional subclasses of T lymphocytes bearing different Ly antigens. I. The generation of functionally distinct T cell subclasses is a differentiative process independent of antigen, *J. Exp. Med.* **141**:1376–1389.

Chatenoud, L., 1989, Monoclonal antibodies, *Curr. Opin. Immunol.* **2**:246–248.

Chatenoud, L., and Bach, J. F., 1990, Monoclonal antibodies to CD3 as immunosuppressants, *Sem. Immunol.* **2**:437–477.

Chatenoud, L., and Bach, J. F., 1984, Antigenic modulation—A major mechanism of antibody action, *Immunol. Today* **5**:20–25.

Chatenoud, L., Baudrihaye, M. F., Kreis, H., Goldstein, G., Schindler, J., and Bach, J. F., 1982, Human *in vivo* antigenic modulation induced by the anti-T cell OKT3 monoclonal antibody, *Eur. J. Immunol.* **12**:979–982.

Chatenoud, L., Baudrihaye, M. F., Chkoff, N., Kreis, H., and Bach, J. F., 1983, Immunologic follow-up of renal allograft recipients treated prophylactically by OKT3 alone, *Transplant. Proc.* **15**:643–645.

Chatenoud, L., Baudrihaye, M. F., Chkoff, N., Kreis, H., Goldstein, G., and Bach, J. F., 1986a, Restriction of the human *in vivo* immune response against the mouse monoclonal antibody OKT3, *J. Immunol.* **137**:830–838.

Chatenoud, L., Jonker, M., Villemain, F., Goldstein, G., and Bach, J. F., 1986b, The human immune response to the OKT3 monoclonal antibody is oligoclonal, *Science* **232**:1406–1408.

Chatenoud, L., Ferran, C., Legendre, C., Franchimont, P., Reuter, A., Kreis, H., and Bach, J. F., 1988, Clinical use of OKT3: The role of cytokine release and xenosensitization, *J. Autoimmun.* **1**:631–640.

Chatenoud, L., Ferran, C., Legendre, C., Franchimont, P., Reuter, A., Kreis, H., and Bach, J. F., 1989, Systemic reaction to the anti-T-cell monoclonal antibody OKT3 in relation to serum levels of tumor necrosis factor and interferon-gamma, *N. Engl. J. Med.* **320**:1420–1421.

Chatenoud, L., Legendre, C., Ferran, C., Bach, J. F., and Kreis, H., 1991, Corticosteroid inhibition of the OKT3-induced cytokine-related syndrome. Dosage and kinetics prerequisites, *Transplantation* **51**:334–338.

Cobbold, S. P., Jayesuriya, A., Nash, A., Prospeno, T. D., and Waldmann, H., 1984, Therapy with monoclonal antibodies by elimination of T-cell, *Nature* **312**:548–551.

Colonna, J. O., Goldstein, L. I., Brems, J. J., Vargas, J. H., Brill, J. E., Berquist, W. J., Hiatt, J. R., and Busuttil, R. N., 1987, A prospective study on the use of monoclonal anti-T3-cell antibody (OKT3) to treat steroid-resistant liver transplant rejection, *Arch. Surg.* **122**:1120–1123.

Cosimi, A. B., 1983, Anti-T cell monoclonal antibodies in transplantation therapy, *Transplant. Proc.* **15**:583–589.

Cosimi, A. B., Burton, R. C., Colvin, B., Goldstein, G., Delmonico, F. L., Laquaglia, M. P., Tolkoff-Rubin, N., Rubin, R. H., Herrin, J. T., and Russel, P. S., 1981, Treatment of acute renal allograft rejection with OKT3 monoclonal antibody, *Transplantation* **32**:535–539.

Dialynas, D. P., Quan, Z. S., Wall, K. A., Pierres, J., Quintans, M., Loken, R., Pierres, M., and Fitch, F. W., 1983a, Characterization of the murine T cell surface molecule, designated T4, identified by monoclonal antibody GK1.5: Similarity of L3T4 to the human Leu-3/74 molecule, *J. Immunol.* **131**:2445–2451.

Dialynas, D. P., Wilde, D. B., Marrack, P., Pierres, A., Wall, K. A., Harran, W., Otten, G., Loken, M. R., Pierres, M., Kappler, J., and Fitch, F. W., 1983b, Characterization of the murine antigenic determinant, designated L3T4a by functional T cell clones appears to correlate primarily with class II MHC antigen reactivity, *Immunol. Rev.* **74**:29–56.

Dillman, R. O., and Royston, I., 1985, Monoclonal antibodies in the therapy of malignant diseases, in: *Handbook of Monoclonal Antibodies* (S. Ferrone and M. P., Dietrich, eds.), Noyes Publications, Park Ridge, N.J., pp. 436–472.

Ferran, C., Sheehan, C., Dy, M., Schreiber, R., Mérite, S., Landais, P., Noël, L. H., Grau, G., Bluestone, J., Bach, J. F., and Chatenoud, L., 1990, Cytokine related syndrome following injection of anti-CD3 monoclonal antibody: Further evidence for transient *in vivo* T cell activation, *Eur. J. Immunol.* **20**:509–515.

Ferran, C., Sheehan, K., Schreiber, R., Bach, J. F., and Chatenoud, L., 1991, Anti-TNF abrogates the cytokine related anti-CD3 induced syndrome, *Transplant. Proc.* **23**:849–850.

Garchon, H. J., Blancher, A., Champonier, F., and Bach, J. F., 1983, Production of human monoclonal antibodies against tetanus toxoid, *Rev. Fr. Transfus. Immunohematol.* **26**:147–151.

Giorgi, J. V., Burton, R. C., Barrett, L. V., Delmonico, G., Goldstein, G., and Cosimi, A. B., 1983, Immunosuppressive effect and immunogenicity of OKT11A monoclonal antibody in monkey allograft recipients, *Transplant. Proc.* **15**:639–642.

Gordon, R. D., Tzakis, A. G., Iwatsuki, S., Todo, S., Esquivel, C. O., Marsh, J. W., Stieber, A., Makowka, L., and Starzl, T. E., 1988, Experience with orthoclone OKT3 in liver transplantation, *Am. J. Kidney Dis.* **11**:141–144.

Greenstein, J. L., Kappler, J., Marrack, P., and Burakoff, S. J., 1984, The role of L3T4 in recognition of Ia by a cytotoxic, H-2D^{d}-specific T cell hybridoma, *J. Exp. Med.* **159**:1213–1224.

Gutstein, N. L., Seaman, W. E., Scott, J. H., and Wofsy, D., 1986, Induction of immune tolerance by administration of monoclonal antibody to L3T4, *J. Immunol.* **137**:1127–1132.

Hayward, A. R., and Schreiber, M., 1989, Neonatal injection of CD3 antibody into nonobese diabetic mice reduces the incidence of insulitis and diabetes, *J. Immunol.* **143**:1555–1559.

Hirsch, R., Eckhaus, M., Auchincloss, H., Sachs, D. H., and Bluestone, J. A., 1988, Effects of *in vivo* administration of anti-T3 monoclonal antibody on T cell function in mice, *J. Immunol.* **140**:3766–3772.

Hirsch, R., Gress, R. E., Pluznik, D. H., Eckhaus, M., and Bluestone, J. A., 1989, Effect of *in vivo* administration of anti-T3 monoclonal antibody on T cell function in mice. II. *In vivo* activation of T cells, *J. Immunol.* **142**:737–743.

Hirsch, R., Bluestone, J. A., DeNenno, L., and Gress, R. E., 1990, Anti-CD3 F(ab')2 fragments are immunosuppressive *in vivo* without evoking either the strong humoral response or morbidity associated with whole mAb, *Transplantation* **49**:1117–1123.

Jaffers, G. J., Fuller, T. C., Cosimi, B., Russell, P. S., Winn, H. J., and Colvin, R. B., 1986, Monoclonal antibody therapy, *Transplantation* **41:**572–578.

Jonker, M., and Den Brok, J. H. A. M., 1987, Idiotype switching of CD4-specific monoclonal antibodies can prolong the therapeutic effectiveness in spite of host anti-mouse IgG antibodies, *Eur. J. Immunol.* **17:**1547–1553.

Jonker, M., Goldstein, G., and Balner, H., 1983a, Effects of *in vivo* administration of monoclonal antibodies specific for human T cell subpopulations on the immune system in a rhesus monkey model, *Transplantation* **35:**521–526.

Jonker, M., Malissen, B., and Mawas, C., 1983b, The effect of *in vivo* application of monoclonal antibodies specific for human cytotoxic T cells in rhesus monkeys, *Transplantation* **35:**374–378.

Jonker, M, Neuhaus, P., Zurcher, C., Fucello, A., and Goldstein, G., 1985, OKT4 and OKT4A antibody treatment as immunosuppression for kidney transplantation in rhesus monkeys, *Transplantation* **39:**247–253.

Jonker, M., and Nooij, F. J. M., van Suylichem, P., Neuhaus, P., and Goldstein, G., 1986, The influence of OKT8F treatment on allograft survival in rhesus monkeys, *Transplantation* **4:**431–435.

Kaplan, H. S., Olsson, L., and Raubitschek, A., 1982, Monoclonal human antibodies: A recent development with wide-ranging clinical potential, in: *Monoclonal Antibodies in Clinical Medicine* (A. J. McMichael and J. W. Fabre, eds.), Academic Press, New York, pp. 17–35.

Kelley, V. E., Naor, D., Tarcic, N., Gaulton, G. N., and Strom, T. B., 1986, Anti-interleukin 2 receptor antibody suppresses delayed type hypersensitivity to foreign and syngeneic antigens, *J. Immunol.* **137:**2122–2124.

Kelley, V. E., Gaulton, G. N., and Strom, T. B., 1987, Inhibitory effects of anti-interleukin 2 receptor and anti-L3T4 antibodies on delayed type hypersensitivity: The role of complement and epitope, *J. Immunol.* **138:**2771–2775.

Kirkman, R. L., Araujo, J. L., Busch, G. J., Carpenter, C. B., Milford, E. L., Reinherz, E. L., Schlossman, S. F., Strom, T. B., and Tilney, N. L., 1983, Treatment of acute renal rejection with monoclonal anti-T-12 antibody, *Transplantation* **36:**620–626.

Kirkman, R. L., Barrett, L. V., Gaulton, G. N., Kelley, V. E., Ythier, A., and Strom, T. B., 1985, Administration of an anti-interleukin 2 receptor monoclonal antibody prolongs cardiac allograft survival in mice, *J. Exp. Med.* **162:**358–362.

Kreis, H., Chkoff, N., Vigeral, Ph., Chatenoud, L., Lacombe, M., Campos, H., Pruna, A., Goldstein, G., Bach, J. F., and Crosnier, J., 1985, Therapeutic use of monoclonal antibodies in kidney transplantation, *Adv. Nephrol.* **14:**389–407.

Kremer, A. B., Barnes, L., Hirsch, R., and Goldstein, G., 1987, Orthoclone OKT3 monoclonal antibody reversal of hepatic and cardiac allograft rejection unresponsive to conventional immunosuppressive treatments, *Transplant. Proc.* (Suppl. 1)**19:**54–57.

Kupiec-Weglinski, J. W., Diamantstein, T. Tilney, N. L., and Strom, T. B., 1986, Therapy with monoclonal antibody to anti-interleukin-2 receptor spares T suppressor cells and prevents or reverses acute allograft rejection in rats, *Proc. Natl. Acad. Sci. USA* **83:**2624–2627.

Kurrle, R., Seyfert, W. Trautwein, A., and Seiler, F. R., 1986, T cell activation by CD3 antibodies: in: *Leukocyte Typing II*, Volume I (E. L. Reinherz *et al.*, eds.), Springer Verlag, New York, pp. 137–146.

Lanier, L. L., and Weiss, A., 1986, Presence of Ti (WT31) negative T lymphocytes in normal blood and thymus, *Nature* **324:**268–270.

Ledbetter, J. A., Rouse, R. V., Micklem, H. S., and Herzenberg, L. A., 1980, T cell subsets defined by expression of Lyt-1,2,3 and Thy-1 antigens. Two parameters, immunofluorescence and cytotoxicity analysis with monoclonal antibodies modify current views, *J. Exp. Med.* **152:**280–298.

Michaelides, M., Hogarth, P. M., and McKenzie, I. F. C., 1981, The immunosuppressive effect of monoclonal anti-Lyt-1.1 antibodies *in vivo, Eur. J. Immunol.* **121:**1005–1012.

Milstein, C., 1982, Monoclonal antibodies from hybrid myelomas. Theoretical aspects and some general comments, in: *Monoclonal Antibodies in Clinical Medicine* (A. J. McMichael and J. W. Fabre eds.), Academic Press, New York, pp. 3–16.

Ortho Multicenter Transplant Study Group, 1985, A randomized chemical trial of OKT3 monoclonal antibody for acute rejection of cadaveric renal transplants, *N. Engl. J. Med.* **313:**337–342.

Reinherz, E. L., 1985, A molecular basis for thymic selection: Regulation of T11 induced thymocyte expansion by the T3-Ti antigen/MHC receptor pathway, *Immunol. Today* **6:**75–79.

Reinherz, E. L., and Schlossman, S. F., 1980, The differentiation and function of human T lymphocytes, *Cell* **19:**821–827.

Reinherz, E. L., Meuer, S., Fitzgerald, K. A., Hussey, R. E., Levine, M., and Schlossman, S. F., 1982, Antigen recognition by human T lymphocytes is linked to surface expression of the T3 molecular complex, *Cell* **30:**735–743.

Riechmann, L., Clark, M., Waldmann, H., and Winter, G., 1988, Reshaping human antibodies for therapy, *Nature* **332:**323–327.

Shapiro, M. E., Kirkman, R. L., Reed, M. H., Puskas, J. D., Mazoujian, G., Letvin, N. L., Carpenter, C. B., Milford, E. L., Waldmann, H. A., Strom, T. B., and Schlossman, S. F., 1987, Monoclonal anti-IL-2 receptor antibody in primate renal transplantation, *Transplant. Proc.* **19:**594–598.

Shaw, S., 1987, Characterization of human leukocyte differentiation antigens, *Immunol. Today* **8:**1–3.

Shizuru, J. A., Edwards, C. T., Bank, B. A., Gregory, A. K., and Fathman, C. G., 1988, Immunotherapy of the non-obese diabetic mouse treatment with an antibody to T helper lymphocytes, *Science* **240:**659–662.

Sikora, K., Alderson, T., Phillips, J., and Watson, D. J., 1982, Human hybridomas from malignant gliomas, *Lancet* **1:**11–14.

Soulillou, J. P., LeMauff, B., Olive, D., Delaage, M., Peyronnet, P., Hourmant, M., Mawas, C., Hirn, M., and Jacques, Y., 1987, Prevention of rejection of kidney transplants by monoclonal antibody directed against interleukin 2 receptor, *Lancet* **1:**1339–1342.

Springer, T. A., Dustin, M. L., Kishimoto, T. K., and Marlin, S. D., 1987, The lymphocyte function associated LFA-1, CD2 and LFA-3 molecules: Cell adhesion receptors of the immune system, *Annu. Rev. Immunol.* **5:**223–252.

Starzl, T. E., and Fung, J. J., 1986, orthoclone OKT3 in treatment of allografts rejected under cyclosporin–steroid therapy, *Transplant. Proc.* **18:**937–941.

Swain, S. L., 1983, T cell subsets and the recognition of MHC class, *Immunol. Rev.* **74:**129–142.

Swain, S. L., Dialynas, D. P., Fitch, F. W., and English, M., 1984, Monoclonal antibody to L3T4 blocks the function of T cells specific for class 2 major histocompatibility complex antigens, J. Immunol. 132:118–1123.

Tite, J., Sloan, A., and Janeway, C. A., Jr., 1986, The role of L3T4 in T cell activation: L3T4 may be both an Ia-binding protein and a receptor that transduces a negative signal, J. Mol. Cell. Immunol. 2:179–187.

Uchiyama, T., Broder, S., and Waldmann, T. A., 1981, A monoclonal antibody reactive with activated and functionally mature human T cells, J. Immunol. 126:1393–1397.

Villemain, F., Jonker, M., Bach, J. F., and Chatenoud, L., 1986, Fine specificity of antibodies produced in rhesus monkeys following in vivo treatment with anti-T cell murine monoclonal antibodies, Eur. J. Immunol. 16:945–949.

Waldor, M. K., Sriram, S., Hardy, R., Herzenberg, L. A., Lanier, L., Lim, M., and Steinman, L., 1985, Reversal of experimental allergic encephalomyelitis with monoclonal antibody to a T-cell subset marker, Science 227:415–417.

Wilde, D. B., Marrack, P., Kappler, J., Dialynas, D., and Fitch, F. W., 1983, Evidence implicating L3T4 in class II MHC antigen reactivity: Monoclonal antibody GK1.5 (anti-L3T4a) blocks class II MHC antigen-specific proliferation, release of lymphokines and binding by cloned murine helper T lymphocyte lines, J. Immunol. 131:2178–2183.

Wofsy, D., 1985, Strategies for treating autoimmune disease with monoclonal antibodies, West. J. Med. 143:804–810.

Wofsy, D., and Seaman, W. E., 1985, Successful treatment of autoimmunity in NZB/NZW F$_1$ mice with monoclonal antibody to L3T4, J. Exp. Med. 161:378–391.

Wofsy, D., and Seaman, W. E., 1987, Reversal of advanced murine lupus in NZB/NZW F$_1$ mice by treatment with monoclonal antibody to L3T4, J. Immunol. 138:3247–3253.

Wofsy, D., Ledbetter, J. A., Hendler, L. P., and Seaman, W. E., 1985a, Treatment of murine lupus with monoclonal anti-T cell antibody, J. Immunol. 143:852–857.

Wofsy, D., Mayes, D. C., Woodcock, J., and Seaman, W. E., 1985b, Inhibition of humoral immunity in vivo by monoclonal antibody to L3T4: Studies with soluble antigens in intact mice, J. Immunol. 135:1698–1701.

Woodcock, J., Wofsy, D., Eriksson, E., Scott, J. H., and Seaman, W. E. 1986, Rejection of skin grafts and generation of cytotoxic T cells by mice depleted of L3T4+ cells, Transplantation 42:636–642.

Immune Response Modifiers of Biological Origin

Chapter 15

IMMUNOTOXINS

David C. Blakey

1. INTRODUCTION

Immunotoxins are covalent conjugates of monoclonal antibodies directed against cell-specific antigens and potent toxins of bacterial or plant origin. Bacterial toxins that have been used to prepare immunotoxins include diphtheria toxin and *Pseudomonas aeruginosa* exotoxin A (reviewed in Blakey *et al.*, 1988a; Wawrzynczak and Davies, 1990). Such immunotoxins may have limited clinical use in patients, however, due to the presence of preexisting neutralizing antibodies to those toxins either as a result of previous bacterial infection or immunization. The majority of work has thus concentrated on the use of toxins or ribosomal-inactivating proteins (RIPs) from plants. Toxins include ricin and abrin from the seeds of *Ricinus communis* and *Abrus precatorius*, respectively. They consist of two polypeptide chains, A and B, each having a molecular weight of approximately 30 kDa, which are linked by a single disulfide bond. Individually, the A and B chains are virtually devoid of cytotoxic action, both being required to exert potent cytotoxic effects. The B-chain subunit contains two binding sites that recognize galactose containing glycoproteins and glycolipids present on the surface of virtually all cell types (Robertus, 1988). Following binding via the B chain, the toxin is taken into the cell by receptor-mediated endocytosis, and the A chain, by an ill-defined mechanism, crosses a cell membrane to reach the cytosol. The A chain then inactivates the 60S ribosomal subunit, thereby terminating protein synthesis and killing the cell. Endo and Tsurugi (1987) have shown that the A chains are specific N-glycosidases that remove an adenine residue from adenosine 4324 in the 28S rRNA of the 60S ribosomal complex. The extreme potency of these toxins results from the fact that entry of very few molecules of A chain into the cytoplasm, perhaps just one, appears sufficient to kill the cell (Eiklid *et al.*, 1980).

Several plants have been found to contain A-chain-like proteins called RIPs (reviewed in Stirpe and Barbieri, 1986). Examples of RIPs include gelonin, saporin, and pokeweed antiviral protein from the seeds of *Gelonium multiflorum*, *Saponaria officinalis*, and *Phytolacca americana*, respectively. As with the isolated A chains of the toxins, these RIPs are not themselves toxins because they lack a B chain by which to bind to cells. They all inactivate

David C. Blakey • ICI Pharmaceuticals, Macclesfield SK10 4TG, Cheshire, England.

Immunopharmacology in Autoimmune Diseases and Transplantation, edited by Hans Erik Rugstad *et al.* Plenum Press, New York, 1992.

eukaryotic ribosomes in a similar fashion to the A chains of abrin and ricin and with a similar potency.

2. PREPARATION AND CYTOTOXIC PROPERTIES OF IMMUNOTOXINS *IN VITRO*

Most intact toxin conjugates have been prepared by attaching the toxin to the antibody using a noncleavable thioether linkage. This minimizes the risk of release of free intact toxin, which would lead to nonspecific toxicity (reviewed in Wawrzynczak and Thorpe, 1987). In contrast, immunotoxins prepared with the A-chain subunits of toxins or with RIPs are generally linked using heterobifunctional cross-linking agents that introduce a cleavable disulfide bond between the A chain and antibody (Fig. 1). This is because A-chain immunotoxins prepared with a disulfide linkage are consistently more potent than their thioether-linked counterparts, suggesting that reductive release of free A chain is an important step in the cytotoxic process (Wawrzynczak and Thorpe, 1987). The most widely

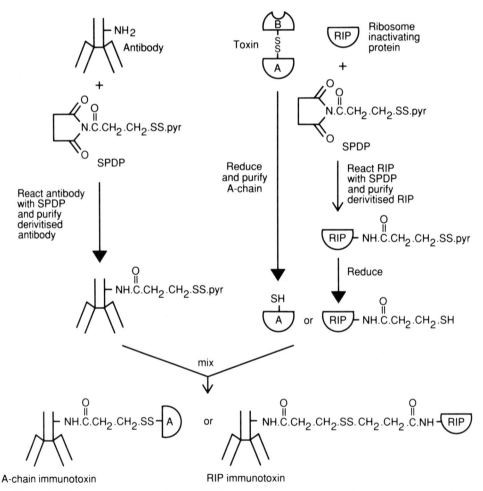

FIGURE 15.1.   Preparation of A-chain and RIP immunotoxins using the SPDP reagent. Pyr = pyridyl.

used agent for this purpose is N-succinimidyl 3-(2-pyridyldithio)propionate (SPDP) (Fig. 1). Free antibody and A chain are removed from the immunotoxin preparation using a combination of gel filtration and affinity chromatography or ion-exchange procedures (reviewed in Blakey et al., 1988a; Lambert and Blattler, 1988). The in vitro cytotoxic potency of the resulting immunotoxins are generally determined by measuring the inhibition of radiolabeled leucine into protein of target cells after exposure to varying concentrations of immunotoxin (Neville and Marsh, 1988).

Intact toxin immunotoxins are extremely potent cytotoxic agents in vitro for cells with the appropriate target antigen often matching or even surpassing the potency of the native toxin. However, due to the presence of galactose-binding sites in the B chain, they can also bind to nontarget cells, which leads to significant nonspecific toxicity both in vitro and in vivo (Blakey et al., 1988a). In vitro this problem can be diminished by the addition of excess galactose or lactose. In contrast, A chain and RIP immunotoxins possess virtually complete specificity in vitro because they do not have a B chain by which to bind nonspecifically to cells. Unfortunately, however, these immunotoxins, unlike their intact toxin counterparts, have variable cytotoxic potency. It is thought that this is because the B chain, in addition to its binding function, also helps the A chain to reach the cytosol of the cell. In support of this hypothesis, addition of free B chain can potentiate the potency of weakly active A-chain-type immunotoxins in vitro (McIntosh and Thorpe, 1984). The potency of A-chain-type immunotoxins is determined by a number of factors including the affinity and valency of the antibody and the nature of the molecule recognized by the antibody which in turn influences the rate and route of entry of the immunotoxin (Blakey et al., 1988a). Carboxylic ionophores and lysosomotropic amines can in some instances potentiate the cytotoxicity of A-chain immunotoxins and are thought to act by interfering with the intracellular processing of the immunotoxins, possibly diverting them to cellular compartments that favor escape of the A chain into the cytosol (Blakey et al., 1988a; Casellas and Jansen, 1988). Some A-chain-type immunotoxins are, however, extremely toxic to target cells (Table I) and have potencies matching their intact toxin counterparts (Bjorn and Villemez, 1988). The extreme potency and high specificity of these A chain and RIP

TABLE I.   Examples of Potent A Chain and RIP Immunotoxins

Immunotoxin	Antigen recognized	Target cell	Cytotoxicity IC_{50} (M)	Reference
OX7-ricin A chain	Thy1.1	Mouse AKR-A lymphoma	2.7×10^{-11}	Blakey et al. (1987a)
OKT1-Saporin	CD5	Human T-lymphocytes	3×10^{-10}	Siena et al. (1988)
HD6-deglycosylated ricin A chain	CD22	Human Burkitt's lymphoma line, Daudi	1.4×10^{-11}	Ghetie et al. (1988)
R17 217-recombinant ricin A chain	Mouse transferrin receptor	L1210 murine lymphocytic leukemia	3×10^{-11}	Bjorn and Groetsema (1987)
C-19-ricin A	Carcinoembryonic antigen	Human adenocarcinoma cell line, LoVo	3.1×10^{-10}	Levin et al. (1982)
260 F9-ricin A	Unidentified breast tumor-associated antigen	Human breast adenocarcinoma line, MCF-7	1×10^{-10}	Bjorn et al. (1985)

immunotoxins *in vitro* suggest that these reagents might be capable of specific deletion of cell populations *in vivo* while having minimal toxicity.

3. PROPERTIES OF A-CHAIN AND RIP IMMUNOTOXINS *IN VIVO*

The antitumor activity of A-chain and RIP immunotoxins has been examined in a number of animal models (reviewed in Blakey *et al.*, 1988a; Griffin *et al.*, 1988). The results of early studies were disappointing even when immunotoxins of high potency were used. For example, an OX7-ricin A-chain immunotoxin specifically inhibited protein synthesis by 50% (IC_{50}) in Thy1.1 expressing AKR-A lymphoma cells at a concentration of 2.7×10^{-11} M (Table I), but when injected intravenously at a dose corresponding to one-twentieth of its LD_{50}, it only extended by nine days the medium survival of mice injected intraperitoneally with 10^6 AKR-A cells one day earlier (Blakey *et al.*, 1987a). This corresponded to eradication of only about 99% of the tumor cells in the peritoneal cavity. Several factors have been identified that reduce the potency of immunotoxins *in vivo* and means to circumvent these have been found or are being sought.

Immunotoxins prepared with ricin A chain are rapidly removed from the blood stream due to hepatic entrapment (Fig. 2). This is because ricin A chain is a glycoprotein containing terminal mannose and fucose sugars that can be recognized by receptors present on liver parenchymal and nonparenchymal cells (Blakey *et al.*, 1988b; Blakey and Thorpe, 1988a). This problem can be overcome by chemically destroying the terminal sugar residues on ricin A chain (Thorpe *et al.*, 1985; Blakey *et al.*, 1988b). Immunotoxins prepared with chemically deglycosylated ricin A chain have longer blood half-lives (Fig. 2) (Blakey *et al.*,

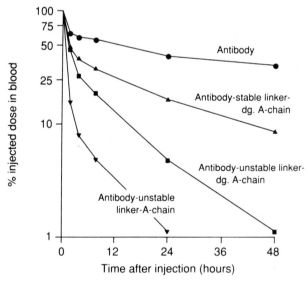

FIGURE 15.2. Blood clearance rates of various immunotoxins in mice. The monoclonal antibody OX7 was attached to native or chemically deglycosylated ricin A-chain, using either the SPDP (unstable linker) or SMPT (stable linker) coupling reagents. After radio-iodination, the blood clearance of the intact immunotoxins was determined in mice by SDS gel analysis of plasma samples taken at various time intervals after injection, as described previously (Blakey *et al.*, 1987b).

1987b) and improved antitumor activity (Thorpe *et al.*, 1988). Similarly, recombinant ricin A chain expressed in *Escherichia coli* (O'Hare *et al.*, 1987) is devoid of carbohydrate and immunotoxins prepared with recombinant ricin A chain have improved antitumor activity compared with their native ricin A-chain counterparts and have long blood half-lives (Griffin *et al.*, 1987; Wawrzynczak *et al.*, 1991).

A more general problem associated with A chain and RIP immunotoxins prepared with conventional heterobifunctional cross-linking agents is that they break down prematurely *in vivo* to release free antibody (Blakey *et al.*, 1987b; Griffin *et al.*, 1988). This is a problem because first it reduces the amount of immunotoxin available to locate and kill the target cells, and second the released free antibody can compete with the immunotoxin for the target antigen. New coupling reagents have been synthesized which introduce hindered disulfide linkages between the antibody and the A chain or RIP which reduce this problem (Worrell *et al.*, 1986; Thorpe *et al.*, 1987) (Fig. 2). Ricin A-chain immunotoxins prepared with one of these linkers, 4-succinimidyl-oxycarbonyl-α-methyl-α(2-pyridyldithio) toluene (SMPT), have improved antitumor activity compared with their unhindered disulfide-linked counterparts (Thorpe *et al.*, 1988).

Antigenic heterogeneity has been observed with many types of tumor cells (Woodruff, 1983) and so may represent a major problem for immunotoxins in cancer therapy. Tumor cells from tumors that developed after immunotoxin therapy in the AKR-A tumor model were sometimes found to lack or have low levels of the target Thy1.1 antigen. These animals therefore died due to outgrowth of a tumor cell population lacking the target antigen and thus being resistant to the immunotoxins (Thorpe *et al.*, 1988). In the same studies tumor cells surviving immunotoxin therapy *in vivo* were also identified that were resistant to the immunotoxin *in vitro* even though they had normal levels of the Thy1.1 antigen. These mutant tumor cells were fully sensitive to ricin, and thus deficient internalization of the immunotoxin was suggested as a possible reason for their resistance. By using cocktails of immunotoxins directed against two or more antigens, it may be possible to overcome the problems of antigenic heterogeneity and the appearance of tumor cell mutants (Yu *et al.*, 1990). Alternatively, immunotoxin therapy could be combined with other forms of therapy that do not rely on target antigen expression for their efficacy (Pearson *et al.*, 1989, 1990).

In the majority of clinical situations immunotoxins will have to reach target cells in extravascular sites if they are to be effective. It remains to be determined whether a relatively large immunotoxin molecule of molecular weight of approximately 180 kDa will be able to overcome the physiological barriers in tumors and gain sufficient access to such cells at nontoxic doses (Jain, 1989). Access to extravascular sites may be improved by the use of antibody or toxin fragments to reduce the size of the immunotoxin since the rate of extravasation from the blood into extravascular tissue is inversely proportional to the size of the protein (Nakamura *et al.*, 1968). Alternatively, access may be improved by using agents that increase the blood supply to the target site. Smyth *et al.* (1987) recently demonstrated that β-adrenergic blocking agents could increase the blood supply to a human tumor xenograft in a mouse and result in an improved therapeutic effect with an antibody–drug conjugate.

Finally, both the antibody and toxin portion of immunotoxins have been found to be immunogenic in patients, resulting in the formation of neutralizing antibodies (Spitler *et al.*, 1987; Byers *et al.*, 1988). In animal models and in recent clinical trials, use of immunosuppressive agents (e.g., cyclosporine, cyclophosphamide) has been found to reduce this problem (Spitler *et al.*, 1989; Pai *et al.*, 1990). The use of human or humanized monoclonal antibodies may also help to reduce the problem of immunogenicity (LoBuglio *et al.*, 1989).

4. CLINICAL TRIALS OF IMMUNOTOXINS IN CANCER

Two clinical trials have been published that have used immunotoxins to treat patients with T- and B-cell leukemias and lymphomas. Both used an immunotoxin prepared by coupling native ricin A chain to T101 antibody using the SPDP reagent (Laurent *et al.*, 1986; Hertler *et al.*, 1988). The T101 antibody reacts with a 65-kDa glycoprotein (CD5) expressed on the cell membrane of mature T cells, most T-cell-derived lymphoid neoplasias, and B cell chronic lymphocytic leukemias (Laurent *et al.*, 1988). Six patients received 10–45mg/m^2 of immunotoxin over a two day to four week period. The only systemic toxicity noted was mild fevers in three patients. All patients had a drop in their white blood cell count, ranging from 25–50% of initial values but prolonged remissions were not achieved. This lack of sustained benefit can be accounted for by the fact that first the T101 immunotoxin was only weakly cytotoxic to fresh leukemia cells in the absence of enhancing agents and second the immunotoxin had a very short half-life, probably resulting, at least in part, from hepatic entrapment and instability (Laurent *et al.*, 1988). Clinical trials have also been reported in which immunotoxins were used to treat patients with malignant melanoma, colorectal carcinoma, and breast carcinoma (Spitler *et al.*, 1987; Spitler, 1988; Gould *et al.*, 1989). The melanoma and colorectal trials used mouse monoclonal antibodies recognizing either the high-molecular-weight antigen present on melanoma cells or the GP72 antigen expressed on colorectal carcinoma, osteogenic sarcoma, and ovarian carcinoma cells, respectively. Both immunotoxins were prepared with SPDP and native ricin A chain. They were relatively potent, inhibiting 50% of protein synthesis in target cells at concentrations of 1–5 $\times$ 10^{-10} M and both were capable of causing significant inhibition of tumors in appropriate human tumor xenograft models.

Twenty-two patients were treated in a phase 1 trial with the antimelanoma immunotoxin (XomaZyme^R-Mel) by intravenous infusion over a 4–5 day period with 3.2–300 mg immunotoxin total dose. The major toxic side effects were a fall in serum albumin (20/22 patients) associated with weight gain and edema, a decreased voltage on EKG (16/22), sinus tachycardia (14/22), malaise/fatigue (15/22), and fever (14/22). All these side effects were transient and reversible after cessation of therapy. One patient in the trial had a complete response and has remained free of detectable tumor for 26 months. However, the survival of the group as a whole was not significantly different from a historic control group given conventional chemotherapy. In a subsequent phase 2 trial in which a dose of 0.4mg/kg per day for 5 days was selected, 3 of 46 patients had partial responses (Spitler *et al.*, 1989).

Sixteen patients were treated in a phase 1 trial with the anticolorectal immunotoxin (XomaZyme^R 791) and were given intravenous infusions over 5 days of between 0.02–0.2 mg immunotoxin/kg per day. The side effects were similar to those for XomaZyme^R-Mel. In addition, proteinuria was seen starting at study day 5 to 10 and resolving between days 30 to 45, and four patients experienced transient mental changes. Two of the 16 patients showed decreases in large, and disappearance of small, liver metastases, as judged by CT scans 2 to 3 months posttherapy.

As in the T101-ricin A-chain trials, XomaZyme^R-Mel was found to be cleared very rapidly from the bloodstream of patients. Approximately two thirds of the injected dose cleared with a half-life of 10–18 min and the remaining third cleared with a half-life of 1.5–5 hr. By using deglycosylated ricin A chain, recombinant ricin A chain, or RIPs devoid of carbohydrate and more stable cross-linking agents, the blood clearance of these immunotoxins might be slowed, and thus more substantial antitumor effects might be seen.

The antibreast immunotoxin used to treat patients with breast carcinoma utilized recombinant ricin A chain, and as expected the immunotoxin had much longer pharmacokinetics (Weiner *et al.*, 1989). In addition to the toxicities seen with other ricin A-chain immunotoxins, this immunotoxin resulted in neuropathies. The antibody (260F9) used in the immunotoxin bound to Schwann cells and this is thought to be the explanation for this toxicity.

In all three trials, neutralizing antibodies were produced against both the antibody and A-chain component, which effectively prevented re-treatment. If this problem can be overcome (see Section 3), improved therapeutic activity might be seen either by redosing with the same immunotoxin or re-treating with a second immunotoxin directed against a different tumor-associated antigen.

5. IMMUNOTOXINS IN TRANSPLANTATION

5.1. Bone Marrow Transplantation

Bone marrow transplantation (BMT) is used to treat hematological disorders such as aplastic anemia and leukemia as well as to replace the bone marrow of patients whose hematopoietic system has been compromised by intensive radiochemotherapy in the treatment of malignant disease (Blakey *et al.*, 1988a; Vallera, 1988).

Allogeneic BMT generally uses bone marrow from a major histocompatibility complex–human leukocyte antigen-matched sibling donor. A life-threatening disease called graft-versus-host disease (GVHD) can occur following transplantation if differences in HLA and non-HLA antigens cause immunocompetent T cells from the donor graft to respond against recipient antigens. A cocktail of three intact ricin anti-T-cell immunotoxins prepared with antibodies T101, UCHT1, and TA1, which bind CD5, CD3, and CD11a determinants, respectively, have been used to destroy those T cells in donor marrow responsible for GVHD in both HLA-matched and -nonmatched recipients (Filipovich *et al.*, 1987; Vallera, 1988). An equimolar mixture of 600 ng immunotoxin/ml effectively inhibited T-cell activity while having minimal pluripotent stem cell toxicity. In these studies, no cases of severe grade 3–4 GVHD were seen following transplantation of the immunotoxin pretreated bone marrow, indicating that such pretreatment was useful for preventing GVHD. However, the elimination of immunocompetent T cells has also led to an increased incidence of graft rejection/failure and leukemic relapse (Vallera, 1988). One explanation for the increased graft failure is that the elimination of T cells prevents secretion of factors having a direct effect on hematopoiesis such as granulocyte–macrophage colony-stimulating factor (GM-CSF). In a murine model, addition of recombinant GM-CSF to T-cell-depleted marrow has been found to increase the incidence of engraftment (Blazar *et al.*, 1988). Increased leukemic relapse may result from the absence of donor T cells that can respond to residual recipient leukemia cells in the immunocompromised patient. Systemic treatment with immunotoxins directed against these leukemic cells may reduce this problem (see Section 4).

Immunotoxins may also be useful in allogeneic bone marrow transplantation in the treatment of patients who develop GVHD. Kernan *et al.* (1988) have described the use of an anti-CD5–SPDP-ricin A-chain immunotoxin (XomaZyme-H65) to treat an 8-year-old girl who developed steroid-resistant grade 3–4 acute GVHD following allogeneic HLA-matched BMT. The patient received 0.05 mg immunotoxin/kg per day by intravenous infusion (30 min) for 14 days. After two days of treatment, CD5-positive T cells could no longer be detected in the bloodstream and a complete clinical response was seen. After cessation of therapy the number of CD5-positive T cells slowly rose, achieving normal levels four months later, but this did not result in reoccurrence of acute GVHD. Thus, a transient depletion of CD5-positive cells using an immunotoxin successfully treated a patient with life-threatening acute GVHD. This study has been extended to a further 35 patients using doses between 0.05–0.33 mg immunotoxin/kg per day. Five of 25 patients who received at least seven doses of immunotoxin and could be evaluated at day 15 had complete responses. Good response was associated with a shorter time between BMT and immunotoxin therapy (Byers et al., 1988). The major side effects seen were similar to those described for the melanoma and colorectal carcinoma clinical trials with the exception that six patients had renal dysfunction that reversed in most cases when immunotoxin therapy was discontinued. Thus, immunotoxins appear to have utility both for preventing occurrence of and treating GVHD in patients undergoing allogeneic BMT.

In autologous BMT a portion of the patient's own marrow is removed before giving the patient intensive radiochemotherapy and is returned on completion of the treatment, thus circumventing GVHD. However, the bone marrow may contain residual malignant cells that have to be eliminated prior to its reinfusion if relapse is not to occur. Filipovich et al. (1985) have used intact ricin immunotoxins prepared with monoclonal antibodies T101, TA1, and UCHT1 recognizing CD5, CD11a, and CD3, respectively, to purge residual leukemic cells from autologous bone marrow of seven patients with T-lineage acute lymphocytic leukemia (ALL)/lymphoma prior to its cryopreservation. A total concentration of 600 ng immunotoxin/ml was used and 100–200 mM lactose was added to minimize nonspecific toxicity due to B-chain binding. Similarly, Gorin et al. (1985) used a T101–ricin A-chain immunotoxin to purge bone marrow of leukemic cells in four patients with T-lineage ALL/lymphoma. In both studies prompt engraftment occurred in all patients, the rate of hematopoietic recovery was nearly normal, and one patient remained in prolonged remission for over one year. The success of this approach, however, is hard to evaluate because relapse may be due either to a failure of the radiochemotherapy to kill all the malignant cells in the patient or a failure of the immunotoxin to kill all the tumor cells in the bone marrow.

5.2. Organ Transplantation

Immunotoxins may be useful in the prevention of graft rejection in man after organ transplantation. Class II-expressing passenger leukocytes present in the donor organ are thought to play a significant role in the induction of transplantation immunity (Snell, 1957; Wiley, 1988). An immunotoxin prepared with ricin A chain and a monoclonal antibody (13.4) recognizing the mouse I-E^K determinant has been shown to specifically kill Ia-bearing rat spleen cells and was capable of completely inhibiting the rat mixed lymphocyte reaction, an in vitro model of transplant rejection (Nakahara et al., 1985). Similarly, an immunotoxin prepared with the same antibody and intact ricin, in the presence of lactose (100 mM), removed cells capable of stimulating a mixed lymphocyte islet cell culture while at the same time not altering the hormone-secreting function of the remaining cells when challenged with glucose. Preliminary studies were reported to suggest that the immunotoxin treatment of islets allowed their successful transplantation across MHC barriers in a rodent model (Shizuru et al., 1986). Wiley et al. (1988) showed that an immunotoxin prepared with ricin A chain and a monoclonal antibody (OX4) directed against rat class II MHC molecules could specifically remove cells capable of stimulating the rat mixed lymphocyte reaction. However, administration of the immunotoxin to isolated rat pancreases by hypothermic perfusion did not prolong their survival when allografted across a MHC barrier. The immunotoxin used in this study had relatively low potency (IC$_{50}$ in rat mixed lymphocyte reaction = 5×10^{-9} M), and thus insufficient immunotoxin may have been infused to exert a significant effect. The amount of immunotoxin infused could not be increased since even at the dose used, acinar cell toxicity was seen, probably as a result of ricin toxicity due to the presence of contaminating ricin B chain.

The experiments reported to date suggest that immunotoxins may be useful for elimination of class II-expressing passenger leukocytes in organ transplants prior to engraftment. An alternative approach, if the organ was to be transplanted across a MHC barrier, would be to select an immunotoxin, based on the tissue typing of the donor and recipient, that recognized an MHC class II antigen on donor cells that was absent on the recipient's cells. This should allow the specific deletion of donor cells possessing class II in the organ transplant after engraftment while leaving the class II-bearing cells of the recipient unharmed.

An alternative use for immunotoxins in transplantation therapy would be to deplete selectively the T-helper subpopulation that interacts with the class II molecules and leads to the cascade of transplant rejection. Support for this idea comes from the finding that injection of mice with the monoclonal antibody L3T4, which recognizes a determinant present on the surface of mouse T-helper lymphocytes, allows islets of Langerhans to be transplanted across a MHC barrier in mice without additional immunosuppression (Shizuru et al., 1987). T-helper cell depletion in man could be accomplished with a pan-T-cell immunotoxin of the type described by Byers et al. (1988) for use in treatment of GVHD or more selectively by using an immunotoxin directed against the CD4 determinant on T-helper cells. Since transient removal of the T-helper cell population leads to indefinite allograft survival in animal models (Shizuru et al., 1987), the period of T-cell depletion and thus immunosuppression may only need to be relatively short-lived.

6. IMMUNOTOXINS IN AUTOIMMUNE DISEASE

Monoclonal antibodies directed against determinants on T-helper cells have been shown to be capable of achieving some therapeutic benefit in a number of animal models of autoimmune disease (Siram and Ranges, 1987; Shizuru et al., 1988) and in man in the treatment of rheumatoid arthritis (Herzog et al., 1987). Recently, Byers and co-workers have used an anti-CD5–ricin A-chain immunotoxin (ZomaZyme-H65) to treat patients with severe rheumatoid arthritis. Approximately 50% of patients responded and 20–40% of these had prolonged remissions lasting over one year following a single five- to nine-day course of therapy (Caperton et al., 1989). Thus, as in organ transplantation, immunotoxins that delete the T-helper cell population may be useful in the treatment of autoimmune disease (Blakey and Thorpe, 1988b). Identification of antigens present on a subset of T-helper cells involved in the autoimmune disease would reduce the problem of nonspecific immunosuppression. One possibility in rheumatoid arthritis is to target the very late activation antigen-1, which has been shown to be present on T-helper cells in the synovium but absent from T-helper cells in the peripheral blood (Hemler et al., 1986).

An alternative therapeutic approach would be to use immunotoxins to kill antigen-presenting cells implicated in the autoimmune disease state. An immunotoxin directed against self-MHC class II determinants would be extremely nonspecific and would lead to general immunosuppression since class II determinants are also expressed on B cells. However, it is possible that antigen-presenting cells involved in autoimmunity may possess specific antigens that, if identified, could be used as targets to deplete these cells specifically.

Finally, in autoimmune diseases where autoantibodies have an important role in the etiology of the disease state, it may be possible to use the autoantigens that evoke the immune response to target toxins specifically to the B-cell population responsible for production of autoantibodies and thus result in clinical benefit. Rennie et al. (1983)

demonstrated that *in vitro* thyroglobulin linked to ricin A chain specifically suppressed the thyroglobulin autoantibody response of lymphocytes from patients with Hashimoto's thyroiditis. In another study, Killen and Lindstrom (1984) coupled ricin to the acetylcholine receptor (ACHR) and demonstrated that this conjugate, in the presence of lactose, could specifically kill ACHR-reactive lymphocytes responsible for causing experimental autoimmune myasthenia gravis in rats. Using the same experimental model, Deshambo and Krolick (1986) demonstrated that an immunotoxin prepared with ricin A chain and polyclonal anti-idiotypic antibodies generated against polyclonal antibodies to the ACHR could selectively kill anti-ACHR-reactive B lymphocytes *in vitro*. Transfer of such immunotoxin-treated ACHR-responsive lymphocytes to sublethally irradiated naive recipient rats followed by antigen challenge with ACHR demonstrated that secondary anti-ACHR antibody response was selectively inhibited for as long as 74 days postantigen challenge *in vivo* (Brown and Krolick, 1988). Thus, by using the autoantigen or appropriate anti-idiotypic antibodies, it may be possible to prepare immunotoxins that can selectively deplete autoantibody-producing B cells *in vivo* without causing general immunosuppression.

7. CONCLUSIONS

Immunotoxins prepared with RIPs or A chains of plant toxins have been shown to be capable of potent and specific cytotoxic effects *in vitro* and they result in impressive antitumor effects in animal tumor models once hepatic clearance and instability have been minimized. Although the results of initial clinical trials with immunotoxins to treat malignant disease have been disappointing, the immunotoxins used were far from optimal (e.g., low cytotoxic potency, rapid hepatic clearance, and poor stability). Thus, further clinical trials are required with immunotoxins having high potency and increased ability to localize to tumor cells *in vivo* before conclusions can be drawn concerning their utility in cancer therapy. In bone marrow transplantation, immunotoxins have been shown to be clinically useful both for preventing and treating GVHD. The latter result suggests that immunotoxins may have a role to play in modulating the immune response *in vivo* and thus may have utility in organ transplantation and treatment of autoimmune disease.

REFERENCES

Bjorn, M. J., and Groetsema, G., 1987, Immunotoxins to the murine transferrin receptor: Intercavitary therapy of mice bearing syngeneic peritoneal tumors, *Cancer Res.* **47:**6639.

Bjorn, M. J., Ring, D., and Frankel, A., 1985, Evaluation of monoclonal antibodies for the development of breast cancer immunotoxins, *Can. Res.* **45:**1214.

Bjorn, M. J., and Villemez, C. L., 1988, Immunotoxins: Selection of cell-surface antigens and their corresponding monoclonal antibodies, in: *Immunotoxins* (A. E. Frankel, ed.), Kluwer Academic Publishers, Boston, pp. 255–277.

Blakey, D. C., and Thorpe, P. E., 1988a, Prevention of carbohydrate-mediated clearance of ricin-containing immunotoxins by the liver, in: *Immunotoxins* (A. E. Frankel, ed.), Kluwer Academic Publishers, Boston, pp. 457–473.

Blakey, D. C., and Thorpe, P. E., 1988b, Treatment of malignant-disease and rheumatoid arthritis using ricin A-chain immunotoxins, *Scand. J. Rheumatol.* **76:**279–287.

Blakey, D. C., Wawrzynczak, E. J., Stirpe, F., and Thorpe, P. E., 1987a, Antitumor activity of a panel of anti-Thy1.1 immunotoxins made with different ribosome-inactivating proteins, in: *Membrane-Mediated Cytotoxicity*, Volume 45, UCLA Symposia (NS), p. 195.

Blakey, D. C., Watson, G. J., Knowles, P. P., and Thorpe, P. E., 1987b, Effects of chemical deglycosylation of ricin A-chain on the *in vivo* fate and cytotoxic activity of an immunotoxin composed of ricin A-chain and anti-Thy1.1 antibody, *Cancer Res.* **47:**947.

Blakey, D. C., Wawrzynczak, E. J., Wallace, P. M., and Thorpe, P. E., 1988a, Antibody toxin conjugates: A perspective, in: *Monoclonal Antibody Therapy; Progress in Allergy*, Volume 45 (H. Waldmann, ed.), S. Karger, Basel, pp. 50–90.

Blakey, D. C., Skilleter, D. N., Price, R. J., and Thorpe, P. E., 1988b, Uptake of native and deglycosylated ricin A-chain immunotoxins by mouse liver parenchymal and non-parenchymal cells *in vitro* and *in vivo*, *Biochim. Biophys. Acta* **968:**172.

Blazar, B. R., Widmer, M. B., Soderling, C. C. B., Urdal, D. L., Gillis, S., Robinson, L. L., and Vallera, D. A., 1988,

Augmentation of donor bone marrow engraftment in histocompatible murine recipients by granulocyte/macrophage colony-stimulating factor, *Blood* **71:**320.

Brown, R. M., and Krolick, K. A., 1988, Selective idiotype suppression of an adoptive secondary anti-acetylcholine receptor antibody response by immunotoxin treatment before transfer, *J. Immunol.* **140:**893.

Byers, V., Henslee, P., Kernan, N., Blazer, B., Gingrich, R., Phillips, G., Antin, J., Mischak, R., O'Reilly, R., and Scannon, P., 1988, Therapeutic response to a pan-T-lymphocyte monoclonal antibody-ricin A-chain immunotoxin in steroid refractory graft versus host disease (GVHD), in: *Abstracts of First International Conference on Immunotoxins*, Durham, North Carolina, p. 50.

Caperton, E., Byers, V., Shepard, J., Ackerman, S., and Scannon, P. J., 1989, Treatment of refractory rheumatoid arthritis (RA) with anti-lymphocyte immunotoxin, American College of Rheumatology Meeting, Cincinnati, Ohio.

Casellas, P., and Jansen, F. K., 1988, Immunotoxin enhancers, in: *Immunotoxins* (A. E. Frankel, ed.), Kluwer Academic Publishers, Boston, pp. 351–369.

Deshambo, R. M., and Krolick, K. A., 1986, Selective *in vitro* inhibition of an antibody response to purified acetylcholine receptor by using anti-idiotypic antibodies coupled to the A-chain of ricin, *J. Immunol.* **137:**3135.

Eiklid, K., Olsnes, A., and Pihl, A., 1980, Entry of lethal doses of abrin, ricin and modeccin into the cytosol of HeLa cells, *Exp. Cell Res.* **126:**321.

Endo, Y., and Tsurugi, K., 1987, RNA N-glycosidase activity of ricin A-chain. Mechanism of action of the toxin lectin ricin on eukaryotic ribosomes, *J. Biol. Chem.* **262:**8128.

Filipovich, A. H., Ramsay, N. K., Hurd, D., Stony, R., Youle, R., Vallera, D. A., and Kersey, J. H., 1985, Autologous bone marrow transplantation (BMT) for T cell leukemia and lymphoma using marrow cleaning with anti-T cell immunotoxins, Autologous BMT Meeting, University Degli Studi di Parma, Parma, Italy.

Filipovich, A. H., Vallera, D. A., Youle, R. J., Haake, R., Blazar, B. R., Neville, D. M., Ramsay, N. K., McGlave, P., and Kersey, J. H., 1987, Graft versus host disease prevention in allogeneic bone marrow transplantation. A pilot study using immunotoxins for T-cell depletion in donor bone marrow, *Transplantation* **44:**62.

Ghetie, M-A., May, R. D., Till, M., Uhr, J. W., Ghetie, V., Knowles, P. P., Relf, M., Brown, A., Wallace, P. M., Janossy, G., Amlot, P., Vitteta, E. S., and Thorpe, P. E., 1988, Evaluation of ricin A-chain immunotoxins directed against CD19 and CD22 antigens on normal and malignant human B-cells as potential reagents for *in vitro* therapy, *Cancer Res.* **48:**2610.

Gorin, N. C., Donay, L., Laporte, J. P., Lopez, M., Zittoun, R., Rio, B. David, R., Stachowiak, J., Jansen, J., Cazellas, P., Poncelet, P., Liance, M. C., Voisin, G. A., Salmon, J., Le Blanc, G., Deloux, J., Nijman, A., and Duhamel, G., 1985, Autologous bone marrow transplantation with marrow decontaminated by immunotoxin T101 in the treatment of leukemia and lymphoma: First clinical observations, *Cancer Treat. Rep.* **69:**953.

Gould, B. J., Borowitz, M. J., Groves, E. S., Carter, P. W., Douglas, A., Weiner, L. M., and Frankel, A. E., 1989, Phase I study of an anti-breast cancer immunotoxin by continuous infusion: Report of a targeted toxin effect not predicted by animal studies, *J. Natl. Cancer Inst.* **81:**775.

Griffin, T. W., Richardson, C., Houston, L. L., Le Page, D., Bogden, A., and Raso, V., 1987, Antitumor activity of intraperitoneal immunotoxins in a nude mouse model of human malignant mesothelioma, *Cancer Res.* **47:**4266.

Griffin, T. W., Morgan, A. C., and Blythman, H. E., 1988, Immunotoxin therapy: Assessment by animal models, in: *Immunotoxins* (A. E. Frankel, ed.), Kluwer Academic Publishers, Boston, pp. 433–455.

Hemler, M. E., Glass, D., Coblyn, J. S., and Jennie, G. J., 1986, Very late activation antigens on rheumatoid synovial fluid T-lymphocytes, *J. Clin. Invest.* **78:**696.

Hertler, A. A., Schlossman, D. M., Borowitz, M. J., Laurent, G., Jansen, F. K.,. Schmidt, C., and Frankel, A. E., 1988, A phase 1 study of T101 ricin A-chain immunotoxin in refractory chronic lymphocytic leukemia, *J. Biol. Resp. Modifiers* **7:**97.

Herzog, C. H., Walker, C. H., Pichler, W., Aeschlimann, A., Wassmer, P., Stockinger, H., Knapp, W., Rieber, P., and Muller, W., 1987, Monoclonal anti-CD4 in arthritis, *Lancet* **2:**1461.

Jain, R. K., 1989, Delivery of novel therapeutic agents in tumors: Physiological Barriers and Strategies, *J. Natl. Cancer Inst.* **81:**570.

Kernan, N. A., Byers, V., Scannon, P. J., Mischak, R. P., Brochstein, J., Flomenberg, N., Dupont, B., and O'Reilly, R. J., 1988, Treatment of steroid-resistant acute graft vs. host disease by *in vivo* administration of an anti-T-cell ricin A-chain immunotoxin, *J. Am. Med. Assoc.* **259:**3154.

Killen, J. A., and Lindstrom, J. M., 1984, Specific killing of lymphocytes that cause experimental autoimmune myasthenia gravis by ricin toxin–acetylcholine receptor conjugates, *J. Immunol.* **133:**2549.

Lambert, J. M., and Blattler, W. A., 1988, Purification and biochemical characterization of immunotoxins, in: *Immunotoxins* (A. E. Frankel, ed.), Kluwer Academic Publications, Boston, pp. 323–350.

Laurent, G., Pris, J., Farcet, J. P., Carayon, P., Blythman, H., Casellas, P., Poncelet, P., and Jansen, F. K., 1986, Effects of therapy with T101 ricin A-chain immunotoxin in two leukemia patients, *Blood* **67:**1680.

Laurent, G., Frankel, A. E., Hertler, A. A., Schlossman, D. M., Casellas, P., and Jansen, F. K., 1988, Treatment of leukemia patients with T 101 ricin A-chain immunotoxins, in: *Immunotoxins* (A. E. Frankel, ed.), Kluwer Academic Publishers, Boston, pp. 483–491.

Levin, L. V., Griffin, T. W. , Haynes, L. R., and Sedor, C. J., 1982, Selective cytotoxicity for a colorectal carcinoma cell line by a monoclonal anti-carcinoembryonic antigen antibody coupled to the A-chain of ricin, *J. Biol. Resp. Modifiers* **1:**149.

LoBuglio, A. F., Wheeler, R. H., Trang, J., Haynes, A., Rogers, K., Harvey, E. B., Sun, L., Ghrayeb, J., and Khazaeli, M. B., 1989, Mouse/human chimeric monoclonal antibody in man: Kinetics and immune response, *Proc. Natl. Acad. Sci. USA* **86:**4220.

McIntosh, D. P., and Thorpe, P. E., 1984, Role of B-chain in the cytotoxic action of antibody-ricin and antibody-abrin conjugates, in: *Receptor-Mediated Targeting of Drugs* (G. Gregoriadis *et al.*, eds.), NATO ASI Series A Vol. 82, Plenum Press, New York, pp. 105–118.

Nakahara, K., Kaplan, D., Bjorn, M., and Fathman, C. G., 1985, The effectiveness of anti-Ia-immunotoxins in the suppression of MLR, *Transplantation* **40:**62.

Nakamura, R. M., Spiegelberg, H. L., Lee, S., and Weigle, W. O., 1968, Relationship between molecular size and intra- and extravascular distribution of protein antigens, *J. Immunol.* **100:**376.

Neville, D. M., and Marsh, J. W., Jr., 1988, Methods for quantifying immunotoxin efficacy, in: *Immunotoxins* (A. E. Frankel, ed.), Kluwer Academic Publishers, Boston, pp. 393–404.

O'Hare, M., Roberts, L. M., Thorpe, P. E., Watson, G. J., Prior, B., and Lord, M. J., 1987, Expression of ricin A-chain in *Escherichia coli*, *FEBS Lett.* **216:**73.

Pai, L. H., FitzGerald, D. J., Tepper, M., Schacter, B., Spitalny, G., and Pastan, I., 1990, Inhibition of antibody response to *Pseudomonas* exotoxin and an immunotoxin containing *Pseudomonas* exotoxin by 15-deoxyspergualin in mice, *Cancer Res.* **50:**7750.

Pearson, J. W., FitzGerald, D. J. P., Willingham, M. C., Wiltrout, R. H., Pastan, I., and Longo, D. L., 1989, Chemoimmunotoxin therapy against a human colon tumor (HT-29) xenografted into nude mice, *Cancer Res.* **49:**3562.

Pearson, J. W., Hedrick, E., Fogler, W. E., Bull, R. L., Ferris, D. K., Riggs, C. W., Wiltrout, R. H., Sivam, G., Morgan, A. C., Groves, E., and Longo, D. L., 1990, Enhanced therapeutic efficacy against an ovarian tumor xenograft of immunotoxins used in conjunction with recombinant α-interferon, *Cancer Res.* **50:**6379.

Rennie, D. P., Wright, J., McGregor, A. M., Wheetman, A. P., Hall, R., and Thorpe, P., 1983, An immunotoxin of ricin A-chain conjugated to thyroglobulin selectively suppresses the anti-thyroglobulin autoantibody response, *Lancet* **2:**1338.

Robertus, J. D., 1988, Toxin structure, in: *Immunotoxins* (A. E. Frankel, ed.), Kluwer Academic Publishers, Boston, pp. 11–24.

Shizuru, J. A., Ramakrishnan, S., Hunt, T., Merrell, R. C., and Fathman, C. G., 1986, Inhibition of rat mixed lymphocyte pancreatic islet cultures with anti-Ia immunotoxin, *Transplantation* **42:**660.

Shizuru, J. A., Gregory, A. K., Tien-Bao Chao, C., and Fathman, C. G., 1987, Islet allograft survival after a single course of treatment of recipient with antibody to L3T4, *Science* **237:**278.

Shizuru, J. A., Taylor-Edwards, C., Banks, B. A., Gregory, A. K., and Fathman, C. G., 1988, Immunotherapy of the nonobese diabetic mouse: Treatment with an antibody to T-helper lymphocytes, *Science* **240:**659.

Siena, S., Lappi, D. A., Bregni, M., Formosa, A., Villa, S., Soria, M., Bonadonna, G., and Gianni, A. M., 1988, Synthesis and characterization of an antihuman T-lymphocyte saporin immunotoxin (OKT1-SAP) with *in vivo* stability into non-human primates, *Blood* **72:**756.

Siram, S., and Ranges, G. E., 1987, Immunotherapy of autoimmune disease with T-cell subset specific antibodies, *Concepts Immunopathol.* **4:**275.

Smyth, M. J., Pietersz, G. A., and McKenzie, I. F. C., 1987, Use of vasoactive agents to increase tumor perfusion and the antitumor efficacy of drug-monoclonal antibody conjugates, *J. Natl. Cancer Inst.* **78:**1367.

Snell, G. D., 1957, The homograft reaction, *Annu. Rev. Microbiol.* **2:**439.

Spitler, L. E., 1988, Clinical studies: Solid tumors, in: *Immunotoxins* (A. E. Frankel, ed.), Kluwer Academic Publishers, Boston, pp. 493–514.

Spitler, L. E., del Rio, M., Khentigan, A., Wedel, N. I., Brophy, N. A., Miler, L. L., Harkonen, W. S., Rosendorf, L. L., Lee, H. M., Mischak, R. P., Kawahata, R. T., Stondemire, J. B., Frandkin, L. B., Bautista, E. E., and Scannon, P. J., 1987, Therapy of patients with malignant melanoma using a monoclonal antimelanoma antibody ricin A-chain immunotoxin, *Cancer Res.* **47:**1717.

Spitler, L. E., Mischak, R., and Scannon, P., 1989, Therapy of metastatic malignant melanoma using xomaZyme Mel, a murine monoclonal anti-melanoma ricin A-chain immunotoxin, *Nucl. Med. Biol.* **16:**625.

Stirpe, F., and Barbieri, L., 1986, Ribosome-inactivating proteins up to date, *FEBS Lett.* **195:**1.

Thorpe, P. E., Detre, S. I., Foxwell, B. M. J., Brown, A. N. F., Skilleter, D. N., Wilson, G., Forrester, J. A., and Stirpe, F., 1985, Modification of the carbohydrate in ricin with metaperiodate-cyanoborohydride mixtures. Effects on toxicity and *in vivo* distribution, *Eur. J. Biochem.* **147:**197.

Thorpe, P. E., Wallace, P. M., Knowles, P. P., Relf, M. G., Brown, A. N. F., Watson, G. J., Blakey, D. C., and Newell, D. R., 1988, Improved antitumor effects of immunotoxins prepared with deglycosylated ricin A-chain and hindered disulphide linkages, *Cancer Res.* **48:**6396.

Vallera, D. A., 1988, Immunotoxins for *ex vivo* bone marrow purging in human bone marrow transplantations, in: *Immunotoxins* (A. E. Frankel, ed.), Kluwer Academic Publishers, Boston, pp. 515–535.

Wawrzynczak, E. J., and Davies, A. J. S., 1990, Strategies in antibody therapy of cancer, *Clin. Exp. Immunol.* **82:**189.

Wawrzynczak, E. J., and Thorpe, P. E., 1987, Methods for preparing immunotoxins: Effect of the linkage on activity and stability, in: *Immunoconjugates: Antibody Conjugates in Radioimaging and Therapy of Cancer* (C. W. Vogel, ed.), Oxford University Press, New York, pp. 28–55.

Wawrzynczak, E. J., Cumber, A. J., Henry, R. V., and Parnell, G. D., 1991, Comparative biochemical, cytotoxic and pharmacokinetic properties of immunotoxins made with native ricin A-chain, ricin A_1 chain and recombinant ricin A-chain, *Int. J. Cancer* **47:**130.

Weiner, L. M., O'Dwyer, J., Kitson, J., Comis, R. L., Frankel, A. E., Bauer, R. J., Konrad, M. S., and Groves, E. S., 1989, Phase I evaluation of an anti-breast carcinoma monoclonal antibody—260F9—recombinant ricin A-chain immunotoxin, *Cancer Res.* **49:**4062.

Wiley, K. N., Powell, C. S., Henry, L., Clark, A., and Fox, M., 1988, An A-chain ricin immunotoxin targeted against rat class II major histocompatibility complex molecules, *Transplantation* **45:**1113.

Woodruff, M. F. A., 1983, Cellular heterogeneity in tumors, *Br. J. Cancer* **47:**589.

Worrell, N. R., Cumber, A. J., Parnell, G. D., Mirza, A., Forrester, J. A., and Ross, W. C. J., 1986, The effect of linkage variation on pharmacokinetics of ricin A-chain antibody conjugates in normal rats, *Anti-Cancer Drug Des.* **1:**179.

Yu, Y. H., Crews, R. J., Cooper, K., Ramakrishnan, S., Houston, L.L., Leslie, D. S., George, S. L., Lider, Y., Boyer, C. M., Ring, D. B., and Bast, R. C., Jr., 1990, Use of immunotoxins in combination to inhibit clonogenic growth of human breast carcinoma cells, *Cancer Res.* **50:**3231.

Chapter 16

INTERFERONS, THYMIC HORMONES, AND INTERLEUKINS

Eric M. Veys

1. INTRODUCTION

Efficient functioning of the immune system relies on a network of complex interactions among various cell types and soluble mediators. Regulatory abnormalities in this network can result in autoimmunity, characterized by the emergence of lymphocyte clones and the synthesis of antibodies directed against the host's own tissue. Although different pathogenic mechanisms may be involved in autoimmune diseases, many of their characteristics are common to most of these diseases. The considerable variety of factors associated with autoimmunity explain the diversity among the autoimmune diseases. Finally, even patients suffering from the same autoimmune disorder may show a great range of clinical symptoms and serological abnormalities. Consequently, the question can be raised of whether or not the classification of autoimmune diseases actually used in medical practice will be profoundly modified by increase of knowledge of the disease mechanisms. Although the etiology of these disorders is largely unknown, immunologic, hormonal, environmental, and genetic factors have been implicated. Adherence to endothelial cells in postcapillary venules (high endothelial venules: HEV) is an indispensable initial step before cellular infiltration into the target organs can occur in autoimmune diseases (Igughi and Ziff, 1986; Matsubara and Ziff, 1987). Several cytokines influence the adherence of lymphocytes to endothelium: interleukin-1 (IL-1), tumor necrosis function (TNF), and lipopolysaccharide (LPS) (Oppenheimer-Marks and Ziff, 1987). Other cytokines such as interferon gamma (IFN-γ) increases both adherence and the migration of T cells.

Current evidence indicates that the presence of IL-1 in the synovial environment may play a crucial role in the pathogenesis of rheumatoid arthritis (RA) (Dinarello, 1986). Chondrocytes and synoviocytes respond to IL-1 *in vitro* by a release of PGE_2, collagenase, proteoglycanase and plasminogen activator and by a stimulation of synovial cell proliferation

Eric M. Veys • Department of Rheumatology, Ghent University Hospital, University of Ghent, B-9000 Ghent, Belgium.

Immunopharmacology in Autoimmune Diseases and Transplantation, edited by Hans Erik Rugstad *et al.* Plenum Press, New York, 1992.

and cartilage resorption (Krakauer *et al.*, 1985; Kunkel *et al.*, 1986). Muscle wasting, fever, acute-phase response, and osteoporosis are other characteristics of the disease that are affected by IL-1.

A deficiency of IL-2 secretion and IL-2 responsiveness was described in patients with autoimmune rheumatic diseases and in models of autoimmune disease in various inbred strains of mice (Wofsy *et al.*, 1981; Miyasaka *et al.*, 1984). IL-2 deficiency may contribute to down-regulation of natural killer cell activity, which has a concomitant release effect on B-cell function, resulting in autoantibody production (Smith and Talal, 1982; Combe *et al.*, 1985).

IFN-γ is known to increase the rate of biosynthesis and membrane density of Ia in cells that have normal basal expression of Ia, such as Ia$^+$ monocytes and thymic epithelium (Basham and Merigan, 1983; Virelizier *et al.*, 1984; Berrih *et al.*, 1985). IFN-γ also induces *de novo* expression of Ia in other cell types such as Ia$^-$ macrophages, vascular endothelium, and fibroblasts. Consequently, IFN-γ enhances the activation of specific T helper cells and the immunity that is dependent on T helper cells (Frasca *et al.*, 1985; Cowing and Frohman, 1986).

If the antigen is a viral product expressed on the membrane of an infected cell, IFN-γ inducing an aberrant Ia expression will produce a T helper cell activation from which the host will benefit. If the antigen presented by the newly Ia$^+$ cell is an autologous cell membrane molecule, one that is unique to a particular tissue and of which the host T helper cells are not tolerant, IFN-γ can trigger an autoimmune attack. Several recent reports have described a decreased level and activity of IFN-γ in the rheumatoid joint environment, both *in vitro* and *in vivo* (Chin *et al.*, 1983; Husby and Williams, 1985; Firestein and Zvaifler, 1987). It is still unknown whether these findings are due to a defective production or to a physiological down-regulation of IFN-γ in RA. Consequently, it is not clear whether the pharmacological administration of IFN-γ to RA patients would reduce the disease activity or induce an exacerbation.

In this chapter the rationale for using thymic hormones and IFN-γ is reviewed and the clinical studies performed in RA with these agents are analyzed. It is obvious that a final conclusion about the efficacy of thymic hormones and IFN-γ in the treatment of RA cannot be drawn as yet; large trials using other modes of administration and other dosages are mandatory before a beneficial effect of these compounds can be confirmed or disproven.

2. THYMIC HORMONES

Different thymic hormones have been isolated; four of them are well-defined and have been more or less purified during the last decade (Table I) (Goldstein *et al.*, 1966; Goldstein, 1968; Bach and Dardenne, 1973; Trainin *et al.*, 1985). Only two have been used in clinical trials in order to evaluate their activity in RA (Goldstein, 1968; Bach and Dardenne, 1973). The complete 49 amino acid sequence of thymopoietin has been determined and the pentapeptide thymopentin (Arg-Lys-Asp-Val-Tyr) (TP-5), corresponding to residues 32–36 of thymopoietin, has been shown to retain the biological activity of the native molecule (Goldstein *et al.*, 1979). Thymulin, formerly designated FTS (facteur thymique sérique) and isolated from porcine serum, has been purified from human serum. Its amino acid sequence has been determined (Glu-Ala-Lys-Ser-Glu-Gly-Gly-Ser-Asu) (Bach, 1983) and the synthetic peptide has been shown to be fully biologically active (Pleau *et al.*, 1977).

The rationale for considering thymic hormones as a mode of treatment for RA is based on the fact that in some *in vitro* assays and *in vivo* models (Goldstein, 1978) the activity of these compounds has been found to mimic that of levamisole. Like levamisole, thymic hormones have been shown to affect T-cell maturation (Goldstein and Lau, 1980), to

TABLE I. Well-defined Thymic Hormones

	Molecular weight	Amino acid sequence synthesis	Reference
Thymosin fraction V		−	Goldstein (1966)
α1	3108	+	
β4	4982	+	
Thymopoietin	5562	+	Goldstein (1968)
Thymic humoral factor	3200	−	Trainin (1985)
Thymulin	857	+	Bach (1973)

improve autoimmune disease in NZB/W mice (Lau et al., 1980), to decrease the autoantibodies in aged mice (Gershwin et al., 1979), and to restore some immune deficiencies in animals and children (Aiuti et al., 1980). Other effects of thymic hormones on T cells have been demonstrated, such as they influence the T-cell proliferation as shown in the phytohemagglutinin (PHA)-induced model in animals and in men (Bach, 1983; Goldstein and Audhya, 1984). As for cytotoxicity and delayed hypersensitivity, thymic hormones are active in different models; the allogenic cytotoxicity in athymic mice, the anti-trinitrophenol (TNP) cytotoxicity on normal thymocytes, the graft-versus-host reaction in normal mice, and the stimulation of delayed-type hypersensitivity in athymic mice. Thymic hormones stimulate T helper cell functions in some systems such as the antibody production in aging mice, the induction of IgA synthesis in ataxia–telangiectasia and in variable immune deficiencies, the production of IL-2 on normal thymocytes and on nude mouse spleen cells, and the increase in anti-DNA IgA autoantibodies in young B/W female mice.

Thymic hormones enhance T suppressor cells, retarding the skin allograft rejection in normal mice, reducing the antibody formation to sheep red blood cells in normal mice and to DNA in B/W male mice, depressing the T-cell-mediated cytotoxicity and the delayed-type hypersensitivity in normal mice and stimulating the con A-induced suppression in systemic lupus erythematosus (SLE) patients and in normal subjects. Recent data, based on the structure of thymopoietin analogues, suggest that there are at least two types of distinct thymopoietin receptors on mature T cells (Audhya et al., 1984) that might correspond to distinct receptors on helper and suppressor T cells. The effect of thymulin and thymopoietin applies to both helper and suppressor functions with a predilection for suppressor T cells at high dosage (Bach, 1987). Skin graft survival can be prolonged (Kaiserlian et al., 1981) and delayed-type hypersensitivity abrogated (Erard et al., 1979) by injecting thymic hormones. Finally, thymopoietin stimulates the release of IFN and IL-2 by mitogen-stimulated cells in in vitro systems (Diezel et al., 1984; Duchateau et al., 1987), but in this instance the nature of the cells and the receptor has not yet been defined (Goldstein, 1987).

2.1. Thymic Hormones in Autoimmune Diseases

Several experimental data seem to indicate that thymic hormones could improve the evolution of autoimmune diseases. Thymopentin inhibits the development of the hemolytic anemia induced in mice with rat erythrocytes (Lau et al., 1980). Thymulin also decreases the severity of hemolytic anemia in NZB mice and prevents Sjögren's syndrome in NZB and B/W mice (Bach et al., 1980). The effect on anti-DNA antibody production in (NZB/NZW) F1 mice and an immune complex glomerulonephritis is more controversial (Bach et al., 1980; Israel-Biet et al., 1983). Thymulin also prevents the onset of experimental allergic encephalomyelitis in the guinea pigs and may eventually cure an already established disease (Nagai et al., 1982).

These encouraging experimental data were not extended to clinical use in humans in autoimmune diseases other than RA.

2.2. Thymic Hormones in the Treatment of RA

Thymic hormones have been the subject of several clinical trials in which TP-5 (Veys et al., 1982, 1984b; Malaise et al., 1985) has been analyzed more extensively than Thy (Amor et al., 1987). None of the schedules used in these studies appeared to dramatically improve the activity of the rheumatic disease. To some extent both compounds (TP-5 and Thy) were found to exert a comparable action. Slow intravenous injections (over 10 min) of TP-5 50 mg three times per week induced a significant decrease in disease activity over the short term (three weeks), but once the drug administration was interrupted, a relapse occurred within four weeks. These positive results, contrasting with the negative ones obtained in other studies, are accounted for by the fact that the intravenous injections were performed slowly (10 min), allowing the drug to reach the cell receptors in higher quantities than with conventional injections, since the half-life of the molecule in human serum is only 30 sec (Malaise et al., (1985).

In long-term assays, the beneficial effects observed in small studies using TP-5 10 mg subcutaneously (SC) (Veys et al., 1984b) and Thy 5 mg SC (Amor et al., 1987) three times per week cannot be denied. That in itself could be sufficient to justify more extensive analysis of these schemes in larger multicenter studies, even if it seems difficult to conceive that a medium dosage can exert some clinical activity, whereas lower and higher dosages cannot.

Although other schemes appear to be inefficient, the absence of adverse reactions should incite us to try out every single therapeutic application of the thymic compounds in the treatment of RA. The biological parameters did not vary significantly in the reviewed trials; rheumatoid factor activity, immunoglobulin levels, and T-cell subsets were not influenced by TP-5 or Thy using the schedules described in these studies. Unfortunately, investigators have failed to compare the immunological characteristics of responders to thymic hormones with those of nonresponders, with the exception of Amor et al. (1987) who found that patients with a high CD4/CD8 ratio respond better to Thy treatment.

3. INTERFERONS

Interferon, initially identified as a cell protector from the cytopathic effect of viruses, was shown to be a potent antiproliferative agent and a modulator of humoral and cellular immunity. Macrophage activation and enhancement of natural killer cell function also are part of the spectrum of interferon activity. Actually, it has become clear that interferon is not a single molecule, but a family of proteins: interferon alpha, interferon beta and interferon gamma. The third compound, IFN-γ, possesses the most potent immunoregulatory activity. IFN-γ increases the rate of biosynthesis and the membrane density of Ia molecules in cells having a normal basal expression of Ia such as Ia$^+$ monocytes and thymic epithelium. IFN-γ also induces de novo expression of Ia in other cell types, notably Ia$^-$ macrophages (Bottazzo et al., 1983), vascular endothelium, fibroblasts (Pober et al., 1983), mammary duct epithelium, intestinal epithelium (Scheynius et al., 1986), mast cells, astrocytes (Fiers et al., 1985), thyroid follicular cells, and keratinocytes (Basham et al., 1984). By increasing the density of the Ia expression on the membrane of Ia$^+$ antigen-presenting cells, it enhances the activation of specific T helper cells and consequently also the T-helper-cell- dependent immunity; in other words it increases the normal immunity.

The potentially detrimental effect of IFN-γ lies in the induction of Ia expression by cells that are normally Ia$^+$ and thus incapable of antigen presentation to T helper cells. If the antigen is a viral product expressed on the membrane of an infected cell, the aberrant Ia expression induced by IFN-γ will be followed by an activation of T helper cells, resulting in a potential benefit for the host. If the antigen presented by the newly formed Ia$^+$ cells is an autologous cell membrane molecule, one that is unique to a particular tissue and not tolerated by the host T helper cells, the end result could be an autoimmune attack on the IFN-γ-induced Ia$^+$ tissue (Cowing and Frohman, 1986).

The last hypothesis is in conflict with recent clinical studies indicating that r-IFN-γ has some efficacy in the treatment of RA (Wolfe et al., 1986; Cannon et al., 1987; Lemmel et al., 1988; Veys et al., 1988). Interferons exert regulatory actions especially directed to the monocyte; they inhibit IL-1-induced prostaglandin release from human peripheral monocytes (Browning and Ribolini, 1987). Interferons may have a beneficial effect in RA because of their involvement in the lipo-oxygenase and cyclo-oxygenase limbs of the eicosanoid pathway as well as that of arachidonic acid itself (Boraschi et al., 1987). Additional areas have to be considered: IFN-γ inhibits the effect of IL-4 on B-cell proliferation, the secretion of IgG$_1$ and IgG$_3$ antibodies, the response to polyclonal type antigens, and the induction of class II antigens on B cells (Coffman and Carty, 1986; Mond et al., 1986).

3.1. Interferons in Autoimmune Diseases

The therapeutic effects of murine IFN on in vitro models of autoimmune diseases have been discouraging. An acceleration of autoimmune disease was reported with IFN-α/β (Heremans et al., 1978; Sergiescu et al., 1979) and IFN-γ (Engleman et al., 1981). These early experiments were performed with crude IFN preparations and the role of other contaminating cytokines cannot be discounted. Further, a recent publication showed that in the (NZB/NZW) F1 model, recombinant murine IFN-γ increased the incidence of glomerulonephritis in this animal model and that monoclonal antibody to IFN-γ delayed the appearance of anti-DNA activity and the onset of the disease (Jacob et al., 1987). Experimental autoimmune thyroiditis in mice was found to be induced by administration of IFN-γ (Remy et al., 1987). In vivo studies on mice revealed that IFN-γ increased the severity of diabetes induced with multiple low doses of the B-cell toxin, streptozotocin (Campbell et al., 1988). These data suggest that IFN-γ plays a key role in the onset of autoimmune diseases by inducing class II major histocompatibility (MHC) expression in situ.

Not all available evidence points in the direction of a potentiating role of IFN-γ on the immune response. Indeed, in a cutaneous delayed-type hypersensitivity reaction in rats, using dinitro-fluorobenzame as antigen, antibodies against IFN-γ were shown to enhance the development of the reaction and to inhibit the class II antigen expression on keratinocytes (Skoglund et al., 1988). In vitro, IFN-γ was shown to suppress anti-DNA antibody and immunoglobulin synthesis on human peripheral blood monocytes from SLE patients (Braude et al., 1988). In view of the contradictory data mentioned above, the use of interferons may be contraindicated in patients with certain autoimmune diseases. Indeed, IFN-γ has been shown to induce an exacerbation of multiple sclerosis accompanied by an increase of circulating monocytes bearing class II surface antigens (Panitch et al., 1987). Antibodies against IFN-γ improved glomerulonephritis in mice, suggesting possible usefulness of such antibodies in SLE.

In vitro studies have shown that IFN-α and -β could have an antagonistic effect on IFN-γ-induced class II expression on macrophages and endothelial cells (Ling *et al.*, 1985; Manyak *et al.*, 1988); consequently, a beneficial effect of treatment with IFN-α and -β can be expected in diseases in which class II MHC expression is increased.

The published data must be interpreted with caution as long as the role of the different cytokines in the pathogenesis of autoimmune diseases is not definitely known, especially in view of the systemic and local role of these molecules on the target organs.

3.2. IFN-γ in the Rheumatoid Joint Environment

In vivo and *in vitro* observations and experiments seem to suggest that little or no IFN-γ is present in or produced by the rheumatoid synovium. Rheumatoid synovial tissue explants, which actively produce prostaglandins and collagenase, do not produce IFN-γ (Chin *et al.*, 1983). Immunofluorescence studies of rheumatoid synovial tissue show little IFN-γ (Husby and Williams, 1985). Mononuclear cells from RA synovial fluid produce much less IFN-γ when stimulated by IL-2 than stimulated peripheral blood mononuclear cells or synovial fluid cells from gouty arthritis patients (Combe *et al.*, 1985). In contrast to some data obtained with bioassays, the determination of IFN-γ in synovial fluid from RA patients using specific radioimmunoassays gave much lower values than in other inflammatory joint effusions (Firestein and Zvaifler, 1986).

These *in vivo* data are in accordance with *in vitro* experiments, showing a physiological down-regulation or an intrinsic defect in IFN-γ production in RA. IFN-γ production in the autologous mixed lymphocyte reaction is decreased at physiological concentrations of prostaglandins (10^{-8}M) and is almost entirely eliminated at pharmacological concentrations (10^{-6}M) (Firestein and Zvaifler, 1986). The proliferation of isolated lymphocytes infected by the Epstein-Barr virus is depressed by autologous T cells and by macrophages. This regulation is modulated by IFN-γ and by nonspecific cytotoxic cells. Finally, infected B cells are eliminated by specific cytotoxic T cells. If RA B cells are infected by the Epstein-Barr virus, their proliferation continues out of regulation and is not prevented by rheumatoid cells (Lotz *et al.*, 1986, 1987). The defect is multifactorial, but is largely due to a failure of lymphokine production, including IFN-γ, by rheumatoid T cells (Lotz *et al.*, 1985; Hasler *et al.*, 1983).

Low levels of synovial fluid interferon may represent a form of physiological down-regulation to protect the joint; pharmacological administration of IFN-γ could consequently induce an exacerbation of the disease activity in RA. However, the low levels of IFN-γ in a rheumatoid joint environment could be due to an intrinsic defect in IFN-γ production in RA; pharmacological administration in this instance could perhaps succeed in reducing disease activity.

In the literature some other arguments can be found to support the rationale for using IFN-γ in the treatment of RA. Some authors reported a decreased natural killer cell activity in RA patients who were shown to be good responders to a levamisole treatment (Barada *et al.*, 1982). As levamisole, IFN-γ was shown to enhance the natural killer cell activity in different models (Nakamura *et al.*, 1984). Finally, we were able to show an increase of the serum IFN-γ levels in patients treated with levamisole (150 mg once weekly for more than six months) 24 and 48 hr after drug intake (Veys *et al.*, 1984a, 1987).

3.3. IFN-γ in the Treatment of RA

Some conclusions regarding the efficacy of IFN-γ in the treatment of RA can be drawn from the four controlled studies published so far (Wolfe *et al.*, 1986; Lemmel *et al.*, 1988;

Cannon et al., 1987, 1990; Veys et al., 1988). From the schedules and dosages used in these studies (subcutaneous injections, 50–100 μg, 2, 3, or 5 days per week), it appears that the compound does not increase disease activity as was initially postulated by some authors. Although a dramatic improvement could not be obtained using these schedules, some encouraging results were reported that were strengthened by the absence of major adverse reactions. More dose range studies and larger multicenter trials are required to find out whether or not the pharmacological administration of IFN-γ is capable of improving disease activity in RA. The optimal dosages, schedules, and route of administration have not yet been established and further fundamental investigations are mandatory to acquire a better knowledge of the mode of action of the compound in the pathogenesis of the disease.

The short-term effect described in the first two studies (Wolfe et al., 1986; Lemmel et al., 1988) led to the hypothesis that IFN-γ activity could be similar to that of nonsteroidal anti-inflammatory drugs; but these positive results could not be confirmed in the one-month evaluation of the long-term studies (Cannon et al., 1987; Veys et al., 1988). The long-term effect suggests that IFN-γ could have some beneficial action on the course of the disease, but a better understanding of the properties of IFN and of the nature of the disease itself is essential to elucidate the paradox of IFN in RA.

4. SUMMARY AND PROSPECTS

Although the primary cause of rheumatoid arthritis is unknown, genetic predisposition and abnormalities of the immune system have been considered as possible etiologic factors. The tissue destruction results from the inflammatory response, but the abnormality that actually initiates RA is unknown. An infectious agent could be capable of triggering the disease process but so could a primary malfunction of the immune system. We cannot say for sure that better knowledge of the etiology and the pathogenic mechanism of the disease will result in a cure or that we will have an exact understanding of the pathogenesis after a cure has been discovered empirically. Since our understanding of the disease and of the agents biologically involved in the regulation of the immune response is far from complete, we need to be aware that unexpected data can be found.

Based on their capability to improve autoimmunity in aged animals, to restore impaired immune function in other experimental models, and to stimulate T suppressor function, thymic hormones were considered as potentially beneficial to the natural course of RA. Several clinical studies were performed with thymopoietin (thymopentin) and thymulin. Different modes of administration were analyzed. No definite conclusion can be drawn about the potency of thymic hormones to influence the course of the disease. The absence of adverse reactions can perhaps justify other studies, once the bioavailability of the compounds are better assessed, and other assays are available to monitor the influence of these compounds on the immune response.

From the fact that IFN-γ is a potent stimulator of different aspects of the immune response, it might be predicted that the pharmacological administration of this agent would induce an exacerbation of disease activity in RA. However, early studies indicate that IFN-γ may have a beneficial effect in RA.

Initially, short-term assays were performed with daily subcutaneous injections of IFN-γ (50 or 100 μg). As some encouraging results were obtained, two double-blind long-term studies were started. Although the results were less spectacular, they clearly showed that IFN-γ administered subcutaneously (100 μg) at first once daily and then twice weekly, did not induce a disease exacerbation after three months in the one study and after six months in the other study. Further large trials using other schedules and perhaps other modes of administration need to be performed to establish whether or not IFN-γ can be considered as a therapeutic agent in RA.

Although the role of IL-1 in the pathogenesis of RA is well documented, no inhibitory effect of known antirheumatic drugs has been firmly established as yet, and in the rheumatology world new compounds capable of inhibiting IL-1 are eagerly awaited. The deficiency of the IL-2 production and the response to IL-2 described in RA, together with a deficiency of IFN-γ, inducing a defective natural killing activity, may be one mechanism responsible for B-cell hyperactivity and for persistent immunoglobulin, autoantibody, and rheumatoid factor production in RA. If this hypothesis is substantiated, biological molecules regulating the cell–cell interactions could be used as therapeutic agents by restoring the immune balance, preventing the perpetuation of antigens, and consequently influencing the initiation phase of autoimmunity.

REFERENCES

Aiuti, F., Businco, L., Rossi, P., and Quinti, I., 1980, Response to thymopoietin pentapeptide in patients with Di George syndrome, *Lancet* 1:91–95.

Amor, B., Dougados, M., Mery, C., de Gery, A., Kahan, A., Dardenne, M., Chatenoud, L., Simon-Lavoine, N., Choay, J., and Bach, J. F., 1987, Nonathymulin in rheumatoid arthritis: Double-blind placebo-controlled trials, in: *Immune Regulation by Characterized Polypeptides*, UCLA Symposia on Molecular and Cellular Biology, Volume 41 (G. Goldstein, J. F. Bach, and H. Wigzell, eds.), Alan R. Liss Inc, New York, pp. 231–244.

Audhya, T., Heavner, G. A., Kroon, D. J., and Goldstein, G., 1984, Cooperativity of thymopoietin 32–36 (the active site) and thymopoietin 38–45 in receptor binding. *Regul. Pept.* 9:155–161.

Bach, J. F., 1983, Thymic hormones, in: *Clinical Immunology and Allergy* (J. F. Bach, ed.), W.B. Saunders, Philadelphia, pp. 3, 133–141.

Bach, J. F., 1987, The role of thymic hormones in T-cell differentiation: An overview, in: *Immune Regulation by Characterized Polypeptides*, UCLA Symposia on Molecular and Cellular Biology, New Series, Volume 41 (G. Goldstein, J. F. Bach, and H. Wigzell, eds.), Alan R. Liss Inc, New York, pp. 245–258.

Bach, J. F., and Dardenne, M., 1973, Studies on thymus products, II. Demonstration and characterization of a circulating thymic hormone, *Immunology* 25:353–366.

Bach, M. A., Droz, D., Noel, D. H., Blanchard, D., Dardenne, M., and Peking, A., 1980, Effect of long-term treatment with circulating thymic factor on murine lupus, *Arthritis Rheum.* 23:1351–1358.

Barada, F. A., O'Brien, W., and Horwitz, D. A., 1982, Defective monocyte cytotoxicity in rheumatoid arthritis. A correlation with disease activity and reversal by levamisole, *Arthritis Rheum.* 25:10–16.

Basham, T. Y., and Merigan, T. C., 1983, Recombinant interferon gamma increases HLA-DR synthesis and expression, *J. Immunol.* 130:1492–1494.

Basham, T. Y., Nickoloff, B. J., Merigan, T. I., and Morhenn, V. B., 1984, Recombinant gamma interferon induces HLA-DR expression on cultured human keratinocytes, *J. Invest. Dermatol.* 83:88–90.

Berrih, S., Arenzana-Seisdedos, F., Cohen, S., Devos, R., Charron, D., and Virelizier, J. L., 1985, Interferon gamma modulates HLA Class II antigen expression on cultured human thymic epithelial cells, *J. Immunol.* 135:1165–1171.

Boraschi, D., Censini, S., Bartalini, M., Ghiara, P., and Di Simplicio, P., and Tagliabur, A., 1987, Interferons inhibit LTC4 production in murine macrophages, *J. Immunol.* 138:4341–4346.

Bottazzo, G. F., Pujoll-Borell, R., and Hanafusa, T., 1983, Role of aberrant HLA-DR expression and antigen presentation in induction of endocrine autoimmunity, *Lancet* 2:1115–1118.

Braude, I. A., Kochberg, M. C., Arnett, F. C., and Waldmann, T. A., 1988, In vitro suppression of anti-DNA antibody and immunoglobulin synthesis in systemic lupus erythematosus patients by human gamma-interferon, *J. Rheumatol.* 15:438–444.

Browning, J., and Ribolini, A., 1987, Interferon blocks interleukin-1-induced prostaglandin release from human peripheral monocytes, *J. Immunol.* 138:2857–2863.

Campbell, I. L., Oxbrow, L., Koulmanda, M., and Harrison, L. C., 1988, IFN-γ induces islet cell MHC antigens and enhances autoimmune streptozotocin-induced diabetes in the mouse, *J. Immunol.* 140:1111–1116.

Cannon, G. W., Emkey, R. D., Denes, A., Cohen, S. A., Saway, P. A., Wolfe, P., Jaffer, A. M., Weaver, A. L., Cogen, L., Gulinello, J., Kennedy, S. M., and Schindler, J. D., 1990, Prospective two-year follow-up of recombinant interferon-γ in rheumatoid arthritis, *J. Rheumatol.* 17:304–310.

Cannon, G. W., Schindler, J. D., Emkey, R. D., Denes, A., Cohen, S. A., and Wolfe, F., 1987, Double-blind trial of recombinant interferon-gamma versus placebo in rheumatoid arthritis (abstract), *Arth. Rheum.* (suppl.) 30(no. 4):518.

Chin, R., Chiou, S., Multz, C. V., and Allison, A. C., 1983, The absence of gamma interferon and the presence of high levels of inflammatory mediators in the supernatants of rheumatoid arthritis synovial explants (abstract 3828), *Fed. Proc.* 42:949.

Coffman, R. L., and Carty, J., 1986, A T-cell activity that enhances polyclonal IgE production and its inhibition by interferon-gamma, *J. Immunol.* 136:949–954.

Combe, B., Pope, R. M., Fischbach, M., Darnell, B., Baron, S., and Talal, N., 1985, Interleukin-2 in rheumatoid arthritis:

Production of and response to interleukin-2 in rheumatoid synovial fluid, synovial tissue and peripheral blood, *Clin. Exp. Immunol.* **59**:520–528.

Cowing, C. C., and Frohman, M. A., 1986, Gamma interferon, Class II histocompatibility antigens, and autoimmunity, in: *Biologically Based Immunomodulators in the Therapy of Rheumatic Diseases* (S. H. Pincus,, D. S. Pisetsky, and L. J. Rosenwasser, eds.), Elsevier, New York, pp. 349–355.

Diezel, W., Waschke, S. R., and Forner, K., 1984, Induction and augmentation of mitogen-induced immune interferon production in human lymphocytes by a synthetic thymopoietin pentapeptide, *Biomed. Biochem. Acta* **43**:K6.

Dinarello, C. A., 1986, Multiple biological properties of recombinant human interleukin-I (beta), *Immunobiology* **172**:301–312.

Duchateau, J., Collet, H., and Bolla, K., 1987, Influence of thymopentin on candidin-induced proliferation and PWM-induced IgG production of human lymphocytes, in: *Immune Regulation by Characterized Polypeptides*, UCLA Symposia on Molecular and Cellular Biology, New Series (G. Goldstein, J. F. Bach, and H. Wigzell, eds.), Alan R. Liss Inc., New York, pp. 83–91.

Engleman, E. G., Sonnenfeld, G., Dauphinee, M., Greenspan, J. S., and Talal, N., 1981, Treatment of NZB/NZW F1 hybrid mice with *Mycobacterium bovis* strain BCG or type II interferon preparations accelerates autoimmune disease, *Arthritis Rheum.* **24**:1396–1402.

Erard, D., Charriere, J., Auffredou, M. T., Galanaud, P., and Bach, J. F., 1979, Regulation of contact sensitivity to DNFB in the mouse: Effects of adult thymectomy and thymic factor, *J. Immunol.* **123**:1573–1576.

Fiers, W., Endler, B., Reske, K., Wekerle, H., and Fontana, A., 1985, Astrocytes as antigen presenting cells. I. Induction of Ia antigen expression on astrocytes by T-cells via immune interferons and its effect on antigen presentation, *J. Immunol.* **134**:3785–3793.

Firestein, G. S., and Zvaifler, N. J., 1986, Interferon and rheumatoid arthritis, in: *Biologically Based Immunomodulators in the Therapy of Rheumatic Diseases* (S. H. Pincus, D. S. Pisetsky, and L. J. Rosenwasser, eds.), Elsevier, New York, pp. 369–378.

Firestein, G. S., and Zvaifler, N. J., 1987, Peripheral blood and synovial fluid monocyte activation in inflammatory arthritis. II. Low levels of synovial fluid and synovial tissue interferon suggest that gamma interferon is not the primary macrophage activating factor, *Arthritis Rheum.* **30**:864–871.

Frasca, D., Adorini, L., Landolfo, S., and Doria, G., 1985, Enhancing effect of IFN-gamma on helper T-cell activity and IL-2 production, *J. Immunol.* **134**:3907–3911.

Gershwin, M. E., Kruse, W., and Goldstein, G., 1979, The effect of thymopoietin 32–36 and ubiquitin on spontaneous immunopathology of New Zealand mice, *J. Rheumatol.* **6**:610–620.

Goldstein, A. L., Slater, F. D., and White, A., 1966, Preparation, assay and partial purification of a thymic lymphocytopoietic factor, *Proc. Natl. Acad. Sci. USA* **56**:1010–1017.

Goldstein, G., 1968, The thymus and neuromuscular function. A substance in thymus which causes myositis and myasthenic neuromuscular block in guinea pigs, *Lancet* **2**:119–122.

Goldstein, G., 1978, Mode of action of Levamisole, *J. Rheumatol.* (Suppl. 4) **5**:143–148.

Goldstein, G., 1987, Overview of immunoregulation by thymopoietin, in: *Immune Regulation by Characterized Polypeptides*, UCLA Symposia on Molecular and Cellular Biology, Volume 41 (G. Goldstein, J. F. Bach, and H. Wigzell, eds.), Alan R. Liss Inc., New York, pp. 51–59.

Goldstein, G., and Audhya, T., 1984, Thymopoietin and splenin: Contrasts and similarities, in: *Regulation of the Immune System*, UCLA Symposia on Molecular and Cellular Biology, New Series (E. Sergarz, H. Cantor, and L. Chess, eds.), Alan R. Liss Inc., New York, pp. 315–323.

Goldstein, G., and Lau, C. Y., 1980, Thymopoietin and immunoregulation, in: *Polypeptide Hormones* (R. F. Beers and E. Basset, eds.), Raven Press, New York, p. 459.

Goldstein, G., Scheid, M. P., Boyse, E. A., Schlesinger, D. H., and Van Wauwe, J., 1979, A synthetic pentapeptide with biological activity characteristic of the thymic hormone thymopoietin, *Science* **204**:1309–1310.

Hasler, F., Bluestein, H. G., Zvaifler, N. J., and Epstein, L. B., 1983, Analysis of the defects responsible for the impaired regulation of Epstein-Barr virus-induced β cell proliferation by rheumatoid arthritis lymphocytes. Diminished gamma-interferon production in response to autologous stimulation, *J. Exp. Med.* **157**:173–188.

Heremans, H., Billiau, A., Colombati, A., Hilgers, J., and Desomer, P., 1978, Interferon treatment of NZB mice: Accelerated progression of autoimmune disease, *Infect. Immun.* **21**:925–930.

Husby, G., and Williams, R. C., 1985, Immunohistochemical studies of interleukin-2 and gamma interferon in rheumatoid arthritis, *Arthritis Rheum.* **28**:174–181.

Igughi, T., and Ziff, M., 1986, Electron microscopic study of rheumatoid synovial vasculature. Intimate relationship between T-cell endothelium and lymphoid aggregation, *J. Clin. Invest.* **77**:355–361.

Israel-Biet, D., Noek, L. H., Bach, M. A., and Bach, J. F., 1983, Marked reduction of DNA antibody production and glomerulopathy in thymulin treated (NZB & NZW)F1 mice by FTS-Zn) or cyclosporin A, *Clin. Exp. Immunol.* **54**:359–365.

Jacob, C. O., Van Der Meide, P. H., and McDevitt, B. O., 1987, *In vivo* treatment of (NZB/NZW) F1 lupus-like nephritis with monoclonal antibody to γ-interferon, *J. Exp. Med.* **166**:798–803.

Kaiserlian, D., Dujic, A., Dardenne, M., Bach, J. F., Blanot, D., and Bricas, E., 1981, Prolongation of murine skin grafts by FTS and its synthetic analogues, *Clin. Exp. Immunol.* **45**:338–343.

Krakauer, T., Oppenheim, J. J., and Jasin, H. E., 1985, Human interleukin-I mediates cartilage matrix degradation, *Cell. Immunol.* **91**:92–99.

Kunkel, S. L., Chensue, S. W., and Phan, S. K., 1986, Prostaglandins as endogenous mediators of interleukin-I production, *J. Immunol.* **136**:186–192.

Lau, C. Y., Freestone, J. A., and Goldstein, G., 1980, Effect of thymopoietin pentapeptide (TP-5) on autoimmunity. I. TP-5 suppression of induced erythrocyte autoantibodies in C$_3$H mice, *J. Immunol.* **125**:1634–1638.

Lemmel, E. M., Brackertz, D., Franke, M., Gaus, W., Hartz, P. W., Machalke, K., Mielke, H., Obert, H. I., Peter, H. M., Sieper, J.,

Sprekeler, R., and Stierle, H., 1988, Results of a multicenter placebo-controlled double-blind randomized phase III clinical study on treatment of rheumatoid arthritis with recombinant interferon-gamma, *Rheumatol. Int.* **8:**87–93.

Ling, P. D., Warren, M. D., and Vogel, S. N., 1985, Antagonistic effect of IFN-beta on the IFN-gamma induced expression of Ia antigen in murine macrophage, *J. Immunol.* **135:**1857–1863.

Lotz, M., Tsoukas, C. D., Fong, S., Carson, D. A., and Vaughan, J. H., 1985, Regulation of Epstein-Barr virus infection by recombinant interferon. Selected sensitivity to IFN-gamma, *Eur. J. Immunol.* **15:**520–525.

Lotz, M., Tsoukas, C. D., Robinson, C. A., Dinarello, C. A., Carson, D. A., and Vaughan, J. H., 1986, Basis for defective responses of rheumatoid arthritis synovial fluid lymphocytes to anti-CD3 (T3) antibodies, *J. Clin. Invest.* **78:**713–721.

Lotz, M., Tsoukas, C. D., Curd, J. G., Carson, D. A., and Vaughan, J. H., 1987, Effect of recombinant human interferons on rheumatoid arthritis B-lymphocytes activated by Epstein-Barr virus, *J. Rheumatol.* **14:**42–45.

Malaise, M. G., Hauwaert, C., Franchimont, P., Danneskiold-Samsoe, B., Bach-Andersen, R., Gröss, D., Gerber, H., Gerschpacher, H., Stocker, H., and Bolla, K., 1985, Treatment of active rheumatoid arthritis with slow intravenous injections of thymopentin. A double-blind placebo-controlled randomized study, *Lancet* **1:**832–836.

Manyak, C., Tse, H., Fischer, P., Coker, L., Sigal, H., and Koo, G. C., 1988, Regulation of class II MHC molecules on human endothelial cells, *J. Immunol.* **140:**3817–3821.

Matsubara, T., and Ziff, M., 1987, Basement membrane thickening of postcapillary venules and capillaries in rheumatoid synovium, *Arthritis Rheum.* **30:**18–30.

Miyasaka, N., Nakamura, T., Russell, I. J., and Talal, N., 1984, Interleukin-2 deficiencies in rheumatoid arthritis and systemic lupus erythematosus, *Clin. Immunol. Immunopathol.* **31:**109–117.

Mond, J., Carmen, J., Sarma, C., Chara, J., and Finkelman, F. D., 1986, Interferon-gamma suppresses B-cell stimulation factor (BSF-1) induction of class II MHC determinants on B-cells, *J. Immunol.* **137:**3534–3537.

Nagai, Y., Osanai, T., and Sakakibara, K., 1982, Intensive suppression of allergic encephalomyelitis (EAE) by serum thymic factor and therapeutic implication for multiple sclerosis, *J. Exp. Med.* **52:**213–224.

Nakamura, M., Manser, T., Pearson, G. D. N., Daley, M. J., and Gefter, M. L., 1984, Effect of gamma-interferon on the immune response *in vivo* and on gene expression *in vitro*, *Nature* **307:**381–386.

Oppenhelmer-Marks, N., and Ziff, M., 1987, Measurement of lymphocyte migration through endothelial cell monolayer *in vitro*: Role of inflammatory factors, *Arthritis Rheum.* **30:**S83.

Panitch, H. S., Hirsch, R. L., Haley, A. S., and Johnson, K. P., 1987, Exacerbation of multiple sclerosis in patients treated with gamma interferon, *Lancet* **1:**893–894.

Pleau, J. M., Dardenne, M., Blouquit, Y., and Bach, J. F., 1977, Structural study of circulating thymic factor: A peptide isolated from pig serum. II. Amino acid sequence, *J. Biol. Chem.* **252:**8045.

Pober, J. S., Collins, T., Gimbrone, Jr., M. A., Cotran, R. S., Gitlin, J. D., Fiers, W., Clayberger, C., Krensky, A., Burakoff, S. J., and Reiss, C. S., 1983, Lymphocytes recognize human vascular endothelial and dermal fibroblast Ia antigens induced by recombinant immune interferon, *Nature* **305:**726–729.

Remy, J. J., Salaero, J., Bechet, M., and Charreire, J., 1987, Experimental autoimmune thyroiditis induced by recombinant interferon-γ, *Immunol. Today* **8:**73.

Scheynius, A., Johansson, C., and Van Der Meide, P. H., 1986, In vivo induction of Ia antigens on rat keratinocytes by gammainterferon, *Br. J. Dermatol.* **115:**543–549.

Sergiescu, D., Cerutti, I., Efthymiou, E., Kahan, A., and Chany, C., 1979, Adverse effects of interferon treatment on the life span of NZB mice, *Biomed. Exp.* **31:**48–51.

Skoglund, C., Scheynius, A., Holmdahl, R., and Van Der Meide, P. H., 1988, Enhancement of DTH reaction and inhibition of expression of class II transplantation antigens by in vivo treatment with antibodies against γ-interferon, *Clin. Exp. Immunol.* **71:**428–432.

Smith, J. B., and Talal, N., 1982, Significance of self recognition and interleukin-2 for immunoregulation, autoimmunity and cancer, *Scand. J. Immunol.* **16:**269–278.

Trainin, N., Handzel, Z. T., and Pech, T. M., 1985, Biochemical and clinical properties of thymic humoral factor, *Thymus* **7:**137–142.

Veys, E. M., Huskisson, E. C., Rosenthal, M., Vischer, T. L., Mielants, H., Thrower, P. A., Scott, J., Ott, H., Scheijgrond, H., and Symoens, J., 1982, Clinical response to therapy with thymopoietin pentapeptide (TP-5) in rheumatoid arthritis, *Ann. Rheum. Dis.* **41:**441–443.

Veys, E. M., Hermanns, Ph., Mielants, H., and Verbruggen, G., 1984a, Mechanism of flu-like syndrome induced by levamisole can be the base of its mode of action in rheumatoid arthritis, in: *Advances in Inflammation Research*, Volume 6 (K. D. Rainsford and G. P. Velo, eds.), Raven Press, New York, pp. 239–250.

Veys, E. M., Mielants, H., Verbruggen, G., Spiro, T., Newdeck, E., Power, D., and Goldstein, G., 1984b, Thymopoietin pentapeptide (thymopentin, TP-5) in the treatment of rheumatoid arthritis. A compilation of several short- and long-term clinical studies, *J. Rheumatol.* **11:**462–466.

Veys, E. M., Luyten, F., Mielants, H., and Verbruggen, G., 1987, Side-effects of levamisole: Recent aspects, in: *Studies in Major Organ Systems*, Part 2 (K. D. Rainsford and G. P. Velo, eds.), MTP Press, Lancaster, pp. 235–243.

Veys, E. M., Mielants, H., Verbruggen, G., Grosclaude, J. P., and Meyer, W., 1988, Interferon-gamma in rheumatoid arthritis. A double-blind study comparing human interferon gamma with placebo, *J. Rheumatol.* **15:**570–574.

Virelizier, J. L., Perez, N., Arenzana-Seisdedos, F., and Devos, R., 1984, Pure interferon gamma enhances class II HLA antigens on human monocyte cell lines, *Eur. J. Immunol.* **14:**101–108.

Wofsy, D., Roths, J. B., Murphy, E. D., Dauphinee, M. J., Kipper, S. B., and Talal, N., 1981, Deficient interleukin-2 activity in MRL/Mp and C57BL/6J mice bearing the lp2 gene, *J. Exp. Med.* **154:**1671–1680.

Wolfe, F., Cathey, M. A., Hawley, D. J., Basler, J. P., and Schindler, J., 1986, Clinical trial with R-IFN-gamma in rheumatoid arthritis, in: *Biologically Based Immunomodulators in the Therapy of Rheumatic Diseases* (S. H. Pincus, D. S. Pisetsky, and L. J. Rosenwasser, eds.), Elsevier, New York, pp. 379–396.

Chapter 17

STRATEGY IN IMMUNOSUPPRESSION

Jean-François Bach

1. INTRODUCTION

Seven different types of immunosuppressive agents are presently available for clinical use with acceptable benefit/toxicity ratio:

- Corticosteroids
- Thiopurines (azathioprine, 6-mercaptopurine)
- Alkylating agents (cyclophosphamide, chlorambucil)
- Methotrexate
- Cyclosporine
- Antilymphocyte sera
- Anti-T-cell monoclonal antibodies

All these agents are widely used alone or in combination. The problem is often posed of the selection of the best agent or of the best association in a given clinical condition. We shall discuss here the rationale of such selection.

Several notions should be taken into consideration:

1. The mechanisms of the immune response is supposed to bring the desired clinical improvement.
2. The duration of treatment needed, which depends on the natural history of the disease.
3. The severity of the underlying medical condition and correspondingly the benefit expected from immunosuppressive therapy, which is an essential factor for the evaluation of the risk/benefit ratio.
4. The cellular target of the various immunosuppressive agents and their intrinsic toxicity (independent of the side effects secondary to the immunosuppression, which are met with all active immunosuppressants).

We shall discuss successively these four topics.

Jean-François Bach • Immunology Clinic, Necker Hospital, 75743 Paris Cedex 15, France.

Immunopharmacology in Autoimmune Diseases and Transplantation, edited by Hans Erik Rugstad *et al.* Plenum Press, New York, 1992.

2. IMMUNOLOGIC MECHANISMS

Immunosuppressive agents are essentially administered in organ or bone marrow transplantation and in autoimmune diseases. One should realize that very diverse mechanisms may operate in these different conditions.

One may assume that antibodies play the central role in antireceptor autoantibody-mediated disease (myasthenia gravis and Graves' disease), in autoimmune cytopenias, and in immune complex diseases (glomerulonephritis and systemic lupus). Conversely, T cells probably play the central role in acute or chronic graft versus host disease, some autoimmune diseases such as active chronic hepatitis, biliary cirrhosis, type 1 diabetes, psoriasis, and probably rheumatoid arthritis.

The case of organ allografts is more complex. T cells are likely to play a predominant role in acute rejection where antibodies are also probably involved. The situation is still less clear in many diseases where the pathogenic mechanisms remain elusive (such as multiple sclerosis or Crohn's disease).

One would thus like to know more about the precise underlying mechanisms. It would be important to determine with more accuracy the role of the various T-cell subsets and their mode of action (lymphokine release, direct cytotoxicity).

This discussion is important to select the most adapted immunosuppressive agent. Antibody production is most sensitive to alkylating agents and to some degree to thiopurines and corticosteroids used at high dosage. Cell-mediated immunity is most sensitive to cyclosporine and antilymphocyte antibodies (polyclonal or monoclonal) and to a lesser degree to azathioprine and corticosteroids.

One should theoretically base the selection of the agent to use in a given disease on these considerations. It should be realized, however, that the selectivity of action of the immunosuppressive agents is not an absolute as mentioned above. Thus, cyclosporine may inhibit *de novo* antibody production (primary immune response) while it is much less efficient, although often partially so, on established antibody production. Additionally, cyclosporine may improve the clinical course of patients with supposedly antibody-mediated disease (such as myasthenia gravis and lupus) without altering antibody titer (Bach and Feutren, 1985).

The case of steroids is particularly complex. It is interesting to note that at sufficient doses corticosteroids are active in most states of hyperimmunity. Their mode of action in individual cases remains obscure but probably involves to a large extent nonimmunological effects (notably an anti-inflammatory action).

These reservations urge caution in any dogmatic approach and favor pragmatism.

3. DURATION OF DISEASE

The duration of a disease is usually unpredictable. Chronic autoimmune diseases may resolve even in severe forms as shown in lupus (Bach *et al.*, 1986) and multiple sclerosis. In fact, self-limiting immunological diseases are common, such as rheumatic fever or membranous glomerulonephritis (Barbanel and Noël, 1979). This notion of self-limitation is crucial because it justifies the use of acute intense immunosuppression in some cases.

Conversely, in many other settings the hyperimmune reaction is chronic, sometimes indefinite. This is the case of rheumatoid arthritis, multiple sclerosis, or allografting. Even in these cases, however, the immunologic activity is not constant and remissions are observed between exacerbation phases.

The case of type I diabetes is apparently unique but could have many equivalents. The disease is diagnosed at a late stage of its natural history, when more than 80% of the beta cells have been destroyed (Bach, 1988). Immunosuppression can still be active but only if administered within 6–8 weeks after initiation of insulinotherapy (Feutren et al., 1986). Ultimately, all beta cells are destroyed and there is no point in giving immunosuppressive agents; hence, the urgency to begin immunosuppression, which also applies to a number of other diseases where the lesions develop rapidly or at least may be completed within a few days or weeks. This is certainly the case for rheumatic fever and allograft rejection episodes and perhaps also for a number of autoimmune diseases such as multiple sclerosis.

Another reason to treat patients at an early stage of the disease is the progressively increasing resistance of the immune response to immunosuppression. This has been well demonstrated for type I diabetes in NOD mice using a model of disease recurrence on islet grafts (Wang et al., 1988). Of course, this pressure to treat early is balanced by the less severe medical status at early stages, which generates hesitation in using aggressive therapy.

4. SEVERITY OF THE DISEASE: THE RISK–BENEFIT RATIO

The nature of expected benefit from immunosuppression varies immensely according to patients. In some cases, immunosuppression is mandatory. This is the case with heart allograft recipients (even if one may perform a second graft) or of very severe devastating autoimmune diseases (for example, some forms of systemic lupus). In these conditions major risks may be taken, but this must not represent an excuse not to search insistently for the least toxic protocols.

In other cases, the benefit is not immediately life-saving but may be at the origin of major clinical improvement with prevention of very severe outcome. One then has the difficult task of achieving the delicate balance between the disease and drug risks. The potential benefit of immunosuppression is great in type I diabetes or in multiple sclerosis, but these are very chronic conditions and only moderate risks can be accepted.

Additionally, one should try to make a fair assessment of the individual drug toxicity depending on the individual disease or patient. Thus patients with rheumatoid arthritis are abnormally sensitive to cyclosporine-induced nephrotoxicity due to the concomitant use of nonsteroidal anti-inflammatory agents.

5. RISKS OF INTENSE OR CHRONIC IMMUNOSUPPRESSION

Evaluating the potential risks of a given immunosuppressive protocol is not always an easy task since the hazards in question, essentially, infections and malignancies, are highly dependent on the dosage, duration of treatment, and individual patients. It is difficult to extrapolate from one protocol using a given drug to another one using different drugs or the same drug but in different pharmacological conditions. The assessment is complicated by the frequent use of drug combinations. As far as infections are concerned, one should emphasize the point that steroids are the main promoter of bacterial infections and that thiopurine and cyclosporine, when used alone at moderate doses, usually do not favor the onset of infections.

6. DRUG COMBINATION

Combinations of several immunosuppressive agents may have several distinct objectives:

1.   decreasing the individual toxicity of each drug for an equivalent global immuno-
     suppression

2.   increasing the immunosuppressive activity due to complementary mode of action (synergy)

3.   actively preventing the deleterious effect of a given agent (for example, low-dose conventional immunosuppression to prevent immunization against xenogeneic antilymphocyte antibodies (Chatenoud et al., 1986).

It is fair to recognize that only the first of these objectives has been fully reached.

It is indeed increasingly apparent that associating two or three immunosuppressive agents with similar overall activity used at low doses may bring a satisfactory state of immunosuppression, comparable to or better than that afforded by each agent given at full dosage. Several examples of such associations are currently used in organ transplantation [notably cyclosporine plus corticoids (double association) or cyclosporine plus azathioprine plus corticosteroids (triple association)]. The efficacy of such associations is difficult to compare in a rigorous methodological way with that of individual therapy, but the increasing success of organ transplantation using this approach has confirmed its value. The risk, however, of overimmunosuppression is heightened and the current tendency is to decrease the dosage of each agent and to avoid some particularly hazardous associations such as antilymphocyte antibodies plus cyclosporine, which are reported to induce a high risk of lymphomas (Touraine et al., 1983). This risk explains the so far limited use of immunosuppressive drug combinations in autoimmune disease.

The search for pharmacological synergy has provided some interesting results experimentally: steroids have been reported to potentiate the action of a number of other immunosuppressive agents such as azathioprine and antilymphocyte globulin (Simmons et al., 1968; Floersheim, 1969). The reality of the synergy is not, however, totally convincing and has not been proven in humans.

More interesting is the consecutive use of different agents with distinct modes of action. One may assume that drugs such as azathioprine and cyclosporine are particularly efficient on chronic immune responses, but that their action is limited in cases of hyperimmune response. When this hyperimmune response is cell-mediated (like in organ allograft rejection), one may use steroids or antilymphocyte antibodies (monoclonal or polyclonal). High-dose cyclophosphamide (bolus doses) may be efficient in the case of humoral hyperimmune responses, as is done in systemic lupus.

The prevention of side effects caused by drug combination is interesting but limited. So far, the prevention of xenosensitization after administration of antilymphocyte antibodies has only been achieved by using cyclosporine and azathioprine–steroid combination (Chatenoud et al., 1986).

7. CONCLUSIONS

Such are the main lines of strategy of clinical immunosuppression. Three lines of thinking have been used as main guidelines:

• sufficient activity with the constant fear of giving too much drug and creating an unnecessary and dangerous state of overimmunosuppression
• selectivity of action adapted to the clinical condition under treatment
• decrease of side effects that appear relatively easily accessible for individual direct drug toxicity but more difficult to achieve for infections and malignancies (overimmunosuppression).

In fact, the two major problems today are probably the difficulty in establishing a profound state of immunosuppression with nontoxic drugs, as needed in the first months following organ transplantation, and avoiding the risk of tumors in long-term treatment (in autoimmune diseases and transplantation).

Progress will come from discovery of new agents but also from further investigation of experimental models and better clinical handling of the presently available drugs, helped by constantly improved pharmacological and immunological monitoring. Pharmacological monitoring today is essentially based on blood level determination. It is only performed for cyclosporine, although it is available for other agents such as steroids and antilymphocyte antibodies, and to a lesser extent for azathioprine and cyclophosphamide. Presently, immunological monitoring is still unfortunately only feasible in the case of monoclonal antibodies. Much effort should be devoted to circumvent these limitations.

REFERENCES

Bach, J. F., 1988, Mechanisms of autoimmunity in insulin-dependent diabetes mellitus, *Clin. Exp. Immunol.* **72:**1–8.

Bach, J. F., and Feutren, G., 1985, Contrasting effects of cyclosporine on humoral and cell-mediated immunity in patients with autoimmune diseases, in: *Autoimmune Diseases* (R. Schindler, ed.), Springer Verlag, Berlin, pp. 33–38.

Bach, J. F., Jacob, L., Feutren, G., and Tron, F., 1986, The questionable role of anti-DNA antibodies in the pathogenesis of systemic lupus erythematosus, *Ann. NY Acad. Sci.* **475:**231–240.

Barbanel, C., and Noël, L. H., 1979, Membranous glomerulonephritis, in: *Nephrology* (J. Hamburger, J. Crosnier, and J. P. Grünfeld, eds.), Wiley, New York, pp. 489–506.

Chatenoud, L., Baudrihaye, M. F., Chkoff, N., Kreis, H., Goldstein, G., and Bach, J. F., 1986, Restriction of the human *in vivo* immune response against the mouse monoclonal antibody OKT3, *J. Immunol.* **137:**830–838.

Feutren, G., Papo, L., Assan, R., Vialettes, B., Karsenty, G., Vexiau, P., Du Rostu, H., Rodier, M., Sirmai, J., Lallemand, A., and Bach, J. F., 1986, Cyclosporin increases the rate and length of remissions in insulin-dependent diabetes of recent onset, *Lancet* **1:**119–124.

Floersheim, G. L., 1969, A study of combined treatment with chemical immunosuppressants and antilymphocytic serum to prolong skin allograft survival, *Transplantation*, **8:**392–402.

Simmons, R. L., Ozerkis, A., and Hoehn, R. J., 1968, Antiserum to lymphocytes: Interaction with chemical immunosuppressants, *Science* **160:**1127–1130.

Touraine, J. L., El Yafi, S., Bosi, E., Chapuis-Cellier, C., Ritter, J., Blanc, N., Dubernard, J. M., Poutel-Lenoble, C., Chevallier, M., Creyssel, R., and Trager, J., 1983, Immunoglobulin abnormalities and infectious lymphoproliferative syndrome (ILPS) in cyclosporine-treated transplant patients, *Transpl. Proc.* **15,** no. 4 (Suppl. 1) 2798–2804.

Wang, Y. M., McDuffie, M., Nomikos, I. N., Hao, L., and Lafferty, K. J., 1988, Effect of cyclosporine in immunologically mediated diabetes in nonobese diabetic mice, *Transplantation* **46:**101S–106S.

Chapter 18

IMMUNOSUPPRESSIVE DRUGS

The Need for Therapeutic Drug Monitoring

Hans Erik Rugstad

1. VALUE AND LIMITATIONS OF THERAPEUTIC DRUG MONITORING OF IMMUNOSUPPRESSIVE DRUGS

During the past two decades there has been enormous progress in our understanding of the relationships between dosage schedules, serum (or whole blood) concentrations, and pharmacological effects of a large number of drugs. Unfortunately, the concept of using drug levels for guidance in pharmacotherapy has also led to a rather pointless controversy. It has suffered almost as much from the unrealistic claims of some uncritical advocates as from the negativity of skeptics. However, it has become clear that in the case of many, but by no means all drugs, information about their concentration in biological fluids is helpful for their optimal use in many therapeutic situations.

I shall concern myself with theoretical considerations of importance for evaluation of the value and limitations of therapeutic drug monitoring (TDM) of immunosuppressive drugs and give clinical data that support these theoretical considerations. I will discuss cyclosporine A (CyA), for which TDM is widely used; azathioprine (plus 6-mercaptopurine and metabolites), for which TDM is possibly used to a lesser degree than it should be; methotrexate, for which TDM is used mainly to avoid toxicity; and briefly comment further on possibilities for monitoring alkylating agents and glucocorticoids used for immunosuppression. The prerequisites for a plasma concentration effect relationship are given in Table I.

All these requirements are hardly met for any drug. How are these conditions fulfilled with regard to immunosuppressive drugs? Relatively little is known about the determining factors of drug response, both efficacy and adverse reactions, for immunosuppressive drugs. It is not known if therapeutic responses and toxic effects are best related to (1) peak concentrations, (2) time above a threshold concentration, or (3) area under the concentration time curve (AUC). In addition, for immunosuppressive drugs there are special difficulties: Endpoint for efficacy is difficult to determine both in organ transplantation and

Hans Erik Rugstad • Department of Clinical Pharmacology, The National Hospital, University of Oslo, N-0027 Oslo 1, Norway.

Immunopharmacology in Autoimmune Diseases and Transplantation, edited by Hans Erik Rugstad *et al.* Plenum Press, New York, 1992.

TABLE I.   Prerequisites for a Plasma (Blood) Concentration–Effect Relationship

Specific and sensitive analytical methods
Drug effect dependent on concentration at receptor
Development of tolerance at receptor site should not be an important problem
Drug active per se (active metabolites?)
Plasma (blood) concentration varies with time according to a defined pharmacokinetic model; time for dosing and
   sampling known
Accurate recording of drug effects

in autoimmune diseases. Also, therapeutic effects and toxic reactions may be delayed for days and weeks, and factors other than drug action may be of great importance, for example, warm ischemia time and tissue compatibility of transplanted organs.

The pharmacokinetics of some immunosuppressive drugs are not known in detail. Moreover, information on the possible relationship between clinical events and drug levels of alkylating agents and azathioprine (plus 6-mercaptopurine and metabolites) is largely gained from studies of cancer chemotherapy and may not be relevant for immunosuppression. There have been few attempts to relate measured drug concentrations and biological effects in autoimmune disease, and relatively little is known about influence of age and hepatic and renal disease on drug effects and kinetics.

Despite the fact that we lack knowledge of many aspects of immunosuppressive drugs, monitoring may be important: Many of these drugs have steep dose–response curves and low therapeutic indices. The drugs may have a high incidence of adverse reactions that may be life-threatening. There is considerable interindividual variation in pharmacokinetics, and some drugs show dose-dependent pharmacokinetics. Polypharmacy is the rule for these patients; it is common to combine two or three immunosuppressive drugs in organ-transplanted patients. In addition, analgesics, anti-inflammatory drugs, and antibiotics are often used. Drug interactions at the pharmacokinetic level are therefore common. The patients often have altered kidney or liver function. Measurements of drug levels in blood or plasma reduces the variation due to pharmacokinetic factors and may contribute to improvement of immunosuppressive drug therapy.

2. CYCLOSPORINE A

The pharmacology of CyA is described in Chapter 12 of this book. Only aspects of therapeutic drug monitoring will be discussed here. CyA is a very efficacious immunosuppressant without being cytostatic, and in contrast to alkylating agents it has a reversible mode of action. In high doses it may be nephrotoxic. CyA is a very lipophilic polypeptide dependent on metabolism in the cytochrome P-450 enzyme system in the liver for its elimination. Its metabolism shows great variation between patients and can be induced or inhibited by other drugs. For the reasons given above, one would therefore presume that monitoring of CyA might be useful. Indeed, CyA is the only immunosuppressive drug that is monitored routinely. One reason for TDM of CyA is the fact that a given dose or dosing regimen produces widely variable blood or plasma concentrations of cyclosporine in different patients. TDM assesses the interindividual variations in drug absorption, distribution, metabolism, and elimination that prevent blood concentrations being estimated from dose alone. TDM assists the clinician to compensate for demographic factors affecting CyA concentrations such as increased clearance in children. TDM of CyA is used (1) to avoid low trough concentrations of CyA, which are frequently associated with organ rejection, (2) to avoid excessive CyA concentrations, which may be associated with overimmunosuppression and occasionally nephrotoxicity, and (3) to monitor compliance.

Low trough concentrations of CyA may result from malabsorption of the drug secondary to the lack of sufficient bile or due to diarrhea. Concomitant use of other drugs such as phenytoin and rifampicin will increase clearance of CyA by induction of drug-metabolizing enzymes and result in low CyA concentrations. High blood concentrations may result from time-dependent improvements in cyclosporine absorption or inhibition of microsomal liver enzymes responsible for CyA metabolism, for example, ketoconazole.

Despite the fact that TDM of CyA has been used extensively almost for a decade, there are still many questions to be asked. When and how should CyA be measured? Should metabolites be measured? Where should CyA be measured—whole blood or plasma? Which level should one aim at? Is the desired level dependent on disease? Is the level dependent on concomitant medication? Is the level dependent on time after transplantation?

2.1. Program for Monitoring CyA

When should CyA be monitored? An organized program of monitoring blood concentrations of CyA should start immediately after initiation of therapy. CyA monitoring is especially important in the early postoperative period during which it is necessary to measure CyA blood concentrations daily or every second day. This intensive monitoring should continue until the clinical condition and cyclosporine dosage are stable and for at least two weeks. One should not put too much emphasis on one single determination, but study the trend. If one concentration is outside the range aimed at, a new sample should be drawn the next day. If two or more samples follow the same trend, a dose adjustment may be justified. In stable patients more than six months posttransplant, blood level determination every other month is usually sufficient. Reasons for additional determinations are dose adjustment, insufficient effect, additional drug therapy, altered function of liver or heart, and adverse or toxic reactions. CyA level is only one among several critical factors such as liver and renal function, infection, and so on and can never replace clinical judgment.

2.2. Assay Methods, Significance of Metabolites, and Biological Specimen

Several methods for CyA concentration measurements are presently in use. They include radioimmunoassay (RIA), high performance liquid chromatography (HPLC), and fluorescence polarization immunoassay (FPIA). Polyclonal antibodies to CyA, used with RIA ("original" RIA from Sandoz, Switzerland) or FPIA (TDx kit, Abbott Ltd.), have varying degrees of cross-reactivity to CyA metabolites. However, two new RIA kits with monoclonal antibodies were introduced early in 1987 by Sandoz. One of these monoclonal antibodies is unspecific with considerable cross-reactivity with several metabolites, and the other is highly specific for the parent compound. The specific monoclonal antibody used in the Sandimmun kit from Sandoz with tritiated tracer is also used with iodinated tracer in the Cyclotrac SP kit from Incstar. Despite the fact that they use the same antibody, the two methods show some variation in CyA results. An analytical CyA kit for FPIA has been available from Abbott with a specific antibody since 1990. The monoclonal antibody used by Abbott in this kit is different from that used by Sandoz and Incstar. Cross-reactivity for some metabolites is greater than for the Sandoz antibody.

Possible immunosuppressive and toxic effects of the numerous CyA metabolites have not been completely investigated, but in clinical use of CyA such effects are of minor importance. A specific method for the parent drug should therefore usually be employed. However, determination of metabolite level may be used diagnostically in certain situations with impaired liver function or rejection of a cardiac transplant. Most studies of the relationship between blood/plasma levels of CyA and its effects up to now have been based on nonspecific methods.

Comparisons of CyA monitoring in whole blood and plasma are complicated by the fact that CyA and its metabolites are unevenly distributed between red blood cells and plasma and this distribution is temperature dependent. Studies using different analytical techniques and with different biological specimens can therefore not readily be compared. A thorough comparison of CyA levels in blood and plasma in 66 renal transplant recipients followed for six months using HPLC, RIA, and FPIA with polyclonal unspecific antibodies and specific and nonspecific monoclonal antibodies, have recently been done by Lindholm and Henricsson (1990). A strong correlation was observed between the results obtained with HPLC and specific monoclonal RIA ($r = 0.98$). The highest values for CyA concentrations in blood were found with nonspecific monoclonal RIA (Sandoz), followed by polyclonal FPIA and polyclonal RIA (mean ratio versus specific monoclonal RIA was 3.3, 2.9, and 2.4, respectively). Specific monoclonal RIA had 7% higher values than HPLC. The concentrations in blood were, on the average, three times higher than those in plasma, with large variations. The monoclonal FPIA method has been evaluated for TDM of CyA in whole blood after kidney, heart, and liver transplantation by Winkler et al. (1992). They found the method to be convenient and precise. The results obtained in patient samples averaged about 10% higher than those obtained with RIA using specific antibody. As expected, in patients with high metabolite accumulation resulting from severe liver dysfunction, the FPIA measurements were considerably higher than specific RIA methods and should be interpreted cautiously. The large interindividual variations in ratios between the results using different media and different assay methods makes it necessary to evaluate each method separately.

The HPLC method has the advantage that it estimates parent CyA and several different drug metabolites separately. Limitations remain for routine use of HPLC, such as the requirement for laborious sample preparations, complex instrumentation, and relatively lengthy per sample analysis time. Present-day clinical practice usually depends on the drug estimated by RIA using kits distributed by Sandoz or Incstar or FPIA (TDx kit from Abbott). Experience with the new kits using the monoclonal-specific antibodies is limited compared with the use of the traditional, polyclonal antibody kit. But there is little doubt that determination of the parent drug only will be an advantage especially in liver and heart transplantation. In these circumstances the levels of CyA metabolites may be more than ten times higher than the levels of the parent drug. The new specific methods make it possible to ensure a certain minimal level of the parent drug in situations with high levels of metabolites. In addition, the new monoclonal antibodies give better performance with regard to specificity, sensitivity, and reproducibility.

The RIA and FPIA have several advantages, such as the possibility of rapidly processing large number of samples, simplicity, and ready standardization and computer analysis of data. Because of the simplicity and flexibility for clinical application, low detection limit, good precision, and accuracy compared with HPLC in detection of CyA, the new specific RIA and FPIA methods have been extensively applied in the clinical areas.

Lindholm and Henricsson (1989) studied the protein binding of CyA in plasma of 66 renal transplant recipients. Analysis was performed with a recently developed method of equilibrium dialysis in steel chambers. Among the 1,848 samples, the free fraction ranged from 0.5 to 4.2%, with a median of 1.30%.

The authors conclude that monitoring of free fraction may prove useful in special situations, for example, in patients with dyslipoproteinemias, but do not recommend routine measurement of unbound CyA.

Where? There has been considerable controversy regarding the appropriate material for CyA determination, whether one should use whole blood or serum or plasma. The major problems with plasma or serum is the observation that the distribution of drug between plasma and blood cells is temperature dependent. When the temperature is lowered from 37°C to 21, the drug diffuses from plasma into blood cells, reaching equilibrium after 2 hr. If one wishes to use plasma or serum, the blood sample is usually allowed to stand at 21° for at least 2 hr.

There is not one single proportional factor one can use to calculate from plasma to blood. Obviously, the distribution between red blood cells and plasma varies from patient to patient and with time elapsed since transplant. Factors of importance are hematocrit, blood lipids, and uneven distribution of CyA itself and metabolites between red blood cells and plasma.

Only good clinical studies relating whole blood or plasma levels to clinical effect and toxicity can show which is the better. Presently, it seems fair to conclude that one can use either one. Increasing numbers of centers are using whole blood; in any case, it is easier and less time-consuming to use whole blood. Recently, consensus with regard to the determination of trough concentrations of CyA in whole blood is that use of parent-drug-specific techniques is the method of choice in most instances (see reports from consensus meetings by Shaw *et al.*, 1990, and Kahan *et al.*, 1990).

2.3. Pharmacokinetic Considerations

Therapeutic drug monitoring of CyA almost always utilizes trough samples, that is, drawn immediately before the next dose is administered. It is uncertain whether a specific peak CyA value is necessary for rejection prophylaxis. Furthermore, TDM by peak value is impractical, because the time to peak after oral administration varies between 1 and 8 hr, thus requiring a full pharmacokinetic profile to determine it with certainty. It is important to be aware of the influence of dosing interval on the trough values. If CyA is given once daily, a trough concentration after 24 hr will be considerably lower than if the same daily dose is divided in two and trough level is measured 12 hr after last dose.

2.4. Therapeutic Range

It appears that the therapeutic window differs among patients. This variability is probably partly due to factors such as individual CyA pharmacodynamics. It is also conceivable that optimal CyA level varies with factors such as disease (organ transplant or autoimmune disease), time after transplant, immunological activity, and concomitant disease. In addition, the therapeutic window is imperfect, so some patients experience rejection in spite of apparently adequate drug levels while others develop nephrotoxicity in the face of low levels. Nephrotoxicity may occur in the absence of toxic CyA drug levels, probably due to synergistic injuries to the allograft by rejection, donor ischemia, procurement injury, and drugs such as amphotericin B and nonsteroidal anti-inflammatory drugs.

Organ rejection is less common when whole blood levels (specific method) are greater than 100 ng/ml.

Only carefully conducted large clinical trials correlating drug levels and clinical events can give the answer to which level one should aim at. For reasons discussed above, the optimal level will vary according to the analytical method used (specific measuring parent drug only or nonspecific including metabolites), choice of biological specimen, whole blood or plasma, and drugs used in addition to CyA. Kahan and co-workers (1984), using plasma and unspecific RIA in a series of 118 consecutive recipients of cadaveric renal allograft, found that serum trough levels provide a useful monitoring index.

Maiorca and co-workers (1985) used whole blood trough levels and an unspecific RIA method in 33 kidney transplant patients and found that levels between 200 and 500 ng/ml provided efficient immunosuppression while reducing the incidence of toxicity. However, since more centers are using whole blood and specific methods, I will mainly discuss studies where the parent drug has been measured in whole blood.

Optimal CyA levels are difficult to establish in organ transplant patients, but most centers would aim at values between 200 and 300 ng/ml in whole blood determined with a specific method in the postoperative period (Table II). The patients should be kept at that level for two weeks and then have a gradual reduction in whole blood concentrations, down to between 50 and 100 ng/ml after six months. These are values for renal transplant patients using triple therapy, that is, small doses of glucocorticoids and azathioprine in addition to CyA. Slightly higher levels should be the aim for heart transplant patients (Table II). Results of TDM with specific methods in whole blood in renal transplant patients have been reported for 52 patients by Kwan et al. (1987), for 45 patients by Kasiske et al. (1988), and for 125 patients by Uchida et al. (1988). A very large study on cyclosporine concentrations in relation to its therapeutic effect and toxicity after renal transplantation has recently been concluded by Lindholm and co-workers (1990). These authors followed 66 consecutive kidney transplant recipients for six months after transplantation. CyA was analyzed by HPLC in plasma, specific and nonspecific monoclonal RIA in whole blood, and polyclonal RIA and polyclonal FPIA in whole blood and plasma. Their results suggest that specific analysis of CyA in whole blood offers the best guidance.

Laufer et al. (1988) reported favorable results in 52 cardiac transplant patients monitored with a specific method in whole blood, aiming at a level of 100–150 ng/ml after six months. Lindberg, Geiran, and Frøysaker (personal communication, 1990) at the department of thoracic surgery, The National Hospital of Norway, used whole blood determinations with a specific RIA method aiming at the values given in Table II for monitoring 51 consecutive heart transplant recipients from November 1987 to February 1990. At that time 48 of these 51 patients were alive. Tredger et al. (1988) found a very good correlation between specific RIA and HPLC in whole blood monitoring of 15 liver transplant patients.

Oldhafer et al. (1988) used whole blood and both an unspecific RIA method and HPLC for CyA determinations in a study of 34 liver transplant patients and concluded that specific measurements of CyA blood concentration are important in order to ensure immunosuppressive levels in liver transplant patients. According to their report it appears that a level of 100–200 ng/ml in whole blood gives sufficient immunosuppression in these patients. Krom et al. (1989) used HPLC whole blood determinations in 100 liver transplant patients and aimed at trough levels of 250–350 ng/ml when CyA was used with corticosteroid and trough levels of 80–120 ng/ml after addition of azathioprine 2 mg/kg.

For autoimmune diseases the therapeutic window is more uncertain. Mihatsch et al. (1988) gives the following recommendations based on experience with the drug in patients with autoimmune diseases: The initial dose should not exceed 5 mg/kg body weight; the dose

TABLE II. Recommended Whole Blood Cyclosporine Levels (Specific Method) in Renal and Heart Transplant Recipients on Triple Therapy[a]

Days post transplant	CyA (ng/ml)
Renal	
0–14	200–300
15–30	150–250
30–60	100–200
60–180	50–150
>180	50–100
Heart	
0–40	200–300
40–80	150–200
>80	100–150

[a]Small doses of azathioprine and prednisolone in addition to CyA.

should be reduced if blood CyA levels are over 200 ng/ml in whole blood (specific method); a dose reduction is recommended if serum creatinine values exceed 30% of pretreatment values, or if other signs of CyA toxicity, such as hepatotoxicity, hypertension, and so on occur. By strict adherence to these suggestions, it should be possible to treat patients for a prolonged period without irreversible renal morphological lesions.

One fundamental observation supports the value of therapeutic drug monitoring of CyA: An optimal drug concentration in blood correlates better with therapeutic effect and toxicity than administered doses.

3. AZATHIOPRINE AND 6-MERCAPTOPURINE

For more than 20 years azathioprine (AZA) has been a main immunosuppressive agent in organ transplantation and in a variety of conditions that are considered to be autoimmune in character such as rheumatoid arthritis, chronic active hepatitis, pemphigus vulgaris, and systemic lupus erythematosus. AZA, the imidazolyl derivative of 6-mercaptopurine (6-MP), is rapidly converted to 6-MP, which is thought to be responsible for most of the immunosuppressive effects *in vivo*. 6-MP acts as a purine antagonist that interferes with biochemical processes involving endogenously occurring purines and their nucleoside and nucleotide metabolites.

The modes of action of AZA, which is primarily used in immunosuppression, and 6-MP, mainly used in treatment of leukemia, are described in Chapter 9 in this book and only the TDM aspects of these substances will be discussed here. AZA and 6-MP are prodrugs; they have no intrinsic immunosuppressive activity, and 6-MP undergoes extensive metabolism along several pathways to form intracellular active metabolites. There is a lack of information about possible relationships between drug levels and clinical events of AZA, 6-MP, and their metabolites when used as immunosuppressants.

The measurement of AZA, 6-MP, and their metabolites presents many analytical difficulties, partly caused by instability in serum and during extraction. Advances in HPLC technology and the use of dithiotreitol (DTT) as a protective agent to keep thiol groups in the reduced state have made specific and sensitive assays possible. It is now feasible to determine these drugs in biological fluids and their metabolites in human lymphocytes and red blood cells in clinically relevant concentrations. For an excellent review, see Lennard (1989).

Lin et al. (1980) determined the plasma pharmacokinetics of AZA and its primary metabolite 6-MP after both intravenous and oral dosing in renal transplant patients. After an oral dose, no AZA was detected using an assay with a lower limit of sensitivity of less than 0.5 ng/ml plasma. The wide variations in 6-MP plasma values observed after both intravenous and oral dosing probably reflect important differences in the disposition and metabolism of 6-MP.

AZA metabolism to red cell 6-thioguanine nucleotide (6-TGN, an active metabolite) was studied by Lennard et al. (1984). Red cell 6-TGN concentrations varied over a ten-fold range. The preliminary finding indicated that elevated red cell 6-TGN concentrations, above the control range, could be associated with bone marrow depression. Maddocks et al. (1986) described that severe bone marrow depression following a short course of AZA therapy was found to be associated with elevated 6-TGN concentrations in red cells 12 days after the drug was withdrawn. AZA usually shows minimal side effects except for those caused by immunosuppression and granulocytopenia. TDM of AZA may therefore be more important in order to secure therapeutic effect than for avoidance of adverse reactions. Lennard and Lilleyman (1987) thus found a higher risk of relapse in leukemic children with high levels of the enzyme thiopurine methyltransferase (TPMT) responsible for S-methylation and thereby reduction of 6-MP activity. High levels of TPMT may render an individual more insensitive to the immunosuppressive effects of 6-MP; inheritance of low TMPT activity may be a risk factor for elevated 6-TGN and bone marrow failure. There are many potential reasons for variable 6-MP metabolism but one, TPMT, is genetic and predictable.

Measurement of 6-MP concentrations alone for therapeutic monitoring of clinical events during immunosuppressive therapy with AZA seems questionable. The variable metabolism of 6-MP to 6-TGN may be of clinical importance and it is probable that the immunosuppressive effects depend on the amount and persistence of thiopurine nucleotides in target cells. Also, metabolite concentrations and enzyme activities in red blood cells may reflect those within (or in equilibrium with) the target cells. Therefore, clinical investigation of dosage strategies based on pharmacokinetic monitoring of 6-MP and the corresponding thiopurine nucleotides may be warranted in patients treated perorally with AZA or 6-MP. Therapeutic drug monitoring might be of importance to detect very poor absorbers of these drugs and patients deviant in metabolism of 6-MP.

4. METHOTREXATE

An extraordinary wide range of doses and serum levels has been employed for methotrexate (MTX), from oral doses of 7.5 mg per week in patients with rheumatoid arthritis up to intravenous infusions of 80 g/m^2 over 24 hr followed by citrovorum factor in sarcoma patients. Serum concentration measurements are required in high-dose therapy to avoid toxicity. In immunosuppression, MTX is usually administered orally and in low or intermediate doses, although high-dose therapy has been tried in rheumatoid arthritis patients resistant to disease-modifying drugs. After oral administration of doses less than 30 mg/m^2, plasma drug profiles are highly variable due to differences in the rate and extent of absorption. With higher doses, the absorptive mechanisms are saturated and proportionately less drug is bioavailable. After intramuscular or subcutaneous injection, virtually all of the drug is absorbed at a relatively rapid rate. In the field of immunosuppression, methotrexate levels may be of value for patients with renal dysfunction and to measure absorption in patients receiving low and intermediate doses.

Hendel (1985) has reviewed the clinical pharmacokinetics of MTX. He and later Schrøder and Fogh (1988) and several others focused on erythrocyte content of polyglutamates of MTX as a measure of steady-state MTX levels in target cells. The finding by Refsum *et al.* (1989) that psoriasis patients on low-dose MTX (25 mg weekly) had a significant and transient increase in fasting plasma homocysteine levels within 48 hours after dose is interesting and possibly of value as a sensitive and responsive parameter of antifolate treatment. Methotrexate polyglutamate levels in erythrocytes and plasma homocysteine levels may prove useful in monitoring MTX therapy of autoimmune disorders, but at present studies correlating such measurements to clinical events are lacking.

5. ALKYLATING AGENTS

Cyclophosphamide, chlorambucil, and busulfan are the only alkylating agents regularly used to treat immune disorders. These agents have been commonly used in bone marrow transplantation to condition the graft recipient but less frequently in other transplant procedures. Cyclophosphamide is widely used in certain autoimmune and chronic inflammatory diseases. Beneficial results have been reported with chlorambucil in disorders with altered immune reactivity, such as vasculitis associated with rheumatoid arthritis and autoimmune hemolytic anemia with cold agglutinins. Only possibilities for pharmacological monitoring will be discussed here since the alkylating agents are described in Chapter 11.

Cyclophosphamide is inactive and exerts its biological activities through alkylating metabolites generated by microsomal enzymes, mainly in the liver. The oxazaphosphorine ring of the parent drug opens and acrolein and phosphoramide mustard are formed. Subsequently, several active metabolites are formed. Phosphoramide mustard especially is of importance for efficacy, whereas acrolein seems to be responsible for hemorrhagic cystitis.

Cyclophosphamide may be administered either parenterally or orally. Characterization of the disposition kinetics of the active metabolites has been delayed by analytical difficulties. Arndt *et al.* (1988) have published a method for HPLC determination of cyclophosphamide and its alkylating metabolites. Hadidi *et al.* (1988) described a thin-layer chromatography method that can quantitate cyclophosphamide and its four principal urinary metabolites. Chlorambucil pharmacokinetics have been studied by Bank *et al.* (1987), using a HPLC method. Also, Workman *et al.* (1989) have used a HPLC method for chlorambucil analogues. In humans, chlorambucil is extensively metabolized to phenylacetic acid mustard. This metabolite seems to have similar cytotoxic activity to chlorambucil. It is therefore important that both the parent compound and the metabolite are determined when trying to correlate plasma concentrations with therapeutic activity and toxicity. However, samples have to be derivatized prior to the gas liquid chromatography (GC) step. Chlorambucil itself seems to have adequate and reliable absorption after oral administration. However, there is a lack of data regarding the active metabolite phenylacetic mustard. Also, there are no data available for correlating alkylating activity in plasma with the therapeutic effect in immunosuppression or adverse reactions.

Grochow *et al.* (1989) described a method for HPLC analysis of busulfan suitable for therapeutic drug monitoring and studied correlation of drug levels and veno-occlusive disease in patients undergoing bone marrow transplantation. They found that all six patients who developed veno-occlusive disease out of a total of 30 patients undergoing bone marrow transplantation had a busulfan AUC greater than the mean. Previously, Mouridtsen *et al.*

(1978) showed a significant correlation between nadir leukocyte count and integrated concentration of metabolites of cyclophosphamide. It thus seems probable that TDM of alkylating agents may be useful for prevention of adverse reactions. Methods are now available for studies of possible correlations between concentrations of active species of alkylating agents and therapeutic effect in immunosuppression. Clinical correlation between kinetic data and efficacy and/or toxicity also awaits studies evaluating the time course of specific cytotoxic metabolites of these alkylating agents.

6. GLUCOCORTICOIDS

Prednisolone is the most widely used glucocorticoid in immunosuppression. Reliable RIA methods with little cross-reactivity to endogenous steroids suitable for TDM are available. High doses of prednisolone given perorally are generally well absorbed and the extent of bioavailability shows less variation than most other drugs used in immunosuppression.

Prednisolone is bound to transcorten, which is a high-affinity, low-capacity binding protein for glucocorticoids and to albumin, which has a low affinity but high capacity for binding of such steroids. Prednisolone is metabolized in the liver. Rifampicin and possibly several other strong inducers of the hepatic microsomal mono-oxygenase enzyme system will decrease serum levels of prednisolone. Differences in pharmacokinetics may be important for the degree of prednisolone side effects, as demonstrated in renal transplant patients by Bergrem et al. (1985). They found that cushingoid patients had a significantly higher peak prednisolone serum concentration, a longer elimination half-life, and a larger area under the time-concentration curve of total and free (i.e., not protein bound) prednisolone. Therapeutic drug monitoring of glucocorticoids is not widely used. If altered drug response is experienced or suspected, a practical compromise would be to measure the concentration of total prednisolone and the corresponding free fraction 10 hr after tablet intake, that is, in the elimination phase. This would give information on unusually high or low concentrations relative to other subjects on the same dose as suggested by Bergrem et al. (1983).

7. PHARMACOKINETIC INTERACTIONS OF IMMUNOSUPPRESSIVE DRUGS

With the use of combination therapy for immunosuppression as well as a wide range of symptomatic therapies, for example, analgesics and antibiotics for the treatment of patients with immunopathies or organ transplants, the field of immunopharmacology practices polypharmacy to an extreme degree. The risk of a drug interaction under these conditions is high. The pharmacological characteristics of some drugs, such as steep dose–response curves, low therapeutic indices, and severe toxicities, suggest that even small changes in the pharmacokinetic profile of the affected drug might significantly alter its toxicity or efficacy. Interactions at the pharmacokinetic level may make it necessary or desirable to measure levels of immunosuppressive drugs in blood or plasma. Cockburn and Krupp (1989) have given an updated review of drug interactions with cyclosporine A. Also, for some other immunosuppressive drugs there are important pharmacokinetic interactions; for example, allopurinol impairs the elimination of 6-mercaptopurine. Salicylate, sulfa, and probenecid may modify the excretion of methotrexate. Inducers and inhibitors of liver microsomal enzymes may have unpredictable overall effects on the activation of cyclophosphamide.

Awareness on the part of the clinician and more extensive pharmacokinetic investigations will be needed to recognize, document, and avoid potentially harmful pharmacokinetic drug interactions involving immunosuppressive drugs.

8. CONCLUSION

The optimal schedules for immunosuppressive drugs are difficult to establish. On one hand, the therapeutic effect is difficult to assess, due to the absence of objective signs and because of the delayed time frame in which to detect inadequate therapy. On the other hand, these drugs cause toxic side effects capable of increasing morbidity. There is a relative agreement on the value of TDM of CyA. It is an enigma that TDM is not used for other immunosuppressive drugs since analytical methods are now available. Even if a therapeutic window of a drug is unknown, TDM may be of great value to reduce the variation caused by pharmacokinetic factors such as detecting patients with decreased or erratic absorption, decreased protein binding, or altered elimination. Consideration of the kinetics of immunosuppressive drugs in planning treatment could lead to more rational, safer, and possibly more efficacious use. I suggest that TDM should be more widely used to solve specific problems in individual patients treated with immunosuppressive drugs. Pharmacokinetic studies should accompany clinical trials with immunosuppressive drugs. Data should be related to the degree of therapeutic response and to the type and degree of toxicity. Pharmacokinetic studies should be conducted in a wide range of patients including patients with hepatic or renal dysfunction.

REFERENCES

Arndt, C. A. S., Balis, F. M., McCully, C. L., Colvin, O. M., and Poplack, D. G., 1988, Cerebrospinal fluid penetration of active metabolites of cyclophosphamide and ifosfamide in rhesus monkeys, *Cancer Res.* **48**:2113–2115.

Bank, B. B., Kanganis, D., Liebes, L. F., and Silber, F., 1989, Chlorambucil pharmacokinetics and DNA binding in chronic lymphocytic leukemia lymphocytes, *Cancer Res.* **49**:554–559.

Bergrem, H., Jervell, J., and Flatmark, A., 1985, Prednisolone pharmacokinetics in cushingoid and non-cushingoid kidney transplant patients, *Kidney Int.* **27**:459–464.

Cockburn, I. T. R., and Krupp, P., 1989, An appraisal of drug interactions with Sandimmun, *Transplant Proc.* **21**:3845–3850.

Grochow, L. B., Jones, R. J., Brundrett, R. B., Braine, H. G., Chen, T-L., Saral, R., Santos, G. W., and Colvin, O. M., 1989, Pharmacokinetics of busulfan: Correlation with veno-occlusive disease in patients undergoing bone marrow transplantation, *Cancer Chemother. Pharmacol.* **25**:55–61.

Hadidi, A-H. F. A., Coulter, C. E. A., and Idle, J. R., 1988, Phenotypically deficient urinary elimination of carboxyphosphamide after cyclophosphamide administration to cancer patients, *Cancer Res.* **48**:5167–5171.

Hendel, J., 1985, Clinical pharmacokinetics of methotrexate in psoriasis therapy, *Dan. Med. Bul.* **32(6)**:329–337.

Kahan, B. D., 1985, Individualization of cyclosporine therapy using pharmacokinetic and pharmacodynamic parameters, *Transplantation* **40**:457–476.

Kahan, B. D., Wideman, C. A., Reid, M., Gibbons, S., Jarowenko, M., Flechner, S., and Van Buren, C. T., 1984, The value of serial serum trough cyclosporine levels in human renal transplantation, *Transplant. Proc.* **16(5)**:1195–1199.

Kahan, B. D., Shaw, L. M., Holt, D., Grevel, J., and Johnston, A., 1990, Consensus document: Hawk's Cay meeting on therapeutic drug monitoring of cyclosporine, *Clin. Chem.* **36(8)**:1510–1516.

Kasiske, B. L., Heim-Duthoy, K., Venkateswara Rao, K., and Awni, W. M., 1988, The relationship between cyclosporine pharmacokinetic parameters and subsequent acute rejection in renal transplant recipients, *Transplantation* **46**:716–722.

Krom, R. A. F., Wiesner, R. H., Rettke, S. R., Ludwig, J., Southorn, P. A., Hermans, P. E., and Taswell, H. F., 1989, Symposium on liver transplantation. Part 1, *Mayo Clin. Proc.* **64(1)**:84–94.

Kwan, J. T. C., Foxall, P. J. D., Townend, J. N., Thick, M. G., Bending, M. R., and Eisinger, A. J., 1987, Therapeutic range of cyclosporin in renal transplant patients by specific monoclonal radioimmunoassay, *Lancet* **2**:962–963.

Laufer, G., Laczkovixs, A., Wollenek, G., Schreiner, W., Kober, I., and Wolner, E., 1988, Incidence and severity of acute cardiac allograft rejection with two different low-dose cyclosporine maintenance protocols, *Ann. Thorac. Surg.* **46**:382–388.

Lennard, L., 1989, Cytotoxic agents: 6-Mercaptopurine, 6-thioguanine and related compounds, in: *Sulphur-containing Drugs and Related Organic Compounds. Chemistry, Biochemistry and Toxicology*, Volume 3, Part B, *Metabolism and Pharmacokinetics of Sulphur-containing Drugs* (L.A. Damani, ed.), Ellis Horwood Limited, Chichester, pp. 9–46.

Lennard, L., and Lilleyman, J. S., 1987, Are children with lymphoblastic leukaemia given enough 6-mercaptopurine? *Lancet* **2:** 785–787.

Lennard, L., Brown, C. B., Fox, M., and Maddocks, J. L., 1984, Azathioprine metabolism in kidney transplant recipients, *Br. J. Clin. Pharmacol.* **18:**693–700.

Lin, S.-N., Jessup, K., Floyd, M., Wang, T.-P. F., VanBuren, C. T., Caprioli, R. M., and Kahan, B. D., 1980, Quantitation of plasma azathioprine and 6-mercaptopurine levels in renal transplant patients, *Transplantation* **29:**290–294.

Lindholm, A., and Henricsson, S., 1989, Intra- and inter-individual variability in the free fraction of cyclosporine in plasma in recipients of renal transplants, *Ther. Drug Monit.* **11:**623–630.

Lindholm, A., and Henricsson, S., 1990, Comparative analyses of cyclosporine in whole blood and plasma by radioimmunoassay, fluorescence polarization immunoassay and high pressure liquid chromatography, *Ther. Drug Monit.* **12:**344–352.

Lindholm, A., Dahlqvist, R., Groth, C. G., and Sjöqvist, F., 1990, A prospective study of cyclosporine concentrations in relation to its therapeutic effect and toxicity after renal transplantation, *Br. J. Clin. Pharmacol.* **30:**443–452.

Maddocks, J. L., Lennard, L., Amess, J., Amos, R., and Meyrick Thomas, R., 1986, Azathioprine and severe bone marrow depression, *Lancet* **1:**156.

Maiorca, R., Christinelli, L., Scolari, F., Sandrini, S., Savoldi, S., Brunori, G., Prati, E., Lojaconi, L., Salerni, B., and Tonini, G., 1985, Cyclosporine toxicity can be minimized by careful monitoring of blood levels, *Transplant. Proc.* **17** (Suppl.2):54–59.

Mihatsch, M. J., Thiel, G., and Ryffel, B., 1988, Hazards of cyclosporine A therapy and recommendations for its use, *J. Autoimmunity* **1:**533–543.

Mouridtsen, H. T., Witten, J., Frederiksen, P. L., and Hulsbaek, I., 1978, Studies on the correlation between rate of biotransformation and haematological toxicity of cyclophosphamide, *Acta Pharmacol. Toxicol.* **43:**328–330.

Oldhafer, K. J., Schumann, G., Wonigeit, K., Oellerich, M., Ringe, B., and Pichlmayr, R., 1988, Cyclosporine A monitoring by radioimmunoassay (RIA) and high-performance liquid chromatography (HPLC) after liver transplantation: Influence of route of administration and of liver function on the 2RIA:HPLC ratio, *Transplant. Proc.* **20** (Suppl. 3):361–365.

Refsum, H., Helland, S., and Ueland, P. M., 1989, Fasting plasma homocysteine as a sensitive parameter of antifolate effect: A study of psoriasis patients receiving low-dose methotrexate treatment, *Clin. Pharmacol. Ther.* **46:**510–520.

Schröder, H., and Fogh, K., 1988, Methotrexate and its polyglutamate derivatives in erythrocytes during and after weekly low-dose oral methotrexate therapy of children with acute lymphoblastic leukemia, *Cancer Chemother. Pharmacol.* **21:**145–149.

Shaw, L. M., Yatscoff, R. W., Bowers, L. D., Freeman, D. J., Jeffery, J. R., Keown, P. A., McGilveray, I. J., Rosano, T. G., and Wong, P.-Y., 1990, Canadian consensus meeting on cyclosporine monitoring: Report of the consensus panel, *Clin. Chem.* **36**(10):1841–1846.

Tredger, J. M., Steward, C. M., and Williams, R., 1988, Blood cyclosporine concentrations in liver transplant recipients: Assay method and influence of changed hepatic and renal function, *Transplant. Proc.* **20** (Suppl. 3):391–393.

Uchida, K., Yamada, N., Orihara, A., Tominaga, Y., Tanaka, Y., Hayashi, S., Kondo, T., Morozumi, K., Satake, M., Taira, N., Haba, T., Kato, H., Asano, H., Kano, T., and Takagi, H., 1988, Minimal low dosage of cyclosporine therapy in renal transplantation by careful monitoring of high-performance liquid chromatography whole blood trough levels, *Transplant. Proc.* **20** (Suppl. 2):394–401.

Winkler, M., Schumann, G., Petersen, D., Oellerich, M., and Wonigeit, K., 1992, Monoclonal fluorescence polarization immunoassay evaluated for monitoring cyclosporine in whole blood afater kidney, heart, and liver transplantation, *Clin. Chem.* **38**(1):123–126.

Workman, P., Oppitz, M., Donaldson, J., and Lee, F. Y. F., 1987, High-performance liquid chromatography of chlorambucil analogues, *J. Chromatogr.* **422:**315–321.

Chapter 19

IMMUNOPHARMACOLOGICAL TREATMENT DURING PREGNANCY AND LACTATION

Monika Østensen

1. INTRODUCTION

Connective tissue diseases have a predilection for the female sex and often affect women of childbearing age. The concurrence of pregnancy and connective tissue disease may represent a hazard both to mother and child. Underlying disease processes will add to the physiological changes of pregnancy and in some cases aggravate symptoms in the pregnant patient. This is a risk in systemic lupus erythematosus (SLE), mixed connective tissue disease (MCTD), and progressive systemic sclerosis (PSS). On the other hand, the fetus may be affected by maternal systemic disease and/or vasculopathy of the placenta associated with connective tissue disease. Placental transfer of maternal autoantibodies may cause neonatal disease from SLE (Lockshin, 1985). Thus both patient and clinician have to face special demands resulting from the interaction between pregnancy and a complex disease process.

Table I compiles data from the literature on pregnancy in connective tissue diseases. The survey shows that pregnancy has little influence on the course of most connective tissue diseases except for rheumatoid arthritis (RA), which improves during pregnancy. In contrast, maternal connective tissue disease may compromise the outcome for the fetus, as in SLE and MCTD.

As connective tissue diseases may run an active course during and after pregnancy, the clinician frequently has to decide on drug treatment during pregnancy and lactation. In this chapter, the available information on immunosuppressive or antirheumatic disease-modifying drugs in the pregnant and lactating patient will be presented and some guidelines for treatment will be discussed.

Monika Østensen • Department of Rheumatology, University Hospital of Trondheim, 7006 Trondheim, Norway. *Immunopharmacology in Autoimmune Diseases and Transplantation*, edited by Hans Erik Rugstad et al. Plenum Press, New York, 1992.

245

TABLE I. Interactions between Pregnancy and Some Connective Tissue Diseases

Disease	Number of pregnancies reported	Effect of pregnancy on disease	Effect of disease on pregnancy	Fetal risks
Systemic lupus erythematosus	ca. 1200	None	Renal complications	Abortion, stillbirth, prematurity
Mixed connective tissue disease	ca. 50	None	Renal complications	Abortion, stillbirth, prematurity
Dermato/polymyositis	13	Probably none	None specific	Abortion, stillbirth, prematurity
Progressive systemic sclerosis	76	Probably none	Cardiac, pulmonary, renal complications	Abortion, stillbirth, prematurity
Rheumatoid arthritis	ca. 425	Remission in ca. 70%	None specific	None specific

1.1. Drug Disposition in the Gravida

Normal pregnancy is associated with profound biological changes that may influence the absorption, distribution, biotransformation, and excretion of drugs (Bogaert and Thiery, 1983). Changes include an increase in total body water, modifications of hepatic drug handling, and increase of renal excretion. The changes in the concentrations of plasma proteins, fatty acids, and other substances may affect the binding of drugs. Experimental, mainly *in vitro*, studies have shown decreased protein binding of many drugs during pregnancy (Perucca and Crema, 1982). This means that more drug will be available in the free, pharmacologically active form. As other factors such as distribution and excretion also change, this may not necessarily imply an altered response to a drug.

1.2. Placental Transfer of Drugs

The basic mechanisms by which drugs cross the placenta are diffusion, facilitated diffusion, active transport, and special transfer processes. The main pathway is simple diffusion, which depends on the molecular weight, stereochemistry, and degree of dissociation and lipid solubility of a substance. In general, lipid-soluble, nonionic, small molecules will easily cross the placenta (Levy and Hayton, 1973). Some drugs may be bound to macromolecules in the placenta, thereby inhibiting their transfer. Occasionally, biotransformation of drugs occurs by placental enzymes (Juchau *et al.*, 1980).

In mothers suffering from systemic diseases, the composition of plasma proteins is modified not only because of pregnancy, but also due to the disease process. In addition, the vasculature of the placenta may be altered as shown, for example, in patients with SLE (Abramowsky *et al.*, 1980). This may interfere with maternal and fetal blood flow in the placenta and thereby alter the rate of drug transfer.

1.3. Drug Disposition in the Fetus

Drugs that have crossed the placenta will equilibrate with the fetal tissues. Both drug protein binding and hepatic breakdown differ from the maternal organism and depend on the stage of fetal development (Levy and Hayton, 1973). Therefore, harmful effects of drugs will depend on the state of pregnancy at which they are given. Unfortunately, possible effects on postnatal development are not known for most drugs given during pregnancy.

1.4. Drug Excretion in Breast Milk

Most drugs taken by a lactating woman will appear in breast milk. The factors that influence the concentration of a given drug in milk are much the same as those mentioned for transplacental transfer. The slightly acidic pH in milk favors the passage of more alkaline drugs. In general, the amounts of drugs secreted into milk and finally ingested by the child are very small (Lewis and Hurden, 1983).

2. CORTICOSTEROIDS

The corticosteroids most commonly used for immunosuppression are prednisone and prednisolone. Betamethasone and dexamethasone have special indications and are rarely given for immunosuppression. Transplacental passage varies for the different corticosteroids. Similar levels of dexamethasone are found in mother and fetus (Osathanondh et al., 1977). Cortisol crosses the placenta and most is converted to inactive cortisone by fetal enzymes (Murphy et al., 1974). Prednisone is converted to its active metabolite prednisolone by the liver. The transplacental transfer of prednisolone is limited. The maternal : cord blood ratio of the drug found were 8:1 and 10:1 (Beitins et al., 1972). The placenta converts prednisolone to the metabolically inactive prednisone, which is poorly reconverted by the fetal liver. Prednisolone or prednisone are therefore the most appropriate glucocorticoids for the treatment of pregnant women.

2.1. Animal Studies

Treatment with corticosteroids in a number of animal species (mouse, chicken, rat, rabbit, monkeys) produces various deleterious effects in the offspring (Sidhu, 1983). In many of those studies, the doses used were very high and exceeded the therapeutic doses in humans.

2.2. Human Studies

Over the last decades, a large number of women have been treated for various medical reasons with corticosteroids during pregnancy. There have been scattered reports of cleft palate, masculinization of female infants, growth retardation, and adrenal suppression in children born to women taking high doses of steroids during pregnancy.

In 1960, Bongiovanni and McPadden reviewed the world literature and found two newborns with cleft palate and one with adrenocortical failure among 260 women who had been treated with cortisone or its analogues during pregnancy. Serment et al. (1968), in a review of 530 corticosteroid-treated pregnancies, noted an overall malformation rate of 2%, which did not differ from the control population. Cleft palate was found in two cases and seemed related to high doses of steroids in the first trimester, a finding also made by others (Popert, 1962).

Increased frequencies of perinatal infection after antepartum exposure to cortico-steroids have been anticipated by some authors, but seem to occur rather infrequent (Schmidt *et al.*, 1984). Infection with cytomegalovirus has been reported in newborns of steroid-treated mothers (Coté *et al.*, 1974).

The influence of corticosteroids on intrauterine growth has been controversial. Some authors have demonstrated an increased incidence of low-birth-weight babies (Reinisch and Simon, 1978) while others were unable to find any growth retardation in infants exposed to corticosteroids *in utero* (Logaridis *et al.*, 1983). Similar inconsistencies are apparent for the incidence of stillbirth and prematurity. Increased frequency of stillbirth and premature delivery were related by some authors (Warrel and Taylor, 1968; Schatz *et al.*, 1975) to antenatal corticosteroids. Yet renal disease, present before or during pregnancy in many of the patients treated with corticosteroids, increases per se the risk for premature delivery. In many of the reports, the possible influence of the underlying disease for which cor-ticosteroids were given has not been delineated. There is also a lack of controlled studies showing the frequency of a quoted adverse event in an untreated population.

2.3. Corticosteroids in Autoimmune Diseases

Numerous reports exist about the use of corticosteroids in pregnant patients with SLE (for review see Meehan and Dorsey, 1987). Among larger recent series is the report of Hayslett and Lynn (1980) on 65 pregnancies in 47 SLE patients with nephropathy. Most of their patients were treated with either corticosteroids alone or combined with azathioprine during pregnancy. No birth defect occurred in the offspring. Another group of 11 SLE patients with renal disease had 18 pregnancies during ongoing treatment with cor-ticosteroids. No corticosteroid-related congenital anomaly was detected (Houser *et al.*, 1980). In two other series, treatment with prednisolone doses ranging from 5 to 100 mg daily in 62 SLE pregnancies did not increase the rate of birth defects (Zulman *et al.*, 1980; Varner *et al.*, 1983).

Prednisone doses varying between 40 to 60 mg daily administered to six pregnant SLE patients, together with 75 mg of aspirin, did not produce harmful effects in the neonates in the study of Lubbe *et al.* (1983). In a recent prospective study, 11 of 28 SLE patients took prednisone throughout pregnancy, but had normal babies (Lockshin *et al.*, 1984). In the large prospective study of Mintz *et al.* (1986), comprising 102 pregnancies in SLE patients, prednisone was given to all patients throughout pregnancy with doses ranging between 10 to 60 mg daily (up to 300 mg daily in a few patients with serious disease flare-ups. There was one congenital heart block but no other malformation occurred. However, 20 neonates were growth retarded, but their mothers had taken the same average dose of prednisone as the mothers of normal weight children.

2.4. Lactation

Prednisone, prednisolone, and methylprednisolone (Coulam *et al.*, 1982) are excreted into human breast milk. Minute amounts of prednisone have been detected in milk after oral doses of 10, 20, and 120 mg of prednisone (Katz and Duncan, 1975; Berlin *et al.*, 1979; Sargraves *et al.*, 1981). After oral doses of 10–80 mg of prednisolone, the milk:plasma ratio was about 0.1 for doses of 20 mg or less and 0.2 for higher doses (Ost *et al.*, 1985).

2.5. Conclusion

There is no evidence for an overall increase of malformations, prematurity, or growth retardation caused by corticosteroids given during pregnancy. High-dose corticosteroid administration during early pregnancy slightly increases the risk of cleft palate development. In late pregnancy, intrauterine exposure to steroids may influence the susceptibility for infection, requiring careful perinatal control. Adrenal insufficiency in the newborn, though theoretically possible, has rarely been reported after antenatal corticosteroid exposure.

Some autoimmune diseases like SLE are clearly associated with increased fetal wastage. Suppression of disease activity by corticosteroids may improve pregnancy outcome. Prednisone or prednisolone may be utilized in the lowest effective dose to control disease activity satisfactorily. Regular follow-ups should test for the development of bacterial infection, hypertension, and diabetes mellitus. Contact with virus-infected individuals should be avoided by steroid-treated patients.

If large doses of steroids are necessary, antacids may be prescribed simultaneously. However, to patients with markedly reduced creatinine clearance, aluminum- and magnesium-containing antacids should not be prescribed since both metals may accumulate in tissues. Possible fetotoxic effects of cimetidine are still disputed. Therefore, its use during pregnancy should be limited to cases of overt gastrointestinal bleeding (Corazza et al., 1982).

Breast-feeding may be permitted in patients treated with 20 mg/day or less of prednisone or prednisolone or no more than 8 mg/day of methylprednisolone (Anderson, 1987). As peak milk concentrations appear after about 1 to 2 hr after an oral dose, exact timing of breast-feeding is advantageous.

3. AZATHIOPRINE

Azathioprine is a purine analogue and interferes with the synthesis of nucleic acids. Azathioprine is no longer used as an antitumor agent, but is now classified as an exclusively immunosuppressive drug. Azathioprine and its active metabolite 6-mercaptopurine cross the placenta in humans, but only very low levels (1–5%) appear in fetal plasma after 24 hr (Saarikoski and Seppala, 1973). However, the fetal liver is unable to convert it to its active form. Theoretically, the fetus should be protected from the effects of azathioprine in early pregnancy since it lacks the enzyme inosinate pyrophosphorylase, which converts azathioprine to thiosinic acid, which is the metabolite acting on dividing cells.

3.1. Animal Studies

Azathioprine is teratogenic in animals when given in large doses (equivalent to > 6 mg/kg body weight per day) and produces skeletal and central nervous system anomalies (Githens et al., 1965; Rosenkrantz et al., 1967; Williamson and Karp, 1981).

3.2. Azathioprine in Human Pregnancy

Most knowledge about azathioprine during gestation has been derived from treatment of renal transplant recipients. Additional experience comes from studies of patients with SLE. The use in other autoimmune diseases is limited.

Estimates of the frequency of birth defects in women taking azathioprine during pregnancy ranges from no increase to up to 9% compared with the general population. Rudolph *et al.* (1979) accumulated data from renal transplant centers in North America. A total of 440 pregnancies in renal allograft recipients treated with corticosteroids and azathioprine was analyzed. No predominant or frequent birth defect was found. Similar data have been recorded from more recent studies of renal transplant recipients (Penn *et al.*, 1980; Hadi *et al.*, 1986). In a European survey on transplant recipients (Registration Committee of the European Dialysis and Transplant Association, 1980), birth anomalies were present in 7 of 103 children. Mothers of abnormal babies had taken significantly higher doses of azathioprine (2.64 mg/kg versus 2.02 mg/kg) than those with healthy babies. Intrauterine exposure to azathioprine may occasionally cause slight suppression of the bone marrow as shown by decreased leukocyte counts and thrombocytopenia at birth (Davison *et al.*, 1985). Adjustment of the maternal leukocyte count during pregnancy by dose reduction avoids neonatal depression of hemopoiesis.

An analysis of 40 pregnancies in SLE patients treated with corticosteroids and azathioprine confirmed that there is no increased risk of congenital malformations (Meehan and Dorsey, 1987).

Antepartum exposure to azathioprine can cause transient gaps, breaks, and deletions in the chromosomes of lymphocytes, which disappear spontaneously after 5 to 32 months (Price *et al.*, 1976; Juchau *et al.*, 1980), although this is not mandatory (Sharon *et al.*, 1974). In one series, 11 of 16 children tested had chromosome aberrations that had disappeared by one year of age. Three infants had normal chromosomes (Juchau *et al.*, 1980). Current information about the general progress in infancy and early childhood of the offspring of patients treated with azathioprine during pregnancy has been reassuring (Coté *et al.*, 1974; Juchau *et al.*, 1980).

3.3. Lactation

By a highly sensitive high-pressure liquid chromatography (HPLC) method, small amounts of 6 mercaptopurine were found in the milk of a nursing mother and a second lactating patient who did not breast-feed (Bennett, 1988). No harmful effects were observed in three children exposed to azathioprine or its metabolites via breast milk (Bennett, 1988).

3.4. Conclusion

The available data on azathioprine during pregnancy suggest no increased risk of congenital anomalies in the offspring of treated mothers. Acute flare-ups of connective tissue disease can represent a serious threat to the welfare of mother and child as reported in SLE and MCTD. Several authors have therefore recommended treating active disease as in the nonpregnant state, including immunosuppressive drugs such as azathioprine and prednisone. As the significance of even low concentrations of azathioprine or its metabolites in milk is unknown, breast-feeding should be avoided.

4. CYCLOSPORINE A

Cyclosporine A (CyA) is a new immunosuppressive agent that has been successfully used to prevent allograft rejection. In recent years, it has also been employed for the treatment of various autoimmune and collagen diseases with partly encouraging results (Førre et al., 1988). There now exist some data on the outcome of pregnancy in allograft recipients who have been treated with CyA at some stage of gestation (Cockburn et al., 1989). Most of these patients were concomitantly treated with prednisone or methylprednisolone.

CyA crosses the placenta, but there are divergences in the literature concerning the amount of drug transfer. In part, this may be due to different methods employed for the detection of CyA [radioimmunoassay (RIA) versus HPLC] in body fluids. Measurements of CyA in cord blood have detected no drug (Klintmalm et al., 1984; Grischke et al., 1986), concentrations equal to and less than maternal serum concentration (Endler et al., 1987). CyA has also been demonstrated in substantial amounts in amniotic fluid and in placental tissue (Flechner et al., 1985). In the few cases where CyA was present in newborn infants, serum concentrations fell rapidly to zero a few days after delivery (Cockburn et al., 1989).

4.1. Animal Studies

CyA is embryotoxic and fetotoxic when given to pregnant animals in doses two to five times greater than used in humans. When animals are treated with doses equivalent to human doses, no teratogenicity has been observed (Mason et al., 1985).

4.2. Human Studies

Experience on CyA during human pregnancy are based on published and unpublished single case reports (Cockburn et al., 1989). The majority of patients were treated with CyA to prevent allograft rejection. A total of 51 pregnancies in 48 mothers and an additional 11 pregnancies conceived from CyA-treated fathers have been reported (Cockburn et al., 1989). Eight abortions occurred, six elective and two spontaneous. Forty-three pregnancies concluded in live deliveries. Fifteen of the infants were premature, whereas 18 were born at term. In ten cases, no data were given on the length of the gestation. The birth weight was recorded for 29 children and was on average 2093 g. Abnormalities recorded in neonates included physiological jaundice, thrombocytopenia (Klintmalm et al., 1984), leukopenia, hypoglycemia in combination with mild disseminated coagulation, asphyxia (Grischke et al., 1986), and elevated serum creatinine (Cockburn et al., 1986). One infant died three days postpartum after convulsions; autopsy demonstrated complete absence of the corpus callosum. Two other neonates had birth defects: one bilateral cataracts and one mild hypoparathyroidism. Hypoplasia of one leg and foot in an infant exposed to CyA in utero has recently been reported (Pujals et al., 1989). Postnatal development was unremarkable in 19 of 20 children where recorded (Cockburn et al., 1989).

In a recent report, Pickrell and Sawers (1988) noticed growth retardation in 9 of 16 infants born to mothers treated with CyA during pregnancy. This observation was confirmed by others (Williams et al., 1988; Varghese et al., 1988). The 11 children fathered by CyA-treated men were all healthy and had a mean birth weight of 2730 g. Chromosome analysis has been performed in three infants. No chromosome aberrations have been detected.

4.3. Lactation

CyA has been detected by RIA in breast milk taken immediately after delivery in amounts < 2% of the maternal dose (Lewis et al., 1983; Flechner et al., 1985). A milk:plasma ratio varying between 1:4.5 and 1:8.5 was found in another study (Ziegenhagen *et al.*, 1988). Unfortunately, no details on the detection method of CyA were given in this study. There are no reports on children exposed to CyA via breast milk.

4.4. Conclusion

At present, there are insufficient data to draw conclusions on possible teratogenicity of CyA. However, the incidence of fetal growth retardation seems to be increased. So far, there is no evidence that the drug infers complications such as nephrotoxicity or facial changes for the neonatal period. However, in absence of more data, CyA should not be given to pregnant women with autoimmune diseases. Since the effect of the drug on the suckling infant is not known, breast-feeding should be avoided in women treated with CyA.

5. CYTOSTATIC DRUGS

Severe collagen and autoimmune diseases may require treatment with immunosuppressive drugs that are antitumor agents. The decision to use drugs with potentially serious side effects should be limited to systemically ill patients or for the reason of corticosteroid sparing in cases of refractory types of RA, juvenile rheumatoid arthritis (JRA), dermatopolymyositis, SLE, and forms of generalized vasculitis such as polyarteritis nodosa and Wegener's granulomatosis. The cytostatic drugs most often used in the aforementioned conditions are cyclophosphamide and chlorambucil.

5.1. Cyclophosphamide

Cyclophosphamide (CP) is an alkylating agent and one of the most-used antitumor agents. Experience with CP and pregnancy is based exclusively on reports in cancer patients. CP is embryotoxic and teratogenic in a number of animal species including mice, rats, rabbits, and monkeys (Mirkes, 1985). In man, seven children with congenital malformations have been reported after first trimester exposure to CP (Briggs *et al.*, 1986; Greenberg and Tanaka, 1964). Concomitant irradiation therapy was given in five patients and multiagent chemotherapy in one case (Nicholson, 1968; Toledo *et al.*, 1971). In contrast, no malformations were observed in three children born after second- and third-trimester treatment with CP (Haerr and Pratt, 1985) combined with other antitumor agents. Such therapy resulted in one premature male child with pancytopenia at birth (Pizzuto *et al.*, 1980). Recently, multiple congenital anomalies were described in a child born after intravenous cyclophosphamide pulse therapy of a SLE mother at days 15 and 46 of gestation (Kirshon *et al.*, 1988).

CP has been demonstrated in human breast milk in one patient (Wiernik and Duncan, 1971) up to 6 hr after an intravenous dose. However, the concentrations were not specified. Another report found leukopenia and thrombocytopenia in an infant breast-fed by a mother who was treated with 6 mg/kg per day of CP (Durodola, 1979).

5.2. Chlorambucil

Chlorambucil is an alkylating agent that has been used with success in connective tissue diseases like RA, JRA, SLE, and Behçet's syndrome. In cancer patients, first-trimester exposure to chlorambucil resulted in two male fetuses with agenesis of one kidney and ureter (Shotton and Monie, 1963; Steege and Caldwell, 1980). Multiple cardiovascular anomalies were detected in another infant who died three days after birth who was exposed to chlorambucil at gestational week 10 (Thompson and Conklin, 1983). When given during late pregnancy, chlorambucil did not cause malformations in four cases (Nishimura and Tanimura, 1976). No data exist on the transfer of chlorambucil to human breast milk.

Chlorambucil has been shown to cause chromosome damage in human lymphocytes related to dose and duration of therapy (Palmer et al., 1984).

5.3. Methotrexate

Methotrexate (MTX) is a folic acid antagonist. During the last ten years, MTX has been used increasingly for the treatment of psoriatic arthritis, RA, SLE, and recently JRA (Christophidis, 1984). Small doses given once a week are sufficient to control disease activity in those conditions.

References describing the use of MTX during pregnancy are limited to patients on cancer treatment or MTX employed for attempted abortion. In those cases, MTX was given daily and usually in much higher doses than those applied for rheumatic diseases. First-trimester exposure to MTX in eight pregnancies resulted in three malformed infants with cranial abnormalities in all of them (Milunsky et al., 1968). In seven cases, MTX was given during late pregnancy (Nicholson, 1968; Sieber and Adamson, 1975) in doses varying from 30 mg to 1.3 g; five normal children were born. One infant with pancytopenia (Meehan and Dorsey, 1987) and one newborn with desquamative fibrosing alveolitis have been described (Walden and Bagshawe, 1979). Recently, Kozlowski et al. (1990) reported on ten pregnancies in eight RA patients who were on low-dose oral MTX during the first trimester of pregnancy. Two elective and three spontaneous abortions occurred, and five children were born at term without congenital malformations. These children developed physically and mentally normally to a mean age of 11.5 years. No increased incidence of congenital malformation has been found in offspring of women treated with MTX prior to conception (Rustin et al., 1984). A slight increase in chromosome aberrations has been demonstrated in patients treated with MTX (Sieber and Adamson, 1975).

After a dose of 22.5 mg/day, low concentrations of MTX (.26 μg/dl) have been detected in human breast milk (Johns et al., 1972).

5.4. Conclusion

The antitumor agents cyclophosphamide, chlorambucil, and high-dose methotrexate markedly increase the risk of fetal abnormalities when given during early pregnancy. Data on fetal effects from low-dose MTX therapy are still insufficient. The risk for congenital malformation is less for intrauterine exposure in late pregnancy. However, it still may result in bone marrow suppression in the neonate. Second-generation effects including fertility or the incidence of cancer after intrauterine exposure to cytostatic drugs have not been sufficiently clarified. Antitumor agents given during pregnancy increase the risk for acquiring viral or bacterial infections both for mother and child.

As the significance of even small amounts of an antitumor agent in breast milk for the nursing infant is uncertain, breast-feeding should be avoided. It is not known if the above mentioned also applies to the low doses of MTX employed in rheumatic patients. At the present stage of knowledge, cytostatic drugs should not be prescribed for pregnant or lactating patients with connective tissue disease. Patients of childbearing age who need antitumor agents should be informed of the necessity of safe birth control before the start of treatment. Attempts to become pregnant should be delayed until three to four months after cessation of therapy. Termination of pregnancy may be offered in cases of the concurrence of pregnancy and antitumor treatment.

6. ANTIRHEUMATIC DISEASE-MODIFYING DRUGS

6.1. Sulfasalazine

Sulfasalazine (SASP) previously has been used almost exclusively in the treatment of inflammatory bowel disease (IBD). Recently, its efficacy in certain rheumatic conditions such as rheumatoid arthritis and ankylosing spondylitis has been rediscovered (Pinals, 1986). As a consequence, SASP is now increasingly employed as a first choice among antirheumatic disease-modifying drugs. Reports regarding its use during and after pregnancy originate exclusively from experience in patients with IBD.

SASP and its principal metabolites cross the placenta (Hensleigh and Kauffman, 1977) and achieve fetal blood levels close to maternal levels (Jarnerot et al., 1981). However, the bilirubin-displacing ability of SASP and its metabolites has been demonstrated to be small (Jarnerot et al., 1981a,b).

Willoughby and Truelove (1980) studied 216 pregnancies in patients with ulcerative colitis. Maintenance therapy with SASP either alone (22 pregnancies) or in combination with steroids (32 pregnancies) did not increase congenital malformations or cause pathological jaundice of the newborns. A large national survey (Mogadam et al., 1981) examined the effect of SASP and steroids on fetal outcome in pregnant women with IBD. Comparing 287 treated pregnancies with 244 not receiving drug treatment, no increase in birth defects, pathological jaundice, or small-for-gestational-age babies were detected.

Lactation

SASP passes poorly to human breast milk (Azad Khan and Truelove, 1979). However, about 40% of its metabolite sulfapyridine has been demonstrated, resulting in very low doses transferred to the child by breast milk (Jarnerot and Into-Malmberg, 1979). Watery diarrhea in two breast-fed infants have been ascribed to SASP's split product, 5-aminosalicylic acid (Nelis, 1989).

6.2. Gold Compounds

Intramuscular gold preparations such as sodium aurothiomalate and aurothioglucose have been used for the treatment of rheumatoid arthritis for decades (Tozman and Gottlieb, 1987). Recently, oral gold (triethylphosphine gold, Auranofin) has been introduced for the treatment of selected cases of RA, psoriatic arthritis, and JRA.

6.2.1. Human Studies

The knowledge of the effects of gold preparations on the human fetus is limited. Aurothiomalate crosses the placenta and has been demonstrated in placental tissue (Rocker and Henderson, 1976), fetal liver and kidney (Møller-Madsen *et al.*, 1987), and in cord serum (Cohen and Orzel, 1981). Gold concentrations in cord serum of a healthy neonate whose mother had been treated with 100 mg of aurothiomalate monthly throughout pregnancy equaled maternal serum levels (Cohen and Orzel, 1981).

Uneventful pregnancies concluding in the delivery of healthy children have been reported in women receiving gold therapy (Freyberg, 1972). One case of multiple fetal malformations in a mother who received 20 mg of aurothiomalate weekly during the first 20 weeks of pregnancy has been reported (Rogers *et al.*, 1980). No abnormalities were detected in the offspring of 26 patients treated with gold throughout pregnancy for bronchial asthma. Except for two children with hip abnormality, no deformities were observed in an additional 43 patients who had terminated gold therapy in early to mid-pregnancy (Miyamoto *et al.*, 1974). In a follow-up study of seven children who had been exposed to doses of aurothiomalate ranging between 15 to 166.5 mg *in utero*, no congenital malformations or psychological disorders were detected after a mean follow-up of 7.7 years (Tarp and Graudal, 1985).

Oral gold (Auranofin) crosses the placenta. To date, little is known about its effect on the human fetus. Six women who received Auranofin while pregnant delivered normal children (Tozman and Gottlieb, 1987).

6.2.2. Lactation

Small amounts of gold have been detected in human breast milk after doses of 370, 50, and 70 mg of aurothiomalate, respectively (Bell and Dale, 1976; Østensen *et al.*, 1986). Minute amounts of gold have also been detected in the serum and urine of nursing infants after both aurothiomalate and aurothioglucose exposure (Blau, 1973; Rooney *et al.*, 1987). However, in a recent study measuring gold excretion into milk continuously over a 20-week period, no gold was detected in the serum or urine of the nursing infant at any time (Rooney *et al.*, 1987). No data exist about the passage of Auranofin into human breast milk.

6.3. Antimalarial Drugs

Aminoquinolone compounds such as chloroquine phosphate and hydroxychloroquine sulfate are used to treat conditions like SLE, RA, and JRA. The literature states that the recommended doses for malaria prophylaxis of 500 mg chloroquine phosphate or 300 mg of chloroquine base weekly are not teratogenic for the human fetus (Wolfe and Cordero, 1985). However, the doses used for the treatment of rheumatic conditions by far exceed this regimen.

Chloroquine crosses the placenta and has been demonstrated in the eyes and ears of fetal mice and rats (Ullberg *et al.*, 1970; Dencker and Lindquist, 1975). Malformations of the inner ear and other abnormalities were reported after intrauterine exposure to 500 mg daily of chloroquine in three siblings born of a mother with SLE (Hart and Naunton, 1964). In another report, a woman had taken 200–300 mg of chloroquine base over three years and throughout two pregnancies. Her two children had retinal degeneration (Paufique and Magnard, 1969). Three other reports on children born after intrauterine exposure to chloroquine and hydroxychloroquine did not find any fetal abnormalities (Fraga *et al.*, 1974; Ross and Garatsos, 1974; Suhonen, 1983). Two series on chloroquine (250–500 mg daily) and hydroxychloroquine (200–400 mg daily) given to pregnant SLE patients (Parke, 1988) and RA patients (MacKenzie, 1983) stated the absence of teratogenicity in the offspring. The effects of chloroquine and hydroxychloroquine on pregnancy outcome were analyzed in

24 pregnant women (11 with SLE, 3 with RA, and 3 on malaria prophylaxis) (Levy *et al.*, 1991). Of a total of 27 pregnancies, 14 resulted in full-term pregnancies, 6 in elective abortions, 4 in spontaneous abortions, and 3 in stillbirths. No congenital malformations or developmental or intellectual abnormalities were detected in the 14 live children.

Lactation

Small amounts of chloroquine and hydroxychloroquine have been detected in human breast milk (Soares *et al.*, 1959; Østensen *et al.*, 1985). In one study, the amount of chloroquine sulfate ingested by a nursing infant was calculated to be about 0.55% of a 300-mg daily dose consumed by the mother (Ette *et al.*, 1987). In another report, 2% of the maternal hydroxychloroquine dose was estimated to be ingested by the breast-fed infant per day (Nation *et al.*, 1984).

6.4. Penicillamine

Except for the treatment of Wilson's disease and cystinuria, penicillamine is used as a second-line drug in RA, JRA, and psoriatic arthritis. Penicillamine crosses the placenta and has been detected in the urine of an infant born to a mother who had been treated for cystinuria with 1200 mg daily throughout pregnancy (Crawhall *et al.*, 1967). In animals, high doses of penicillamine given during gestation interfere with collagen and cartilage synthesis in the fetus. In humans, three cases of connective tissue abnormalities have been reported in infants born to mothers treated for cystinuria or RA with doses up to 2 g daily during gestation (Mjølnerød *et al.*, 1971; Solomon *et al.*, 1977; Linares *et al.*, 1979). By contrast, no abnormalities were detected in 50 children born to 27 mothers with Wilson's disease and 7 with cystinuria treated with 0.5–2.0 g/day during early gestation or throughout pregnancy (Maracek and Graf, 1976; Scheinberg and Sternlieb, 1975; Gregory and Mansell, 1983). In a further report on 19 pregnant RA patients treated with penicillamine, the only congenital abnormality observed was a ventricular septum defect (Lyle, 1978).

Lactation

The excretion of penicillamine into breast milk has not been investigated. No harmful effects were observed in a nursing child of a mother who ingested 1500 mg of penicillamine daily during a lactation period of three months (Gregory and Mansell, 1983).

6.5. Conclusion

Available data from the literature indicate no increased risk of teratogenicity for SASP and aurothiomalate. The issue remains controversial for antimalarials, Auranofin, and penicillamine, and these drugs should therefore probably be avoided during gestation. However, termination of pregnancy seems not justified when they have been used close to or early in pregnancy.

It appears from the scanty information presented in the literature that most antirheumatic disease-modifying drugs are present in only small amounts in milk. Breast-feeding may probably be allowed during treatment with sulfasalazine and aurothiomalate. The lack of data warrants caution against breast-feeding with Auranofin- and penicillamine-treated mothers. The concentrations of antimalarials excreted into milk are so low that they do not protect the nursing infant from malaria. However, possible accumulation of anti-malarials in the juvenile retina cannot be excluded. Therefore, antimalarials should not be given to lactating mothers.

7. DRUGS DURING PREGNANCY AND LACTATION: GENERAL RECOMMENDATIONS

Disease activity is one of the most important factors that control the outcome of pregnancy in connective tissue disease. The aim of any treatment during pregnancy is to control the disease process satisfactorily for the benefit of mother and child. The basic rules for prescribing during pregnancy and lactation should follow the recommendations suggested by Hawkins (1983):

1. Regard every female patient with connective tissue disease of childbearing age as a potential antenatal patient. If treatment with potent immunosuppressive drugs is required, discuss family planning with the patient.
2. Assess the real need for medication during pregnancy and lactation carefully in each patient.
3. Review all drug regimens during pregnancy and lactation to see how good control of the disease process can minimize risks.
4. Use agents that have been widely employed in pregnancy and lactation without evident harmful effects on the child.

REFERENCES

Abramowsky, C. R., Vegas, M. E., Swinehart, G., and Gyves, M. T., 1980, Decidual vasculopathy of the placenta in systemic lupus erythematosus, N. Engl. J. Med. 303:668–672.

Anderson, P. O., 1987, Corticosteroid use by breast-feeding mothers, Clin. Pharm. 6:445.

Azad Khan, A. K., and Truelove, S. C., 1979, Placental and mammary transfer of sulphasalazine, Br. Med. J. 2:1553.

Beitins, I. Z., Bayard, F., Ances, I. G., Kowarski, A., Migeon, C. J., 1972, The transplacental passage of prednisone and prednisolone in pregnancy near term, J. Pediatr. 81:936–945.

Bell, R. A. F., Dale, I. M., 1976, Gold secretion in maternal milk, Arthritis Rheum 19:1374.

Bennett, P. N., ed., 1988, Drugs and Human Lactation, Elsevier, Amsterdam, pp. 286–287.

Berlin, C. M., Jr., Kaiser, D. G., and Demers, L., 1979, Excretion of prednisone and prednisolone in human milk, Pharmacologist 21:264.

Blau, S. P., 1973, Metabolism of gold during lactation, Arthritis Rheum. 16:777–778.

Bogaert, M. C., and Thiery, M., 1983, Pharmakokinetics and pregnancy, Eur. J. Obstet. Gynecol. Reprod. Biol. 16:229–235.

Bongiovanni, A. M., and McPadden, A. J., 1960, Steroids during pregnancy and possible fetal consequences, Fertil. Steril. 11:181–186.

Briggs, G. G., Freeman, R. K., Yaffe, S. J., eds., 1986, in: Drugs in Pregnancy and Lactation, 2nd Edition, Williams and Wilkins, Baltimore, pp. 112–113.

Christophidis, N., 1984, Methotrexate, Clin. Rheum. Dis. 10:401–415.

Cockburn, I., Krupp, P., and Monka, C., 1989, Present experience of Sandimmun in pregnancy, Transplant. Proc. 21:3730–3732.

Cohen, D., Orzel, J., 1981, Infants of mothers receiving gold therapy, Arthritis Rheum. 24:104–105.

Corazza, G. R., Gasbarrini, G., Di Nisio, Q., and Zulli, P., 1982, Cimetidine in peptic ulcer therapy during pregnancy, Clin. Trials J. 19:91–93.

Coté, C. J., Meuwissen, H. J., Pickering, R. J., 1974, Effects on the neonate of prednisone and azathioprine administered to the mother during pregnancy, J. Pediatr. 85:324–328.

Coulam, C. B., Mayer, T. P., Jiang, N. S., and Zinck, H., 1982, Breast feeding after renal transplantation, Transplant Proc. 13:605–609.

Crawhall, J. C., Scowen, E. F., Thompson, C. J., 1967, Dissolution of cystine stones during D-penicillamine treatment of a pregnant patient with cystinuria, Br. Med. J. 1:216–218.

Davison, J. M., Dellagrammatikas, H., and Parkin, J. M., 1985, Maternal azathioprine therapy and depressed haemopoiesis in the babies of renal allograft patients, Br. J. Obstet. Gynaecol. 92:233–239.

Dencker, L., Lindquist, N. G., 1975, Distribution of labeled chloroquine in the inner ear, Arch. Otolaryngol. 101:185–188.

Durodola, J. I., 1979, Administration of cyclophosphamide during late pregnancy and early lactation: A case report, J. Natl. Med. Assoc. 71:165–166.

Endler, M., Derfler, K., Schaller, A., and Nowotny, C., 1987, Schwangerschaft und Geburt nach Nierentransplantation unter Cyclosporin A, Gebrutsch u. Frauenheilk. 660–663.

Ette, E. I., Essien, E. E., Ogonor, J. I., and Brown-Awala, E. A., 1987, Chloroquine in human milk, J. Clin. Pharmacol. 27: 499–502.

Flechner, S. M., Katz, A. R., Rogers, A. J., van Buren, C., Kahan, B. D., 1985, The presence of cyclosporine in body tissues and fluids during pregnancy, Am. J. Kidney Dis. 5:60–63.

Førre, Ø, Waalen, K., Rugstad, H. E., Berg, K. J., Solbu, D., Kåss, E., 1988, Cyclosporine A in rheumatoid arthritis, Springer Semin. Immunopathol. 10:263–277.

Fraga, A., Mintz, G., Orozco, J., Orozco, J. H., Sterility and fertility rates, fetal wastage and maternal morbidty in systemic lupus erythematosus, J. Rheumatol. 1:293–298.

Freyberg, R., 1972, Gold therapy for rheumatoid arthritis, in: Arthritis and allied conditions (J. L. Hollander, ed.), Lea and Febiger, Philadelphia, pp. 455–482.

Githens, J. H., Rosenkrantz, J. G., Tunnock, S. M., 1965, Teratogenic effects of azathioprine, J. Pediatr. 66:959–961.

Greenberg, L. H., and Tanaka, K. R., 1964, Congenital anomalies probably induced by cyclophosphamide, J. Am. Med. Assoc. 188:423–426.

Gregory, M. C., and Mansell, M. A., 1983, Pregnancy and cystinuria, Lancet 2:1158–1160.

Grischke, E., Kaufmann, M., Dreikorn, K., Linderkamp, O., Kubli, F., 1986, Erfolgreiche Schwangerschaft bei Nierentransplantation und Cyclosporin A, Geburtshilfe Frauenheilk. 46:176–179.

Hadi, H. A., Stafford, C. R., Williamson, J. R., Fadel, H. E., and Devoe, L. D., 1986, Pregnancy outcome in renal transplant recipients, South. Med. J. 79:959–964.

Haerr, R. W., and Pratt, A. T., 1985, Multiagent chemotherapy for sarcoma diagnosed during pregnancy, Cancer 56:1028–1033.

Hart, C. N., and Naunton, R. F., 1964, The ototoxicity of chloroquine phosphate, Arch. Otolaryngol. Head Neck Surg. 80:407–412.

Hawkins, D. F., 1983, Prescribing in pregnancy, in: Drugs and Pregnancy (D. F. Hawkins, ed.), Churchill Livingstone, Edinburgh, pp. 41–52.

Hayslett, J. P., and Lynn, R. I., 1980, Effect of pregnancy in patients with lupus nephropathy, Kidney Int. 18:207–220.

Hensleigh, P. A., and Kauffman, R. E., 1977, Maternal absorption and placental transfer of sulfasalazine, Am. J. Obstet. Gynecol. 127:443–444.

Houser, M. T., Fish, A. J., Tagatz, G. E., Willams, P. P., and Michael, A. F., 1980, Pregnancy and systemic lupus erythematosus, Am. J. Obstet. Gynecol. 138:409–413.

Jarnerot, G., and Into-Malmberg, M. B., 1979, Sulphasalazine treatment during breast feeding, Scand. J. Gastroenterol. 14: 869–871.

Jarnerot, G., Into-Malmberg, M. B., Esbjoerner, E., 1981a, Placental transfer of sulphasalazine and sulphapyridine and some of its metabolites, Scand. J. Gastroenterol. 16:693–697.

Jarnerot, G., Andersen, S., Esbjoerner, E., Sandstroem, B., Brodersen, R., 1981b, Albumin reserve for binding of bilirubin in maternal and cord serum under treatment with sulphasalazine, Scand. J. Gastroent. 16:1049–1055.

Johns, D. G., Rutherford, L. D., Keighton, P. C., Vogel, C. L., 1972, Secretion of methotrexate into human milk, Am. J. Obstet. Gynecol. 112:978–980.

Juchau, M. R., Chao, S. T., and Omiecinski, C. J., 1980, Drug metabolism by the human fetus, Clin. Pharmacol. 5:320–339.

Katz, F., and Duncan, B. R., 1975, Entry of prednisone into human milk, N. Engl. J. Med. 293:1154.

Kirshon, B., Wasserstrum, N., Willis, R., Herman, G. E., and McCabe, E. R. B., 1988, Teratogenic effects of first-trimester cyclophosphamide therapy. Obstet. Gynecol. 72:462–464.

Klintmalm, G., Althoff, P., Appleby, G., and Segerbrandt, E., 1984, Renal function in a newborn baby delivered of a renal transplant patient taking Cyclosporine, Transplantation 38:98–99.

Kozlowski, R. D., Steinbrunner, J. V., MacKenzie, A. H., Clough, J. D., Wilke, W. S., and Segal, A. M., 1990, Outcome of first trimester exposure to low-dose methotrexate in eight patients with rheumatic disease, Am. J. Med. 88:589–592.

Levy, G., and Hayton, W. L., 1973, Pharmacokinetic aspects of placental drug transfer, in: Fetal Pharmacology (L. Boreus, ed., Raven Press, New York, pp. 29–39.

Levy, M., Buskila, D., Gladman, D. D., Urowitz, M. B., and Koren, G., 1991, Pregnancy outcome following first trimester exposure to chloroquine, Am. J. Perinatol. 8:174–178.

Lewis, G. J., Lamont, C. A. R., Lee, H. A., and Slapak, M., 1983, Successful pregnancy in a renal transplant recipient taking cyclosporine A, Br. Med. J. 286:603.

Lewis, P. J., and Hurden, E. L., 1983, Drugs and breast feeding, in: Drugs and Pregnancy (D. F. Hawkins, ed., Churchill Livingstone, Edinburgh, pp. 204–228.

Linares, A., Zarranz, J. J., Rodriguez-Alarcon, J., and Diaz-Perez, J. L., 1979, Reversible cutis laxa due to maternal D-penicillamine treatment, Lancet 2:43.

Lockshin, M. D., 1985, Lupus pregnancy, Clin. Rheum. Dis. 11:611–632.

Lockshin, M. D., Reinitz, E., Druzin, M. L., Murrman, M., and Estes, D., 1984, Case-control prospective study demonstrating absence of lupus exacerbation during or after pregnancy, Am. J. Med. 77:893–898.

Logaridis, T. E., Doran, T. A., Scott, J. G., Gare, D. G., and Comtesse, C., 1983, The effect of maternal steroid administration on fetal platelet count in immunologic trobocytopenic purpura, Am. J. Obstet. Gynecol. 145:147–151.

Lubbe, W. F., Palmer, S. J., Butler, W. S., Liggins, G. C., 1983, Fetal survival after prednisone suppression of maternal lupus-anticoagulant, Lancet 1:1361–1363.

Lyle, W. H., Penicillamine in pregnancy, Lancet 1:606.

MacKenzie, A. H., 1983, Antimalarial drugs for rheumatoid arthritis (Oral gold symposium), Am. J. Med. 75:48–58.

Maracek, Z., and Graf, M., 1976, Pregnancy in penicillamine treated patients with Wilson's disease, N. Engl. J. Med. 295:841–842.

Mason, R. J., Thomson, A. W., Whiting, P. H., Gray, E. S., Brown, P. A. J., Catto, G. R. D., Simpson, J. G., 1985, Cyclosporine-induced fetotoxicity in the rat, Transplantation 39:9–12.

Meehan, R. T., Dorsey, J. K., 1987, Pregnancy among patients with systemic lupus erythematosus receiving immunosuppressive therapy, J. Rheumatol. 14:252–258.

Mjølnerød, O. K., Rasmussen, K., Dommerud, S. A., and Gjeruldsen, S. T., 1971, Congenital connective tissue defect probably due to D-penicillamine treatment in pregnancy, Lancet 1:673–675.

Milunsky, A., Graef, J. W., Gaynor, M. F., 1968, Methotrexate-induced congenital malformations, J. Pediatr. 72:790–795.

Mintz, G., Niz, J., Gutierrez, G., Garcia-Alonso, A., and Karchmer, S., 1986, Prospective study of pregnancy in systemic lupus erythematosus. Results of a multidisciplinary approach, J. Rheumatol. 13:732–739.

Mirkes, P. E., 1985, Cyclophosphamide teratogenesis: A review, Teratogen. Carcinogen. Mutagen. 5:75–88.

Miyamoto, T., Miyaji, S., Horiuchi, Y., Hara, M., Ishihara, K., 1974, Gold therapy in bronchial asthma—special emphasis upon blood levels of gold and its teratogenicity, Nippon Noika Gakkai Zaashi 63:1190.

Mogadam, M., Dobbins, W. O., Korelitz, B. I., and Ahmed, S. W., 1981, Pregnancy in inflammatory bowel disease: Effect of sulfasalazine and corticosteroids on fetal outcome, Gastroenterology 80:72–76.

Møller-Madsen, B., Danscher, G., Uldbjerg, N., and Allen, J. G., 1987, Autometallographic demonstration of gold in human fetal liver and placenta, Rheumatol. Int. 7:47–48.

Murphy, B. E. P., Clark, S. I., Donald, I. R., Pinsky, M., and Vedady, D., 1974, Conversion of maternal cortisol to cortisone during placental transfer to the human fetus, Am. J. Obstet. Gynecol. 118:538–541.

Nation, R. L., Hackett, L. P., Dusci, L. J., and Ilett, K. F., 1984, Excretion of hydroxychloroquine in human milk, Br. J. Clin. Pharmacol. 17:368–369.

Nelis, G. F., 1989, Diarrhoea due to 5-aminosalicylic acid in breast milk, Lancet 1:383.

Nicholson, H., 1968, Cytotoxic drugs in pregnancy, J. Obstet. Gynaecol. Br. Commonw. 75:307–312.

Nishimura, H., and Tanimura, T., 1976, Information on prenatal hazards of drugs, in: Clinical aspects of the teratogenicity of drugs, Elsevier, New York, pp. 100–121.

Osathonondh, A., Tuchinsky, D., Kamali, H., Fencl, M. D., Taeusch, H. W., 1977, Dexamethasone levels in treated pregnant women and newborn infants, J. Pediatr. 90:617–620.

Ost, L., Wettrell, G., Bjørkheim, I., and Rane, A., 1985, Prednisolone excretion in human milk, J. Pediatr. 106:1008–1011.

Østensen, M., Brown, N. D., Chiang, P. K., Aarbakke, J., 1985, Hydroxychloroquine in human breast milk, Eur. J. Clin. Pharmacol. 28:357.

Østensen, M., Skavdal, K., Myklebust, G., Tomassen, Y., Aarbakke, J., 1986, Excretion of gold into human breast milk, Eur. J. Clin. Pharmacol. 31:251–252.

Palmer, R. G., Dore, C. J., and Denman, A. M., 1984, Chlorambucil-induced chromosome damage to human lymphocytes is dose dependent and cumulative, Lancet 1:246–249.

Parke, A. L., 1988, Antimalarial drugs, systemic lupus erythematosus and pregnancy, J. Rheumatol. 15:607–610.

Paufique, L., and Magnard, P., 1969, Retinal degeneration in two children following preventive antimalarial treatment of mother during pregnancy, Bull. Soc. Opththalmol. Fr. 69:466–467.

Penn, I., Makowski, E. L., and Harris, P., 1980, Parenthood following renal transplantation, Kidney Int. 18:221–233.

Perucca, E., and Crema, A., 1982, Plasma protein binding of drugs during pregnancy, Clin. Pharmacokin. 7:336–352.

Pickerell, M. D., and Sawers, R., 1988, Pregnancy after renal transplantation: Severe intrauterine growth retardation during treatment with cyclosporine A, Br. Med. J. 296:825.

Pinals, R. S., 1986, Sulfasalazine in the rheumatic diseases: An old agent reborn, Postgrad. Adv. Rheumatol. 2:3–12.

Pizzuto, J., Aviles, A., Noriega, L., Niz, J., Morales, M., and Romero, F., 1980, Treatment of acute leukemia during pregnancy: Presentation of nine cases, Cancer Treat. Rep. 64:679–683.

Popert, A. J., 1962, Pregnancy and adrenocortical hormones, Br. Med. J. 1:967–972.

Price, H. V., Salaman, J. R., Laurence, K. M., and Langmaid, H., 1976, Immunosuppressive drugs and the foetus, Transplantation 21:294–298.

Pujals, J. M., Figueras, G., Puig, J. M., Lloveras, J., Aubia, J., Masramon, J., 1989, Osseous malformation in baby born to woman on cyclosporine, Lancet 1:667.

Registration Committee of the European Dialysis and Transplant Association, 1980, Successful pregnancies in women treated by dialysis and kidney transplantation, Br. Obstet. Gynaecol. 87:839–845.

Reinisch, J. M., and Simon, N. G., 1978, Prenatal exposure to prednisone in humans and animals retards intrauterine growth, Science 202:436–438.

Rocker, I., and Henderson, W. J., 1976, Transfer of gold from mother to fetus, Lancet 2:1246.

Rogers, J. G., Anderson, R., Chow, C. W., Gillam, G. L., and Marman, L., 1980, Possible teratogenic effects of gold, Aust. Paediatr. J. 16:194–195.

Rooney, T. W., Lorber, A., Veng-Pedersen, P., Herman, R. A., Meehand, R. Hade, J., Hade, A., and Furst, D. E., 1987, Gold pharmacokinetics in breast milk and serum of a lactating woman, J. Rheumatol. 14:1120–1122.

Rosenkrantz, J. G., Githens, J. H., Cox, S. M., and Kellum, D. L., 1967, Azathioprine and pregnancy, Am. J. Obstet. Gynecol. 97:387–394.

Ross, J. B., and Garatsos, S., 1974, Absence of chloroquine-induced ototoxicity in a fetus, Arch. Dermatol. 109:573.

Rudolph, J. E., Schweizer, R. T., and Bartus, S. A., 1979, Pregnancy in renal transplant patients, Transplantation 27:26–29.

Rustin, G. J. S., Booth, M., Dent, J., Salt, S., Rustin, F., Bagshawe, K. D., 1984, Pregnancy after cytotoxic chemotherapy for gestational trophoblastic tumours, Br. Med. J. 288:103–106.

Saarikoski, S., and Seppala, M., 1973, Immunosuppression during pregnancy: Transmission of azathioprine and its metabolites from the mother to the fetus, Am. J. Obstet. Gynecol. 115:1100–1106.

Sargraves, R., Kaiser, D., and Sharpe, G. L., 1981, Prednisone and prednisolone concentrations in the milk of a lactating mother, Drug Intell. Clin. Pharm. 15:484.

Schatz, M., Patterson, R., Zeitz, S., O'Rourke, J., and Malam, H., 1975, Corticosteroid therapy for the pregnant asthmatic patient, J. Am. Med. Assoc. 233:804–807.

Scheinberg, H., and Sternlieb, I., 1975, Pregnancy in penicillamine treated patients with Wilson's disease, N. Engl. J. Med. 293:1300–1302.

Schmidt, P. L., Sims, M. E., Strassner, H. T., Paul, R. H., Mueller, E., and McCarth, D., 1984, Effect of antepartum glucocorticoid administration upon neonatal respiratory distress syndrome and perinatal infection, Am. J. Obstet. Gynecol. 178: 178–186.

Serment, H., Charpin, J., Tessier, G., and Felce, A., 1968, Corticothérapie et grossesse, Bull. Féd. Soc. Gynécol. Obstét. Franc. 20:159–161.

Sharon, E., Jones, J., Diamond, H., and Kaplan, D., 1974, Pregnancy and azathioprine in systemic lupus erythematosus, Am. J. Obstet. Gynecol. 118:25–28.

Shotton, D., and Monie, I. W., 1963, Possible teratogenic effect of chlorambucil on a human fetus, J. Am. Med. Assoc. 186:74–75.

Sidhu, R. K., 1983, Corticosteroids in pregnancy, in: Drugs and Pregnancy. Human Teratogenesis and Related Problems (D. F. Hawkins, ed.), Churchill Livingstone, Edinburgh, pp. 116–127.

Sieber, S. M., and Adamson, R. H., 1975, Toxicity of antineoplastic agents in man: Chromosomal aberrations, antifertility effects, congenital malformations, and carcinogenic potential, Adv. Cancer Res. 22:57–155.

Soares, R., Pauline, E., and Pereina, J. P., 1959, Concentration and elimination of chloroquin by the placental circulation and milk in patients receiving chloroquin salt, Bull. Trop. Dis. 56:412.

Solomon, L., Abrams, G., Dinner, M., and Berman, L., 1977, Neonatal abnormalities associated with D-penicillamine treatment during pregnancy, N. Engl. J. Med. 296:54–55.

Steege, J. F., and Caldwell, D. S., 1980, Renal agenesis after first trimester exposure to chlorambucil, South. Med. J. 73:1414–1415.

Suhonen, R., 1983, Hydroxychloroquine administration in pregnancy, Arch. Dermatol. 119:185–186.

Tarp, U., and Graudal, H., 1985, A follow-up study of children exposed to gold compounds in utero, Arthritis Rheum. 28:235–236.

Thompson, J., and Conklin, K. A., 1983, Anesthetic management of a pregnant patient with scleroderma, Anesthesiology 59: 69–71.

Toledo, T. M., Harper, R. C., and Moser, R. H., 1971, Fetal effects during cyclophosphamide and irradiation therapy, Ann. Intern. Med. 74:87–91.

Tozman, E. C. S., and Gottlieb, N. L., 1987, Adverse reactions with oral and parenteral gold preparations, Med. Toxicol. 2:177–189.

Ullberg, S., Lindquist, N. J., and Sjøstrand, S. E., 1970, Accumulation of chorioretinotoxic drugs in the fetal eye, Nature 227:1257–1258.

Varghese, Z., Lui, S. F., Fernando, O. N., Sweny, P., and Moorhead, J. F., 1988, Pregnancy after renal transplantation. Br. Med. J. 296:1400–1401.

Varner, M. W., Meehan, R. T., Syrop, C. H., Strottmann, M. P., and Goplerud, C. P., 1983, Pregnancy in patients with systemic lupus erythematosus, Am. J. Obstet. Gynecol. 145:1025–1040.

Walden, P. A. M., and Bagshawe, K. D., 1979, Pregnancies after chemotherapy for gestational trophoblast tumours, Lancet 2:1241.

Warrell, D. W., and Taylor, R., 1968, Outcome for the fetus of mothers receiving prednisolone during pregnancy, Lancet 1:117–118.

Wiernik, P. H., and Duncan, J. H., 1971, Cyclophosphamide in human milk, Lancet 1:912.

Williams, P. F., Brons, I. G. M., Evans, D. B., Robinson, R. E., and Calne, R. Y., 1988, Pregnancy after renal transplantation, Br. Med. J. 296:1400.

Williamson, R. A., and Karp, L., 1981, Azathioprine teratogenicity: Review of the literature and case report, Obstet. Gynecol. 58:247–250.

Willoughby, C. P., and Truelove, S. C., 1980, Ulcerative colitis and pregnancy, Gut 21:469–474.

Wolfe, M. S., and Cordero, J. F., 1985, Safety of chloroquine in chemosuppression of malaria during pregnancy, Br. Med. J. 290:1466–1467.

Ziegenhagen, D. J., Crombach, G., Dieckman, M., Zehntner, E., Wienand, P., and Baldamus, C. A., 1988, Schwangerschaft unter Ciclosporin-Medikation nach Nierentransplantation, Dtsch. Med. Wschr. 113:260–263.

Zulman, J. I., Talal, N., Hoffman, C. S., and Epstein, W. V., 1980, Problems associated with the management of pregnancies in patients with systemic lupus erythematosus, J. Rheumatol. 7:37–49.

Part III

IMMUNOTHERAPY IN AUTOIMMUNE DISEASE

Chapter 20

SYSTEMIC LUPUS ERYTHEMATOSUS AND RELATED SYNDROMES

Alfonso Monereo, Munther Andrawes Khamashta,
Juan José Vazquez, and *Graham Robert Vivian Hughes*

1. INTRODUCTION

Systemic lupus erythematosus (SLE) is a chronic disorder with an autoimmune background in which tissue damage is mediated by immune complexes. It is a multisystem disease with a very heterogeneous clinical profile. Classification criteria established by the American Rheumatism Association (Tan *et al.*, 1982) provide a useful guide for the clinician.

The etiology is still unclear. Most authors support a multifactorial origin including genetic, hormonal, and environmental factors (Decker *et al.*, 1979; Steinberg and Klinman, 1988). Whatever the etiology, there are profound immunological disturbances including polyclonal activation of B lymphocytes, production of a variety of antinuclear and other antibodies, and disorders in T-cell immunoregulation. B-lymphocyte activation, resulting in polyclonal hypergammaglobulinemia, is a frequent finding. A correlation of the disease activity with the increase of IgG and IgA secreting cells in peripheral blood is reported (Blaese *et al.*, 1980). Recent studies also suggest primary B-cell hyperactivity (Sakane, 1988).

The antibody specificities found in SLE are numerous. Some are associated with specific manifestations of the disease, such as anti-Ro (directed against RNA polymerase) with cutaneous lupus and congenital heart block, or antiphospholipid antibodies with thromboses, fetal loss, and thrombocytopenia (Hughes *et al.*, 1986), or antibodies against nuclear ribonucleoprotein (anti-RNP) with the presence of mixed connective tissue disease. A pathogenic role is not proved in all of them. Immune complexes play a central role in the pathogenesis of SLE. They deposit in diverse tissues, activate complement, and lead to an

Alfonso Monereo and Juan José Vazquez • Department of Internal Medicine, La Paz Hospital, 28002 Madrid, Spain. *Munther Andrawes Khamashta and Graham Robert Vivian Hughes* • Lupus Arthritis Research Laboratory, The Rayne Institute, St. Thomas' Hospital, London SE1 7EH, England.

Immunopharmacology in Autoimmune Diseases and Transplantation, edited by Hans Erik Rugstad *et al.* Plenum Press, New York, 1992.

inflammatory reaction, leading to tissue damage. Clearance of immune complexes in SLE is also impaired, due in part to a deficit in complement receptors (CR1) on the cellular surface (Steinberg and Klinman, 1988).

Many alterations in T-cell function have been described in SLE such as decreased T suppressor cells and abnormalities in their function (e.g., a decrease in proliferating response to specific antigens and decrease of interleukin production). B- and T-cell disorders are more prominent in patients with active disease.

The heterogeneity of SLE makes it difficult to plan pharmacological treatment. Treatment has to be planned on an individual basis. Some general principles must be considered:

1. SLE has active periods alternating with symptom-free periods.
2. There is no cure, so treatment goals are focused to relieve the symptoms and organ damage during active disease and avoid new flare-ups of clinical activity and progression of organ damage already established.
3. It may affect almost every organ with a wide spectrum of severity. An aggressive approach is not indicated for abnormal immunological findings in an oligosymptomatic patient (Hughes, 1982). Immunosuppressives may be indicated in those with severe visceral or hematological involvement.

Finally, there are some biological parameters that may help the clinician to determine the degree of disease activity. The finding of these activity indexes is not per se an indication of treatment, but provide valid information in specific situations. These activity indexes are ESR, anti-DNA antibody titer, circulating immune complexes, lymphocytopenia, complement fractions C3 and C4, and total complement activity (Hughes, 1975; Morrow *et al.*, 1982).

The main pharmacological agents and therapeutic regimens are discussed in this chapter.

2. NONSTEROIDAL ANTI-INFLAMMATORY DRUGS

Nonsteroidal anti-inflammatory drugs (NSAIDs) are useful first-line agents in treating symptoms such as arthralgia, arthritis, and occasionally serositis. To obtain an antipyretic or analgesic effect, low doses of aspirin (e.g., 300 mg every 4–6 hr) may be enough, but in general NSAIDs have replaced aspirin.

Generally, NSAIDs are well tolerated. The toxic effects are well known and most are shared by all the agents. Gastrointestinal blood loss due to microbleeding may develop in patients treated with aspirin and other NSAIDs. High-dose aspirin may induce hepatotoxicity, which seems to be especially frequent in patients with SLE (Travers and Hughes, 1978). Treatment should be stopped in cases of hepatic enzyme elevation four to six times above the normal range. Hepatotoxicity is less frequent if another derivate such as diflunisal, which lacks the orthoacetyl ring, is used (Hughes, 1979). NSAIDs may reversibly reduce the glomerular filtration rate (Ter Borg *et al.*, 1989), though sulindac may be an exception. In practice, this effect of NSAIDs may have been exaggerated. The majority of SLE patients at some time receive NSAIDs, and clinically significant renal deterioration has been very unusual. Idiosyncratic reactions including interstitial nephritis, fever, rash, and even aseptic meningitis have been described in SLE patients treated with ibuprofen.

NSAIDs highly bind to plasma proteins, displacing other molecules such as warfarin and sulfonylureas. They also decrease the renal elimination of chlorpropamide, methotrexate, and lithium.

3. ANTIMALARIALS

The use of antimalarials in SLE goes back over 30 years. In 1954, Dubois reported good results in patients with mild to moderate disease and predominantly cutaneous involvement. The mechanism of action of antimalarials in SLE remains undefined. Many effects have been studied and reviewed (Lanham and Hughes, 1982; Dubois and Wallace, 1987) (Table I).

The antimalarials most frequently used in SLE are quinacrine (Atabrine) (an acridine compound), chloroquine, hydroxychloroquine, and aminodiaquine (4 aminoquinolines). They are water-soluble compounds, and thus well absorbed orally. Plasma levels increase after 2 to 4 hr, reaching maximum levels in 8–12 hr. Between three to five weeks, plasma levels and urinary elimination stabilize (Lanham and Hughes, 1982). Urinary excretion is both in unaltered form and as metabolites.

The main clinical use of antimalarials is in cases of mild to moderate disease. The best response is observed in cutaneous lesions, polyarthralgia, pleuritic pain, and low-grade pericardial inflammation. It also ameliorates symptoms like malaise and lethargy. The initial response rate is high, but relapses are frequent. Up to 80% of patients need maintenance doses or re-treatment. Their use is especially beneficial during steroid withdrawal once the disease activity is in remission (Dubois and Wallace, 1987).

Our first choice is hydroxychloroquine in an initial dose of 200 mg. Improvement may take up to three months. If no response is obtained, the daily dose can be raised to 400 mg. In some circumstances, another antimalarial with no retinotoxic effect may be added, such as quinacrine (50–100 mg/day) (Dubois and Wallace, 1987). To maintain remission, low doses (e.g., 1 or 2 tablets per week) may be required. Maintenance therapy seems to reduce the frequency of new flare-ups (Rudnicki et al., 1975; The Canadian Hydroxychloroquine Study Group, 1991).

Toxic effects such as malaise and dizziness frequently appear when starting treatment, but usually improve spontaneously. Skin pigmentation changes are frequent. The most important toxicity is on the retina, which occurs when high doses are taken (more than 500 mg/day) and less frequently with hydroxycloroquin doses around 200 mg/day. Retinal toxicity usually occurs after two to three years of treatment, although great variability may be seen (7 months to 10 years). The main determinant seems to be the daily dose, although risk increases with cumulative doses higher than 300 g (Lanham and Hughes, 1982). The first change seen in the fundus is pigmentation with a fine granulated pattern best seen in the

TABLE I. Antimalarials: Mechanism of Action

Anti-inflammatory effects
    Stabilization of lysosomal membrane of inflammatory cells
    Inhibition of chemotaxis and phagocytosis
    Decreased prostaglandin synthesis by inhibiting phospholipase A and C
    Decreased activity of cholinesterase and hyaluronidase
    Decreased enzymatic lysis of cartilage mucopolysaccharides
Immunomodulator effects
    Inhibition of in vitro lymphocyte transformation
    Decreased response to phytohemagglutinin and other specific antigens
    Decreased antigen–antibody complex formation and increase in their dissociation (dose-dependent effect)
    Decreased production of mononuclear accessory factors for monocyte functions
    Decreased production of immunoglobulin-secreting cells
    Selective inhibition of interleukin secretion by monocytes
    Bind DNA bases stabilizing them and decreasing protein synthesis
    Block DNA-anti DNA reaction and inhibit SLE phenomenon

macular region. Macular edema and loss of the foveolar reflex may be found. In the most severe cases of toxicity, a characteristic bull's-eye retinal lesion is seen. Visual loss occurs late in the course of treatment, starting with reading difficulties, missing words or letters, or blacked-out areas in the visual field. Other symptoms are photophobia, blurred distance vision, and light flashes. In the visual field central or paracentral scotomata may be found. Examination before treatment and six-month interval fundoscopic tests are necessary.

4. CORTICOSTEROIDS

Corticosteroids act as anti-inflammatory and immunoregulating agents (Kehrl and Fauci, 1983). As anti-inflammatory agents, steroids block the increased permeability of the basal membrane and the transit of immune complexes through it. They also reduce adhesiveness and chemotaxis of macrophages and polymorphonuclear cells, decreasing their accumulation in the inflammatory focus. In addition, they stabilize and protect lysosomal membranes, avoiding liberation of enzymes.

As immunoregulating agents, steroids act on monocytes, reducing bactericidal capacity and production of soluble factors such as interleukins. They reduce B-lymphocyte responses and protein synthesis, especially IgG. On cellular immunity, they act at different levels, including cell proliferation and response to lymphokines, decreased cytotoxic reactions, and inhibition of T helper production.

Steroids are used in high doses (1–1.5 mg/kg per day of prednisone or methylprednisolone) in patients with severe visceral disease. They are also indicated in less severe but nevertheless active disease (arthritis, fever, serositis) unresponsive to NSAIDs alone or combined with antimalarials. In the latter case they are used in low doses, the minimum dose sufficient to control the symptoms.

In severe visceral disease, initial doses of prednisone or methylprednisolone range between 1 to 1.5 mg/kg per day administered parenterally. Initially, the total daily dose in three or four fractions is recommended to achieve maximal effects. This dose is maintained until unequivocal signs of improvement appear, normally in one to two weeks. Gradual reduction of the daily dose is carried out over the next several weeks or months until a low maintenance dose is reached. For long-term maintenance therapy, alternate-day steroids are an alternative, although opinions differ as to their value in sparing long-term side effects.

The increased tendency to infection associated with steroid therapy is now the leading cause of death in SLE patients (Rosner *et al.*, 1982). These infections include gram-negative bacilli, *Staphylococcus*, tuberculosis, *Listeria*, fungus (especially *Candida*), virus (herpes), and protozoa (*Toxoplasma* and *Pneumocystis carinii*). For prophylaxis against reactivation of tuberculosis, patterns of treatment vary widely. Some advocate the use of prophylactic treatment with 12 months of isoniazid therapy in those developing a positive Mantoux reaction (Bass *et al.*, 1986).

5. STEROID PULSE THERAPY

Use of steroid pulses were initiated during the 1970s in renal transplant rejection. The aim of this treatment is to obtain immunosuppressive and anti-inflammatory effects without appearance of the secondary effects of high-dose steroids. There are dose-dependent steroidal effects that could be responsible for a qualitative difference with this treatment modality, such as inhibition of granulocyte aggregation, decreased expression of IL-2 receptor in T lymphocytes, induction of prolonged alteration of T killer activity, and enhancement of monocyte Fc receptor-mediated phagocytic activity (Kimberly, 1988).

Treatment consists of intravenous infusion of 1 g of prednisone in 500 ml of saline over 4 hr. This dose is usually administered once a day for a period of three days. It has been used in thrombocytopenia, hemolysis, cerebritis, pleuropericarditis, subacute cutaneous lupus, and intra-alveolar hemorrhage (Evanson et al., 1980). Response is variable (Mackworth-Young et al., 1984). However, patients with rapid and recent renal function deterioration show comparably better results with this regimen (Kimberly et al., 1981). In extrarenal lupus, steroid pulses have variable success in neurological disease and thrombocytopenia refractory to other treatments (Evanson et al., 1980; Lurie and Kahalch, 1982; Mackworth-Young et al., 1984). The use of pulse steroid therapy has been advocated for safer splenectomy in severe refractory thrombocytopenia (Dubois and Wallace, 1987).

In general, pulse steroids are well tolerated (Kimberly, 1982) and lacking in the classic secondary effects of long-term steroid treatment. However, harmful secondary effects, including psychosis, hallucinations, focal neurologic symptoms, convulsions, acute pulmonary edema, or precipitation of congestive heart failure, arrhythmias, and sudden death, have been described (Wollheim, 1984).

6. IMMUNOSUPPRESSIVES

Originally employed in the treatment of neoplastic diseases, immunosuppressives are now widely used for the treatment of autoimmune diseases, especially in severe forms of SLE. The main cytostatic agents used as immunosuppressives in SLE are:

1. Azathioprine. This is a purine analogue that blocks adenine and guanine synthesis, suppressing nonspecific inflammation. Humoral and cell-mediated immunity are also affected, the latter to a greater degree (Balow et al., 1987).
2. Cyclophosphamide. This is an alkylating agent that decreases cellular replication by cross-linking DNA bases. Cyclophosphamide also inhibits antibody production and acts nonspecifically on inflammation and T-mediated immunity (Steinberg, 1986).
3. Methotrexate. This drug works by blocking the dihydrofolate reductase enzyme, the precursor of tetrahydrofolic, a carbon group supplier in biosynthesis. It also blocks the formation of DNA synthesis. It acts mainly on cellular immunity (Balow et al., 1987).

The use of immunosuppressives in SLE recently has been reviewed (Lieberman and Schatten, 1988). In addition to their use in severe disease and as steroid-sparing agents, they are also indicated in some manifestations that are known to respond better to immunosuppressives such as diffuse proliferative glomerulonephritis. It is important to consider that these lesions must be at least partially reversible. The response has to be periodically evaluated with objective parameters and terminated if no demonstrable response is obtained in a reasonable period of time.

A practical approach to the clinical use of these cytostatic agents includes the following recommendations (Clements and Davis, 1986): Regular blood checks, initially every 7–14 days, and subsequently every 2–4 weeks once the treatment response is achieved. Leukocyte counts below 3500 (or granulocytes less than 1000) or platelets less than 100,000 per mm^3 demands a temporary withdrawal. At the first sign of infection, a leukocyte count should be obtained and treatment withheld if leukopenia is present. In the presence of a positive Mantoux reaction, isoniazid chemoprophylaxis may be indicated. Attenuated vaccines should not be used during treatment, as an adequate response will not be obtained.

Azathioprine is less toxic than cyclophosphamide and has wider therapeutic uses, for example, in patients with discoid lupus resistant to antimalarials, some moderate forms of proliferative glomerulonephritis, and in some patients with membranous glomerulonephritis (Steinberg, 1986; Lieberman and Schatten, 1988).

Cyclophosphamide is used in situations of progressive renal disease, with severe pulmonary, hematological, and central nervous system involvement. Improvement is seen after ten days of treatment. Standard doses are 1–2 mg/kg per day.

Immunosuppressives associated with corticosteroids delay the progression to terminal renal failure in patients with lupus nephritis (Donadio *et al.*, 1978; Carette *et al.*, 1983). Different approaches to treatment include pulses of cyclophosphamide, the most effective in preventing progression to renal failure (Austin *et al.*, 1986; Balow *et al.*, 1987). This therapy consists of administering one cyclophosphamide pulse (1 g/m^2 intravenously) every one to three months. Favorable results have also been described with this regimen in refractory extrarenal lupus (McCune *et al.*, 1987).

Methotrexate is also used is SLE treatment. A good response has been observed in patients resistant to steroid and azathioprine treatment (Davidson *et al.*, 1987). The dose is 7.5–15 mg weekly.

Immunosuppressive agents are all marrow-toxic and are all associated with an increase in infections. Leukopenia may appear 7 to 14 days after a single dose, recovering in 21 to 25 days (Clements and Davis, 1986). The risk of infection increases significantly when the leukocyte count falls below 2000.

Azathioprine can produce hypersensitivity hepatitis with cholestasis and jaundice and idiosyncratic reactions with fever, rash, and leukopenia. Azathioprine toxicity is enhanced with the simultaneous use of allopurinol and in the presence of liver disease (Steinberg, 1986). It is the least teratogenic, and some authors proclaim it is safe during pregnancy. It is not known whether it increases the risk of neoplasms in SLE.

Cyclophosphamide produces important urologic toxicity due to its metabolite acrolein. Hemorrhagic cystitis, chronic cystitis, and urothelial carcinoma are the major manifestations. When high pulse doses are used, acute bladder toxicity may be prevented by maintaining a high urinary volume. Recently, the use of sodium 2-mercaptoethamine sulfonate has been shown to reduce the severity of acute cystitis. Cyclophosphamide causes infertility, though potentially reversible when used before puberty. It also increases the incidence of neoplasms, particularly hematopoietic and cutaneous, and it is teratogenic.

Methotrexate is hepatotoxic. Its use should be avoided in patients with liver disease. During treatment, serum transaminase levels must be monitored and liver biopsy performed if serious hepatotoxicity is suspected (Clemens and Davis, 1986). Cyclophosphamide may also produce oral ulcers and acute interstitial pneumonia. It is the most teratogenic agent.

7. OTHER THERAPEUTIC MEASURES

Omega-3 fatty acid dietary supplementation is currently used in SLE patients (Clark *et al.*, 1989, Thörner *et al.*, 1990). This treatment was inspired by studies in the NZB/W mouse experimental model, showing a prolonged survival with fish oil dietary supplementation (Prickett *et al.*, 1981). Beneficial effects of omega-3 fatty acid dietary supplementation are believed to be due to a reduction of inflammatory metabolites, modulating the inflammatory activity, and to a potential decrease of the SLE-related accelerated atherosclerosis.

Plasmapheresis is used to remove substances such as autoantibodies or immune complexes directly implicated in the pathogenesis of autoimmune diseases (Klippel, 1984).

Beneficial effects of plasmapheresis appear to be transitory and followed by rebound effect. It has to be used in combination with steroids and cyclophosphamide (Jones, 1984) or synchronized with pulses of cyclophosphamide (Barr *et al.*, 1988). The synergistic effect of these combinations is based on an enhancement of the cytotoxic effect. In SLE there are no precise indications for the use of plasmapheresis. It is most frequently used in active disease resistant to steroids and immunosuppressives (Jones, 1984).

Danazol is a synthetic androgen derivate, which has been used with good results in idiopathic thrombocytopenic purpura, autoimmune hemolytic anemia, and in cases of SLE (Morley *et al.*, 1982). Androgens favor immune complex elimination and exert an immuno-regulatory action on T-lymphocyte populations. Oddly, however, it has been found to cause frequent rashes in SLE.

Total lymphoid irradiation, widely used in the treatment of Hodgkin's disease, has been used in cases of nephritis with atrophy and scarring, with clinical improvement (Strober *et al.*, 1987). Lymphoid irradiation causes a reduction of B-lymphocyte activity. There are no precise indications.

Still under consideration are cyclosporine A (Camsonne *et al.*, 1986) and monoclonal antibodies directed against immunocompetent cells (Wolfsy and Seaman, 1987). As an alternative in drug-resistant lupus nephritis, high-dose intravenous gammaglobulin has been reported to be successful (Lin *et al.*, 1989; Akashi *et al.*, 1990). Possible mechanisms of action are delineated elsewhere (Lin *et al.*, 1989); clinical efficacy and indications are still undetermined.

Treatment of clinical manifestations associated with the presence of antiphospholipid antibodies requires anticoagulation (Hughes *et al.*, 1986). The duration of this treatment may need to be prolonged in the presence of persistently high antiphospholipid antibody levels because of the risk of the occurrence of new thrombotic events upon withdrawal (Asherson *et al.*, 1985). Thrombosis despite anticoagulation treatment has been also described, and for these cases immunosuppressive treatment has been recommended (Harris *et al.*, 1985). In the case of repeated fetal loss, there are reports of success using treatment with 40 mg of prednisone plus low doses of aspirin (75 mg/day) (Branch *et al.*, 1985). Monitoring of anticardiolipin antibody levels is necessary. The isotype and titers of the anticardiolipin antibody seem to have prognostic value and may be a useful guide during treatment (Harris *et al.*, 1986). The recent observation that these antibodies may have direct effects on platelet membranes (Khamashta *et al.*, 1988) suggests that trials of antiplatelet regimens may be indicated in patients with thrombosis associated with the antiphospholipid antibody syndrome.

REFERENCES

Akashi, K., Nagasawa, K., Mayumi, T., Yokota, E., Oochi, N., and Kusaba, T., 1990, Successful treatment of refractory systemic lupus erythematosus with intravenous immunoglobulins, *J. Rheumatol.* **17**:375–379.

Asherson, R. A., Chan, J. K. H., Harris, E. N., Gharavi, A. E., and Hughes, G. R. V., 1985, Anticardiolipin antibody, recurrent thrombosis and warfarin withdrawal, *Ann. Rheum. Dis.* **44**:823–825.

Austin, H. A., Klippel, J. H., Balow, J. E., Le Riche, G. N., Steinberg, A. D., Plotz, P. H., and Decker, J., 1986, Therapy of lupus nephritis. Controlled trial of prednisone and cytotoxic drugs, *N. Engl. J. Med.* **316**:614–619.

Bakke, A. C., Kirkland, P. A., Kitridou, R. C., Quismorio, F. P., Rea, T., Ehresmann, G. R., and Horwitz, D. A., 1983, T lymphocyte subsets in systemic lupus erythematosus, *Arthritis Rheum.* **26**:745–750.

Balow, J. E., Austin, H. A., Tsokos, G. C., Antonovych, T. T., Steinberg, A. D., and Klippel, J. H., 1987, Lupus nephritis, *Ann. Intern. Med.* **106**:79–94.

Barr, W. G., Hubbell, E. A., and Rabinson, J. A., 1988, Plasmapheresis and pulse cyclophosphamide in systemic lupus erythematosus, *Ann. Intern. Med.* **108**:152–153.

Bass, J. B., Farer, L. S., Hopewell, P. C., Jacobs, R. F., 1986, Treatment of tuberculosis and tuberculosis infection in adults and children, *Am. Rev. Respir. Dis.* **134**:355–363.

Blaese, R. M., Grayson, J., and Steinberg, A. D., 1980, Increased immunoglobulin-secreting cells in blood of patients with active systemic lupus erythematosus, *Am. J. Med.* **69:**345–350.

Branch, W. D., Scott, J. R., Kochenour, N. K., and Hershgald, E., 1985, Obstetric complications associated with the lupus anticoagulant, *N. Engl. J. Med.* **313:**1322–1326.

Camsonne, R., Troussard, X., Le Porrier, M., Macro, M., and Moulin, M. A., 1986, Efficacité de la ciclosporine dans le lupus á manifestation hématologique corticoïde-dependant et résistant á la splénectomie, *La Presse Médicale* **15:**76.

The Canadian Hydroxychloroquine Study Group, 1991, A randomized study of the effect of withdrawing hydroxychloroquine sulfate in systhemic lupus erythematosus, *N. Engl. J. Med.* **324:**150–154.

Carette, S., Klippel, J. H., Decker, J. J., Austin, H. A., Plotz, P. H., Steinberg, A. D., and Balow, J. E., 1983, Controlled studies of oral immunosuppressive drugs in lupus nephritis. A long-term follow-up, *Ann. Intern. Med.* **99:**1–8.

Clark, W. F., Parbtani, A., Huff, M. W., Reid, B., Holub, B. J., and Falardeau, P., 1989, Omega 3 fatty acid dietary supplementation in systemic lupus erythematosus, *Kidney Int.* **36:**653–660.

Clements, P. J., and Davis, J., 1986, Cytotoxic drugs: Their clinical application to the rheumatic diseases, *Sem. Arthritis Rheum.* **15:**231–254.

Davidson, J. R., Graziano, F. M., and Rothenberg, R. J., 1987, Methotrexate therapy for severe systemic lupus erythematosus, *Arthritis Rheum.* **30:**1195–1196.

Decker, J. L., Steinberg, A. D., Reinertsen, J. L., Plotz, P. H., Balow, J. E., and Klippel, J. H., 1979, Systemic lupus erythematosus: Evolving concepts, *Ann. Intern. Med.* **91:**587–604.

Donadio, J. V., Holley, K. E., Ferguson, R. H., and Ilstrup, D. M., 1978, Treatment of diffuse proliferative lupus nephritis with prednisolone and combined prednisone and cyclophosphamide, *N. Engl. J. Med.* **229:**1151–1155.

Dubois, E., 1954, Quinacrine (Atabrine) in treatment of systemic and discoid lupus erythematosus, *Arch. Intern. Med.* **94:**131–141.

Dubois, E., and Wallace, J., 1987, Management of discoid and systemic lupus erythematosus, in: *Dubois' Lupus Erythematosus*, 3rd Ed. (E. Dubois and J. Wallace, eds.), Lea and Febiger, Philadelphia, pp. 501–564.

Evanson, S., Passo, M. H., Aldo-Benson, M. A., and Benson, M D., 1980, Methylprednisolone therapy for nonrenal lupus erythematosus, *Ann. Rheum. Dis.* **39:**377–380.

Harris, E. N., Gharavi, A. E., and Hughes, G. R. V., 1985, Antiphospholipid antibodies, *Clin. Rheum. Dis.* **11:**591–609.

Harris, E. N., Chan, J. K. H., Asherson, R. A., Aber, V., Gharavi, A. E., and Hughes, G. R. V., 1986, Thrombosis, recurrent fetal loss and thrombocytopenia: Predictive value of the anticardiolipin test, *Arch. Intern. Med.* **146:**2153–2156.

Hughes, G. R. V., 1975, Anti-nucleic acid antibodies in SLE. Clinical and pathological significance, *Clin. Rheum. Dis.* **1:**545–559.

Hughes, G. R. V., 1979, Systemic lupus erythematosus: Treatment and prognosis, *Br. Med. J.* **2:**1019–1022.

Hughes, G. R. V., 1982, The treatment of SLE: The case for conservative management, *Clin. Rheum. Dis.* **8:**299–313.

Hughes, G. R. V., Harris, E. N., and Gharavi, A. E., 1986, The anticardiolipin syndrome, *J. Rheumatol.* **13:**486–489.

Jones, J. V., 1984, Plasmapheresis in SLE, *Clin. Rheum. Dis.* **8:**243–259.

Khamashta, M. A., Harris, E. N., Gharavi, A. E., Derue, G., Gil, A., Vazquez, J. J., and Hughes, G. R. V., 1988, Immune mediated mechanism for thrombosis: Antiphospholipid antibody binding to platelet membranes, *Ann. Rheum. Dis.* **47:**849–854.

Kehrl, J. H., and Fauci, A. S., 1983, The clinical use of glucocorticoids, *Ann. Allergy* **50:**2–10.

Kimberly, R. P., 1982, Pulse methylprednisolone in SLE, *Clin. Rheum. Dis.* **8:**261–277.

Kimberly, R. P., 1988, Systemic lupus erythematosus: Treatment. Corticosteroids and anti-inflammatory drugs, *Rheum. Dis. Clin. North Am.* **14:**203–221.

Kimberly, R. P., Lockshin, M. D., Sherman, R. L., McDougal, J. S., Inman, R. D., and Christian, C. L., 1981, High-dose intravenous methylprednisolone pulse therapy in systemic lupus erythematosus, *Am. J. Med.* **76:**817–824.

Klippel, J. H., 1984, Apheresis. Biotechnology and the rheumatic diseases, *Arthritis Rheum.* **27:**1081–1085.

Kovarsky, J., 1983, Clinical pharmacology and toxicology of cyclophosphamide: Emphasis on use in rheumatic diseases, *Sem. Arthritis Rheum.* **12:**359–372.

Lanham, J., and Hughes, G. R. V., 1982, Antimalarial therapy in SLE, *Clin. Rheum. Dis.* **8:**279–298.

Lieberman, J. D., and Schatten, S., 1988, Systemic lupus erythematosus: Treatment. Disease modifying therapies, *Rheum. Dis. Clin. North Am.* **14:**223–243.

Lin, C. Y., Hsu, H. C., and Chiang, H., 1989, Improvement of histological and immunological change in steroid and immunosuppressive drug-resistant lupus nephritis by high dose intravenous gammaglobulin, *Nephron* **53:**303–310.

Lurie, C., and Kahalch, M. B., 1982, Pulse corticosteroid therapy for refractory thrombocytopenia in systemic lupus erythematosus, *J. Rheumatol.* **9:**311–314.

Mackworth-Young, C. G., Morgan, S. H., and Hughes, G. R. V., 1984, Intravenous methylprednisolone in the treatment of systemic lupus erythematosus, *Scand. J. Rheumatol.* (Suppl.) **54:**16–18.

McCune, W. J., Golbus, J., Zeldes, W., Bohlke, P., and Fox, D. A., 1987, Treatment of refractory systemic lupus erythematosus with monthly intravenous cyclophosphamide (Abstr), *Arthritis Rheum.* **30**(Suppl. 4):85.

Morley, K. D., Parke, A., and Hughes, G. R. V., 1982, Systemic lupus erythematosus: Two patients treated with danazol, *Br. Med. J.* **284:**1431–1432.

Morrow, J. W., Isenberg, D. A., Todd-Pokropek, A., Parry, H. F., Snaith, M. L., 1982, Useful laboratory measurements in the management of SLE, *Q. J. Med.* **202:**125–128.

Prickett, J. D., Robinson, D. R., and Steinberg, A. D., 1981, Dietary enrichment with the polyunsaturated fatty acid eicosapenta-noic acid prevents proteinuria and prolongs survival in NZB/NZW F_1 mice, *J. Clin. Invest.* **68:**556–559.

Rosner, S., Ginzler, E. M., Diamond, H. S., Weiner, M., Schlesinger, M., Fries, J. F., Wasner, C., Medsger, T. A., Ziegler, G., Klippel, J. H., Hadler, N. M., Albert, D. A., Hess, E. V., Spencer-Green, G., Grayzel, A., Worth, D., Hahn, B. H., and Barnett, E. V., 1982, A multicenter study of outcome in systemic lupus erythematosus: II. Causes of death, *Arthritis Rheum.* **25:**612–617.

Rudnicki, R., Greham, G., and Rothfield, N., 1975, The efficacy of antimalarials in systemic lupus erythematosus, *J. Rheumatol.* **2:**323–330.

Sakanke, T., Suzuki, N., Takada, S., Veda, Y., Murakawa, Y., Tsuchida, T., Yamauchi, Y., and Kishmoto, T., 1988, B-cell hyperactivity and its relation to distinct clinical features and the degree of disease activity in patients with systemic lupus erythematosus, *Arthritis Rheum.* **31:**345–350.

Steinberg, A. D., 1986, The treatment of lupus nephritis, *Kidney Int.* **30:**769–787.

Steinberg, A. D., and Klinman, D. M., 1988, Systemic lupus erythematosus: Pathogenesis of systemic lupus erythematosus, *Rheum. Dis. Clin. North Am.* **14:**25–41.

Strober, S., Farinas, M. C., Field, E. H., Solovera, J. T., Kiberd, B. A., Myers, B. D., and Hoppe, R. T., 1987, Lupus nephritis after total lymphoid irradiation persistent improvement and reduction of steroid therapy, *Ann. Intern. Med.* **107:**689–690.

Tan, E., Cohen, A., Fries, J., Masi, A., McShane, D., Rothfield, N., Scaller, J., Talal, N., Winchester, R., 1982, The 1982 revised criteria for the classification of systemic lupus erythematosus, *Arthritis Rheum.* **25:**1271–1277.

Ter Borj, E. J., de Jong, P. E., Meijer, S., and Kallemberg, C. G. M., 1989, Renal effects of indomethacin in patients with systemic lupus erythematosus, *Nephron* **53:**238–243.

Thörner, A., Walldius, G., Nilsson, E., Hadell, K., and Gullberg, R., 1990, Beneficial effects of reduced intake of polyunsaturated fatty acids in the diet for one year in patients with systemic lupus erythematosus, *Ann. Rheum. Dis.* **49:**134.

Travers, R., and Hughes, G. R. V., 1978, Salicylate hepatotoxicity in SLE: A common occurrence? *Br. Med. J.* **11:**1532–1533.

Wolfsy, D., and Seaman, W. E., 1987, Reversal of advanced murine lupus in NZB/NZW F_1 mice with monoclonal antibody to L3T4, *J. Immunol.* **138:**3247–3253.

Wollheim, F., 1984, Acute and long-term complications of corticosteroids pulse therapy, *Scand. J. Rheumatol.* (Suppl.) **54:**27–32.

Chapter 21

IMMUNOPHARMACOLOGY OF VASCULITIC SYNDROMES

P. A. Bacon, R. A. Luqmani, D. G. I. Scott, and *D. Adu*

1. INTRODUCTION

The first descriptions of vasculitis were by Kussmaul and Maier in 1866. It may affect any vessel and occur *de novo* or complicate preexisting diseases. Essentially it can be defined as an inflammation of blood vessels. Vasculitis is an important component of the pathology of connective tissue diseases; Bywaters (1976) hypothesized that vascular inflammation was the basis of connective tissue disease.

The systemic vasculitides are multisystem diseases that pose severe problems in clinical management. These are rare diseases with the incidence of systemic vasculitis being difficult to determine with accuracy. Sack *et al.* (1975) reported an annual figure of two per million for polyarteritis nodosa, whereas our data suggested a higher figure of 4.6 for the same disease (Scott *et al.*, 1982).

Classifications of vasculitis have been based on vessel size, organ involvement, pathology, and etiology when known (Zeek, 1952). There is strong evidence to suggest an immunopathological etiology for at least some of these diseases. As Fan *et al.* (1980) stressed in their extensive review, however, vascular inflammation may be the end result of many different causes, and any single immunological abnormality can produce a spectrum of clinical problems that often overlaps with that produced by other immunological events. A clinically based classification, which is a guide to therapeutic intervention, has been suggested (Scott, 1988), but in practice there is often considerable overlap when using any system of classification. It is more appropriate to keep the provisional diagnosis under review, in order to avoid unnecessarily treating patients with only small vessel cutaneous vasculitis, for example, unless they develop any evidence of other organ involvement. In our experience, the most common forms of systemic vasculitis are rheumatoid vasculitis (Ball, 1954; Sokoloff and Bunim, 1957; Kulka, 1959), Wegener's granulomatosis (Wegener, 1936;

P. A. Bacon and *R. A. Luqmani* • Department of Rheumatology, The University of Birmingham, The Medical School, Birmingham B15 2TT, England.   *D. G. I. Scott* • Norfolk and Norwich Hospital, Norfolk, Norwich NR1 3SE, England.   *D. Adu* • Department of Nephrology, Queen Elizabeth Hospital, Birmingham B15 2TJ, England.

Immunopharmacology in Autoimmune Diseases and Transplantation, edited by Hans Erik Rugstad *et al.* Plenum Press, New York, 1992.

Godman and Churg, 1954) and polyarteritis nodosa (Kussmaul and Maier 1866, Frohnert and Scheps, 1967).

With such diversity it is not surprising to find a range of treatments used. Decisions on therapy are difficult, yet they are important since these diseases have a serious prognosis, with a very definite fatality, although the outlook appears much better in recent decades. Baggenstoss *et al.* (1950) first reported the successful use of steroids given to a small number of patients with vasculitis. Since then, there have been many studies using either steroids alone and later steroids in combination with cytotoxic agents, which have shown a reduction (sometimes dramatic) in the short-term mortality of these diseases (Fauci, 1978; Fauci *et al.*, 1989; Leib *et al.*, 1979; Scott and Bacon, 1984). Many series in the literature do not distinguish between different types of vasculitis, but it is clear that the overall outlook has been vastly improved by the use of cytotoxic agents in a variety of forms of necrotizing vasculitis and that one drug in particular, namely cyclophosphamide, stands out as effective therapy for this group of disorders.

2. CYCLOPHOSPHAMIDE

This chapter will discuss the use of cyclophosphamide, in particular, in a variety of forms of necrotizing vasculitis, both idiopathic types such as Wegener's granulomatosis and polyarteritis nodosa (PAN) as well as in vasculitis associated with connective tissue diseases such as rheumatoid arthritis. It will examine the evidence of benefit in these diseases and look at the role of intermittent as opposed to continuous therapy. Side effects will be discussed and the possible mechanism of action of the drug will be briefly considered.

2.1. Use of Cyclophosphamide in Necrotizing Vasculitides

This group includes the syndromes in which serious end-organ damage or death are common in the untreated case. Necrotizing vascular inflammation can involve almost any body system alone or in combination, and there is an overlap in many of the clinical, laboratory, and histological features in these disorders. Indeed, at one time rheumatoid vasculitis and polyarteritis nodosa were thought to be part of the same entity (Ellman and Ball, 1948).

2.1.1. Wegener's Granulomatosis

Wegener (1936) described this condition in three cases of what he took to be an infectious disease with a poor prognosis. The characteristic triad of upper and/or lower respiratory tract necrotizing lesions in association with a focal segmental necrotizing glomerulonephritis and a systemic vasculitis was defined by Godman and Churg (1954). The common features at presentation include constitutional upset, pulmonary involvement, renal disease, evidence of an acute-phase response, low hemoglobin, and raised white cell count and platelets.

Novack and Pearson (1971) were the first to point out that in Wegener's granulomatosis, cyclophosphamide had a dramatic effect. This was later extensively confirmed by the NIH group (Fauci and Wolff, 1973; Wolff *et al.*, 1974). The survival time, in their untreated cases, was five months, and in those treated with steroids alone, 12 months. With continuous low-dose oral cyclophosphamide there was an 80% five-year survival. The same group is now talking about cures in this hitherto uniformly fatal disease (Fauci *et al.*, 1983). In our experience of 22 patients studied over an eight-year period (mean follow-up two years), the overall mortality was 37.5% despite the aggressive use of cytotoxic agents, prednisolone, and plasma exchange. Therefore, the prognosis in this disease remains serious; cyclophosphamide, or other cytotoxic agents, are not a panacea. Earlier referral for therapy is one part of the answer since tissue necrosis inevitably leaves scars and functional impairment.

2.1.2. Limited Wegener's Granulomatosis

Classical Wegener's granulomatosis has long been described as a generalized disease, but sporadic reports in the literature suggest that there are more limited forms of the disease. Carrington and Liebow (1966) described 16 cases with no evidence of renal involvement despite classical histological changes in the lungs. However, at postmortem it was noted that in five of the patients there was microscopic evidence of granulomatous lesions that in life had not manifested in any clinically detectable abnormality. Whether these patients are simply at an early stage of their disease or whether they are in fact a separate *forme fruste* has not yet been established, since long-term follow-up of these cases (apart from one single report) has not been described. In addition, some authors (Anderson and Stravides, 1978; Woodworth *et al.*, 1987) have described the reverse situation, with renal involvement (focal necrotizing glomerulonephritis in each case) predating the appearance of the respiratory tract lesions. A comparison between our group of nine patients with limited Wegener's and 16 with classical Wegener's demonstrated significant differences in their clinical presentation, laboratory features, and outcome. The group with limited disease had significantly less constitutional upset or pulmonary disease; the hemoglobin, white cell count, and platelet count tended to be normal. Although the mortality was low (no deaths after two years' mean follow-up), limited Wegener's can nevertheless be locally very destructive, and in our experience immunosuppressive therapy is required at this stage. We have noted progression to classical Wegener's disease in one patient despite cyclophosphamide and prednisolone treatment.

Recent evidence is emerging that the antibiotic trimethoprim/sulfamethoxazole may be of value in the treatment of the classical form of the disease (DeRemee *et al.*, 1985; West *et al.*, 1987; Axelson *et al.*, 1987). The mechanism of action may be truly anti-infective. If infection is at least in part responsible for the manifestations of the disease, then the most likely site of entry of an organism is the upper respiratory tract. Thus it would be reasonable to postulate that antibiotics have a place in the treatment of limited Wegener's and might even obviate the need for more toxic immunosuppressive therapy. Alternative mechanisms of action, such as radicle scavenging, are also possible. Of the five cases we have treated with trimethoprim/sulfamethoxazole, three responded favorably. The improvement was highlighted when they accidentally ran out of tablets and noticed a return of upper respiratory tract symptoms, which responded to restarting the drug.

2.1.3. Polyarteritis Nodosa

This disease has a similar clinical picture of severe multisystem disease to Wegener's but without the consistent involvement of the upper and lower respiratory tract (Rose and Spencer, 1957). The untreated survival is very poor in many series, particularly in the elderly. The use of steroids on their own improved the one-year survival to 71% in an early study but had much less effect on the long-term survival (Pickering *et al.*, 1960). Leib *et al.* (1979) have demonstrated the important therapeutic role of cytotoxic drugs (using mainly azathioprine). Their series consisted of 64 cases seen over a 22-year period, the treatments being nonrandomized, with cytotoxic agents being used in only the most severely affected group. They were able to demonstrate significantly longer mean survival (149 months) and an 80% five-year survival in the patients given cytotoxic agents compared to 53% on steroids alone (mean survival 63 months) or 12% on no treatment (mean survival 3 months).

Our own experience from Bristol supported this (Scott *et al.*, 1982). The mortality was high in the untreated group from a district general hospital; in some of those who died early in the course of the disease, the diagnosis was made at postmortem. The steroids gave apparent short-term benefit, but there was still a two-thirds mortality. In the small group who were given cyclophosphamide together with steroids, the mortality was only 25%. Comparison of these cases from 1974 to 1980 with our more recent data in our renal and rheumatological units gives a clear view of the overall change in prognosis as well as some factors relating to prognosis (Table I). The former group were largely in a precyclophosphamide era and the majority received steroids alone. The latter two groups all had cyclophosphamide with none having steroid alone. The overall mortality in the first group was 53%; the second group who presented to our nephrology unit with severe renal involvement in the majority, often in renal failure requiring dialysis, had a 40.5% mortality; the final group who presented to the rheumatology unit had much less renal involvement and had no deaths after a mean follow-up of 3.9 years. It is interesting that the main cause of death in the early group was active vasculitis, supplemented by complications of vasculitis such as hypertension. Only one patient died of sepsis but this was the biggest single cause of death in the later renal group. Thus while mortality due to vasculitis has diminished, the problem of sepsis has become more prominent and is related to therapy. The recent series reported from Minneapolis also highlighted the problem of sepsis (Bradley *et al.*, 1989).

TABLE I. Polyarteritis Nodosa[a]

	Pre-1980 (37)[b]	Post-1980	
		Renal (74)	Rheumatology (14)
Age (mean, range)	61 (29–77)	57 (19–77)	51 (34–75)
Sex (male:female)	1.3:1	1.6:1	1:1
Deaths	53%	40.5%	0%
Clinical findings			
Constitutional	>70%	98.6%	85.7%
Cutaneous	51%	28.4%	42.9%
Cardiovascular	56%	28.4%	0%
Pulmonary	65%	56.8%	57.1%
Abdominal	78%	5.4%	25%
Renal	76%	95.9%	25%
Neurological	>24%	12.2%	57.1%
Ophthalmic	5%	16.2%	57.1%
ENT		21.6%	31.3%
Musculoskeletal	62%	37.8%	91%

[a]This table compares our experience before and after 1980. In the post-1980 group we have divided the patients according to whether they presented to the renal or rheumatology departments. The clinical features described are cumulative and were confirmed by histological or radiological examination in most cases. In the pre-1980 group many cases were only diagnosed at post-mortem, whereas all the post-1980 group were diagnosed in life.
[b]Number of patients in the group.

One group of patients appears to have a less favorable response to cyclophosphamide. This is the group of patients with microscopic PAN, a term suggested by Davson and colleagues (1948) and based on careful pathological analysis. In our own patients with microscopic PAN and significant renal impairment, the mortality was 38% despite aggressive therapy (Adu et al., 1987), showing that the situation is still far from ideal in this group. This is not a unique experience since the mortality in the literature ranges from 20 to 50% (Droz et al., 1979; Serra et al., 1984; Savage et al., 1985).

Risk factors for poor outcome include age, significantly elevated serum creatinine (greater than 500 μmole/liter) at onset, oliguria, and the presence of crescents on renal histology.

2.1.4. Rheumatoid Vasculitis

We use the term systemic rheumatoid vasculitis (SRV) to refer to patients with rheumatoid arthritis who have clinical and/or histological evidence of vasculitis, or who have nailfold infarcts in the presence of significant extraarticular features. Cutaneous lesions are one of the most common lesions of SRV (Scott et al., 1981c). In 1948, Ellman and Ball suggested that the necrotizing vasculitis complicating rheumatoid disease was the exact equivalent of polyarteritis nodosa. The histology is identical and the clinical picture bears many similarities (Ball, 1954; Sokoloff and Bunim, 1957). Thus there is a definite overlap between these lesions and systemic necrotizing rheumatoid vasculitis. However, our own investigations suggest that the pathogenesis of the histologically identical lesions of systemic rheumatoid vasculitis is very different from that of PAN. In SRV, high levels of IgG rheumatoid factor and complement-fixing rheumatoid factor-containing immune complexes are found that correlate well with clinical features (Scott et al., 1981a). These are not present in PAN (Allen et al., 1981). Brief improvement is seen following removal of circulating complexes by plasma exchange (Scott et al., 1981b). SRV is a serious condition that is often relapsing and has a significant and cumulative mortality (Scott et al., 1981c). We are not referring here to the isolated finding of typical nail edge/nailfold vasculitis of rheumatoid arthritis that clearly involves small vessels and does not, per se, require cytotoxic therapy. Cytotoxic drugs appear to delay the relapse seen after plasma exchange, with azathioprine being less effective than cyclophosphamide.

In the case of steroids alone, there is some evidence that they may actually be a factor inducing the vasculitis of SRV (Kemper et al., 1957; Vollertsen et al., 1986). Other authors have used cyclophosphamide (Weisman and Zvaiffler, 1975) or chlorambucil (Kahn et al., 1967) with success, but not azathioprine. The only double-blind placebo-controlled study in rheumatoid vasculitis utilized azathioprine and was abandoned due to deaths in both groups (Nicholls et al., 1973). In our experience of over 100 cases, cyclophosphamide is the drug of choice in SRV but no formal study has been performed.

2.1.5. Behçet's Syndrome

Since the original paper by Behçet (1937), diagnostic criteria have been drawn up for this condition that predominantly affects mucous membranes, skin, joints, the uveal tract, and central nervous system (predominantly the brain stem). These have been reviewed by Shimizu (1977), who reported on the prevalence of the disease in Japan (up to 80 cases/100,000 in some areas) and described the vasculitic lesions seen in a series of 81 well-documented cases. Pathological studies have confirmed that it affects blood vessels of all sizes.

Although the initial treatment tended to be with colchicine (Mizushima *et al.*, 1982), this was found to be inferior to the use of chlorambucil (O'Duffy *et al.*, 1984) at 0.2 mg/kg per day with a gradual tapering of the dose. However, since then the latter drug has been reevaluated and not found to be useful in the most significant and common lesion of Behçet's namely the uveitis. Tabbara (1983) reported that in ten male patients with ocular Behçet's, seven were rendered oligospermic and three azoospermic by chlorambucil, without any significant improvement in their eye lesions (75% of their eyes had a visual acuity of 20/200 or worse). In a recent study comparing colchicine with cyclosporine A, it was shown that cyclosporine A was superior in the uveitis of Behçet's (Masuda *et al.*, 1989). It also helped the mucosal and skin manifestations of the disease. It was stressed in this paper, however, that patients with neurological involvement were specifically excluded from this series, presumably due to the neurotoxicity of cyclosporine A making it difficult to assess any new neurological features. A trial of azathioprine compared with placebo in 73 patients with Behçet's (of whom 48 had eye disease) showed that this drug was effective, both in terms of eye disease and the other manifestations (Yazici *et al.*, 1990).

2.1.6. Churg–Strauss Syndrome

In the original description of this disorder in 1957 (Churg and Strauss, 1957), it was shown to be a separate disease from polyarteritis nodosa. There was more of a tendency to involve the upper and lower respiratory tract, as with Wegener's disease, but with asthma as a regular feature. The pathological lesions closely resembled those seen in polyarteritis nodosa, but often showed distinguishing granulomatous features. Later work (Finan and Winkelmann, 1983) could not confirm that granulomata could be used as a distinguishing feature, however, and the disease is considered by many to be a variant of PAN.

Lanham *et al.* (1984) attempted to define it as a triad of asthma, eosinophilia, and a systemic vasculitis involving two or more extrapulmonary organs. In their experience, steroids alone were beneficial, although four of their series of 16 cases were given cytotoxic agents, and three had additional plasma exchange. Chumbley *et al.* (1977) also found that steroids alone were useful. However, their five-year survival is only 62%, suggesting that the long-term prognosis might have been improved by the addition of cytotoxic agents. A recent large study from France (Guillevin *et al.*, 1988) combined data on polyarteritis nodosa and Churg-Strauss syndrome, which the authors considered to be inseparable. In their experience there was no statistically significant treatment benefit from the use of cyclophosphamide in terms of outcome; but the mortality was high in their steroid-only group and they did not use cyclophosphamide as aggressively as we do. In our more limited experience of four cases, there was a poor response to steroids alone, and all our patients have done well on intermittent high-dose cyclophosphamide and prednisolone.

2.1.7. Primary Angiitis of the Nervous System

Originally described by Cravioto and Feigin in 1959, the syndrome of vasculitis limited to the central nervous system has recently been extensively reviewed by Sigal (1987) and also by Calabrese and Mallek (1987). The latter authors proposed diagnostic criteria for the condition that include unexplained neurological features after extensive clinical and laboratory assessment together with evidence of vasculitis on cerebral angiography or histology of central nervous tissue, but without evidence of systemic vasculitis. Their approach to therapy of the eight cases they had managed was very successful (only one death, and no neurological deficit in the remaining seven). This compared favorably with that in the previously reported literature where they cited a 71% mortality and half of the survivors had residual deficits. Treatment regimens were variable, including no treatment, steroids alone, and steroids in combination with cytotoxic drugs. There was no clear relationship between treatment and outcome in these cases, however. In Sigal's review, there was a very strong survival advantage over no treatment (with 36/36 deaths) in those patients given either steroids alone (4/18 deaths) or in combination with cytotoxic drugs (0/6 deaths). There was a greater tendency to improve the neurological features with the addition of cytotoxic agents.

2.1.8. Mucocutaneous Lymph Node Syndrome

Kawasaki (1967) described 50 patients aged between two months and nine years, of whom over half were under the age of two years. He later published in English his further experience of this relatively new disease (Kawasaki *et al.*, 1974), describing his group's experience of over 6000 cases in Japan up to 1973 and a mortality of 1–2% chiefly from cardiovascular causes. The disease has also been recognized in other countries, but not as frequently. This is an acute febrile illness of unknown etiology, which can result in coronary artery aneurysms or ectasia in 15–25% of children with the disease.

The initial treatment was aspirin for the fever and as an antithrombotic agent (Kusakawa, 1983). A Japanese study (Furosho *et al.*, 1984) suggested that high-dose intravenous gamma globulin might prevent the development of coronary artery aneurysms. In a multicenter study of 85 children who were randomized to receive either aspirin or high-dose intravenous gamma globulin (IVGG), they found that the incidence of coronary artery lesions (aneurysm or dilatation) was 42% in the aspirin group, but significantly less (15%) in the IVGG group. This was later confirmed by Newburger *et al.* (1986) in a multicenter, randomized U.S. trial comparing the effect of aspirin alone with aspirin and high-dose IVGG (400 mg/kg per day for four days). A total of 168 children took part in the study, and there was a significant advantage in terms of the frequency of coronary artery abnormalities in the group given IVGG. The rationale for using this was not entirely clear, but they suggested that saturation of Fc receptors on platelets and endothelial cells might prevent endothelial damage. Since then they have gone on to demonstrate endothelial cell abnormalities consistent with their hypothesis in a small group of children (Leung *et al.*, 1989). They showed increased expression of adhesion molecules on skin blood vessel endothelium in untreated subjects, which reverted toward normal after treatment in line with an improvement in clinical response.

Thus IVGG appears to be the treatment of choice in this disease. Aspirin is still considered necessary for its antithrombotic action. It should be stressed that steroids have no effect in this disease, and may be expected to have an adverse effect on outcome.

2.2. Cyclophosphamide Regimens

2.2.1. Pulse versus Continuous Therapy in Rheumatoid Vasculitis

We have experimented with several regimens of cyclophosphamide in order to deliver a large dose of the drug at intervals for maximal efficiency while trying to minimize side effects (Hall *et al.*, 1979; Bacon, 1979). We have devised a regimen of intermittent bolus doses of cyclophosphamide combined with methylprednisolone in our patients that in SRV appears to be more successful than continuous oral regimens (Scott and Bacon, 1984). The protocol for our current regimen is outlined in Table II. The results of the 1984 study of rheumatoid vasculitis showed a higher incidence of early healing in the group given intermittent high-dose cyclophosphamide and prednisolone compared to other treatments. This included

TABLE II. Dose Schedules for High-Dose Intermittent Cyclophosphamide and Prednisolone
with Alterations for Age, Renal Function, and Marrow Toxicity[a]

	Cyclophosphamide 15 mg/kg[a] (up to 1000 mg/bolus)[b]	Prednisolone 10 mg/kg (up to 1000 mg/bolus)
Renal impairment		
For serum creatinine:		
<150 μmole/liter	15 mg/kg	10 mg/kg
150–250 μmole/liter	10 mg/kg	10 mg/kg
251–500 μmole/liter	7.5 mg/kg	10 mg/kg
>500 μmole/liter	5 mg/kg	7 mg/kg
Marrow toxicity	Stop until blood count returns to within normal range; reduce dose by 25%	10 mg/kg
Previous cytotoxic agents	Stop previous drugs; wait two weeks before commencing bolus	10 mg/kg
Age >70 years	10 mg/kg	10 mg/kg

[a]Usual dose.
[b]Each bolus dose is given either as an intravenous infusion in one day (prednisolone followed by cyclophosphamide) or orally as the same total dose as the intravenous regimen, divided over a three-day period. Bolus doses are given at increasing intervals with clinical response.

improvement in mononeuritis multiplex seen in all three patients thus treated. Improvement was apparent within 24 hr in some patients, which compares to the two or more weeks required for improvement with oral therapy (Scott and Bacon, 1984). The incidence of late relapse in patients on intermittent therapy was half that of the patients treated with oral low-dose continuous regimens. In these patients, intermittent cyclophosphamide was usually used to induce remission and they were later put on regular oral maintenance cyclophosphamide or azathioprine in combination with prednisolone at a gradually tapering dose. The latter regimen in particular had a high relapse rate. Our current experience suggests that the use of intermittent oral cyclophosphamide over a longer period diminishes the late relapse rate further. Finally, intermittent cyclophosphamide appeared to affect the survival in these patients. Although the crude mortality was the same for both groups, the patients on intermittent therapy actually had more severe disease.

In Table III we have compared our series of patients with SRV treated before 1980 (pre-1980) with our current patients in Birmingham (post-1980). Although there are some differences in clinical features (e.g., much more cardiovascular and pulmonary involvement in the earlier series), there are some important conclusions to draw from this comparison. First, the relapse rate in our later series is minimal and similar in both treatment groups. It should be noted, in the later series, that of the patients not given high-dose intermittent cyclophosphamide and prednisolone as an initial treatment, five were subsequently treated in this way due to relapse (i.e., the overall relapse rate on intermittent therapy was extremely low). However, the overall mortality is higher on this therapy. This, of course, reflects the fact that many of these patients were severely ill since therapy was not randomized. However, it must be noted that many of the deaths were as a result of infection.

2.2.2. Pulse Therapy in Other Systemic Necrotizing Vasculitides

The intermittent intravenous regimen of cyclophosphamide combined with methylprednisolone has now been extended by our group. Twenty-nine cases of systemic rheuma-

TABLE III. A Comparison of Rheumatoid Vasculitis Treated
before and after 1980 by Our Group[a]

	Pre-1980		Post-1980	
	Pulse C/P	Other	Pulse C/P	Other
N	21	24	11	21
Age (mean, range)	62 (44–77)	61 (38–79)	52 (25–70)	60 (36–75)
Sex (male:female)	0.9:1	1.2:1	0.8:1	0.3:1
Relapse	24%	54%	9%	9.5%
Deaths	24%	29%	36.4%	23.8%
Clinical findings				
Cutaneous	>78%	>70%	72.7%	80.9%
Cardiovascular	34%	18%	0%	4.8%
Pulmonary	38%	30%	9%	9.5%
Peripheral	52%	25%	9%	38.1%
Neuropathy				
CNS	—	—	18.2%	0%
Ophthalmic	14%	12%	0%	0%

[a]We have separated the treatment groups based on their initial management, comparing the outcome and cumulative clinical features (confirmed by biopsy or radiology in most cases). It should be noted that in the post-1980 group, five cases who relapsed on other therapy were subsequently controlled on pulse cyclophosphamide and prednisolone.

toid vasculitis have been treated as well as 15 patients with other systemic necrotizing vasculitis including polyarteritis nodosa, Wegener's granulomatosis, aortitis, and lupus vasculitis. The results in these patients have been compared with those treated with oral cyclophosphamide. It is clear that the mortality in the intravenous group was as low as the best results obtained with oral cyclophosphamide. Interestingly, the late relapse rate was considerably lower in those on the intermittent regimen.

2.2.3. Intermittent Oral versus Intravenous

Recently we extended the idea of intermittent doses to use oral rather than intravenous therapy. The same total dose of cyclophosphamide was used, 15 mg/kg, but spread over three consecutive days (i.e., at 5 mg/kg per day). A single oral dose of prednisolone, ranging from 200 mg down to 60 mg/day (judged by disease severity and progressively diminished), was given with each dose of cyclophosphamide. Thus the total amount of steroid given was reduced each time. This regimen has been given as the initial therapy in the treatment of at least 35 of our patients with a number of necrotizing vasculitides including rheumatoid vasculitis, PAN, and Wegener's granulomatosis. It appears to be associated with a lower mortality and no increase in the relapse rate when compared to the use of continuous oral cyclophosphamide and prednisolone.

With improved prognosis the side effects of these drugs become important. This has been examined for the different regimens. The most prominent side effect is nausea and vomiting but this is usually easy controlled with antiemetics. The mechanism is probably central, but with the oral intermittent regimen, gastric perforation requiring surgery has occurred in two patients. Why this happened is not clear, but these two patients had been on nonsteroidals as well as other drugs. Despite this, we routinely use an H_2-antagonist given at night during the period of the oral intermittent regimen. The other side effects appear to be diminished by the intermittent regimen. The incidence of cystitis was definitely lower, although it is still important to have a high fluid intake on the days of the oral regimen in particular. We have not found it necessary to use methyl cysteine as a bladder protectant in patients on intermittent cyclophosphamide. This is supported by the NIH study of lupus nephritis treated by intermittent bolus cyclophosphamide (Austin *et al.*, 1986). These studies have led us to the conclusion that the intermittent regimen can be a useful way to give these drugs.

The use of repeated boluses of steroid alone may cause problems, particularly in patients with advanced renal failure as evidenced by the group with microscopic polyarteritis. The use of intravenous bolus cyclophosphamide combined with a single dose of methylprednisolone appears to have definite benefits in a wide variety of types of necrotizing vasculitis. It produces rapid improvement and is still the simplest way to initiate therapy in severely ill patients. However, the use of intermittent oral pulses are much easier to manage on a long term from patients' point of view. This appears to diminish the side effects except the gastrointestinal ones, which can be controlled with an antiemetic plus an H_2-antagonist. We have used this both as initial therapy in a range of patients and as longer-term therapy after two or more IV boluses in patients who have severe clinical problems.

2.2.4. Mechanisms of Action of Cyclophosphamide

We have shown benefit from cyclophosphamide in patients with the necrotizing vasculitis of PAN as well as that of SRV. However, the pathogenesis of these two diseases appears different despite their histological similarities. Cyclophosphamide even appears to favorably influence the giant cell arteritis of Takayasu's, which has an entirely different histological appearance. There is thus confusion as to the mechanism of action. In SRV we have demonstrated elevated levels of IgG rheumatoid factors and of complement-fixing immune complexes in patients with active disease (Scott *et al.*, 1981a). Following therapy, levels of both the IgG rheumatoid factor and the immune complexes fall, suggesting immunosuppressant action at the B-cell level with diminished formation of autoantibodies and immune complexes. We have also found increased levels of circulating activated T cells in such patients that again fall with therapy (along with a reduction in IgG rheumatoid factor). By contrast, in PAN, relevant complement-fixing immune complexes are rare (except in the few cases associated with hepatitis B). In addition, we do not find elevated levels of activated T cells in these patients using a variety of markers. Therefore, the mechanism(s) of action of cyclophosphamide in this PAN is unlikely to be through these immunological pathways. *In vitro* experiments using an assay of indium release from cultured endothelial cells as an assay of cytotoxicity does suggest that both lymphocytes and serum can mediate endothelial cell cytotoxicity in SRV. A similar picture with lymphocyte-mediated cellular cytotoxicity is seen in Takayasu's arteritis. Serial data in individual patients with either rheumatoid vasculitis or Takayasu's arteritis show that the fall in *in vitro* cytotoxicity is temporally related to the clinical improvement following cyclophosphamide.

It is likely that the cyclophosphamide is affecting the cells mediating the vascular damage in these diseases rather than the underlying trigger factors. In necrotizing vasculitis, polymorph-mediated damage may be stimulated by either immune complexes or by free radicals (Cochrane and Aikin, 1966; Cochrane, 1968), indicating that polymorphs may also be a target of cyclophosphamide. Lymphocytes of both natural killer lineage and activated cytotoxic CD8+ cells could mediate endothelial cell damage via appropriate receptors, and again they may both be affected by cyclophosphamide. This is in addition to the depressed antibody and immune complex formation following its effect on B cells. Cyclophosphamide may have a direct effect on endothelial cells both to diminish surface receptor expression of adhesion molecules and to diminish cytokine release. A final interesting effect of cyclophosphamide in rheumatoid disease is the way it appears to shift patients across the clinical and immune spectrum (see Figure 21.1). We have previously speculated that there are separate immunopathogenetic mechanisms that form the basis of rheumatoid disease (Bacon, 1979): vasculitis, synovitis, and granulomata (rheumatoid nodules). Oral cyclophosphamide is an effective treatment for rheumatoid synovitis, although the intermittent regimens are less than successful (Hall *et al.*, 1979). In SRV we have observed a number of patients who have developed a flare-up in their joint disease simultaneously with improvement in vasculitis following intermittent bolus cyclophosphamide (Bacon, 1987). It is interesting that the use of steroids and gold for rheumatoid synovitis have on occasion been associated with the development of rheumatoid vasculitis. This is not a universal pathway, since Willkens *et al.* (personal communication) have noted that methotrexate for rheumatoid synovitis can be associated with the development of rheumatoid nodules and our experience is similar. This effect may not depend on preexisting synovitis, since we have seen five patients whose joint disease developed during or soon after the treatment of vasculitis with cyclophosphamide.

2.2.5. Side Effects

Toxic effects of cyclophosphamide are a problem. The bladder toxicity is well known, due chiefly to the effect of acrolein, one of its urinary metabolites. As well as causing hemorrhagic cystitis and bladder fibrosis, it has been associated with bladder carcinoma. Stillwell *et al.* (1988) reviewed their group of 111 patients with Wegener's disease treated with cyclophosphamide. Hemorrhagic cystitis occurred in 17 cases, of whom three later developed

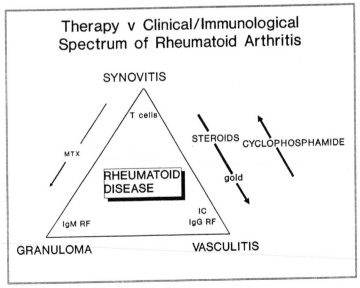

FIGURE 21.1.   This illustrates a model for the ways in which various aspects of therapy for RA can affect the clinical presentation, especially of systemic disease. The best-documented shifts occur with steroids inducing SRV and intermittent cyclophosphamide (for SRV) causing a flare-up in inactive synovitis. Other shifts may come to light, since no current therapy for RA cures the disease. IC, Immune complexes; RF, rheumatoid factor; MTX, methotrexate.

bladder carcinoma. All these cases were given continuous oral therapy, and this is in contrast to the experience of using intermittent high-dose intravenous cyclophosphamide where bladder toxicity is rare (Austin *et al.*, 1986).

Suppression of the immune system inevitably exposes patients to potentially serious infections, and was recently reviewed by Bradley *et al.* (1989). In their 15 patients with various types of vasculitis, treated with daily oral cyclophosphamide and steroids, ten patients developed significant infections, of whom two died. There did not appear to be any clear relationship between dose or degree of leukopenia and the infective episode. Although this paper highlighted the potential for severe infections, the proportion of patients with problems was considerably higher than our own experience and those of others (Fauci *et al.*, 1983).

Long-term effects of cyclophosphamide administration may be even more worrisome. *In vitro* work has demonstrated an increased frequency of hypoxanthine-guanine phosphoribosyl transferase mutants in T-cell clones (Palmer *et al.*, 1988) and of increased sister chromatid exchange in peripheral blood mononuclear cells derived from patients treated with cyclophosphamide (Palmer *et al.*, 1986). The end result of these observed abnormalities of DNA has not been established at a clinical level, but are clearly a cause for concern. Baker *et al.* (1987) described the delayed onset of a variety of malignant diseases including bladder carcinoma in patients with rheumatoid arthritis treated with cyclophosphamide. There appeared to be a relationship to total dose and duration of therapy with the incidence of malignancy.

In view of the potential problems of low-dose oral continuous therapy both in the short and in the long term, we have tended to favor the use of high-dose intermittent cyclophosphamide.

2.2.6. Dose Modifications

Dose modification for renal disease, age, and marrow toxicity induced either by previous (recent) use of other cytotoxic agents or by cyclophosphamide are suggested in Table II, based on our current practice for bolus therapy. Similar reductions in cyclophosphamide dose are recommended when using the low-dose oral continuous regimen.

3. THERAPY OF NONNECROTIZING SYSTEMIC VASCULITIDES

3.1. Giant Cell Arteritis/Polymyalgia Rheumatica

The earliest descriptions of these two conditions (Bruce, 1888; Hutchinson, 1890) were of separate entities, but subsequently the considerable overlap of the two diseases (up to 50% in one series by Goodman in 1979) in many patients has led most workers in this field to regard them as either a single disease or as two ends of a spectrum of disease. They are both characterized by constitutional upset in patients over the age of 50, often with an elevated ESR. In polymyalgia rheumatica there is early morning stiffness and discomfort in the hip and shoulder girdles, whereas giant cell arteritis (GCA) often produces severe headaches, jaw and tongue claudication, and visual loss. The value of temporal artery biopsy before or within one week of commencing steroid therapy (Allison and Gallagher, 1984) is considerable in GCA, but characteristic giant cells may also be seen in cases of PMR [14.3% of cases of pure PMR in one series (Delecoeuillerie *et al.*, 1988)].

The treatment of both syndromes is with prednisolone, although this is felt to have little effect on the underlying pathogenetic mechanisms, which may involve lymphocyte subset changes (CD 4$^+$ cells have been found in affected vessels by Andersson et al. in 1987). This might explain the relapse rate on stopping steroid therapy (Dasgupta et al., 1989). Azathioprine has been used with considerable success in steroid resistant cases (De Silva and Hazelman, 1986).

3.2. Takayasu's Arteritis

In 1908, Takayasu, a Japanese ophthalmologist, first described a curious retinopathy with anastomosis of arteries and veins in a young woman. The condition was later associated with diminished upper limb pulses, and the condition that bears his name was defined. Inada (1977) classified the disease according to which parts of the aorta were affected based on his series of 83 cases over a 15-year period. The disease only affects elastic arteries (i.e., large arteries) and the pathological findings can vary from granulomatous or inflammatory to fibrosis in the late stages (Nasu, 1977).

Therapy of this disease tends to be with prednisolone only. Hall and colleagues (1985) reported a five-year survival of 94% in their series of 32 Caucasian cases. They found a good response to steroids: 16 patients had absent pulses, and with steroids, eight patients had a return of pulses. Nevertheless, 12 patients eventually required reconstructive surgery. The ESR was found to be a useful guide to disease activity, but the duration of therapy required was undetermined. In a series of 20 patients followed for a mean of 4.6 years, results were similar (Shelhamer, 1985). Of the 16 patients given steroids, eight responded well while six had progressive disease. The latter group were given additional cyclophosphamide with benefit in four patients. The authors suggested that cyclophosphamide would be a useful adjunct to cases resistant to steroids alone. Our experience has been similar. Of six patients treated, only two responded to steroids alone, while the other four did well with the addition of high-dose intermittent cyclophosphamide.

4. OTHER IMMUNOSUPPRESSIVE THERAPIES IN VASCULITIS

Many of these are used in a wide variety of settings both within and outside the scope of rheumatology. There are many comprehensive reviews of individual agents (Steinberg et al., 1972; Fauci et al., 1976; Fauci, 1985) and in this chapter we have summarized some of those used in our practice.

4.1. Azathioprine

The usual dose of azathioprine in vasculitis is 1.5–2 mg/kg per day usually combined with prednisolone. Marrow suppression may warrant dosage adjustment and it is our practice to temporarily stop therapy and then reintroduce it at a 25% reduction in the previous dose when the total white cell count and platelet count reach the normal range. Other effects include gastrointestinal intolerance and rarely hepatotoxicity. Although there may be long-term effects, which may include the induction of lymphoid tumors (Rosman, 1973), the drug has been used safely in pregnancy (Schein and Winokur, 1975).

It serves a very useful role in a steroid-sparing capacity in the treatment of resistant polymyalgia rheumatica/giant cell arteritis (De Silva and Hazelman, 1986). Although it was used successfully in the induction of remission of polyarteritis nodosa in the study by Leib *et al.* (1979), azathioprine has been superseded by cyclophosphamide in necrotizing vas-culitides. Many groups are using it as a maintenance therapy, after cyclophosphamide, and this is currently the subject of a controlled, randomized prospective study in our unit.

4.2. Cyclosporine A

This compound has recently been extensively reviewed by Kahan (1989). It originates from *Tolypocladium inflatum Gams* and in recent years has been widely used as an immuno-suppressant agent. Wendling *et al.* (1985) recorded the successful use of cyclosporine A in two patients with giant cell arteritis (one of whom had Takayasu's arteritis) who had failed to respond adequately to steroids alone. Three cases of Wegener's granulomatosis, which were resistant to cyclophosphamide, achieved stabilization of renal function as well as overall clinical improvement (Borleffs *et al.*, 1987; Gremmel *et al.*, 1988). The combination of cyclosporine A with other immunosuppressive agents in clinical practice make it difficult to delineate its own toxic effects, but since it does not damage polymorphonuclear leukocytes or pulmonary alveolar macrophages (Drath and Kahan, 1984), it is less likely to predispose to bacterial and fungal infections.

4.3. Therapeutic Apheresis

The problem with cytotoxic agents is that they are immunosuppressive in a wide variety of ways. More selective therapy might diminish the side effects and aid an understanding of disease mechanisms. Plasmapheresis has the attraction of immediately removing soluble mediators of inflammation from the circulation. It may have a more prolonged effect by improving reticuloendothelial function, and thus immune complex clearance, an effect persisting after the end of the exchange (Lockwood *et al.*, 1979).

Hind *et al.* (1983) were able to demonstrate that patients with rapidly progressive glomerulonephritis who were dialysis-dependent (but did not have antiglomerular basement membrane disease) tended to recover renal function better if steroids and immunosuppres-sive agents were combined with plasma exchange. Unfortunately there was considerable mortality in their group (15/27 of the patients without antiglomerular basement membrane disease), often due to sepsis. It has been well recognized that the combination of plasma exchange with immunosuppressive agents can predispose to a very high risk of serious infections (Wing *et al.*, 1980; Lhote *et al.*, 1988).

In our experience with vasculitis, it had little benefit except in the very short term (Scott *et al.*, 1981b). It has been most extensively investigated with SRV. In this condition, there is a prompt fall in complement-fixing immune complexes and in IgG rheumatoid factor levels associated with clinical improvement during plasma exchange; the IgM rheumatoid factor titers showed little change. Complement levels may actually fall further during exchange. The clinical benefit is largely to halt the development of new lesions. Very little healing of existing lesions occurred during plasma exchange and the relapse rate was high unless cyclophosphamide was added to the regimen. Using bolus intermittent cyclo-phosphamide, there was very little evidence of any additional benefit from adding plasma exchange. Dwosh and colleagues (1983) concluded that there was no benefit over a sham procedure in patients with rheumatoid arthritis despite improvement in laboratory variables. Lymphocyte depletion has been used in the technique of lymphapheresis in a number of centers. A controlled trial from the NIH showed that it was indeed effective in rheumatoid arthritis (Wallace *et al.*, 1981), but less so than the uncontrolled data had suggested (Goldman *et al.*, 1979).

5. CONCLUSIONS

Cyclophosphamide represents a real advance in the therapy of a wide range of vasculitides (particularly the necrotizing vasculitides, which previously had a poor prognosis). Cyclophosphamide is usually combined with steroids and may be used in a variety of ways. Intermittent regimens can be given to increase the dose of cyclophosphamide at any one time, which may produce more rapid benefit. The increased interval between the doses may account for the diminished side effects seen with the intermittent regimens. An intermittent intravenous cyclophosphamide and methylprednisolone combination can be used for seriously ill patients, but the dose needs to be tailored for diminished renal function. An oral intermittent regimen forms a useful and easy to manage maintenance therapy. It should be stressed that the low-dose oral continuous regimens are equally successful in treating vasculitis, but in view of their side effects, we tend to favor the high-dose intermittent regimen. In cases responding well, the duration of total therapy is still undetermined. The risk of relapse must be balanced against the risks of therapy and this will vary for different diseases. The dose interval can be increased in the latter months with the intermittent regimens. Despite all of these advantages, the blanket immunosuppressive effect of cyclophosphamide is clearly a disadvantage. Mathieson *et al.* (1990) have successful used monoclonal antibody therapy in a case of intractable systemic vasculitis, raising the possibility of specifically targeting certain cells such as lymphocytes, which are thought to be responsible for the disease, while sparing other blood cells such as neutrophils, which would reduce the incidence of adverse effects. The future may lie in exploring combinations of cytotoxic drugs with semiselective immunomodulating actions.

REFERENCES

Abdou, N. I., Zweimann, B., and Casella, S. R., 1973, The effects of azathioprine therapy on bone marrow dependent and thymus dependent cells in man, *Clin. Exp. Immunol.* **13**:55–64.

Adu, D., Howie, A. J., Scott, D. G. I., Bacon, P. A., McGonigle, R. J. S., and Michael, J., 1987, Polyarteritis and the kidney, *Q. J. Med.* **62**:221–237.

Allen, C., Elson, C. J., Scott, D. G. I., Bacon, P. A., and Bucknall, R. C., 1981, IgG antiglobulins in rheumatoid arthritis and other arthritides: Relationship with clinical features and other parameters, *Ann. Rheum. Dis.* **40**:127–131.

Allison, M. C., and Gallagher, P. J., 1984, Temporal artery biopsy and corticosteroid treatment, *Ann. Rheum. Dis.* **43**:416–417.

Anderson, C. L., and Stravides, A., 1978, Rapidly progressive renal failure as the primary manifestation of Wegener's granulomatosis, *Am. J. Med. Sci.* **275**:109–112.

Andersson, R., Jonsson, R., Tarkowski, A., Begtsson, B.-A., and Malmvall, B.-E., 1987, T cell subsets and expression of immunological activation markers in the arterial walls of patients with giant cell arteritis, *Ann. Rheum. Dis.* **46**:915–923.

Austin, H. A., Klippel, J. H., Balow, J. E., le Riche, N. G., Steinberg, A. D., Plotz, P. H., and Decker, J. L., 1986, Therapy of lupus nephritis: Controlled trial of prednisolone and cytotoxic drugs, *N. Engl. J. Med.* **314**:614–619.

Axelson, J. A., Clark, R. H., and Ancerewicz, S., 1987, Wegener's granulomatosis and trimethoprim-sulphamethoxazole, *Ann. Intern. Med.* **107**:600.

Bacon, P. A., 1979, Circulating immune complexes in systemic rheumatoid disease, *Rheum. Rehab.* (Suppl.)**18**:11–15.

Bacon, P. A., 1987, Vasculitis—clinical aspects and therapy, *Acta Med. Scand.* (Suppl.) **715**:157–163.

Baggenstoss, A. H., Shick, R. M., and Polley, H. F., 1950, The effect of cortisone on the lesions of periarteritis nodosa, *Am. J. Pathol.* **27**:537–591.

Baker, G. L., Kahl, L. E., Zee, B. C., Stolzer, B. L., Agarwal, A. K., and Medsger, T. A., 1987, Malignancy following the treatment of rheumatoid arthritis with cyclophosphamide. Long-term cases control follow-up study, *Am. J. Med.* **83**:1–9.

Ball, J., 1954, Rheumatoid arthritis and polyarteritis nodosa, *Ann. Rheum. Dis.* **13**:277–290.

Behçet, H., 1937, Uber rezidivierende. Aphthose durch ein Virus versuachte Geschgwurec am Mund, am Auge und an den Genitalien, *Dermatol. Wochenschr.* **105**:1152–1157.

Borleffs, J. C., Derksen, R. H., and Hene, R. J., 1987, Treatment of Wegener's granulomatosis with cyclosporin (letter), *Ann. Rheum. Dis.* **46**:175.

Bradley, J. D., Brandt, K. D., and Katz, B. P., 1989, Infectious complications of cyclophosphamide treatment for vasculitis, *Arthritis Rheum.* **32**:45–53.

Bruce, W., 1888, Senile rheumatic gout, *Br. Med. J.* **2**:811–313.

Bywaters, E. G. L., 1976, Vasculitis in rheumatoid arthritis, in: *Non-articular Forms of Rheumatoid Arthritis* (T. E. W. Feltkamp, ed.), Proceedings of the IV ISRA Symposium, Stafleu's Scientific Publications, Leiden, pp. 82–84.

Calabrese, L. H., and Mallek, J. A., 1987, Primary angiitis of the central nervous system, *Medicine (Baltimore)* **67**:20–39.

Carrington, C. B., and Liebow, A. A., 1966, Limited forms of angiitis and granulomatosis of Wegener's type, *Am. J. Med.* **41**:497–527.

Chumbley, L. C., Harrison, R. A., and DeRemee, R. A., 1977, Allergic granulomatous angiitis (Churg-Strauss syndrome). Report and analysis of 30 cases, *Mayo Clin. Proc.* **52**:477–484.

Churg, J., and Strauss, L., 1957, Allergic granulomatosis, allergic angiitis, and periarteritis nodosa, *Am. J. Pathol.* **27**:277–301.

Cochrane, C. G., 1968, Immunologic tissue injury mediated by neutrophilic leukocytes, *Adv. Immunol.* **9**:97–162.

Cochrane, C. G., and Aikin, B. S., 1966, Polymorphonuclear leukocytes in immunologic reactions. The destruction of vascular basement membrane *in vivo* and *in vitro*, *J. Exp. Med.* **124**:733–752.

Cravioto, H., and Feigin, I., 1959, Noninfectious granulomatous angiitis with a predilection for the nervous system, *Neurology* **9**:599–609.

Dasgupta, B., Duke, O., Timms, A., Pitzalis, C., and Panayi, G. S., 1989, Selective depletion and activation of CD 8+ lymphocytes from peripheral blood of patients with polymyalgia rheumatica and giant cell arteritis, *Ann. Rheum. Dis.* **48**:307–311.

Davson, J., Ball, J., and Platt, R., 1948, The kidney in periarteritis nodosa, *Q. J. Med.* **17**:175–202.

Delecoeuillerie, G., Joly, P., Cohen de Lara, A., and Paolaggi, J. B., 1988, Polymyalgia rheumatica and temporal arteritis: A retrospective analysis of prognostic features and different corticosteroid regimens (11 year survey of 210 patients), *Ann. Rheum. Dis.* **47**:733–739.

DeRemee, R. A., McDonald, T. J., and Weiland, L. H., 1985, Wegener's granulomatosis: Observations on treatment with antimicrobial agents, *Mayo Clin. Proc.* **60**:27–32.

De Silva, M., and Hazelman, B. L., 1986, Azathioprine in giant cell arteritis/polymyalgia rheumatica in a double blind study, *Ann. Rheum. Dis.* **45**:136–138.

Drath, D. B., and Kahan, B. D., 1984, Phagocytic cell function in response to immunosuppressive therapy, *Arch. Surg.* **119**:156–160.

Droz, D., Noel, L. H., Leibowitch, M., and Barbanel, C., 1979, Glomerulonephritis and necrotizing angiitis, in: *Advanced Nephrology*, Volume 8, Year Book Medical Publishers, Chicago, pp. 343–363.

Dwosh, I. L., Giles, A. R., Ford, P. M., Pater, J. L., Anastassiades, T. P., and the Queens University Plasmapharesis Study Group, 1983, Plasmapharesis in rheumatoid arthritis. A double-blind cross over trial, *N. Engl. J. Med.* **308**:1124–1129.

Ellman, P., and Ball, R. E., 1948, Rheumatoid disease with joint and pulmonary manifestations, *Br. Med. J.* **2**:816–820.

Fan, P. T., Davis, J. A., Somer, T., Kaplan, L., and Bluestone, R., 1980, A clinical approach to systemic vasculitis, *Semin. Arthritis Rheum.* **9**:248–304.

Fauci, A. S., 1978, The spectrum of vasculitis, *Ann. Intern. Med.* **89**:660–676.

Fauci, A. S., 1985, Cytotoxic and other regulatory agents, in: *Textbook of Rheumatology*, 2nd edition (W. N. Kelley, E. D. Harris, Jr., S. Ruddy, and C. B. Sledge, eds.), W. B. Saunders, Philadelphia, pp. 833–857.

Fauci, A. S., and Wolff, S. M., 1973, Wegener's granulomatosis: Studies in eighteen patients and a review of the literature, *Medicine (Baltimore)* **52**:535–561.

Fauci, A. S., Dale, D. C., and Balow, J. E., 1976, Glucocorticoid therapy: Mechanisms of action and clinical considerations, *Ann. Intern. Med.* **84**:304–315.

Fauci, A. S., Katz, P., Haynes, B. F., and Wolff, S. M., 1979, Cyclophosphamide therapy of severe systemic necrotizing vasculitis, *N. Engl. J. Med.* **301**:235–238.

Fauci, A. S., Haynes, B. F., Katz, P., and Wolff, S. M., 1983, Wegener's granulomatosis: Prospective clinical and therapeutic experience with 85 patients for 21 years, *Ann. Intern. Med.* **98**:76–85.

Finan, M. C., and Winkelmann, R. K., 1983, The cutaneous extravascular necrotizing granuloma (Churg-Strauss granuloma) and systemic disease: A review of 27 cases, *Medicine (Baltimore)* **62**:142–158.

Frohnert, P. P., and Sheps, S. G., 1967, Long-term follow-up study of periarteritis nodosa, *Am. J. Med.* **43**:8–14.

Furusho, K., Kamiya, T., Nakano, H., Kiyosawa, N., Shinomiya, K., Hayashidera, T., Tamura, T., Hirose, O., Manabe, Y., Yokoyama, T., Kawarano, M., Baba, K., Baba, K., and Mori, C., 1984, High dose intravenous gamma globulin for Kawasaki disease, *Lancet* **2**:1055–1088.

Godman, G. C., and Churg, J., 1954, Wegener's granulomatosis: Pathology and review of the literature, *A.M.A. Arch. Pathol.* **58**:533–553.

Goldman, J. A., Casey, H. L., McIlwain, H., Kirby, J., Wilson, C. H., Jr., and Miller, S. B., 1979, Limited plasmapharesis in rheumatoid arthritis with vasculitis, *Arthritis Rheum.* **22**:1146–1150.

Goodman, B. W., Jr., 1979, Temporal arteritis, *Am. J. Med.* **67**:839–852.

Gremmel, F., Druml, W., Schmidt, P., and Graninger, W., 1988, Cyclosporin in Wegener's granulomatosis, *Ann. Intern. Med.* **108**:491.

Guillevin, L., Le, T. H. D., Godeau, P., Jais, P., and Wechsler, B., 1988, Clinical findings and prognosis of polyarteritis nodosa and Churg-Strauss angiitis: A study in 165 patients, *Br. J. Rheumatol.* **27**:258–264.

Hall, N. D., Bird, H. A., Ring, E. F. J., and Bacon, P. A., 1979, A combined clinical and immunological assessment of four cyclophosphamide regimes in rheumatoid arthritis, *Agents Actions* **9**:97–102.

Hall, S., Barr, W., Lie, J. T., Stanton, A. W., Kazmier, F. J., and Hunder, G. G., 1985, Takayasu arteritis: A study of 32 North American patients, *Medicine (Baltimore)* **64**:89–99.

Hind, C. R. K., Paraskevakou, H., Lockwood, C. M., Evans, D. J., Peters, D. K., and Rees, A. J., 1983, Prognosis after immunosuppression of patients with crescentic nephritis requiring dialysis, Lancet 1:263–265.

Hutchinson, J., 1890, Diseases of the arteries: On a peculiar form of thrombotic arteritis of the aged which is sometimes productive of gangrene, Arch. Surg. 1:323–329.

Inada, K., 1977, Aortitis syndrome, in: Vascular Lesions of Collagen Disease and Related Disorders (Y. Shiokawa, ed.), University Park Press, Baltimore, pp. 143–148.

Kahan, B. D., 1989, Cyclosporine, N. Engl. J. Med. 321:1725–1738.

Kahn, M. F., Bedoiseau, M., and deSeze, S., 1967, Immunosuppressive drugs in the management of malignant and severe rheumatoid arthritis, Proc. R. Soc. Med. 60:130–133.

Kawasaki, T., 1967, Mucocutaneous lymph node syndrome—clinical observation of 50 cases, Jap. J. Allergy 16:178–222.

Kawasaki, T., Kosaki, F., Okawa, S., Shigematsu, I., and Yanagawa, H., 1974, A new infantile acute febrile mucocutaneous lymph node syndrome (MCNS) prevailing in Japan, Pediatrics 54:271–276.

Kemper, J. W., Baggenstoss, A. H., and Slocumb C. H., 1957, The relationship of therapy with cortisone to the incidence of vascular lesions in rheumatoid arthritis, Ann. Intern. Med. 46:831–851.

Kulka, J. P., 1959, The vascular lesions associated with rheumatoid arthritis, Bull. Rheum. Dis. 10:201–202.

Kusakawa, S., 1983, Long-term administrative care of Kawasaki disease, Acta Paediatr. Japan (Overseas Ed.) 25:205–209.

Kussmaul, A., and Maier, R., 1866, Uber eine bisher nicht beschreibene eigenthumliche Arteriener Krankung (periarteritis nodosa). Die mit Morbus Brightii und rapid fortschreitender allgemeiner Muskellahmung einhergeht, Deutsches Arch. Klin. Med. 1:484–517.

Lanham, J. G., Elkon, K. B., Pusey, C. D., and Hughes, G. R. V., 1984, Systemic vasculitis in asthma and eosinophilia: A clinical approach to the Churg-Strauss syndrome, Medicine (Baltimore) 63:65–81.

Leib, E. S., Restivo, C., and Paulus, H. E., 1979, Immunosuppressive and corticosteroid therapy of periarteritis nodosa, Am. J. Med. 67:941–947.

Leung, D., Cotran, R. S., Kurt-Jones, E., Burns, J. C., Newburger, J. W., and Pober, J. S., 1989, Endothelial cell activation and high interleukin-1 secretion in the pathogenesis of acute Kawasaki disease, Lancet 2:1298–1302.

Levy, J., Barnett, E. V., MacDonald, N. S., Klinenburg, J. R., and Pearson, C. M., 1972, The effect of azathioprine on gammaglobulin synthesis in man, J. Clin. Invest. 51:2233–2238.

Lhote, F., Guillevin, L., Leon, A., Brissel, A., Luk, C., Sobel, A., and Simon, P., 1988, Complications of plasma exchange in the treatment of polyarteritis nodosa and Churg-Strauss angiitis and the contribution of adjuvant immunosuppressive therapy: A randomized trial in 72 patients, Artif. Organs 12:27–33.

Lockwood, C. M., Woolledge, S., Nicholas, A., Cotton, C., and Peters, D. K. 1979, Reversal of impaired spenic function of patients with nephritis or vasculitis (or both), N. Engl. J. Med. 300:524–530.

Masuda, K., Nakujima, A., Urayani, A., Naskae, K., Kogure, M., and Inaba, G., 1989, Double-masked trial of cyclosporin vs. colchicine and long-term open study of cyclosporin in Behçet's disease, Lancet 1:1093–1096.

Mathieson, P. W., Cobbold, S. P., Hale, G., Clark, M. R., Oliviera, D. B. G., Lockwood, C. M., and Waldmann, H., 1990, Monoclonal antibody therapy in systemic vasculitis, N. Engl. J. Med. 323:250–254.

Mizushima, Y., Matsuda, T., Ohama, N., Hoshi, K., and Takeuchi, A., 1982, Colchicine and anti-thrombotic drugs in the treatment of Behçet's disease, in: Behçet's Disease: Pathogenetic Mechanisms and Clinical Future (G. Inaba, ed.), Japan Medical Research Foundation Publication No. 18, University of Tokyo Press, pp. 513–517.

Nasu, T., 1977, Pathology of Takayasu's truncoarteritis: A statistical observation of 76 autopsy cases in Japan, in: Vascular Lesions of Collagen Disease and Related Disorders (Y. Shiokawa, ed.), University Park Press, Baltimore, pp. 149–160.

Newburger, J. W., Takahashi, M., Burns, J. C., Beiser, A. S., Chung, K. J., Duffy, C. E., Glode, M. P., Mason, W. H., Reddy, V., Sanders, S. P., Shulman, S. T., Wiggins, J. W., Hicks, R. V., Fulton, D. R., Lewis, A. B., Leung, D. Y. M., Colton, T., Rosen, F. S., and Melish, M. E., 1986, The treatment of Kawasaki's syndrome with intravenous gamma globulin, N. Engl. J. Med. 315:341–347.

Nicholls, A., Snaith, M. L., Maini, R. N., and Scott, J. T., 1973, Controlled trial of azathioprine in rheumatoid vasculitis, Ann. Rheum. Dis. 32:589–591.

Novack, S. NA., and Pearson, C. M., 1971, Cyclophosphamide therapy in Wegener's granulomatosis, N. Engl. J. Med. 284:938–942.

O'Duffy, J. D., Robertson, D. M., and Goldstein, N. P., 1984, Chlorambucil in the treatment of uveitis and meningoencephalitis of Behçet's disease, Am. J. Med. 76:75–84.

Palmer, R. G., Dore, S., and Denman, A. M., 1986, Cyclophosphamide induces more chromosome damage than chlorambucil in patients with connective tissue diseases, Q. J. Med. 59:395-400.

Palmer, R. G., Smith-Burchnell, C. A., Pelton, B. K., Hylton, W., and Denman, A. M., 1988, Use of T cell cloning to detect in vivo mutations induced by cyclophosphamide, Arthritis Rheum. 31:757–761.

Pickering, G., Bywaters, E. G. L., Danielli, J. F., Gell, P. G., Kellgren, J. H., Long, D. A., Neuberger, A., Nicholson, H., Prunty, F. T. G., Robb-Smith, A. H. T., Payling-Wright, G., Conybeare, E. T., and Duthie, J. J. R., 1960, Treatment of polyarteritis nodosa. Results after three years: Report to the Medical Research Council by the Collagen Disease and hypersensitivity panel, Br. Med. J. 1:1399–1400.

Rose, G. A., and Spencer, H., 1957, Polyarteritis nodosa, Q. J. Med. 26:43–81.

Rosman, M., Bertino, J. R., 1973, Azathioprine, Ann. Intern. Med. 79:694–700.

Sack, M., Cassidy, J. T., and Bole, G., 1975, Prognostic factors in polyarteritis, J. Rheumatol. 2:411–420.

Savage, C. O., Winearls, C. G., Evans, D. J., Rees, A. J., and Lockwood, S. M., 1985, Microscopic polyarteritis: Presentation, pathology and prognosis, Q. J. Med. 56:467–483.

Schein, P. S., and Winokur, S. T., 1975, Immunosuppressive and cytotoxic chemotherapy: Long-term complications, Ann. Intern. Med. 82:84–95.

Scott, D. G. I., 1988, Classification and treatment of systemic vasculitis, *Br. J. Rheumatol.* **27**:251–253.

Scott, G. D. I., and Bacon, P. A., 1984, Intravenous cyclophosphamide plus methylprednisolone in the treatment of systemic rheumatoid vasculitis, *Am. J. Med.* **76**:377–384.

Scott, D. G. I., Bacon, P. A., Allen, C., Elson, C. J., and Wallington, T., 1981a, IgG rheumatoid factor, complement and immune complexes in rheumatoid synovitis and vasculitis: Comparative and serial studies during cytotoxic therapy, *Clin. Exp. Immunol.* **43**:54–56.

Scott, D. G. I., Bacon, P. A., Bothamley, J. E., Allen, C., Elson, C. L., and Wallington, T. B., 1981b, Plasma exchange in rheumatoid vasculitis, *J. Rheumatol.* **8**:433–439.

Scott, D. G. I., Bacon, P. A., and Tribe, C. R., 1981c, Systemic rheumatoid vasculitis: A clinical and laboratory study of 50 cases, *Medicine (Baltimore)* **60**:288–297.

Scott, D. G. I., Bacon, P. A., Elliott, P. J., Tribe, C. R., and Wallington, T. B., 1982, Systemic vasculitis in a district general hospital 1972–1980: Clinical and laboratory features, classification and prognosis of 80 cases, *Q. J. Med.* **51**:292–311.

Serra, A., Cameron, J. S., Turner, D. R., Hartley, B., Ogg, C. S., Neild, G. H., Williams, D. G., Taube, D., Brown, C. B., and Hicks, J. A., 1984, Vasculitis affecting the kidney: Presentation, histopathology and long-term outcome, *Q. J. Med.* **53**:181–207.

Shelhamer, J. H., Volkman, D. J., Parrillo, J. E., Lawley, T. J., Johnston, M. M., and Fauci, A. S., 1985, Takayasu's arteritis and its therapy, *Ann. Intern. Med.* **103**:121–126.

Shimizu, T., 1977, Behçet's disease: A systemic inflammatory disease, in: *Vascular Lesions of Collagen Disease and Related Disorders* (Y. Shiokawa, ed.), University Park Press, Baltimore, pp. 201–211.

Sigal, L., 1987, The neurologic presentation of vasculitic and rheumatological syndromes: A review, *Medicine (Baltimore)* **66**:157–179.

Sokoloff, L., and Bunim, J. J., 1957, Vascular lesions in rheumatoid arteritis, *J. Chronic Dis.* **5**:668–687.

Steinberg, A. D., Plotz, P. H., Wolff, S. M., Wong, V. G., Agus, S. G., and Decker, J. L., 1972, Cytotoxic drugs in treatment of nonmalignant diseases, *Ann. Intern. Med.* **76**:619–642.

Stillwell, T. J., Benson, R. C., Jr., deRemee, R. A., McDonald, T. J., and Weiland, L. H., 1988, Cyclophosphamide-induced bladder toxicity in Wegener's granulomatosis, *Arthritis Rheum.* **31**:465–470.

Tabbara, K. K., 1983, Chlorambucil in Behçet's: A reappraisal, *Ophthalmology* **90**:906–908.

Takayasu, M., 1908, A case with peculiar changes of the central retinal vessels, *Acta Soc. Ophthalmol. Japan* **12**:554.

Vollertsen, R. S., Conn, D. L., Ballard, D. J., Ilstrup, D. M., Kazmar, R. E., Silverfield, J. C., 1986, Rheumatoid vasculitis: Survival and associated risk factors, *Medicine (Baltimore)* **65**:365–375.

Wallace, D., Goldfinger, D., Lowe, D., Brachman, M., and Klinenberg, J., 1981, A double blind controlled study of lymphapharesis in rheumatoid arthritis, *Arthritis Rheum.* **24**:S125.

Wegener, F., 1936, Uber generalisierte, septische Gefasserkrankungen, *Verh. Dtsch. Ges. Pathol.* **29**:202–209.

Weisman, M., and Zvaiffler, N. J., 1975, Cryoglobulinaemia in rheumatoid arthritis. Significance in serum of patients with rheumatoid vasculitis, *J. Clin. Invest.* **56**:725–739.

Wendling, D., Hory, B., and Blanc, D., 1985, Cyclosporine: A new adjuvant therapy for giant cell arteritis? *Arthritis Rheum.* **28**:1078–1079.

West, B. C., Todd, J. R., and King, J. W., 1987, Wegener's granulomatosis and trimethoprim-sulphamethoxazole; Complete remission after a twenty-year course, *Ann. Intern. Med.* **106**:840–842.

Wing, E. J., Burns, F. J., Fraley, D. S., Segel, D. P., and Adler, S., 1980, Infectious complications with plasmapharesis in rapidly progressive glomerulonephritis, *J. Am. Med. Assoc.* **244**:2423–2426.

Wolff, S. M., Fauci, A. S., Horn, R. G., and Dale, D. C., 1974, Wegener's granulomatosis, *Ann. Intern. Med.* **81**:513–525.

Woodworth, T. G., Abuelo, J. G., Austin, H. A., III, and Esparza, A., 1987, Severe glomerulonephritis with late emergence of classic Wegener's granulomatosis, *Medicine (Baltimore)* **66**:181–191.

Yazici, H., Pazarali, H., Barnes, C. G., Tuzun, Y., Ozyazgan, Y., Silman, A., Serdaroglu, S., Oguz, V., Yurdakul, S., Lovatt, G. E., Yazici, B., Somani, S., and Muftuoglu, A., 1990, A controlled trial of azathioprine in Behçet's syndrome, *N. Engl. J. Med.* **322**:281–285.

Yu, D. T., Clements, P. J., Peter, J. B., Levy, J., Paulus, H. E., and Barnett, E. V., 1974, Lymphocyte characteristics in rheumatic patients and response to therapy, *Arthritis Rheum.* **17**:37–45.

Zeek, P. M., 1952, Periarteritis nodosa: A critical review, *Am. J. Clin. Pathol.* **22**:777–790.

Chapter 22

IMMUNOTHERAPY IN AUTOIMMUNE LIVER DISEASE

Martin Lombard and *Roger Williams*

1. INTRODUCTION

The liver may be involved in generalized immunoinflammatory reactions or may become the target for an organ-specific immune attack. Specific cell types (e.g., epithelial cells, hepatocytes) may be preferentially affected during such a reaction, giving rise to a number of clinical syndromes. The etiologic agents and pathogenetic mechanisms are still incompletely understood, but nevertheless have allowed clinical trials of immunotherapy to be conducted. In this chapter we discuss the possible immunopathogenetic mechanisms resulting in different patterns of liver disease, the rationale behind specific therapeutic regimens, and the difficulties in assessing these. We also review the data from reported therapeutic trials.

2. AUTOIMMUNE DISEASE INVOLVING BILIARY EPITHELIUM

2.1. Primary Biliary Cirrhosis

Primary biliary cirrhosis (PBC) is a progressive disease of the liver affecting small- and medium-sized bile ducts, resulting in progressive fibrosis and cirrhosis (Kaplan, 1987). It is characterized as an autoimmune disease on the basis of its association with other clinical conditions thought to have an immune basis (e.g., hypothyroidism, arthritis, sicca syndrome), similarities with graft-versus-host disease, and evidence of multiple immunological abnormalities both *in vitro* and *in vivo* (James *et al.*, 1983; Mackay and Gershwin, 1989). These have included presence of autoantibodies, especially mitochondrial antibodies; raised immunoglobulin fractions (particularly IgM); complement activation and appearance of immune complexes in the serum; decreased T-lymphocyte subset populations with suppressor cell function deficits; and lymphocytic infiltration of portal tracts with aberrant expression of human leukocyte antigen (HLA) class II complexes on biliary epithelium. Some of these immunological abnormalities have been found in a proportion of first-degree relatives and an

Martin Lombard and *Roger Williams* • Institute of Liver Studies, King's College School of Medicine, London SE5 8RX, England.

Immunopharmacology in Autoimmune Diseases and Transplantation, edited by Hans Erik Rugstad *et al.* Plenum Press, New York, 1992.

association with the C4b2 component of the major histocompatibility complex (MHC) has been described, although no classical HLA association is known. Thus genetic factors may explain the occasional occurrence of PBC in successive generations. Its female preponderance has been ascribed to genetic immune responsiveness and immunomodulation by estrogens.

The stimulus for formation of antimitochondrial antibodies and induction of periductal cytotoxic T-lymphocyte infiltration in PBC is unknown. The two principal theories concerning the mechanism of autoimmunity include the concepts of modification of "self" molecules and cross-reaction with "external antigens." The aberrant expression of HLA-DR on biliary epithelium surrounded by T-lymphocyte infiltration has been cited in favor of the former mechanism, an unidentified virus being postulated as the initial immune trigger (Ballardini et al., 1984). In contrast, the mitochondrial autoantigens, specifically the M2 subtype, have recently been identified as components of the pyruvate dehydrogenase multienzyme complex located on mitochondrial membranes (Yeaman et al., 1988). The presence of this enzyme complex in mammals, yeast, and bacteria could allow cross-reactivity between bacterial antigens and mammalian cells. Indeed, M2 antibodies have been shown to react with normal colonic bacterial flora, thus supporting the cross-reaction theory. The reasons for specific immunoreactivity against biliary epithelium and whether mitochondrial antibodies have a primary or secondary role in this remain unclear. The chronic nature of the disease could be explained by either persistence of the cross-reacting antigen or T-cell induction of MHC class II antigens on biliary epithelium, propogating a cytotoxic response. Neither explanation can account for the long asymptomatic phase lasting for many years in some patients or for the variation in rate of progression of the disease presenting at similar stages in different individuals.

2.1.1. Immunotherapy in PBC

Therapy in PBC has been aimed at interrupting the T- and B-lymphocyte mechanisms and cooperation essential to an immunoinflammatory reaction. A major difficulty in evaluating treatment in this condition is the variable course and insidious progression referred to above. Reports that asymptomatic patients had a benign prognosis and normal life expectancy have been challenged by subsequent findings that many such patients later become symptomatic and then assume the same prognosis as patients symptomatic at presentation (Beswick et al., 1985; Mitchison et al., 1990). Entry criteria for therapeutic trials have usually required patients to be symptomatic or to have histological evidence of disease beyond stage I, thus excluding patients in whom immunopathogenic mechanisms are at an early stage of development and presumably more easily reversed or controlled. The later superimposition of fibrosis and cholestasis produces a variable spectrum of pathology, making interpatient comparison and serial comparison in individual patients extremely difficult in drug trials involving immunotherapy. In addition, it is unclear which clinical or laboratory parameters most usefully indicate a therapeutic response. Models defining prognostic variables for PBC have indicated that the presence of granulomas in liver biopsies and absence of symptoms correlate with prolonged survival while high bilirubin, low albumin, and presence of cirrhosis correlate with shortened survival (Roll et al., 1983; Christensen et al., 1985; Dickson et al., 1989). Serum bilirubin appears to be the best single prognostic variable and survival can be predicted with some accuracy once this is persistently raised above 80–100 μmole/liter. Patient survival has become the most important measurable parameter for efficacy of treatment, but the insidious nature compounded by the heterogeneity of clinical presentation has bestowed upon therapeutic trials the necessity of recruiting large numbers of patients who can be followed for many years. To date, few controlled clinical studies have satisfied these criteria.

2.1.1a. Drugs with Major Immune-Modulating Effects

Corticosteroids have been administered on an uncontrolled basis to small numbers of patients with PBC for over 30 years. On theoretical grounds, the immunosuppressive and anti-inflammatory effects of prednisolone might be expected to produce a response. Initial reports indicated an improvement in pruritus, general well-being, and liver biochemistry, but disease progression appeared to be unaffected. Only recently have corticosteroids been evaluated in a controlled trial (Mitchison *et al.*, 1989). This study at Newcastle-upon-Tyne involved 36 patients over a three-year period and confirmed the earlier indications of subjective improvement in symptoms in half of the patients on treatment compared to only one on placebo and a trend toward improvement in liver enzymes and immunoglobulins. There was histological follow-up in less than half of the patients but the available data seemed to indicate less progression in the prednisolone group. Photon absorptiometric assessment of bone loss in radius and femur showed no significant difference in the two groups, although mean loss in the steroid-treated group was higher. Effects of steroid on vertebral bone loss was not assessed. This has now become an important consideration as orthotopic liver transplantation is being increasingly used for patients with primary biliary cirrhosis. The combination of high-dose steroids and immobilization in the immediate posttransplant period can be disastrous for an already osteopenic patient.

Azathioprine was evaluated in PBC in the mid-1970s following demonstration of its efficacy in preventing renal allograft rejection. In an uncontrolled study at the Royal Free Hospital London, 22 patients were treated with azathioprine 2 mg/kg per day and reported a subjective improvement that was not reflected in liver biochemistry or histology after two years of treatment, but there was a trend toward improved survival after three years. In a major international controlled study in which 248 patients were randomized to receive azathioprine 1.5 mg/kg per day or placebo for up to six years, a significant improvement in mean survival of 22 months in the treated group was reported (Christensen *et al.*, 1985). The drug was well tolerated at this dose and this treatment regimen has been adopted by some investigators. Reports of hepatotoxicity with azathioprine in patients with liver disease have been confined to doses in excess of 2 mg/kg per day. This remains the only drug to date for which a statistically significant effect on survival in PBC has been reported.

Cyclosporine A has immunosuppressive properties largely targeted on T-cell cytotoxic responses and associated lymphokine function and is effective in preventing liver allograft rejection. An early uncontrolled study of cyclosporine 10 mg/kg per day given to six patients with PBC for eight weeks was abandoned because of deteriorating renal function as assessed by serum creatinine. At King's College Hospital, 19 patients given cyclosporine 3 mg/kg per day showed minimal nephrotoxicity after a median follow-up duration of 22 months. This lower dosage of cyclosporine was also shown to correct the suppressor cell deficit in PBC. Following this report, a multicenter, double-blind, placebo-controlled trial involving 349 patients was conducted over a six-year period. Multivariate analysis of this trial showed that low-dose cyclosporine A prolonged life compared to placebo, and serum bilirubin and symptoms were also improved. Almost 10% of patients on cyclosporine suffered some degree of renal impairment and it remains to be seen whether cyclosporine will be adopted as a treatment in primary biliary cirrhosis. Results of two smaller studies in North America involving 12 patients randomized and followed for 12 months and 36 patients randomized and followed for two years support these findings of symptomatic and laboratory improvement in many patients without gross impairment of renal function at the lower dosage of 3–5 mg/kg per day (Wiesner et al., 1990).

Cyclophosphamide and Chlorambucil, the alkylating agents, have been used in auto-immune arthritis, nephritis, and SLE with reported benefit. At low doses, the predominant effect is thought to be on B-lymphocyte humoral function and this is considered essential to the T-cell cytotoxic response in PBC. The National Institutes of Health in the United States evaluated chlorambucil 0.5–4 mg/kg per day in 13 patients with PBC in comparison with 11 matched patients receiving no therapy for two to four years. Serum albumen, bilirubin, and hepatic enzymes improved in the treated group while they deteriorated in the controls. Circulating immunoglobulin and lymphocyte count were reduced and the average intensity of inflammatory cell infiltrate on liver biopsy decreased significantly. Bone marrow suppression occurred in all 13 patients on chlorambucil and was severe enough to warrant discontinuation in four patients. These investigators counsel against widespread use of this agent in view of its severe side effects and its potential to induce malignancy.

2.1.1b. Drugs with Minor Immune-Modulating Effects

Penicillamine, evaluated in PBC because of its cupruretic activity and the high copper loading consequent upon failure of biliary excretion seen in this condition, also has immunosuppressive properties. Almost 1000 patients have been randomized in seven separate controlled trials to treatment with penicillamine 250–1000 mg daily or placebo following an initial report of improvement in 55 patients given penicillamine compared to 32 patients given placebo. The results in the subsequent trials have been remarkably consistent in showing no significant beneficial effect on symptomatology, hepatic biochemistry, histological progression, or survival. Serious toxicity was reported in up to 30% of patients. Penicillamine was effective in decoppering the liver, underlining the fact that copper plays no role in the pathogenesis of this condition.

Colchicine interferes with collagen synthesis and procollagen transport in the liver and has been shown to decrease fibrosis in carbon tetrachloride-induced cirrhosis in rats. In addition, it has antimitotic and anti-inflammatory effects and *in vitro* pharmacological doses correct the suppressor cell defect found in PBC. Three prospective controlled trials involving 181 patients have now been reported using colchicine 1–1.2 mg/day. There was agreement in the reports that hepatic biochemistry was improved in the treatment group without significant side effects. Serum alkaline phosphatase and aminotransferase were reduced in all three studies up to 50% in the treatment group, and while bilirubin was also reduced or remained stable, it invariably increased in the placebo groups. Colchicine appeared to have no effects on symptoms and in two of the studies did not retard histological progression over a two- to four-year follow-up period. A trend toward improved survival in the treatment group was reported by the Manchester group after four years of treatment and the improved survival was statistically significant in Kaplan's study (see Kaplan, 1989a).

Ursodeoxycholic acid was recently reported to produce dramatic and sustained symptomatic and biochemical improvement in 15 patients followed for two years in an uncontrolled French study (Poupon et al., 1987). These data have been confirmed by several small studies reported in abstract form (James, 1990). No study has included long-term histological or survival data. It has been proposed that improved survival could be predicted on the basis of a reduction in serum bilirubin, an independent prognostic variable in PBC. In the French study there was no effect on immunoglobulins or autoantibody levels, but a formal evaluation of any immune-modulating effect of the drug in PBC has not been undertaken. Theoretically, minor effects may be expected through an alteration in membrane lipid composition because ursodeoxycholic acid reduces serum cholesterol, which can be markedly elevated in PBC. Deterioration of PBC with this treatment has also been reported.

Other agents recently reported to have effects in PBC include estrogens administered to five patients in an uncontrolled pilot study as *estradiol* 0.05 mg daily. This caused reduction of serum gamma-glutamyl transferase in five patients, AST in four, and alkaline phosphatase in three, but serum bilirubin increased in two patients. The investigators postulated a mechanism of action involving suppressor cell function or alterations in biliary membrane composition. In view of other circumstantial evidence possibly implicating estrogens in the pathogenesis of this condition, their administration would seem ill-advised. The opioid antagonist, *nalmefene*, administered to 11 patients with PBC, improved pruritus and fatigue index scores and reduced serum bilirubin levels in half of the patients. All patients experienced an opioid withdrawal reaction, there was no effect on serum enzyme levels, and effects on immunologic parameters were not reported. In a short-term cross-over, double-blind study of nine patients, *rifampicin* 300–450 mg/day produced a dramatic improvement in pruritus without a measurable change in bile acids. Other biochemical and immunologic parameters were not assessed.

Plasmapheresis has been shown to be of benefit in autoimmune thyroid disease and has been evaluated in five patients with PBC. After a mean of 63 treatments per patient, improvements in hypercholesterolemia and pruritus were reported. There was no effect on liver biochemistry or histological progression and effect on immunologic parameters was not assessed.

2.2. Primary Sclerosing Cholangitis

Primary sclerosing cholangitis (PSC) is an uncommon syndrome characterized by inflammation and fibrosis of the intrahepatic and extrahepatic medium-sized and larger bile ducts. It most commonly presents in young men and is frequently associated with inflammatory bowel disease (Wiesner *et al.*, 1985; Schrumpf *et al.*, 1988). Until recently surprisingly little information was available on the natural history of PSC and most data derive from patients who have presented initially with inflammatory bowel disease.

The etiology of this disease is unknown but immunologic factors and recurrent bacterial destructive cholangitis are believed to account for the pathological findings. There are similarities between PSC and the destructive cholangitis associated with either arterial or biliary infusion of chemical agents or with cytomegalovirus and reovirus type 3 infections. Unlike PBC, PSC has not been associated with other organ-specific immune disorders and the presence of autoantibodies to mitochondrial, nuclear, muscle, or liver antigens is reported in less than 10% of cases. Nevertheless, reports of an association between PSC and HLA B8, DR3 phenotype, aberrant expression of HLA class II antigens on biliary epithelium, and elevated circulating immune complexes in serum together with altered T- and B-lymphocyte reactivity have given credence to the notion that it has an autoimmune basis. Further support for this comes from reports, particularly in children, of a syndrome with all of the features of autoimmune chronic active hepatitis but which is steroid-unresponsive and progresses to a condition indistinguishable from PSC on cholangiography (El-Shabrawi *et al.*, 1987).

There has been speculation of cross-reactivity involving colonic and biliary epithelium, although colectomy is not usually followed by any improvement in the liver lesion. No specific cross-reacting or other antigens have been identified and it is unclear why not all patients with chronic ulcerative colitis develop PSC or why in some patients the liver lesion precedes the colitis. In the later stages of PSC, a proportion develop cholangiocarcinoma arising usually in the upper part of strictured bile ducts.

2.2.1. Immunotherapy in PSC

Therapy in PSC has been aimed at treating instances of exacerbating infective cholangitis, improving biliary drainage, inducing cupruresis, and reducing inflammation or fibrosis. There have been few controlled trials of these treatment measures. The reasons for this have much in common with the difficulties encountered in PBC: small numbers of patients and the superimposition of fibrotic, cholestatic, and obstructive pathological processes in the liver. In addition, the effects of inflammatory bowel disease and its treatment on PSC have to be considered. It remains unclear whether there is a long asymptomatic phase in PSC as in PBC because radiographic examination is a relatively crude investigation for slight changes in bile duct caliber and liver biopsy is susceptible to sampling error. Most patients with PSC are symptomatic at presentation and mean survival estimated by life-table analysis in two series was more than a decade. Recently a prognostic model using regression analysis of clinical parameters has been developed for PSC and the complexity of the model serves to underscore the complexity and unpredictable nature of this condition (Wiesner *et al.*, 1989).

2.2.1a.   Immune-Modulating Drugs in PSC.   Corticosteroids, 15–60 mg oral prednisolone daily continued for three to six months, has been reported to improve laboratory tests and subjective well-being in precirrhotic PSC, but there have never been controlled trials to substantiate this report and anecdotal reports indicate no benefit. In a recent study, the Mayo Clinic group compared combined therapy of colchicine 1.2 mg/day and prednisolone 40 mg/day, reducing to a maintenance of 10 mg/day in 12 patients, to 12 matched patients given no treatment. In the treatment group significant improvements in serum bilirubin, alkaline phosphatase, and AST, all of which were reduced by approximately 50%, were observed over a 12-month period. The results were all the more impressive because 80% of the patients had advanced (stage III or IV) disease at entry on liver biopsy. This study was abandoned recently because of significant osteoporosis in the treatment group.

Following anecdotal reports of improved biliary drainage in PSC with biliary lavage, two small controlled studies compared endoscopic retrograde biliary lavage combined with either oral or nasobiliary corticosteroids. In the first of these, Tytgat's group from Amsterdam perfused the biliary system of eight patients with PSC and recurrent cholangitis for up to ten weeks. Three of these patients were simultaneously treated with 15 mg of oral prednisolone daily, which was continued for 12 months, and the other five had prednisolone added to the perfusion solution. In seven patients, normalization of temperature and bilirubin during treatment was associated with serial reduction in serum alkaline phosphatase and radiographic improvement in some patients. In a later study at the Royal Free Hospital London, 11 consecutive patients without recurrent cholangitis were randomized to receive biliary lavage with normal saline 1 liter/day for two weeks (5 patients) or lavage with normal saline containing hydrocortisone 100 mg/liter (6 patients). These investigators reported a tendency for liver function tests to deteriorate during lavage but return to baseline levels at three months. No radiographic improvement was observed in any patient although one in either group had less pruritus. Half of the patients receiving hydrocortisone had adverse reactions of fluid retention or paranoid ideation.

Penicillamine 750 mg daily in 39 patients was compared with placebo in 31 patients at the Mayo Clinic over a 36-month period (La Russo *et al.*, 1988). No effect of treatment was observed on clinical, biochemical, histological, or radiographic parameters and there was no difference in survival or overall progression between the two groups. Twenty percent of the patients in the treated group developed severe side effects necessitating discontinuation.

2.2.1b.   Other Agents in PSC.   There have been no controlled trials of *azathioprine* in PSC. A report of a single patient in whom radiographic changes became normal after nine months of azathioprine 150 mg/day were countered by a subsequent report in another patient of deterioration and possible predisposition to cholangitis. In both cases biliary drainage was also used and the effect of the drug is impossible to interpret. Kaplan's group in Boston have reported clinical and histological improvement in two patients with PSC treated with intermittent low-dose *methotrexate* 15 mg/week for one and six years (Kaplan *et al.*, 1989b) and have since undertaken a double-blind placebo-controlled trial of this agent in PSC. Reports of hepatotoxicity associated with use of this drug in other conditions are worrisome, although recent studies suggest that many liver biopsies in patients with psoriasis are abnormal before methotrexate therapy. Several centers have recently made preliminary reports of beneficial effects on liver chemistry with *ursodeoxycholic acid* 10–15 mg/kg per day in PSC. Duration of therapy was not long enough to assess the effects on fibrosis or radiographic bile duct caliber.

Percutaneous or endoscopic stenting has a role in the management of this condition in cases where an isolated stricture can be implicated. Surgery is best avoided as orthotopic liver transplantation is being increasingly considered for those patients with advanced disease and previous surgery adds difficulty to the procedure.

3. AUTOIMMUNITY INVOLVING LIVER PARENCHYMAL CELLS

3.1. Autoimmune Chronic Active Hepatitis

Autoimmune chronic active hepatitis (AICAH) is a defined entity comprising a particular pattern of histological features lasting for longer than six months in the absence of serological evidence of viral infection (McFarlane and Eddleston, 1989). It is distinguishable from chronic persistent hepatitis, which rarely progresses to cirrhosis, by the presence of piecemeal necrosis on liver biopsy. It usually though not exclusively affects young females and is associated with raised serum immunoglobulins (usually IgG), a variety of autoantibodies against smooth muscle, DNA, liver, and kidney microsomal membranes (especially in younger patients), and liver-specific membrane lipoproteins (anti-LSP). It is unclear what part, if any, these autoantibodies play in the pathogenesis of the condition. Some of the autoantibodies have been used to define categories within AICAH that have predictable natural history and prognosis and anti-LSP and has been found useful in predicting relapse following steroid withdrawal. The diagnosis of AICAH must exclude other causes of chronic active hepatitis. The occurrence of chronic active hepatitis following viral infection with hepatitis A or B virus and the high antibody titers to other viruses (e.g., measles) in serum of patients with AICAH suggests the triggering of an immune response by a virus with perpetuation due to an immunodeficiency or cross-reacting antigen. It seems likely that in some cases, the diagnosis of AICAH will be revised as diagnostic tests for hepatitis C and other non-A non-B hepatitis viruses become available (see Editorial, 1990). Nevertheless, the dramatic response to immunosuppressive agents in HBsAg⁻ CAH marks it out as a distinct entity.

3.2. Immunotherapy in AICAH

Since many therapeutic trials have now confirmed the efficacy of immunosuppressive therapy in this condition, response to treatment has also been included as a diagnostic criterion and is particularly useful to differentiate AICAH from early PBC in which histological features may resemble a hepatitic pattern. The description of AICAH as an entity coincided with the clinical introduction of corticosteroids in the 1950s so that therapeutic effect was established early. More recent trials in addition to confirming the therapeutic benefit of steroids and azathioprine in this condition have addressed the problems of duration and cessation of therapy and to defining subgroups of patients in whom the disease runs an atypical course.

3.2.1. Corticosteroids and Azathioprine in AICAH

Although specific dosage schemes differ between centers, there is rarely a need for initial treatment with high-dose corticosteroids 0.5–1.0 mg/kg per day to induce remission and good control is achieved with 10–15 mg/day. Early trials were consistent in showing reduction of serum liver enzymes and immunoglobulins and improved survival. The dose of corticosteroid is usually reduced when liver biochemistry normalizes and the addition of azathioprine at this stage (1.5 mg/kg per day) has allowed reduction of maintenance prednisolone to 10 mg/day or less in most patients. Treatment with azathioprine alone is not effective in inducing remission and anecdotal experience suggests that its introduction simultaneous with steroids can be deleterious. Remission of disease and patient well-being can be maintained for many years on this regimen despite the development of cirrhosis in many patients. Several investigators have indicated that this treatment may be inappropriate for asymptomatic patients with little disease activity on histological examination, a proportion of whom never develop clinically overt disease. The concept of "disease activity" has arisen from histological criteria describing the extent of inflammatory infiltration and piecemeal necrosis.

It has been argued that since the dose of corticosteroid, often as little as 5–10 mg daily, required to maintain complete remission is rarely associated with significant side effects, therapy should be lifelong to avoid the hazards of relapse. However, the occurrence of AICAH in older females has highlighted the adverse effect of corticosteroid-induced bone loss and the aggravated fluid retention in cirrhotic patients has given impetus to attempts at steroid withdrawal. In our experience, up to 90% of patients relapse following withdrawal of combined therapy (Hegarty et al., 1983) although in other trials (Mayo Clinic and Royal Free Hospital), the percent relapse was less. Differences in patient selection, diagnostic criteria, and duration of withdrawal may account for some of the discrepancy in the numbers relapsing in these studies. In contrast to the 90% relapse rate in 12 months encountered following withdrawal of corticosteroids and azathioprine from patients at King's College Hospital, withdrawal of azathioprine alone at this center resulted in only 30% relapse during a 36-month follow-up. A subsequent study at King's College showed that remission could be maintained following withdrawal of corticosteroid if the dose of azathioprine were simultaneously increased to 2 mg/kg per day (Stellon et al., 1988). Increases beyond this dosage may be associated with azathioprine-induced hepatotoxicity.

3.2.2. Other Immunosuppressive Agents in AICAH

The success of corticosteroid treatment and the minimizing of its adverse effects by addition of azathioprine has precluded the need to use other agents. Nonetheless, there have been small studies reported using single-agent or combined therapy such as azathioprine, 6-mercaptopurine, 6-thioguanine, penicillamine, chlorambucil, and cyclosporine A (see Schaffner, 1985). None of these agents has been as effective at inducing remission in AICAH as corticosteroids, nor do they appear to be as well tolerated.

REFERENCES

Ballardini, G., Mirakian, R., Bianchi, F. B., Pisi, E., Doniach, D., and Bottazzo, G. F., 1984, Aberrant expression of HLA-DR antigens in bile duct epithelium in primary biliary cirrhosis: Relevance to pathogenesis, *Lancet* 2:1009–1013.

Beswick, D. R., Klatskin, G., and Boyer, J. L., 1985, Asymptomatic primary biliary cirrhosis: A prospective report on long-term follow-up and natural history, *Gastroenterology* 89:267–271.

Christensen, E., Neuberger, J., Crowe, J., Altman, D. G., Popper, H., Portmann, B., Doniack, D., Ranek, L., Tygstrup, N., and Williams, R., 1985, Beneficial effect of azathioprine and prediction of prognosis in primary biliary cirrhosis, *Gastroenterology* 89:1084–1091.

Dickson, E. R., Grambsch, P. M., Fleming, T. R., Fisher, L. D., and Langworthy, A., 1989, Prognosis in primary biliary cirrhosis: Model for decision making, *Hepatology* 10:1–7.

Editorial, 1990, Hepatitis C virus upstanding, *Lancet* 335:1431–1432.

Hegarty, J. E., Nouri-Aria, K. T., Portmann, B., Eddleston, A. L. W. F., and Williams, R., 1983, Relapse following treatment withdrawal in patients with autoimmune chronic active hepatitis, *Hepatology* 3:685–689.

James, O. F. W., 1990, Ursodeoxycholic acid treatment for chronic cholestatic liver disease, *J. Hepatol.* 11:5–8.

James, S. P., Hoofnagle, J. H., Strober, W., and Jones, E. A., 1983, Primary biliary cirrhosis: A model autoimmune disease, *Ann. Intern. Med.* 99:500–512.

Kaplan, M. M., 1987, Primary biliary cirrhosis, *N. Engl. J. Med.* 316:521–528.

Kaplan, M. M., 1989a, Medical treatment of primary biliary cirrhosis, *Sem. Liver Dis.* 9:138–144.

Kaplan, M. M., 1989b, Methotrexate treatment of cholestatic liver disease: Friend or foe? *Q. J. Med.* 72:757–761.

La Russo, N. F., Wiesner, R. H., Ludwig, J., MacCarty, R. L., Beaver, S. J., and Zinsmeister, A. R., 1988, Prospective trial of penicillamine in primary sclerosing cholangitis, *Gastroenterology* 95:1036–1042.

Mackay, I. R., and Gershwin, M. E., 1989, Primary biliary cirrhosis: Current knowledge, perspectives and future directions, *Sem. Liver Dis.* 9:149–157.

McFarlane, I. G., and Eddleston, A. L. W. F., 1989, Chronic active hepatitis, in: *Immunology and Immunopathology of the Liver and Gastrointestinal Tract* (S. Targan and F. Shanahan, eds.), Igaku-Shoin, New York, pp. 281–304.

Minuk, G. Y., Bohme, C. E., Burgess, E., Hershfield, N. B., Kelly, J. K., Schaffer, E. A., Sutherland, L. R., and Van Rosendaal, G., 1988, Pilot study of cyclosporin A in patients with symptomatic primary biliary cirrhosis, *Gastroenterology* 95:1356–1363.

Mitchison, H. C., Bassendine, M. F., Malcolm, A. J., Watson, A. J., Record, C. O., and James, O. F., 1989, A pilot, double blind, controlled 1 year trial of prednisolone treatment in primary biliary cirrhosis: Hepatic improvement but greater bone loss, *Hepatology* 10:420–429.

Mitchison, H. C., Lucey, M. R., Kelly, P. J., Neuberger, J. M., Williams, R., and James, O. F. W., 1990, Symptom development and prognosis in primary biliary cirrhosis, *Gastroenterology* 99:778–784.

Poupon, R., Chretien, Y., Poupon, R. E., Ballet, F., Calmus, Y., and Darnis, F., 1987, Is ursodeoxycholic acid an effective treatment for primary biliary cirrhosis, *Lancet* 1:834–836.

Roll, J., Boyer, J. L., Barry, D., and Klatskin, G., 1983, The prognostic importance of clinical and histologic features in asymptomatic and symptomatic primary biliary cirrhosis, *N. Engl. J. Med.* 308:1–7.

Schaffner, F., 1986, Autoimmune chronic active hepatitis: Three decades of progress, in: *Progress in Liver Diseases*, 8th ed. (H. Popper and F. Schaffner, eds.), Grune & Stratton, London, pp. 485–503.

Schrumpf, E., Fausa, O., Elgjo, K., and Kolmannskog, F., 1988, Hepatobiliary complications of inflammatory bowel disease, *Sem. Liver Dis.* 8:201–210.

Stellon, A. J., Keating, J., Johnson, P., McFarlane, I., and Williams, R., 1988, Maintenance of remission in autoimmune chronic active hepatitis with azathioprine after corticosteroid withdrawal, *Hepatology* 8:781–784.

Wiesner, R. H., La Russo, N. F., Ludwig, J., and Dickson, E. R., 1985, Comparison of the clinicopathologic features of primary sclerosing cholangitis and primary biliary cirrhosis, *Gastroenterology* 88:108–114.

Wiesner, R. H., Grambsch, P. M., Dickson, E. R., Ludwig, J., MacCarty, R. L., Hunter, E. B., Fleming, T. R., Fisher, L. D., Beaver, S. J., and La Russo, N. F., 1989, Primary sclerosing cholangitis: Natural history, prognostic factors and survival analysis, *Hepatology* 10:430–436.

Wiesner, R. H., Ludwig, J., Lindor, K. D., Jorgensen, R. A., Baldus, W. P., Homburger, H. A., and Dickson, E. R., 1990, A controlled clinical trial of cyclosporine in the treatment of primary biliary cirrhosis, *N. Engl. J. Med.* 322:1419–1424.

Yeaman, S. J., Fussey, S. P. M., Danner, D. J., James, O. F. W., Mutimer, D. J., and Bassendine, M. F., 1988, Primary biliary cirrhosis: Identification of two major M2 mitochondrial autoantigens, *Lancet* 1:1067–1070.

Chapter 23

INSULIN-DEPENDENT DIABETES MELLITUS

J. L. Mahon, J. Dupre, and *C. R. Stiller*

1. INTRODUCTION

In insulin-dependent diabetes mellitus (IDDM), or type 1 diabetes, there is selective loss of the beta cells of the pancreas. This leads to insulinopenia, ketosis, and the need for exogenous insulin to sustain life. Although IDDM can occur at any age, it usually arises in the young and as a result is among the most common, major chronic pediatric diseases in the Western world. In Canada, the annual incidence is approximately 9 new cases/100,000 in those under 19 years of age (Ehrlich *et al.*, 1982). Despite provision of parenteral insulin, chronic IDDM is associated with undue morbidity, including micro- and macrovasculopathy and neuropathy (Kolb and Nerup, 1985) and premature mortality (Borch-Johnsen *et al.*, 1986). This has led to a search into the fundamental causes of the disease with the hope of developing curative treatment—in distinction to the existing, problematic one of substitution.

Immunotherapy for IDDM of recent onset represents the first widely explored attempt at such a strategy and it reflects recent developments in animal models of diabetes, immunology, and pharmacology. For now, however, the use of immunoactive agents for human IDDM remains experimental and need to be conducted under close scrutiny in specialized centers. In this chapter we will review relevant pathogenetic aspects of IDDM in humans, consider some studies that have used immunotherapy for newly diagnosed IDDM, and propose future possibilities for this approach to the disease.

2. PATHOGENETIC CONSIDERATIONS RELEVANT TO IMMUNOMODULATION FOR HUMAN IDDM

A current hypothesis accounting for the development of IDDM proposes that pancreatic islets in a genetically predisposed individual sustain an insult that leads to immune-mediated destruction of beta cells. The specific basis for the genetic propensity is not

J. L. Mahon, J. Dupre, and *C. R. Stiller* • University Hospital, The University of Western Ontario, London, Ontario N6A 5A5, Canada.

Immunopharmacology in Autoimmune Diseases and Transplantation, edited by Hans Erik Rugstad *et al.* Plenum Press, New York, 1992.

established. Although this tendency is clearly associated with the human leukocyte antigen (HLA)-D region of the major histocompatibility complex (MHC), many details remain obscure, such as the existence of genes conveying risk that are not within the MHC (Hodge et al., 1981; Bell et al., 1984), the site(s) where and way(s) in which the MHC confers the potential for and protection from disease (Nerup et al., 1987), and the existence of subtypes of IDDM based on MHC differences (Ludviggson et al., 1986). Resolution of these issues may expand the options for immunotherapy for IDDM (for example, monoclonal antibody targeted to a specific MHC product), as well as make it possible to identify those individuals at inevitable risk for developing IDDM who may then be treated before onset of clinical disease.

Just as the basis for genetic risk in IDDM is unclear, so also the nature of the initial insult is not known. Both exogenous (viral infections, chemical agents) and endogenous factors (interleukin 1) have been implicated (Drash, 1986; Diabetes Epidemiology Research International, 1987; Mandrup-Poulsen, 1988). The evidence suggesting a causal relationship between an extraneous event and IDDM is compelling and is supported by low concordance for disease in identical twins (Tattersall and Pyke, 1972), but it is circumstantial in nature. Almost unequivocal descriptions of exposure to external agents causing IDDM in man have been rare (Yoon et al., 1979; Prosser and Karam, 1978). Moreover, the hypothesis of pretranscriptional modification of genes coding for immunoactive proteins has led to the suggestion that monozygotic twins are not truly identical, and thus the concordance rate of just 50% would not need environmental variation to be explained (Eisenbarth, 1987). Nevertheless, it has been estimated that up to 95% of IDDM worldwide is caused by factors in the environment (Diabetes Epidemiology Research International, 1987). This concept receives impetus by creating the treatment option, should it prove true, for disease prevention by reducing the prevalence of risk factors. Such an approach is more appealing than potentially dangerous immunotherapy.

While prospective studies of environmental conditions suspected to be important in individuals developing IDDM are essential in clarifying this relationship and must be continued, they are formidable undertakings. The prospect of an answer in the foreseeable future seems remote, particularly if multiple, nonspecific triggers exist (Nerup et al., 1988). Furthermore, in the event that a precipitant is identified, it is improbable that all cases of IDDM could be prevented. In short, arguments exist for both immunogenetically and environmentally oriented therapeutic strategies for IDDM, making exploration in both directions important.

The contention that beta-cell loss in IDDM is immune-mediated can be taken as virtually proven through observations made over the last 20 years. These include the histopathological finding of mononuclear cell infiltration and selective beta-cell destruction (insulitis) in pancreata of patients with IDDM of recent onset (Gepts, 1965), islet-directed humoral and cellular immune abnormalities preceding (Srikanta et al., 1986) and at the time of diagnosis (Nerup et al., 1971; Wilkin and Armitage, 1986), the association of risk of disease with the MHC, development of insulitis in segmental pancreatic transplants between monozygotic twins discordant for IDDM (Sibley et al., 1985), and the capacity to alter the natural course of beta-cell destruction by immunosuppression. The establishment of this concept of beta-cell destruction by an immune response is a landmark in the understanding of IDDM, however, several questions surround the process to which answers are needed for the development of optimal immunomodulatory treatment.

For example, definition of the primary immune effector event in cellular and molecular terms could create the potential for use of more precisely directed and presumably less toxic agents. At a cellular level, there is experimental and clinical evidence incriminating the cytotoxic T lymphocyte (Sibley et al., 1985; Bottazo et al., 1985), macrophage (Mandrup-Poulsen, 1988), natural killer cell (Woda and Biron, 1986), and B lymphocyte (Lernmark, 1985). On a molecular level, certain humoral factors appear capable of injuring the beta cell such as interleukin 1(IL-1), possibly by induction of free radical formation (Mandrup-Poulsen, 1988) and immunoglobulin directed toward the islet cell (Lernmark, 1985).

A second unresolved group of questions that is pertinent relates to duration and tempo of insulitis before and after onset of the clinical syndrome. Data from first-degree relatives of patients with IDDM show that in this high risk group, subclinical beta-cell loss can last years (Gorsuch et al., 1981). What is not established is whether such a course occurs in the more usual situation, that is, in those without an immediate family history of IDDM. Preliminary findings suggest that this is possible (Maclaren et al., 1985). A protracted period of occult insulitis enlarges the window of time for immunomodulation, but such an approach depends on safe and accurate identification of patients having subclinical beta-cell destruction that inevitably leads to overt diabetes.

Similarly, it is not clear if beta-cell aggression fluctuates in intensity at times other than the apparent amelioration seen during the spontaneous clinical remission shortly after diagnosis. It has been hypothesized that the process accelerates immediately before symptomatic metabolic failure (Nerup et al., 1988). Furthermore, studies in IDDM-discordant identical twins have found evidence of beta-cell dysfunction in conjunction with islet cell cytoplasmic antibodies in the nondiabetic twin, suggesting that loss of beta cells may arrest spontaneously (Heaton et al., 1987). If beta-cell destruction waxes and wanes, then the option of intermittent immunotherapy with reduction in dose-related side effects would arise.

A third question concerning the chronology of insulitis is the duration of immune memory once beta-cell destruction is complete. This seems long-lived based on observations in segmental pancreas transplants between identical twins discordant for IDDM where insulitis, with selective beta-cell killing not attributable to rejection, occurred in the absence of immunosuppression and despite up to 26 years of disease in the recipient (Sibley et al., 1985). If the abnormal immune response is, in effect, lifelong, then not only is there a need for indefinite immunomodulation in newly diagnosed diabetics so treated, but successful pancreatic islet replacement and schemes for in vivo islet cell regeneration must also depend heavily on immunomodulation.

There are other important questions of pathogenesis in IDDM that do not address the process of beta-cell loss but are still relevant to immunotherapy for the disease. The most important of these considers the basis for chronic micro- and microvascular complications. Specifically, "Are these complications a result of loss of beta cells?" Cross-sectional studies (Madsbad, 1983) are equivocal in showing an inverse relationship between beta-cell function and the frequency of complications. Prospective data controlling for other variables that may influence morbidity would support the rationale for attempting to preserve beta-cell function by immunotherapy should this relationship be substantiated. However, the definitive demonstration of cause and effect rests with randomized controlled studies of agents capable of preserving beta-cell function over many years. Two other related questions of subsidiary importance are "Does more normal long-term metabolic control reduce the risk of complications?" and, if so, "Does greater endogenous insulin secretion facilitate metabolic control?" A prospective trial is now in progress that should provide part of the answer, namely, the relationship between glycemic control and development and progression of microvascular morbidity (The Diabetic Control and Complications Group, 1986). If improved glycemic control reduces the likelihood of complications, then the search for immunotherapy that can safely maintain beta cells receives further justification.

3. SELECTED IMMUNOTHERAPEUTIC TRIALS IN IDDM OF RECENT ONSET

It has been nine years since the first accounts of immunotherapy for human IDDM. Most studies over this time have used no controls or have compared very small numbers of subjects to historical or nonrandom, concurrent controls. As of January 1989, at least 11 reported trials have used a randomized, concurrently controlled design (Table I). There are several points to consider when appraising this experience.

First, there has been no comparison of the long-term risk-to-benefit ratio of immunotherapy against that of conventional therapy. This is not a surprise in view of the novelty of immunotherapy for IDDM, as well as the time required (up to 15 years) for chronic complications to develop under conventional therapy. In this second respect, it is likely that the prognosis for a conventionally treated insulin-dependent diabetic has improved (Nerup, 1989) and may continue to do so. This will serve to increase the risk–benefit ratio required of any new treatment before it can supplant existing modalities in clinical practice.

Treatment effect has usually been assessed in terms of clinical response and endogenous insulin secretion. In the case of clinical response, this has taken the form of insulin dose over time and when the effect is deemed to be favorable has been given the name "remission." These responses have been further characterized in some studies by parameters of metabolic control such as glycated hemoglobin (GHb). Treatment effect in respect to endogenous insulin secretion has usually been inferred from connecting-peptide (CP) levels in the peripheral blood, often following a secretogogue (e.g., glucagon or a standardized meal).

In the strictest sense, "remission" means complete absence of clinical and laboratory stigmata of the disease. If this has occurred in IDDM after development of the clinical syndrome, then it appears to be rare. Metabolic studies in diabetics in immunosuppression-

TABLE I. Randomized, Controlled Trials of Immunotherapy for IDDM

Agents (Reference)	Design[a]	Total number of subjects	Treatment effect[b]
Interferon (3)	DB, PC	43	Clear: none
Cyclosporine (4)	DB, PC	122	Clear: enhanced clinical remission rate within 1 year
Cyclosporine (5)	DB, PC	188	Clear: enhanced clinical remission rate and increased CP level within and at 1 year
Cyclosporine (6)	DB, PC	23	Clear: enhanced CP level within and at 1 year
Azathioprine (7)	DB, PC	49	Clear: increased, unstimulated CP level within 6 months
Azathioprine (8)	Not blinded	24	Possible: enhanced clinical remission rate within 1 year and enhanced CP level at 1 year
Prednisone (9)	Not blinded	31	Clear: none
Ciamexone (10)	Not blinded	20	Possible: enhanced clinical remission rate
Cyclosporine, prednisone vs. cyclosporine (11)	Not specified	25	Possible: comparable clinical remission rates at 9 months between cyclosporine alone vs. lower-dose cyclosporine plus prednisone
Azathioprine and corticosteroid (12)	Not blinded	46	Clear: increase CP level within and at 1 year possible: improved metabolic status within and at 1 year
Nicotinamide (13)	DB, PC	16	Possible: prolongation of spontaneous remission

[a]DB, PC, double blind, placebo controlled.
[b]CP, connecting peptide.

References:(3) Koivisto *et al.* (1984); (4) Feutren *et al.* (1986); (5) The CERT group (1988); (6) Skyler (1988); (7) Cook *et al.* (1989); (8) Harrison *et al.* (1985); (9) Mistura *et al.* (1981); (10) Usadel *et al.* (1986); (11) Assan *et al.* (1988); (12) Silverstein *et al.* (1988); (13) Vague *et al.* (1987).

associated noninsulin-receiving states reveal gross abnormalities in blood glucose and endogenous insulin responses to intravenous glucose (Dupre et al., 1987). This, in part, reflects the fact that by the time of clinically apparent beta-cell failure, a large proportion of cells have been destroyed. Thus, while there is sufficient beta-cell recovery in about 20% of diabetics during immunosuppression within the first year to maintain target glycemia on conventional grounds without insulin injections (The Canadian–European Randomized Control Trial Group, 1988), there is no margin to handle extraordinary metabolic stress.

The definition of response based on insulin therapy makes definitive conclusions of efficacy by this criterion impossible in absence of randomly allocated, concurrent controls. This is because of the influence of other factors on blood glucose levels including diet, exercise, and the spontaneous clinical remission experienced by most diabetics within the first year. The potential bias of variation in diet and exercise also makes double-blinding important. Similarly, CP levels increase from the time of diagnosis to the third to sixth month during conventional treatment, which necessitates concurrent, randomized controls for conclusions of efficacy related to endogenous insulin secretion.

Most of the nonrandomized studies will not be considered further here: a comprehensive review is available (Skyler, 1988). The two most systematically investigated immunosuppressants for human IDDM to date have been azathioprine (Aza) and cyclosporine A (CyA) and the remainder of this chapter will focus on these agents.

Initial experience with Aza by Australian (Harrison et al., 1985) and American (Silverstein et al., 1986) groups was promising enough to lead both to undertake larger randomized, controlled trials. In the United States, 46 diabetics were randomized to receive either Aza and a 10-week course of corticosteroid (CS) or no immunosuppression (Silverstein et al., 1988). Patients were not blinded because of the easily perceived side effects of CS. One year after entry, the treated group had significantly higher meal-stimulated CP levels and required less insulin to maintain similar GHb levels in comparison to the control group. Ten immunosuppressed patients discontinued insulin for at least one week within the first year of whom three remained off insulin up to one year; just two control patients temporarily stopped injections prior to one year. There were ten patients with sufficient apparent benefit at one year to justify continued immunosuppression. Over the next two years, Aza was discontinued in seven for reasons of patient choice, noncompliance, headache, or loss of apparent benefit. Other adverse events included the expected but reversible effects related to CS, and the need to discontinue Aza prior to one year in three patients in response to non-life-threatening side effects.

In an Australian study, 49 diabetics were randomized to placebo or Aza treatment (Cook et al., 1989) under double-blinded conditions. Partial remission was defined as normal GHb and fasting capillary glucose $\leq$ 8.0 mM with an insulin dosage of < 0.5 units/day. There was no significant difference between groups in this outcome at 6 and 12 months. There was an effect on fasting CP values in the Aza group insofar as the mean value showed a significant rise from zero to three months, and was also significantly greater than the control group at three and six months. However, no differences were observed between groups in meal-stimulated CP levels over time. Adverse events in the Aza group included a greater incidence of certain skin lesions (herpes, verrucae) and transient episodes of neutropenia.

The clinical experience with CyA for IDDM has evolved contemporaneously to that of Aza, progressing from open, uncontrolled studies (Stiller et al., 1984; Assan et al., 1985; Bougneres et al., 1988) to randomized, placebo-controlled trials. The first randomized, double-blinded, placebo-controlled study of CyA for IDDM was conducted in France (Feutren et al., 1986). One hundred and twenty-two subjects were enrolled. The experimental group received CyA daily and the dose was adjusted according to clinical response, serum creatinine levels, and predose CyA concentrations ("troughs"). A "complete" remission required fasting blood glucose levels < 7.8 mM, postprandial glucose levels < 11.1 mM, and GHb ≤ 7.5% in the absence of exogenous insulin. "Partial" remission required the same metabolic criteria in conjunction with an insulin dosage < 0.25 units/kg per day. In patients followed to nine months, a statistically significant difference existed in the complete remission rate between groups (CyA, 24%; placebo, 6%). When partial and complete remission rates were combined within groups, CyA-treated subjects had significantly higher rates at both six and nine months. CP values were not provided in this report.

In a second double-blinded, placebo-controlled trial of CyA involving centers in Europe and Canada (CERT, 1988), 188 diabetics were randomized. Insulin was given with the objective of maintaining capillary blood glucose levels < 7.8 mM before meals and the dose was minimized as far as possible without exceeding this target. Two definitions of remissions were used. A clinical definition required that patients have target glycemia without exogenous insulin ("noninsulin receiving" or "NIR" remission); a compound definition required a glucagon-stimulated CP (GSCP) level ≥ 0.6 nM or the NIR state. Characteristics of both groups at entry were similar with the important exception of GSCP being significantly higher in the control group. NIR remissions were significantly more frequent in CyA-treated subjects at six (CyA, 39%; placebo, 19%) and 12 (CyA, 24%; placebo, 10%) months. The compound remission rate was also significantly higher in the CyA arm at both time points (6 months: CyA, 52%; placebo, 31%; 12 months: CyA, 33%; placebo, 21%) when adjustment was made for the difference in entry CP level. CP secretion was maintained at approximately the same level in the second six months in the CyA group, resulting in a higher value at one year in comparison to that of the control group.

In this trial, possible interaction of treatment with baseline characteristics was explored by multivariate analysis. Only the duration of clinically overt disease showed an interaction: the efficacy of CyA in terms of NIR remission was confined to patients with short-duration disease (defined as ≤ 6 weeks nocturia and ≤ 2 weeks insulin therapy). The reverse occurred in the placebo group, with a higher spontaneous remission rate in patients having disease of longer duration at entry. A subgroup of patients not different in their baseline characteristics from the study population as a whole was analyzed with respect to the predictive value of islet cell antibodies, insulin autoantibodies, and HLA-DR phenotype for remissions (Mandrup-Poulsen et al., 1989). While antibody positivity was suppressed by CyA treatment, islet cell antibody and insulin autoantibody status prior to entry did not predict clinical remission or beta-cell function after three months under CyA therapy. Similarly, HLA-DR phenotype did not identify patients having a favorable response CyA treatment.

The side effects of CyA therapy in newly diagnosed insulin-dependent diabetics have been consistent across the reported experience. The minor side effects (reversible and non-life-threatening) include hypertrichosis, gum hyperplasia, a nonprogressive anemia, headache, tremor, peripheral paresthesia, and gastrointestinal upset. The cosmetic effects have been unusual reasons for discontinuation of the drug but may be one reason for a preponderance of males in some series. The major side effects (irreversible, potentially life-threatening) include infection, lymphoproliferative disease (LPD), and nephrotoxicity.

In all series to date, life-threatening infections have not been reported, although there has been a nonstatistically significant increase in minor infections among CyA-treated subjects in the controlled trials. Regarding LPD, there have been no reports thus far of this occurring in patients given CyA for IDDM. This is consistent with the very low incidence of LPD among all patients with autoimmune diseases given CyA (B. von Graffenreid, personal communication); however, the long-term risk for such lesions remains unknown. In the absence of the recognition of any new complication or increase in the incidence of significant infection or LPD among CyA-treated patients with autoimmune disease, chronic nephrotoxicity with or without hypertension is the major limitation in the use of CyA for IDDM.

The nephrotoxicity of CyA in recent-onset diabetes can be evident on functional and morphological grounds. A reduction in glomerular filtration rate of approximately 30% as determined by a variety of techniques ranging from relatively insensitive creatinine-based methods (Feutren et al., 1986; CERT, 1988) to more definitive studies of clearance of radioisotopes (CERT, 1988; Feutren, 1988) can occur. This can be accompanied by hyperkalemia, is probably secondary to renal vasoconstriction, and is reversible on discontinuation of CyA (Assan et al., 1988; Dupre et al., 1988). It appears to be a concentration-dependent effect, being a consistent observation in studies where trough levels by the whole blood polyclonal radioimmunoassay of at least 400 ng/ml occurred (Feutren et al., 1986; CERT, 1988) but not seen in one study using 12-hr troughs of < 350 ng/ml (Bougneres et al., 1988).

Morphological nephrotoxicity has been evaluated in the context of conditions of clinical use of CyA and variables of renal function in a series of 90 renal biopsies from newly diagnosed diabetics treated for at least eight months (Feutren, 1988). Biopsies were given a score based on the presence and severity of the lesions on light microscopy that are associated with CyA therapy (interstitial fibrosis, focal tubular atrophy, and arteriolopathy). Structural changes attributed to CyA therapy without doubt were seen in 17 biopsies; they were rated as moderate in severity using a scale of none, minimal, slight, moderate, and severe. The most marked feature in these biopsies was interstitial fibrosis. In 29 further biopsies, changes were rated as slight. It was noted that this degree of abnormality could be seen in up to 10% of normal subjects. The remaining 44 biopsies were normal.

A number of variables were analyzed in relation to the biopsy score in the hope of identifying risk factors for chronic injury. Older age, higher CyA troughs in the first three months, higher elevations in plasma creatinine over baseline, and higher maximum creatinine rises at any time prior to biopsy were associated with moderate morphological changes while cumulative CyA dose and hypertension were not. A multivariate analysis was done to further assess the relationship between these variables and nephrotoxicity: greater maximum creatinine increment over baseline and higher age emerged as the strongest correlates.

A consideration of the results of the trials of Aza and CyA for new onset IDDM has led, and may lead, to further insight with respect to pathogenesis. Completely new questions are also raised. It is clear that immunosuppression alters the natural course of beta-cell destruction. This is the strongest available evidence that loss of beta cells is immune-mediated in human IDDM. The observation that islet cell antibody fails to predict clinical remission is consistent across studies (Silverstein et al., 1988; Cook et al., 1989; Mandrup-Poulsen et al., 1985, 1989) and is an argument against islet cell antibody playing a primary pathogenetic role at this stage of the disease.

It is apparent that immune intervention at the relatively late point of onset of clinical diabetes can still result in near-normal levels of insulin secretion as manifested by CP levels. In about one fifth of patients, this response is sufficient to obtain normal GHb levels without exogenous insulin for most of the first year after diagnosis (CERT, 1988). While the long-term clinical significance of this finding is not apparent and subject to the limitation that CP levels in the peripheral blood represent a semiquantitative measure of endogenous insulin secretion, it can be suggested that in some patients a large, viable but functionally depressed mass of beta cells are present at the time of diagnosis. This is contrary to the contention supported by autopsy findings (Gepts, 1965) that most beta cells are destroyed at the time of presentation and that the improved response is a manifestation of extraordinary insulin secretion by a few remaining cells.

The interaction between duration of clinical disease, timing of immunointervention, and response is a recurrent finding in the trials of CyA (CERT, 1988; Bougneres et al., 1988;

Dupre *et al.*, 1988). In a French open study in children (Bougneres *et al.*, 1988) and the Canadian–European randomized trial (CERT), clinical remission rates exceeding 50% within the first year were obtained in CyA-treated subjects with symptomatic disease of six weeks or less. The findings with respect to short- and long-duration symptoms may have pathogenetic implications. They suggest that beta-cell loss can progress over a period of several weeks, if not days, around the time of overt metabolic failure. Such a tempo is in distinction to the observation of subclinical beta-cell destruction lasting years in patients at high genetic risk for IDDM, but is consistent with the *in vitro* finding of enhanced susceptibility of more active beta cells to IL-1-mediated killing (Spinas *et al.*, 1988) under the presumption that as the islet fails the remaining beta cells work harder. The better outcome with immunosuppression in subjects with a short history of symptoms in comparison to those with a long prodrome leads to the inference that beta-cell failure in patients with a short history is the result of a more aggressive process that includes a greater functional but reversible component.

The loss of clinical response despite preservation of CP secretion by immunosuppression has been observed in three studies (CERT, 1988; Dupre *et al.*, 1988; Silverstein *et al.*, 1988), and if such a course is inevitable under these conditions, is a major limitation to this approach. In the absence of evidence to suggest that CP levels in these circumstances reflect anything other than endogenous insulin secretion, the discrepancy between exogenous insulin requirement and enhanced CP levels points to other factors affecting insulin requirements. Preliminary data indicate that changing insulin action may play a role (Hramiak *et al.*, 1988). Recrudescent but low-grade insulitis despite immunosuppression may also be a factor in relapse: anecdotal descriptions of reversal of relapse through intensification of immunotherapy exist (Dupre *et al.*, 1988; Silverstein *et al.*, 1987). It remains to be clearly demonstrated, however, whether modification of ongoing immunosuppression can maintain or reestablish clinical remissions. Any attempt to do so is limited by the current requirement of defining relapse in the term of hyperglycemia only, and from that inferring insulitis. This may be false given the factor of changing insulin resistance, and draws attention to the lack of definitive markers of active beta-cell destruction.

The interaction between age, immunotherapy, and outcome is unclear, but with the exception of the French open study of CyA in children, several trials using either CyA or Aza suggest no or reduced efficacy in the younger diabetic (Dupre *et al.*, 1988; Silverstein *et al.*, 1988; Cook *et al.*, 1989). The less favorable response in these subjects is consistent with the observation of poorer endogenous insulin secretion in younger patients at the time of diagnosis (Karjalainen *et al.*, 1989), and suggest that insulitis is more malevolent in children. The higher clinical response rate obtained in the French open study may have been a result of the relatively early timing of immunointervention.

The effect of Aza alone on the course of beta-cell destruction is not clear. The main virtue of this agent in comparison to CyA is its lack of nephrotoxicity. This is an important strength because long-term treatment appears to be necessary, and diabetic nephropathy is highly correlated with morbidity and mortality in IDDM making use of potentially nephrotoxic drugs undesirable. The Australian study of Aza (Cook *et al.*, 1989) used the strongest design and showed no clinically significant effect. In attempting to explain the negative finding the authors noted that the patient population was younger than that of other studies, and that an inadequate dose of Aza could not be excluded in view of the lack of an effect on lymphocyte count. The possibility of a type II statistical error also exists. The Florida randomized Aza–Cs trial, on the other hand, demonstrated clinical efficacy provided one is prepared to accept that a treatment bias did not occur.

Comparing these two trials with a view to account for the difference in outcome is speculative. Nevertheless, with the exception of the use of CS, they appear comparable in several ways, including the number and characteristics of the enrolled populations at entry (mean age, duration of symptoms, and mean CP level) and Aza dose. While this might suggest that the addition of CS made the difference, there is enough conflicting data to make the role for CS in recent-onset IDDM unresolved. Studies evaluating CS alone have, at best, suggested enhanced CP secretion only (Elliott et al., 1986); none, including at least one randomized study (Mistura et al., 1981), has demonstrated a favorable clinical response in newly diagnosed diabetics receiving this class of drug. CS therapy has the theoretical disadvantage of increasing beta-cell activity through creation of an insulin-resistant state and with that, as noted above, an increase in the cell's susceptibility to lymphokines. In addition, CS treatment results in discrepancies in insulin therapy between two study groups. This may lead to a difference in outcome that is not a result of CS but is instead a consequence of larger doses of insulin, in light of data suggesting that intensive insulin therapy at diagnosis prolongs endogenous insulin secretion (Shah et al., 1989).

In using Aza and CS concurrently, the Florida trial is one of several that has employed immunotherapeutic combinations. This concept is well-established in organ transplantation and has the theoretical advantage of minimizing individual drug toxicity without loss of efficacy, but also the possible disadvantage of overimmunosuppression. In the case of IDDM there will be an additional rationale for multifaceted strategies if it is established that the abnormal immune response is heterogenous over time. To date, however, no such combination has been convincingly shown to be superior to any single agent in inducing and maintaining clinical remissions.

4. CONCLUSION

Immunotherapy for newly diagnosed IDDM in 1989 is experimental. It seems typical of most developments in therapeutics in that fewer questions are answered than are asked and it has not resulted in immediate, dramatic clinical benefit. Nevertheless, it has afforded for the first time the opportunity of changing the natural course of IDDM at a fundamental and appealing level.

The evolution of this approach from experimental to conventional will depend on developments within the fields of clinical diabetology, epidemiology, experimental diabetes, transplantation, and immunopharmacology. Breakthroughs in any of these areas could quickly transform the role and nature of immunotherapy for IDDM, including the possibility of rendering it obsolete. For the short-term, however, it can be anticipated that it will continue to be pursued with certain emphases.

For example, the interest in the subclinical phase of IDDM has become particularly intense given the relationship between early intervention and outcome. Immunointervention in a few such subjects have been undertaken (Levy-Marchal, 1983; Eisenbarth et al., 1986), but it has been hard to justify the systematic use of potent immunosuppressant drugs in this setting because of difficulty with ascertainment of patients who inevitably develop IDDM. These studies are further limited to the small proportion of subjects at particularly high genetic risk and cannot be reasonably adapted, for the moment, to the more common sporadic case. The ability to easily identify the asymptomatic patient without an immediate family history of IDDM but with unremitting insulitis could provide a major focus for further immunotherapeutic trials.

It is hoped that the criteria for selection of patients receiving immunotherapy will improve. This applies both in the identification of those patients at greatest risk for long-term diabetic complications under conventional therapy and of those most likely to show a favorable response to the proposed treatment.

Finally, it can be expected that the testing of other immunoactive agents including combination protocols and intensive insulin therapy will continue. In particular, the application of semispecific immunotherapy through monoclonal antibodies directed to a variety of targets including the T lymphocyte and its products, as well as use of nonspecific anti-inflammatory agents such as free-radical scavengers, seems likely. These treatments may arise in experimental diabetes and transplantation and, if promising, then be tested in the human diabetic. As always, the definitive evaluation of such therapies will require long-term risk–benefit evaluation using meaningful end points under randomized, controlled conditions.

REFERENCES

Assan, R., Feutren, G., Debray-Sachs, M., Quiniou-Debrie, M. C., Laborie, C., Thomas, G., Chatenoud, L., and Bach, J. F., 1985, Metabolic and immunological effects of cyclosporin in recently diagnosed Type 1 diabetes mellitus, *Lancet* 1:69–71.

Assan, R., Feutren, G., and Sirmai, J., 1988, Cyclosporine trials in diabetes: Updated results of the French experience, *Transplant. Proc.* 20(3S4):178–183.

Bell, G. I., Horita, S., and Karam, J. H., 1984, A polymorphic locus near the human insulin gene is associated with IDDM, *Diabetes* 33:176–83.

Borch-Johnsen, K., Kreiner, S., and Deckert, T., 1986, Mortality of Type 1 diabetes in Denmark: A study of relative mortality in 2930 Danish Type 1 diabetic patients diagnosed from 1933–1972, *Diabetologia* 29:767–72.

Bottazo, G. F., Dean, B. M., McNally, J. M., MacKay, E. H., Swift, P. G., and Gamble, D. R., 1985, In situ characterization of autoimmune phenomena and expression of HLA molecules in the pancreas in diabetic insulitis, *N. Engl. J. Med.* 313:353–60.

Bougneres, P. F., Carel, J. C., Castano, L., Boitard, C., Gardin, J. P., Landais, P., Hors, J., Mihatsch, M. J., Paillard, M., Chaussain, J. L., and Bach, J. F., 1988, Factors determining early remission of type 1 diabetes in children treated with cyclosporin A, *N. Engl. J. Med.* 318:633–670.

The Canadian–European Randomized Control Trial Group (CERT), 1988, Cyclosporin-induced remission of IDDM after early intervention, *Diabetes* 37:1574–1582.

Cook, J. J., Hudson, I., Harrison, L. C., Dean, B., Colmon, P. G., Werther, G. A., Warne, G. L., and Court, J. M., 1989, A double-blind controlled trial of azathioprine in children with newly diagnosed type 1 diabetes, *Diabetes* 38:779–783.

Diabetes Epidemiology Research International, 1987, Preventing IDDM: The environmental challenge, *Br. Med. J.* 295:479–481.

The Diabetic Control and Complications Trial Group, 1986, The diabetic control and complications trial (DCCT), *Diabetes* 35:530–545.

Drash, A. L., 1986, Diabetes mellitus in the child and adolescent, *Curr. Problems Pediatr.* 16:413–466.

Dupre, J., Stiller, C. R., Jenner, M. R., Mahon, J. L., Keown, P., Rodger, N. W., and Wolfe, B., 1987, Responses to nutrients in non-insulin requiring remission of Type 1 diabetes during administration of cyclosporin, *Diabetes* 36(S1):74A.

Dupre, J., Stiller, C. R., Gent, M., Donner, A., von Graffenreid, B., Murphy, G., Heinrichs, D., Jenner, M. R., Keown, P. A., Laupacis, A., Mahon, J., Martell, R., Rodger, N. W., and Wolfe, B. W., 1988, Effects of immunosuppression with Cy in IDDM of recent onset: The Canadian Open Study at 44 months, *Transplant. Proc.* 20(3S4):184–192.

Ehrlich, R. M., Walsh, L. J., Falk, J. A., Middleton, P. J., and Simpson, N. E., 1982, The incidence of IDD in Toronto, *Diabetologia* 22:289–291.

Eisenbarth, G. S., 1987, Genes, generator of diversity, glycoconjugates, and autoimmune beta-cell insufficiency in type 1 diabetes, *Diabetes* 36:355–364.

Eisenbarth, G. S., Srikanta, S., Rabinowe, S. L., Jackson, R. A., Ganda, O. P., and Soeldner, J. S., 1986, Restoration of first-phase insulin secretion by daily prednisone in two islet cell antibody positive nondiabetic individuals, *Transplant. Proc.* 18:805–808.

Elliott, R. B., Pilcher, C. C., and Edgar, B. W., 1986, Long-term outcome of children with IDDM treated ab initio with prednisone, *Pediatr. Adoelsc. Endocrinol.* 15:345–349.

Feutren, G., 1988, Functional consequences and risk factors of chronic cyclosporine nephrotoxicity in Type 1 diabetes trials, *Transplant. Proc.* 20(3S4):356–366.

Feutren, G., Papoz, L., Assan, R., Vialettes, B., Karsenty, G., Vexiau, P., Du Rostu, H., Rodier, M, Sirmai, J., Lallemand, A., and Bach, J. F., 1986, Cyclosporin increases the rate and length of remissions in IDDM of recent onset, *Lancet* 2:119–123.

Gepts, W., 1965, Pathological anatomy of the pancreas in juvenile diabetes mellitus *Diabetes* 14:619–633.

Gorsuch, A. N., Spencer, K. M., Lister, J., McNally, J. M., Dean, B. M., Bottazo, G. F., and Cudworth, A. G., 1981, The natural history of IDDM: The evidence for a long prediabetic period, *Lancet* 2:1363–1365.

Harrison, L. C., Colmon, P. G., Dean, B., Baxter, R., and Martin, F. I., 1985, Increase in remission rate in newly diagnosed Type 1 diabetic subjects treated with azathioprine, *Diabetes* 34:1306–1308.

Heaton, D. A., Millward, B. A., Gray, P., Tun, Y., Hules, C. N., Pyke, D. A., and Leslie, R. D., 1987, Evidence of beta-cell dysfunction which does not lead on to diabetes: A study of identical twins of insulin dependent diabetics, *Br. Med. J.* 294: 145–146.

Hodge, S., Anderson, C., Neiswanger, K., Field, L., Spence, M., Sparkes, R., Crist, M., Terasaki, P., Rimoin, D., and Rotter, J., 1981, Close genetic linkage between diabetes mellitus and Kidd blood group, *Lancet* 2:893–895.

Hramiak, I., Finegood, D., and Dupre, J., 1988, Insulin sensitivity in Cy-treated type 1 diabetics in remission, *Diabetes* 37(S1):16A.

Karjalainen, J., Salmela, P., Ilonen, J., Surcel, H., and Knip, M., 1989, A comparison of childhood and adult type 1 diabetes mellitus, *N. Engl. J. Med.* 320:881–886.

Koivisto, V. A., Aro, A., Cantell, K., et al., 1984, Remissions in newly diagnosed type 1 (insulin-dependent) diabetes mellitus: Influence of interferon as an adjunct to insulin therapy, *Diabetologia* 27:193–197.

Kolb, H., and Nerup, J., 1985, TIDM: Rationale for immune intervention, in: *Cyclosporin in Autoimmune Diseases* (R. Schindler, ed.), Springer-Verlag, Berlin, pp. 117–119.

Lernmark, A., 1985, Molecular biology of IDDM, *Diabetologia* 28:195–203.

Levy-Marchal, C., Czernichow, P., Quiniou, M. C., Shahs, M., and Bach, J. F., 1983, Cyclosporin administration reversed abnormalities in a prediabetic child, *Diabetes* 32(S1):51A.

Ludvigsson, J., Samuelsson, U., Benforts, C., Deschamps, I., Drash, A., Francois, R., Herz, G., New, M., and Schober, E., 1986, HLA-DR3 is associated with a more slowly progressive form of insulin dependent diabetes, *Diabetologia* 29:207–210.

Maclaren, N. K., Horne, G., Spillar, R. P., Barbour, H., Harrison, O., and Duncan, J., 1985, Islet cell autoantibodies in U.S. school children, *Diabetes* 34(S1):335A.

Madsbad, S., 1983, Prevalence of residual B cell function and its metabolic consequences in Type 1 diabetes, *Diabetologia* 24:141–147.

Mandrup-Poulsen, T., 1988, On the pathogenesis of IDDM, *Dan. Med. Bull.* 35:438–460.

Mandrup-Poulsen, T., Nerup, J., Stiller, C. R., Marner, B., Bille, G., Heinrichs, D., Martell, R., Dupre, J., Keown, P. A., Jenner, M. R., Rodger, N. W., Wolfe, B., Graffenreid, B. V., and Binder, C., 1985, Disappearance and reappearance of islet cell cytoplasmic antibodies in cyclosporin-treated insulin dependent diabetics, *Lancet* 1:599–602.

Mandrup-Poulsen, T., Molvig, J., Andersen, H. U., Helqvist, S., and Munck, M., for the Canadian/European Diabetes Study Group, 1990, Lack of predictive value of islet cell antibodies, insulin autoantibodies, and HLA-DR phenotype for remission in Type 1 diabetic patients treated with cyclosporine, *Diabetes* 39:204–210.

Mistura, L., Beccaria, L., Meschi, F., D'Arcais, A., Pellini, C., Puzzovio, M., and Chiumello, G., 1981, Prednisone treatment in newly diagnosed Type 1 diabetic children: 1 year follow-up, *Diabetes Care* 10:39–43.

Nerup, J., 1989, Rationale of immune intervention in type one diabetes, in: *Immunotherapy of Type One Diabetes* (H. Kolb, D. Andreani, and P. Pozzilli, eds.), John Wiley and Sons, Chichester, pp. 5–11.

Nerup, J., Anderson, O. O., Bendixen, G., Egeborg, J., and Poulsen, J. E., 1971, Antipancreatic cellular hypersensitivity in diabetes mellitus, *Diabetes* 20:424–427.

Nerup, J., Mandrup-Poulsen, T., and Molvig, J., 1987, The HLA-IDDM association: Implications for etiology and pathogenesis of IDDM, *Diabetes Metab. Rev.* 3:770–802.

Nerup, J., Mandrup-Poulsen, T., Molvig, J., Helqvist, S., Wogensen, L., and Egeborg, J., 1988, Mechanisms of pancreatic beta-cell destruction in type 1 diabetes, *Diabetes Care* 11(Suppl.1):16–23.

Prosser, P. R., and Karam, J. H., 1978, Diabetes mellitus following rodenticide ingestion in man, *J. Am. Med. Assoc.* 239:1148–1150.

Shah, S. C., Malone, J. I., and Simpson, N. E., 1989, A randomized trial of intensive insulin in newly diagnosed IDDM, *N. Engl. J. Med.* 320:550–554.

Sibley, R. K., Sutherland, D. E., Goetz, F., and Michael, A. F., 1985, Recurrent diabetes mellitus in the pancreas iso- and allograft, *Lab. Invest.* 53:132–144.

Silverstein, J., Riley, W., Spillar, R., Buithieu, M., Barbour, H., Harrison, D., and Alamo, A., 1986, A trial of immunosuppression with Imuran, *Diabetes* 35(Suppl.1):5A.

Silverstein, J., Spillar, R., Maclaren, N., and Decker, P., 1987, Immunotherapy with steroids and azathioprine in IDDM: The importance of steroid induction, *Diabetes* 36(Suppl.1):74A.

Silverstein, J., Maclaren, N., Riley, W., Spillar, R., Radjenovic, D., and Johnson, S., 1988, Immunosuppression with azathioprine and prednisone in recent-onset IDDM, *N. Engl. J. Med.* 319:599–604.

Skyler, J., 1988, Immune intervention studies in IDDM, *Diabetes Metab. Rev.* 3:1017–1035.

Spinas, G. A., Palmer, J. P., Mandrup-Poulsen, T., Andersen, H., Nielsen, J., and Nerup, J., 1988, The bimodal effect of interleukin 1 on rat pancreatic beta-cells—stimulation followed by inhibition—depends upon dose, duration of exposure, and ambient glucose concentration, *Acta Endocrinol.* 119:307–311.

Srikanta, S., Ricker, T., McCulloch, D. K., Soeldner, J. S., Eisenbarth, G. S., and Palmer, J. P., 1986, Autoimmunity to insulin, beta-cell dysfunction, and development of IDDM, *Diabetes* 35:139–142.

Stiller, C. R., Dupre, J., Gent, M., Jenner, M. R., Keown, P. A., Laupacis, A., Martell, R., Rodger, N. W., Graffenried, B. V., and Wolfe, B. M., 1984, Effects of cyclosporine immunosuppression in IDDM of recent onset, *Science* 223:1362–1367.

Tattersall, R. B., and Pyke, D. A., 1972, Diabetes in identical twins, *Lancet* 2:1120–1125.

Usadel, K. H., Teuber, J., Schmeidl, R., Schwedes, U., Bicker, U., and Herz, M., 1986, Management of type 1 diabetes with ciamexone, *Lancet* 2:567.

Vague, P. N., Violettes, B., Lassmann-Vague, V., and Vello, J. J., 1987, Nicotinamide may extend remission phase in ID diabetes, *Lancet* 1:619.

Wilkin, T., and Armitage, M., 1986, Markers for IDDM: Towards early detection, *Br. Med. J.* 293:1323–1326.

Woda, B. A., and Biron, C. A., 1986, Natural killer cell number and function in the spontaneously diabetic BB\ rat, *J. Immunol.* 137:1860–1866.

Yoon, J. W., Austin, M., Ondera, T., and Notkins, A. L., 1979, Virus-induced diabetes mellitus: Isolation of a virus from a pancreas of a child with diabetic ketoacidosis, *N. Engl. J. Med.* 300:1173–1179.

Chapter 24

IMMUNOREGULATORY TREATMENT IN INFLAMMATORY BOWEL DISEASE

Morten H. Vatn

1. INTRODUCTION

Despite common signs and symptoms of ulcerative colitis and Crohn's disease, leaving up to 10–20% of instances unclassified, many important differences are clinically apparent, giving rise to distinct differences in treatment. These differences are most conspicuous with regard to endoscopic and histological pathology. Whereas ulcerative colitis is characterized by colorectal or rectal mucosal involvement, Crohn's disease is primarily a submucosal process involving any part of the gut from the mouth to the anus, in an intermittent manner and with a tendency of abscessa or fistula formation. The structural and anatomical manifestations form the basis for different medical and surgical managements, of which surgery has quite different implications for the prognosis of Crohn's disease compared to ulcerative colitis.

The imbalance in the immunoregulatory system in inflammatory bowel disease (IBD) forms a theoretical rationale for immunoregulatory treatment. Nevertheless, the introduction of immunomodulating drugs has been hampered by difficulties in evaluation of response due to specious results, uncontrolled trials, and the fact that these diseases have a natural fluctuating course and a variety of expressions.

The choice of treatment in idiopathic IBD is based on our experience from controlled clinical trials combined with individual clinical experience. Many individual modifications are necessary during follow-up. Immunoregulatory treatment has to be considered in relation to other forms of drug therapy, considering efficacy, side effects, and clinical state of the patient (Peppercorn, 1990).

Because of differences in pathology, clinical behavior, and prognosis, the two diseases

Morten H. Vatn • Medical Department A, The National Hospital, University of Oslo, N-0027 Oslo 1, Norway.
Immunopharmacology in Autoimmune Diseases and Transplantation, edited by Hans Erik Rugstad *et al.* Plenum Press, New York, 1992.

will generally be discussed separately. An exception to this is similar treatment applied for severe ulcerative and Crohn's colitis, characterized by a fulminant clinical picture and extensive involvement of the colon (Jewell, 1989).

2. ACUTE SEVERE ULCERATIVE COLITIS AND CROHN'S DISEASE

The severity of the disease at the start of treatment has great bearing on the outcome of the illness. It has been shown (Truelove and Witts, 1955) that cortisone-treated patients had a more favorable outcome than the corresponding control patients, at each level of severity, in both first attacks and relapses. The favorable experience with intensive treatment has been reached with intravenous doses of hydrocortisone from 100 mg (Truelove and Witts, 1955) to 300 mg daily (Meyers et al., 1983), corresponding to 20–60 mg daily of methylprednisolone. Experience from controlled trials recommend five- to ten-day courses of intensive treatment (Meyers et al., 1983; Truelove and Jewell, 1974). Observations on the use of higher doses of prednisone (80–160 mg given daily over 11 to 13 days) have been reported (Kristensen et al., 1974), showing good response in 13 of 31 patients with severe ulcerative colitis. Around two thirds of patients with first-attack colitis go into remission, remaining generally symptom-free for at least one to three years on maintenance treatment.

Response to intensive treatment may be reduced if the patient has been treated with steroids prior to the attack (Meyers et al., 1983). Corticotropine 120 units daily, equivalent to 300 mg hydrocortisone, may represent an alternative choice of treatment in those cases; however, data are few. Parenteral nutrition is indicated in a minority of cases, whereas optimal fluid and electrolyte balance is obligate. Antibiotics have been used as supportive agents to steroids (Truelove and Jewell, 1974), but the role of antibacterial treatment is unclear.

Patients showing no improvement during five to ten days of intensive treatment are immediate cases for surgery. Exact determination of time for follow-up before surgery is difficult to set due to the relative significance of all the signs of disease activity. There is evidence, however, that even among patients showing improvement without remission during the five to ten days of intensive treatment, the majority of cases will require urgent surgery within the next six weeks. The speed of dose reduction during remission must be related to the rate of improvement and the duration of high-dose treatment prior to reduction.

Fulminant left-sided colitis often has the same prognosis in the long run as fulminant extensive colitis, in spite of a less severe clinical picture during the attack. Response to high doses of steroids is often poor, and the patients have continual rectal bleeding for weeks or months before surgery. Alternative treatment is steroid or 5-aminosalicylic acid (5-ASA) enema preparations alone or in combination with oral medication.

In severe ulcerative and Crohn's colitis, daily dosages of prednisone at a rate of 0.5–1 mg/kg body weight, mostly 45–60 mg per day in divided doses, are recommended. The duration of high-dose treatment is dependent on the clinical course, but a reduction from 60 to 45 to 30 mg daily with five- to seven-day intervals is often sufficient to maintain improvement. Below 30 mg, a reduction of 5 mg at a time should be performed with one to two weeks treatment on each level. Below 20 mg, a smaller reduction, 2.5 mg at a time, is often necessary along with careful observation of signs of relapse.

Recurrences during this period of dose reduction are treated by a moderate increase of dose to, for example, 30 mg. Then, slower reduction is performed, ending 2.5–5 mg higher than the dose level applied when relapse occurred. If this level is below 20 mg, maintenance treatment may be performed for a longer period, from several weeks to months, before careful reduction is tried. Prerequisites for prolonged periods of treatment at increased dose levels are continual improvement and drug tolerance.

A second recurrence, occurring during "retarded" dose reduction, calls for alternative therapy as a combination of drugs or surgery. Salazopyrine or 5-ASA is combined with oral methylprednisolone in ulcerative colitis and Crohn's colitis from the time of early remission. If not used initially, metronidazole 800 to 1200 mg daily may be combined with the former drugs when relapse occurs.

The common side effects of glucocorticoids may occur during acute-stage treatment with high doses of methylprednisolone. During rapid reduction below 20 mg daily, only moderate cushingoid phenomena are recognizable. Methylprednisolone causes less fluid retention compared with hydrocortisone. Mental problems, insomnia, electrolyte disturbances, and gastroduodenal ulcer may occur during high-dose treatment.

3. CORTICOSTEROIDS IN CHRONIC ACTIVE ULCERATIVE COLITIS

Intestinal signs of active inflammation, endoscopically and histologically, with increased stool frequency or a mixture of blood but without signs of an acute illness with clinical impairment, weight loss, or signs of anemia are characterized as chronic active colitis. This stage may represent the first onset of disease, a relapse from a quiescent stage, or improvement from acute or fulminant colitis. A beneficial effect of oral cortisone (Truelove and Witts, 1955) and prednisone (Lennard-Jones et al., 1960) have been demonstrated by controlled trials. There is a tendency to greater response among patients with a first attack of disease than with a relapse. Corticosteroid therapy has been shown to be superior to sulfasalazine, judged by sigmoidoscopic and clinical assessment during two weeks of follow-up in patients with an attack of ulcerative colitis (Truelove et al., 1962). The optimal dose for outpatients with moderately severe active colitis is 40–60 mg prednisone daily in divided doses, showing clearly superior remission rate compared with 20 mg/day (Baron et al., 1962). The speed of dose reduction is especially critical from around 20 mg/day and downward (Lennard-Jones et al., 1965). It is very often recommended to extend the time of treatment on each dose level and to shorten the distance between dose levels.

When relapse occurs before the quiescent stage is reached, a moderate increase to, for example, 30 mg is often successful. When remission is not obtained with this regimen, alternative treatments with combinations of drugs or surgery is indicated. Prolonged treatment periods of six months or more on 15–20 mg per day, sometimes higher, may be beneficial in some instances without serious side effects, resulting in a gradual and finally stable remission. These cases must be followed with special caution. Any clinical impairment or signs of relapse during this treatment is an indication for surgery. In most instances of active colitis refractory to optimal treatment for three to four months, the patients are in favor of surgery.

Divided doses and a single dose daily has been shown to be therapeutically equivalent. A single dose might cause less adrenal suppression; however, divided doses seem preferable because of fewer abdominal side effects and better patient compliance.

There is no evidence to suggest that previous steroid administration is harmful to the patients who have undergone surgery. On the contrary, it must be regarded as a fundamental error to stop the treatment with steroids too quickly prior to or after surgery. In patients who have been on doses higher than 10 mg daily for weeks or months, treatment should not be ended earlier than three to six weeks after surgery. On the other hand, in patients who have been on high doses for less than two weeks, steroid treatment might be discontinued within five to ten days without signs of adrenal impairment.

4. CORTICOSTEROIDS IN DISTAL ACTIVE ULCERATIVE COLITIS, PROCTITIS, AND PROCTOSIGMOIDITIS

Even though we do not know if differences in localization, distribution, and extent of colitis point to specific etiological or pathogenetic mechanisms, variation in clinical pattern certainly gives reason for alternations in therapeutic strategy. The differential diagnosis between acute or severe colitis and active chronic colitis may be particularly difficult in ulcerative colitis affecting the distal part of the large intestine. This limited involvement of the colon very seldom causes general clinical impairment of the patient, in contrast to the acutely ill patient with acute total colitis. Also, the normal-appearing configuration of haustrae of the transverse and ascending colon on x-ray examination may falsely give the impression of an unaffected large intestine. Only carefully performed distal colonoscopy with biopsies may reveal a severely or acutely affected bowel wall. These circumstances call for special caution during the follow-up of patients with distal colitis and consideration of doses of steroid and sulfasalazine. The continuation of daily bleeding in these patients very often is a reminder of therapeutic resistance and at most of a time-limited response to high doses of treatment.

Topical steroids and 5-ASA preparations have been shown to be quite beneficial for the treatment of distal ulcerative colitis, proctitis, and proctosigmoiditis. The clinical and endoscopic response was 70% after two weeks treatment with 5-ASA preparation enemas, increasing to around 90% response rate after four weeks of treatment (Danish 5-ASA Group, 1987). In poor respondents or at early relapse, both morning and evening doses may be given.

Since a proportion of rectally administered steroids is absorbed, it has been suggested that beneficial effects are due to systemic action. It has, however, been shown that preparations of prednisone enemas resulting in different serum levels were of equal therapeutic efficacy (Lee et al., 1980). Absorption and adrenal suppression vary widely, depending on which preparation is used. By the use of prednisolone-21-phosphate enemas, it was found that the average excretion of radiolabeled prednisolone was between one half and one sixth the amount measured when an equivalent dose was given by mouth (Lee et al., 1971). Prednisone enemas have shown a greater tendency toward adrenal suppression than prednisolone. As much as three fourths of the dose might be absorbed (Halvorsen et al., 1969). Enemas given as foam seem to be superior to regular enemas in many patients with proctitis. Significant improvement of idiopathic proctitis and proctosigmoiditis may also be achieved with prednisolone or 5-ASA suppositories in singular or divided doses.

5. CORTICOSTEROIDS IN QUIESCENT COLITIS

Long-term prophylactic therapy with prednisone has been shown to be inefficient in preventing relapse in patients with ulcerative colitis in remission, in doses between 15 and 100 mg daily. Side effects are often troublesome, and, therefore, in the majority of cases larger doses are not acceptable even if they might be effective.

Many of these patients represent a stage between quiescent and active colitis, sometimes with intermittent symptoms like bleeding. Therefore, any patient with endoscopic or histological signs of activity should not be classified as simple quiescent colitis. They should be followed more closely for the sake of early diagnosis of relapse and change of therapeutic strategy.

6. AZATHIOPRINE IN ULCERATIVE COLITIS

The evidence for the use of azathioprine in the treatment of ulcerative colitis is limited. A significant steroid reduction in combination with 1.5 mg/kg of azathioprine, however, has been demonstrated compared with placebo (Rosenberg et al., 1975) in chronic active colitis. Doses of 2–2.5 mg/kg over a six-month period has shown a steroid-sparing effect in chronic ulcerative colitis (Kirk and Lennard-Jones, 1982). Comparing placebo with azathioprine, both in combination with corticosteroids, showed equivalent numbers of relapses in the two treatment groups (Jewell and Truelove, 1974) for those treated for attack of colitis. The drug may seem useful in patients requiring steroids, refusing surgery, or who are poor surgical risks. If applied, treatment should be given for at least three to six months.

The need for azathioprine in ulcerative colitis will always be limited as colectomy represents a permanent cure of the disease.

7. CROMOGLYCATE IN ULCERATIVE PROCTOCOLITIS

An effect on symptoms and endoscopic and histological appearances has been shown in patients with total quiescent colitis given 2 g daily by mouth over a two- to six-month period (Mani et al., 1976). In active proctitis or colitis, a combination of 100 mg orally three times daily and 200 mg enema twice daily showed an effect on symptoms and sigmoidoscopic and histological findings in 14 of 26 patients. There was a greater eosinophilic count at the start of the trial in those who responded to cromoglycate than in those who did not (Heatley et al., 1975). Favorable results have been reported in uncontrolled studies (Della Cella et al., 1976). Altogether, however, in spite of the promising results, cromoglycate has so far no place in the routine treatment of ulcerative colitis.

8. CORTICOSTEROID THERAPY OF ACUTE AND ACTIVE CROHN'S DISEASE

Corticosteroids are generally beneficial in symptomatic patients with Crohn's disease. Indications for intravenous therapy in acute or severe Crohn's colitis are similar to those in ulcerative colitis. Prednisolone is quite sufficiently absorbed in extensive small bowel involvement, even in nutritional malabsorption (Tanner et al., 1981; Bergrem and Opedal, 1983). Oral therapy with daily doses of 30–60 mg prednisolone has shown good to excellent long-term response. Two large controlled trials (Summers et al., 1979; Malchow et al., 1984) have shown around 80% remission in small bowel Crohn's disease. In the presence of combined small and large bowel involvement, steroid therapy in doses from 1–4 mg/kg body weight of prednisone has been shown to reduce the activity of Crohn's disease over four months (Singleton, 1977).

In conclusion, corticosteroids are obviously effective in most cases of acute or active Crohn's disease. An important question is, due to side effects and relapse rate, when to stop treatment and the speed of tapering before ending the treatment.

9. MAINTENANCE TREATMENT IN CROHN'S DISEASE

One study (Malchow *et al.*, 1984) has shown a mild benefit with prolonged, low-dose steroid maintenance treatment. This group of patients had obtained remission during an initial, high-dose prednisolone regimen. Other studies have failed to demonstrate a benefit of steroids on recurrence (Singleton, 1977; Smith *et al.*, 1978). In addition, a 30-year study of 174 patients with Crohn's disease, managed largely without steroids, showed an annual risk of operation of not more than 11% in the first five years (Cooke *et al.*, 1980) comparable to previous reports on long-term steroid treatment (Sparberg and Kirsner, 1966).

Neither doses of 7.5 mg nor 17.5 mg/day reduced the relapse rate compared with placebo (Summers *et al.*, 1979). Thus, steroids in low or moderate doses do not seem to give protection against relapse once remission is obtained, and abolishing the treatment will not increase the risk of relapse. Increasing the doses of steroids would certainly have increased the frequency of side effects. Also, combined treatment with steroids and salazopyrine have not shown a reduced risk of recurrences (Smith *et al.*, 1978).

10. THE TREATMENT OF RELAPSE OR CHRONIC CROHN'S DISEASE

The first clinical relapse in a patient with Crohn's disease may principally be considered and treated as a first attack. Repeated treatment periods with steroids may be successful, but certain factors are important for the choice of strategy at the next relapse. In addition to general well-being, patients' tolerance to treatment and nutritional status, the time between exacerbations, the localization and extension of disease, and the presence of complications seem to be of special relevance to the therapeutic approach.

If a patient has responded quickly to steroids during a previous attack or if remission has lasted for several years, steroid treatment would be applied at the next attack. There is not enough evidence to claim that steroid response decreases with the number of treatment periods. On the other hand, there is reason to believe that in many patients the disease becomes increasingly aggressive throughout the years, as indicated by follow-up of general Crohn's disease patients (Truelove and Pena, 1976) and follow-up after resection (Mekhjan *et al.*, 1979). This may explain why many patients seem more difficult to treat during later stages. On the other hand, early operation might influence the length of remission (Bergman and Krause, 1976). Continuation of steroid treatment must, therefore, be evaluated against surgery, especially in localized small bowel involvement. Thus, the localization as well as a limited extension of disease in the small intestine may count in favor of a complete small bowel resection, especially if a relapse occurs after many years of remission. This may be the case whether or not previous resection has been performed (Mekhjan *et al.*, 1979). A new trial with steroids will, however, in most instances be carried out, but the possibility of surgery should be brought into discussion and introduced to the patient at this stage. Repeated relapses of Crohn's colitis or extensive small bowel involvement very often respond poorly to repeated steroid treatment with or without combination with salazopyrine (Allan *et al.*, 1977). Supplementation with adjuvant treatment is very often needed, although surgery does represent an alternative in Crohn's colitis.

Complete resection of ileal or ileocolic disease has changed the surgical strategy over time in the direction of smaller but complete resections, in contrast to bypass operations and partial resections, especially of the large bowel. There is little documented evidence from controlled trials for a change of disease course or reduction in relapse rate after steroids when dividing materials into subgroups. There is, however, direct evidence from individual case improvement to continue the strategy of intermittent steroid treatment as long as a stable remission seems possible. In extensive small bowel involvement or short bowel syndrome after resection, the smallest effective dose should be combined with optimal supportive therapy.

When relapse or chronic disease are mainly caused by the occurrence of abscesses or fistulas, intensified treatment such as immunosuppression or surgery should continuously be considered. If relapse occurs at prednisone doses of about 10–15 mg daily, immunosuppressive therapy should be considered in any case.

11. AZATHIOPRINE THERAPY IN ACTIVE CROHN'S DISEASE

Altogether, there is no statistical evidence in favor of an effect of azathioprine alone versus placebo in active Crohn's disease. In most trials and in a lot of case reports, however, a striking effect has been observed in a limited number of individuals. It therefore seems likely that a subset of Crohn's disease patients with active disease do respond to azathioprine beyond the steroid-sparing effect.

12. AZATHIOPRINE THERAPY DURING REMISSION IN CROHN'S DISEASE

The first randomized controlled trial demonstrated a clear benefit from azathioprine during a 24-week study (Willoughby et al., 1971), in contrast to a study of azathioprine in operated and unoperated patients in remission (Watson and Bukowsky, 1974).

The largest trial undertaken so far, including 234 patients, did not demonstrate an effect of azathioprine over a four-month treatment period (Singleton, 1976; Summers et al., 1979) compared with placebo. This study has been criticized for the short observation period, and that all other active compounds were completely withdrawn just a few weeks before the start of the study, which can explain many of the early relapses.

The studies showing an effect superior to placebo in Crohn's disease patients in remission have applied a treatment period exceeding six months after withdrawal of steroid therapy. The effect has been most striking in newly diagnosed cases in daily doses of 1–2.5 mg/kg. In a double-blind withdrawal trial of patients who had been in remission for at least six months (O'Donoghue et al., 1978), the cumulative probability of relapse was nil at six months and 5% at one year among those on azathioprine compared with 25% at six months and 41% at one year among those in the control group.

13. AZATHIOPRINE AND 6-MERCAPTOPURINE AS PREDNISONE-SPARING TREATMENT IN CROHN'S DISEASE

The most striking effects reported in the first uncontrolled studies were decreased in steroid dependency and dramatic healing of fistulas. In a controlled study of the steroid-sparing effect of azathioprine over 26 weeks, reduction or discontinuation of steroids without worsening of symptoms was possible in all ten of the patients receiving active drug, significantly more frequent than in the placebo group (Rosenberg et al., 1975). Two relapses were recorded in the azathioprine-treated group versus seven in the placebo group.

The largest study in terms of patient-years' follow-up included 83 patients with intractable Crohn's disease in a double-blind two-year cross-over study of 6-mercaptopurine

(6-MP) versus placebo over a seven-year period (Present *et al.*, 1977). Clinical improvement, reduction of steroid requirements and closure of fistulas occurred significantly more often among patients treated with 6-MP than in the group receiving placebo. Delayed onset of action for at least four to six months was common.

In an uncontrolled open series (Nyman *et al.*, 1985), the mean observation period exceeding five years, all but one of the treated patients improved, and 11 of 42 went into complete remission during therapy. Also, local and systemic complications decreased significantly. Steroid therapy was reduced or withdrawn in all the patients and the average remission period after withdrawal of all drugs in ten patients was 40 months.

14. SUMMARY OF THE EXPERIENCE WITH AZATHIOPRINE IN CROHN'S DISEASE

These examples illustrate that the main indications for azathioprine in Crohn's disease are maintenance treatment for the sake of keeping patients in remission, treatment of refractory disease or required toxic doses of steroids, or treatment of extraintestinal or intestinal complications. The possibility of a limited effect of azathioprine as monotherapy seems reasonable from analysis of subgroups showing an 18% improvement compared with placebo (Singleton, 1981) and improvement in 8 of 11 patients after additional azathioprine in patients previously refractory to prednisone and salazopyrine (Goldstein *et al.*, 1980).

The present documentation supports the use of azathioprine in conjunction with prednisone. Its use in long-term treatment should be reserved for patients who have responded to a combined treatment with steroids and who have been able to be withdrawn from steroids while continuing the treatment with azathioprine alone.

15. DOSAGE AND FOLLOW-UP OF PATIENTS ON AZATHIOPRINE

The most common initial dose of azathioprine, 50 mg/day, is combined with an individually adjusted dose of steroids. During slow tapering of steroid doses, the dose of azathioprine may be increased to 100 mg daily within a few weeks. Later the dose may have to be increased to 150 or 200 mg/day in special cases. Weekly assessments of blood cell counts are required during the two first months of treatment with azathioprine. In most cases the tolerance is good and further controls may be performed every second or third month. When the dose of steroids is beneath the previous relapse level with no signs of recurrence, the patient is in a state of "preservation," which means that the treatment is effective but the patient is not in remission. Very careful tapering of doses of steroids is necessary. Below the 15-mg level, months of treatment on each dose level may be needed before further reduction. At a sign of recurrence, increased doses may be necessary as for steroid treatment alone. In some patients, low doses of steroids, 7.5–10 mg, must be continued over years as symptomatic treatment. Azathioprine therapy, if tolerated, may be continued for several years, either alone or combined with intermittent or continuous steroid treatment (Present, 1989; Markowitz *et al.*, 1990).

16. SIDE EFFECTS OF AZATHIOPRINE

The most common complications of azathioprine have been bone marrow depression, nausea, fever, and rashes (Sachar and Present, 1978). Toxicity has been reported in 16% of patients in large studies (Singleton *et al.*, 1979) along with 15% developing leukopenia. The appearance of leukopenia seems to be dose-dependent.

Pancreatitis has been reported within the first months in larger series, in 5 of 113 patients (Singleton *et al.*, 1979) in one study and in 4 of 42 patients in another (Nyman *et al.*, 1985).

An increased risk for non-Hodgkin's lymphoma, has never been established in relation to immunosuppressant therapy in inflammatory bowel disease. The only drug-related death among all reported control trials occurred from bone marrow failure after treatment with azathioprine for 11 years (Drucker and Jeejeebhoy, 1970).

17. CYCLOSPORINE A IN THE TREATMENT OF INFLAMMATORY BOWEL DISEASE

Favorable experience with cyclosporine A (CyA) in autoimmune diseases attracted gastroenterologists to apply this new therapeutic agent in therapy-resistant Crohn's disease patients (Dannecker *et al.*, 1985; Marbet *et al.*, 1986; Allam *et al.*, 1987). By administration of CyA, improvement of clinical and chemical parameters has been observed, especially using 10–15 mg/kg daily intravenously. Remission on oral CyA therapy was reported in a few patients (Allison and Pounder, 1984; Bianchi *et al.*, 1984; Dannecker *et al.*, 1985), but not in all patients studied (Bianchi *et al.*, 1984). Controlled trials are in progress. Preliminary reports of ongoing trials (Brynskov *et al.*, 1988) seem to indicate inconsistent response to treatment. Some patients seem to relapse immediately after cessation, whereas others (18%) remain in improved condition during follow-up. A blood concentration of 200 mg/ml has been suggested to be necessary for therapeutic effect (Marbet *et al.*, 1986).

Preliminary results from an ongoing trial (Brynskov *et al.*, 1988) applying 5–7.5 mg/kg daily and reaching a therapeutic interval between 400 and 800 mg/ml in whole blood, do report complete and incomplete malabsorption as a result of CyA in some patients. Other side effects reported are hyperesthesia, hirsutism, nausea and vomiting, transient hyperkalemia, and hypermagnesemia (Allam *et al.*, 1987). These side effects have mostly been considered as mild, usually responding to treatment and seldom severe enough to warrant discontinuation of therapy. Since common side effects such as hypertension, nephrotoxicity, and reduced liver function so far are rarely reported, chances are that CyA may be tolerable in long-term treatment in IBD.

18. OTHER IMMUNOREGULATORY AGENTS

The use of other immunomodulating agents such as nitrogen mustard, cyclophosphamide, levamisole, BCG, and phytohemagglutinin has not been accompanied by a clinical response. Generally, these nonspecific immunoadjuvants seem less promising than the more commonly used immunoregulatory agents. Future research may, however, detect more specific drugs that act on specific immunoregulating mechanisms, for example, suppressor T lymphocytes, in Crohn's disease (Goodacre and Bienstock, 1982; Ginsberg and Falchuk, 1982).

19. IMMUNOREGULATORY TREATMENT OF IBD IN CHILDREN

Growth retardation and delayed sexual development are reported to occur in up to 30% of children and adolescents with Crohn's disease (Kirschner *et al.*, 1978). Also, corticosteroids may contribute to growth failure (Friedman and Strang, 1966); however, growth more often accelerates when disease activity is suppressed by steroids (Whittington *et al.*, 1977). The key to normalization of growth is nutritional support, which should go along with immunoregulatory treatment in active Crohn's disease. Growth retardation is usually not a problem in quiescent stages of disease, but careful nutritional and medical management may be needed. Individually adjusted alternate-day treatment with steroids, shown to produce fewer cushingoid side effects and less adrenal suppression, is especially recommended during maintenance treatment (MacGregor *et al.*, 1969).

There is a general experience that patients with colonic involvement seem less responsive to steroids, are treated for longer periods with higher doses, and thereby suffer more growth suppression and other side effects from steroids. It is also important to bear in mind that especially in children the side effects may outweigh the favorable effects of treatment. The dose levels and duration of treatment with corticosteroids should therefore be determined with special caution.

Azathioprine or 6-MP should be used in steroid-resistant disease or for its steroid-sparing effect (Present *et al.*, 1980). Treatment in primary complicated cases may begin at the same time as corticosteroids, both in a dosage of 1–2 mg/kg daily. If colonic disease is present, initial treatment with sulfasalazine also should be introduced.

The effect of immunosuppressives seems to be more favorable in Crohn's colitis and ileocolitis than in ileitis (Present *et al.*, 1980). Control of blood counts should follow the same guidelines for all age groups.

20. SUMMARY

1. Immunoregulatory treatment is effective in IBD.
2. Corticosteroids are drugs of choice in fulminant and acute colitis.
3. Corticosteroids have an effect in active chronic colitis, but no documented benefit as maintenance treatment in ulcerative colitis or chronic disease in remission.
4. Corticosteroids should be tapered, gradually and individually, after primary improvement of the disease. During systematic follow-up and personal support of the patients with colitis, salazopyrine or 5-ASA is introduced, usually not before the dose of steroids are reduced and not before two weeks of steroid treatment.
5. Initial doses of 45–60 mg/day in fulminant or acute colitis, and 30–45 mg/day in active chronic or relapsing colitis may be applied. Alternate-day treatment seems to produce fewer side effects, which is of special importance in children.
6. Corticosteroids should be the primary choice in ileal involvement of Crohn's disease at the time of onset or relapse.
7. Corticosteroids should be applied as second choice after or in combination with salazopyrine as treatment of active chronic colitis or ileocolitis.
8. Principally, ulcerative and Crohn's colitis are to be treated similarly in the presence of diffuse or extensive inflammation, whereas localized stenosis primarily should be treated with steroids in Crohn's disease, with surgery in ulcerative colitis.
9. Azathioprine or 6-MP are valuable as a steroid-sparing treatment and as maintenance treatment during remission in Crohn's disease, especially after initial resistance to other treatments or in the presence of complications such as fistulas.
10. Whenever azathioprine or 6-MP are tolerated, full therapeutic effect must not be expected until after four to six months. When no side effects have occurred during the first two months, the drugs are usually tolerated for several years.

11. CyA is not generally recommended at the present stage. A beneficial effect of CyA, however, is documented in active Crohn's disease, and the drug may be recommended in complicated disease resistant to other forms of treatment.
12. In all patients subjected to immunoregulatory treatment, the therapeutic benefit should be carefully weighed against the risk of side effects of the drugs. The patients should be systematically followed, with special attention to dose adjustment, duration of treatment, combinations with other drugs, nutritional problems, and psychosocial support.

REFERENCES

Allam, B. F., Tillman, J. E., Thompson, T. J., Crossling, F. T., and Gilbert, L. M., 1987, Effective intravenous cyclosporine therapy in a patient with severe Crohn's disease, Gut 28:1166–1169.

Allan, R., Steinberg, D. M., and Williams, J. A., 1977, Crohn's disease involving the colon; an audit of clinical management, Gastroenterology 73:723–732.

Allison, M. C., and Pounder, R. E., 1984, Cyclosporine for Crohn's disease, Lancet 1:902–903.

Baron, O. H., Connell, A. M., Kanaghinis, T. G., Lennard-Jones, J. E., and Avery, J. F., 1962, Out-patient treatment of ulcerative colitis: Comparison between three doses of oral prednisone, Br. Med. J. 2:441–443.

Bergman, L., and Krause, U., 1976, Postoperative treatment with corticosteroids and salazosulphapyridine (Salazopyrin®) after radical resection for Crohn's disease, Scand. J. Gastroenterol. 11:651–656.

Bergrem, H., and Opedal, I., 1983, Bioavailability of prednisolone in patients with intestinal malabsorption: The importance of measuring serum protein-binding, Scand. J. Gastroenterol. 18:545–549.

Bianchi, P. A., Mondelli, M., Di Polo, F., and Ranzi, T., 1984, Cyclosporine for Crohn's disease, Lancet 1:1242.

Brynskov, J., Freund, L., Rasmussen, S. N., Lauritzen, K. Schaffalitzky de Muckadell, O., Williams, N., MacDonald, A., Tantan, R., Molina, F., and Campanini, M. C., 1989, A placebo-controlled, double-blind, randomized trial of cyclosporine therapy in active chronic Crohn's disease, New Engl. J. Med. 321:845–850.

Cooke, W. T., Mallas, E., and Prior, P., 1980, Crohn's disease: Course, treatment and long-term prognosis, Q. J. Med. 195:363–384.

Danish 5-ASA Group, 1987, Topical 5-Aminosalicylic acid versus prednisolone in ulcerative proctosigmoiditis. A randomized double-blind multicenter trial, Dig. Dis. Sci. 32:598–602.

Dannecker, G., Malchow, H., Niessen, K. H., and Ranke, M. B., 1985, Morbus Crohn: Erse Erfahrung mit Cyclosporin A bei einer adoelscenten, Deutsche Med. Wschr. 10:339–342.

Della Cella, G., Garabaldi, L. R., and Durand, P., 1976, Ulcerative colitis and disodium cromoglycate, Lancet 1:1129.

Drucker, W. R., and Jeejeebhoy, K. N., 1970, Azathioprine: An adjunct to surgical therapy of granulomatous enteritis, Ann. Surg. 172:618–626.

Friedman, M., and Strang, L. B., 1966, Effect of long-term corticosteroids and corticotropine on the growth of children, Lancet 2:568–572.

Ginsberg, C. H., and Falchuk, Z. M., 1982, Defective autologous mixed-lymphocyte reaction and suppression cell generation in patients with IBD, Gastroenterology 83:1–9.

Goldstein, F., Menduke, H., Thornton, J. J., and Abramson, J., 1980, Autoinflammatory drug treatment of Crohn's disease: A prospective evaluation of 100 consecutively treated patients, J. Clin. Gastroenterol. 2:77–85.

Goodacre, R. L., and Bienstock, J., 1982, Reduced suppressor cell activity in intestinal lymphocytes from patients with Crohn's disease, Gastroenterology 82:653–658.

Halvorsen, S., Myren, J., and Aakvaag, A., 1969, On the absorption of prednisolone disodium phosphate after rectal administration, Scand. J. Gastroenterol. 4:581–584.

Heatley, R. V., Calcraft, B. J., Rhodes, J., Owen, E., and Evans, B. K., 1975, Disodium cromoglycate in the treatment of chronic proctitis, Gut 16:559–563.

Jewell, D. P., 1989, Corticosteroids for the management of ulcerative colitis and Crohn's disease, Gastroenterology 18:21–34.

Jewell, D. P., and Truelove, S. C., 1974, Azathioprine in ulcerative colitis. Final report on controlled therapeutic trial, Br. Med. J. 4:627–630.

Kirk, A. P., and Lennard-Jones, J. E., 1982, Control trial of azathioprine in chronic ulcerative colitis, Br. Med. J. 284:1291–1292.

Kirschner, B. S., Vainchet, D., and Rosenberg, L. H., 1978, Growth retardation in inflammatory bowel disease, Gastroenterology 75:504–511.

Kristensen, M., Koudahl, G., Fischerman, K., and Jarnum, S., 1974, High dose prednisone treatment in severe ulcerative colitis, Scand. J. Gastroenterol. 9:177–183.

Lee, D. A. H., Taylor, G. M., and James, V. H. T., 1971, Plasma prednisolone levels and adrenocortical responsiveness after administration of 21-phosphate as a retention enema in proctocolitis, Br. Med. J. 3:84–86.

Lee, D. A. H., Taylor, G. M., and James, V. H. T., 1980, Rectally administered prednisolone—evidence for a predominantly local action, Gut 21:215–218.

Lennard-Jones, J. E., Longmore, A. J., Newell, A. C., Wilson, C. W. F., and Jones, F. A., 1960, Assessment of prednisone, salazopyrine and topical hydrocortisone hemisuccinate used as out-patient treatment for ulcerative colitis, Gut 1:217–222.

Lennard-Jones, J. E, Misiewicz, J. J., Connell, A. M., Baron, J. H., and Jones, F. A., 1965, Prednisone as a maintenance treatment for ulcerative colitis in remission, Lancet 1:188–189.

MacGregor, R. R., Sheagren, J. N., and Lipsett, M. B., 1969, Alternate-day prednisone therapy: Evaluation of delayed hypersensitivity responses, control of disease and steroid side effects, N. Engl. J. Med. 280:1427–1431.

Malchow, H., Ewe, K., and Brandes, J. W., 1984, European cooperative Crohn's disease study (ECCDS): Results of drug treatment, Gastroenterology 86:249–266.

Mani, V., Lloyd, G., Green, F. H. Y., Fox, H., and Turnberg, L. A., 1976, Treatment of ulcerative colitis with oral disodium cromoglycate: A double-blind controlled trial, Lancet 1:439–441.

Marbet, U. A., Gyr, K., and Stalder, C., 1986, Cyclosporin A bei akuten Morbus Crohn: erste Erfahrungen, Schweiz. Med. Wschr. 116:962–963.

Markowitz, J., Rosa, J., Grancher, K., Aiges, H., and Daum, F., 1990, Long-term 6-mercaptopurine treatment in adolescents with Crohn's disease, Gastroenterology 99:1347–1351.

Mekhjian, H. S., Switz, D. M., Watts, H. D., Deren, J. D., Katon, R. M., and Beeman, F. M., 1979, National cooperative Crohn's disease study: Factors determining recurrence of Crohn's disease after surgery, Gastroenterology 77:907–913.

Meyers, S., Sachar, D. B., Goldberg, J. D., and Janowitz, H. D., 1983, Corticotropin versus hydrocortisone in the intravenous treatment of ulcerative colitis, Gastroenterology 85:351–357.

Nyman, M., Hansson, I., and Eriksson, S., 1985, Long-term immunosuppressive treatment in Crohn's disease, Scand. J. Gastroenterol. 20:1197–1203.

O'Donoghue, D. P., Dawson, A. N., Powell-Tuck, J., Brown, R. L., and Lennard-Jones, J. E., 1978, Double-blind withdrawal trial of azathioprine as maintenance treatment for Crohn's disease, Lancet 2:955–957.

Peppercorn, M. A., 1990, Advances in drug therapy for inflammatory bowel disease, Ann. Intern. Med. 112:50–60.

Present, D. H., 1989, 6-Mercaptopurine and other immunosuppressive agents in the treatment of Crohn's disease and ulcerative colitis, Gastroenterology 18:57–71.

Present, D. H., Korelitz, B. I., and Wisch, N., 1980, Treatment of Crohn's disease with 6-mercaptopurine: A long-term, randomized, double-blind study, N. Engl. J. Med. 302:981–987.

Present, D. H., Wisch, N., and Glass, J. L., 1977, The efficacy of immunosuppressive therapy in Crohn's disease: A randomized, long-term, double-blind study, Gastroenterology 72:1114.

Rosenberg, J. L., Wall, A. J., Levin, B., and Kirsner, J. B., 1975, A controlled trial of azathioprine in the management of chronic ulcerative colitis, Gastroenterology 69:96–99.

Sachar, D. B., and Present, D. H., 1978, Immunotherapy in inflammatory bowel disease, Med. Clin. North Am. 62:173–183.

Singleton, J. W., 1976, National cooperative Crohn's disease study (NCCDS): Preliminary results of part I, Gastroenterology 80:938.

Singleton, J. W., 1977, National cooperative Crohn's disease study (NCCDS): Results of drug treatment, Gastroenterology 72:11–33.

Singleton, J. W., 1981, Azathioprine has a very limited role in the treatment of Crohn's disease, Dig. Dis. Sci. 26:368–371.

Singleton, J. W., Law, D. H., and Kelley, M. L., 1979, National cooperative Crohn's disease study: Adverse reactions to study drugs, Gastroenterology 77:870–882.

Smith, R. C., Rhodes, J., Heatley, R. V., Hughes, L. E., Crosby, D. L., Rees, B. I., Jones, H., Evans, K. T., and Lawrie, B. W., 1978, Low dose steroids and clinical relapse in Crohn's disease: A controlled trial, Gut 19:606–610.

Sparberg, M., and Kirsner, B., 1966, Long-term corticoid therapy for regional enteritis: An analysis of 58 courses in 54 patients, Am. J. Dig. Dis. 11:865–880.

Summers, R. W., Switz, D. M., Sessions, J. T., Jr., Becktel, J. M., Best, W. R., Kern, F., and Singleton, J. W., 1979, National cooperative Crohn's disease study: Results of drug treatment, Gastroenterology 77:847–869.

Tanner, A. R., Halliday, J. W., and Powell, L. W., 1981, Serum prednisolone levels in Crohn's disease and coeliac disease following oral prednisolone administration, Digestion 21:310–315.

Truelove, S. C., and Jewell, D. P., 1974, Intensive intravenous regimen for severe attacks of ulcerative colitis, Lancet 1:1067–1070.

Truelove, S. C., and Pena, A. S., 1976, Course and prognosis of Crohn's disease, Gut 17:192–201.

Truelove, S. C., and Witts, L. J., 1955, Cortisone in ulcerative colitis. Final report on a therapeutic trial, Br. Med. J. 2:1041–1048.

Truelove, S. C., Watkinson, G., and Draper, G., 1962, Comparison of corticosteroid and sulphasalazine therapy in ulcerative colitis, Br. Med. J. 2:1708–1711.

Watson, W. C., and Bukowsky, M., 1974, Azathioprine in management of Crohn's disease: A randomized cross-over study, Gastroenterology 142:796.

Whittington, P. F., Barnes, H. W., and Bayless, I. M., 1977, Medical management of Crohn's disease in adolescence, Gastroenterology 72:1338–1334.

Willoughby, J. M. T., Kumar, P. J., and Becket, J., 1971, Controlled trial of azathioprine in Crohn's disease, Lancet 2:944–947.

Chapter 25

DISORDERS OF NEUROMUSCULAR TRANSMISSION

Rolf Nyberg-Hansen and *Leif Gjerstad*

1. INTRODUCTION

Disorders of the neuromuscular transmission process are characterized clinically by variable weakness and abnormal fatigability of skeletal muscles without signs of neural disease. The fluctuant weakness is made worse by activity. Muscle power is, at least in part, restored by rest. The two main disorders of neuromuscular transmission, acquired myasthenia gravis (MG) and the Lambert-Eaton myasthenic syndrome (LEMS), are both autoimmune diseases. LEMS is often associated with carcinoma, especially of the lung (neoplastic LEMS), but also occurs in patients with presumed autoimmune disorders (nonneoplastic LEMS). Fluctuant weakness and fatigability are especially localized to muscles innervated by motor nuclei of the brain stem in MG while the muscles of the shoulder and pelvic girdle are most frequently affected in LEMS. MG is a postsynaptic disorder of neuromuscular transmission while LEMS is caused by a presynaptic membrane defect.

MG may be divided into congenital, neonatal, drug-induced, and acquired forms. *Congenital myasthenia* is due to congenital defects in the neuromuscular transmission process. Different subtypes exist depending on the type of defect. In contrast to other forms of myasthenia, there is no immunological cause for the disease (Engel, 1986b). Immunomodulating therapy therefore has no effect in patients with congenital myasthenia. *Neonatal myasthenia* is a transient disorder occurring in some infants born to mothers with acquired MG. The transient symptoms are probably related to the passive transfer of maternal antibodies against acetylcholine receptors. However, an independent antibody production of the affected infant may occur (Engel, 1986a). *Drug-induced myasthenia* can be caused by different agents either interfering with the presynaptic release of acetylcholine (e.g., botulinum toxin) or by inducing the production of antibodies affecting the postsynaptic membrane (e.g., penicillamine).

Only acquired MG and LEMS will be considered in the following.

Rolf Nyberg-Hansen and *Leif Gjerstad* • Department of Neurology, The National Hospital, University of Oslo, 0027 Oslo 1, Norway.

Immunopharmacology in Autoimmune Diseases and Transplantation, edited by Hans Erik Rugstad *et al.* Plenum Press, New York, 1992.

2. MYASTHENIA GRAVIS

MG was probably first described in 1672 by the Oxford physician Thomas Willis (1672) in his work *De Amina Brutorum* (Guthrie, 1903). The first comprehensive account of the disorder, however, was given by Erb (1879). The term *myasthenia gravis* was coined by Jolly (1895) who called the disease myasthenia gravis pseudoparalytica. Myasthenia gravis alone soon became adopted.

Acquired MG may be divided into ocular and generalized forms. It is a chronic disease with a tendency to remit and to relapse. Spontaneous improvement may occur, particularly during the early phase of the disease. The introduction of modern immunopharmacological treatment regimens in MG has greatly improved the prognosis and enabled most of the patients to lead useful, active lives.

2.1. Pathogenesis

Acquired MG is an antibody-mediated autoimmune disorder with interference of neuromuscular transmission in skeletal muscle by antibodies against nicotinic acetylcholine receptors (ACh-R). Circulating polyclonal antibodies (anti-ACh-R) can be demonstrated in nearly 90% of patients with generalized MG and in 75% of patients having disease limited to the ocular muscles (Engel, 1986a). New techniques may improve the detection in cases with extremely low antibody titers (Ohta *et al.*, 1990). The antibodies appear to be specific to patients with MG and do thus serve a useful diagnostic function. In some patients, autoantibodies against other parts of skeletal muscle occur; however, their role in the pathogenesis remains uncertain (Connor *et al.*, 1990). The role of cell-mediated immune responses in the pathogenesis of MG also remains to be precisely delineated.

The hypothesis that MG was an autoimmune disease was originally formulated by Simpson (1960) who suggested that "myasthenia is an 'auto immune' response of muscle in which an antibody to endplate protein may be formed." Furthermore, an increased incidence of other presumed autoimmune diseases occurs in MG patients. The most common is the association with thyroid diseases.

MG is characterized physiologically by a reduced amplitude of the miniature end plate potential and of the end plate potential itself. The basic abnormality is a decrease in functional ACh-R numbers at neuromuscular junctions where there normally is a high local concentration of receptors at the crests of folds of the postsynaptic membrane. ACh-R is a transmembrane glycoprotein of approximately 250 kDa that is composed of five subunits arranged as a pentamer (two α and one each of β, γ, and δ) and is an integral part of the postsynaptic membrane (McCarthy *et al.*, 1986). Two ACh molecules react with one ACh-R. There is a sustained production of antibodies directed against several different antigenic determinants of the receptor in MG. Blocking antibodies constitute only a minor fraction (Engel, 1986a; Burges *et al.*, 1990). Most of the antibodies are thus directed at determinants other than the ACh binding sites on the two α chains, especially against the main immunogenic region (MIR), which harbors several antigenic determinants. The MIR is located on the α chain but does not contain the binding site for ACh. The biologic half-life of the ACh-R is approximately 10–12 days.

The antibody response in MG is polyclonal, or products of the numbers of clones of B cells activated by the multiple antigenic determinants on ACh-R. The operatively active anti-ACh-R antibody is IgG (IgG_1, IgG_2, and in some cases, IgG_3), although small amounts of IgM and IgA may be found (Vincent and Newsom-Davis, 1980; Lefvert, 1981; Tindall,

1981). They impair neuromuscular transmission mainly by modulation (internalization and degradation) of the ACh-R and by complement-mediated destruction of the postsynaptic membrane. IgG as well as complement C3 and C9 have been identified at the postsynaptic membrane (Engel *et al.*, 1977; Sahashi *et al.*, 1980). Immune complexes may be demonstrated at the neuromuscular junction even when circulating anti-ACh-R antibodies cannot be detected (Engel, 1986a). The result of the autoimmune process is changes in the morphology of the neuromuscular junction with simplification of the normal folded structure of the postsynaptic membrane and reduction of the area harboring ACh-R, thereby leading to a decrease in the number of functional receptors. The basic etiology of the immunoregulatory defect leading to MG is, however, still not yet known.

The titer of anti-ACh-R antibodies seems to correlate roughly with the clinical severity of the disease for the individual patient (Besinger *et al.*, 1981; Limburg *et al.*, 1983; Komiya and Sato, 1988). However, between patients there is little or no correlation between the antibody titer and the severity of the disease or the duration of the symptoms (Lindstrøm *et al.*, 1976; Compston *et al.*, 1980). In general, mean titer values tend to be low in patients with ocular MG, whereas patients with thymoma have significantly higher antibody titers than do nonthymoma patients. The poor correlation between the clinical state of the individual patient and the titer levels may possibly be accounted for by the heterogeneity of the antibodies. Thus, antibodies are directed against several different antigenic determinants of the ACh-R. Furthermore, there may even be antigenic differences between receptors of different muscle groups (Vincent and Newsom-Davis, 1980).

A reduction in anti-ACh-R antibody titer has been shown to correlate roughly with long-term clinical improvement after treatment with corticosteroids, azathioprine, or thymectomy. However, this correlation may be better understood when measurements are made of monoclonal rather than polyclonal antibody levels. The effect of various therapeutic regimens on subgroups of antibodies is not yet known.

The association of thymic abnormalities with MG was first recognized by Weigert (1901), and thymectomy as a method of treatment in MG was adopted after the report of Blalock *et al.* (1939). The thymus gland is abnormal in approximately 75–80% of MG patients, and thymoma is present in 10–15% of all cases. The tumor may be present before MG is evident. In younger patients, thymic hyperplasia is a predominant finding, whereas atrophy tends to occur more frequently in older patients. Some of the anti-ACh-R antibodies are produced in the thymus gland, especially in younger patients. In older patients and in MG patients with thymomas, the role of the thymus in the immune response is less clear (Engel, 1986a).

Younger patients with thymic hyperplasia usually have an intermediate level of anti-ACh-R antibodies. In this age group there is a female preponderance and a strong association with the histocompatibility antigens HLA-A1, -B8, and -DRW3. In patients with onsets of MG after 40 years of age, however, there is a male preponderance. Atrophy of the thymus and a low antibody titer are usually found in this age group in whom there is an association with HLA-A3, -B7, and -DRW2 (Compston *et al.*, 1980; Carlsson *et al.*, 1990). MG patients with thymomas have the highest titer of anti-ACh-R antibodies and show no clear HLA association or sex preponderance.

2.2. Thymectomy

The initial standard treatment of MG is anticholinesterase agents, which was originally reported by Walker (1934). Such drugs ameliorate the myasthenic symptoms by slowing the hydrolysis of ACh. They have to a varying degree beneficial effects in most patients, but normal muscle function is rarely restored. They are of greatest use in mild cases. Pyridostigmine (Mestinon) is most commonly used. It is more long-acting than neostigmine. The dosage is steadily increased until maximum benefit is obtained. Attention must be paid to muscarinic side effects, which often occur. They may partly be overcome by an anticholinergic drug such as atropin.

If the effect of anticholinesterase agents is not satisfactory, early thymectomy is recommended in patients less than approximately 50 years of age (Figure 25.1). Some authors consider early thymectomy indicated irrespective of the effect of the anticholinesterase agents. Younger patients with thymic hyperplasia, an intermediate antibody titer level, and

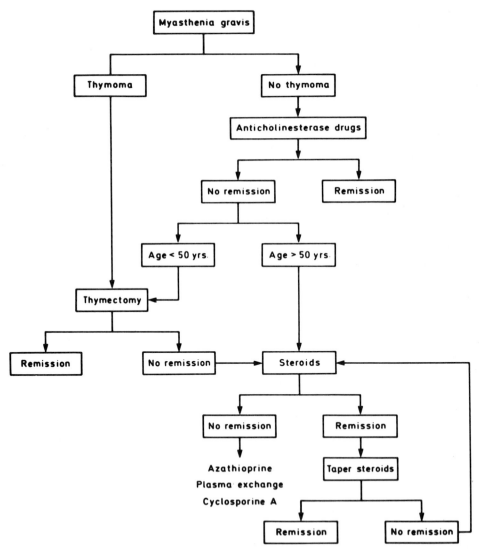

FIGURE 25.1. Decision making in the treatment of myasthenia gravis. In patients without thymoma, thymectomy is recommended if the weakness is generalized and no spontaneous remission occurs in 6–12 months. Thymectomy is controversial and usually not recommended in patients over 50 years of age or in patients with pure ocular myasthenia.

association with HLA-A1, -B8, and -DRW3 seem to respond best to thymectomy, whereas the value of this treatment for those in the older age group is more controversial (Engel, 1986a). Thymectomy usually has a minor effect on the course of the disease in patients over 50 years of age in whom thymic atrophy is a predominant feature. Accordingly, many authors are reluctant to use this form of therapy in patients above this age.

In patients with thymomas, thymectomy should be considered whenever possible. Thymomas are usually benign tumors but may be locally invasive. Patients often fail to show an improvement in their myasthenic symptoms after removal of the tumor.

2.3. Corticosteroids

In view of the immunopathogenesis of MG, the efficacy of various immunosuppressive treatment regimens is now recognized. Corticosteroids are used when the myasthenic symptoms are not adequately controlled by anticholinesterase agents alone or combined with thymectomy (Fig. 25.1). The benefits of long-term treatment with steroids have only become apparent within the last 10–15 years. If the effect of thymectomy is not satisfactory, steroid treatment is usually started after an observation period of approximately 6–12 months after the operation, sometimes even earlier. We prefer to start with an initial dosage of 20 mg prednisolone on alternate days, which is gradually increased by increments of 10 mg on every fourth day until 100 mg on alternate days is reached or a maximum response achieved. With this regimen, the initial deterioration that may occur when the initial prednisolone dosage is high is avoided. The cause of this initial steroid-induced deterioration in MG patients is not clear.

When sustained improvement while receiving 100 mg prednisolone every other day is achieved, the dosage is gradually reduced. Approximately 75% of MG patients show good improvement or remission. Patients over the age of 40 with atrophy of the thymus, low antibody titers, and association with HLA-A3, -B7, and -DRW2 seem to respond best (Compston et al., 1980). The clinical improvement tends to be associated with a fall in the anti-ACh-R antibody titer. However, an appropriate long-term maintenance dosage below approximately 30 mg alternate days is seldom achieved. In the long run, it is hardly possible to avoid side effects such as acne, osteoporosis, weight gain, hypertension, diabetes, or cataracts when a maintenance dosage at this level is used for years. The benefit of prednisolone treatment must therefore be weighed against the side effects.

Prednisolone probably acts by modifying the autoimmune response to ACh-R. Significant clinical improvement correlates with a decrease of antibody titer. The most striking decrease usually occurs in less than three months (Engel, 1986a).

2.4. Azathioprine and Cyclophosphamide

The main indication for immunosuppressive drugs such as azathioprine or cyclophosphamide is progressive generalized MG not controlled by thymectomy and corticosteroids, or limited by the high dosage and/or side effects of these drugs (Fig. 25.1). They allow more sparing use of corticosteroid probably by suppressing different autoantibodies than prednisolone (Pestronk et al., 1989).

Azathioprine in the dosage of 2–2.5 (or 3) mg/kg per day is most commonly used, usually together with steroids. After starting treatment with azathioprine, there is usually a delay of three to six months before improvement occurs (Mertens *et al.*, 1981). This seems to be correlated with a slow decline in antibody titer. Azathioprine appears to act more quickly when given together with prednisolone. This combination probably has a synergistic effect in MG as in other immunologic disorders. When using azathioprine, particular emphasis should be paid to drug toxicity on hematopoietic tissue.

2.5. Plasma Exchange

The role of plasma exchange in the treatment of MG has been controversial. It is often beneficial, but the improvement is transient. The procedure lowers the anti-ACh-R antibody titer, and clinical improvement follows a reduction of antibody levels after a lag of one to two days. However, after 2–6 weeks a rise in antibody titer occurs and is usually associated with clinical deterioration. In the long run, plasma exchange seems to be effective only when used together with immunosuppressive drugs (Fig. 25.1). However, it has a definite place in the short term such as acute management of myasthenic crises, prevention of impending crises or preparation of patients for surgery such as thymectomy. Furthermore, intermittent exchanges may be of value in selected, severely affected patents together with steroids and azathioprine or cyclosporine A (CsA).

2.6. Cyclosporine A

The use of corticosteroids and azathioprine may be limited by side effects and/or a lack of optimal response. Some recent studies indicate that the rapidly acting immunosuppressive drug CsA (Borel *et al.*, 1977) may be an alternative in such patients (Fig. 25.1) (Nyberg-Hansen and Gjerstad, 1985, 1988a,b; Tindall *et al.*, 1987, 1988; Schalke *et al.*, 1988). Results from these recent studies seem promising.

CsA seems to act specifically and reversibly on T cells, predominantly on T helper cells, presumably by inhibiting the synthesis and release of lymphokines, especially interleukin 2 (Shevach, 1985). Although the major immunologic response in MG is antibody mediated, sustained production of antibodies to ACh-R is T-cell dependent. The effect of CsA in MG may be a suppression of T helper cell activation of B cells producing anti-ACh-R antibodies (Muraguchi *et al.*, 1983), or induction of suppressor cells that inhibit antibody production by primed lymphocytes (McIntosh and Drachman, 1984).

CsA in combination with prednisolone probably has a synergistic effect in MG as in other immunological disorders, thus allowing more sparing use of prednisolone. In addition, CsA may potentiate the effect of prednisolone by reducing the clearance of this drug (Øst, 1984).

Drug toxicity may prove to be the limiting factor in the use of CsA, especially nephrotoxicity (Bennett and Pulliam, 1983). The maintenance dosage should therefore be kept as low as possible, preferably 5 mg/kg per day or less and trough levels of CsA in whole blood should not exceed 200–250 μg/liter. Renal function should be carefully monitored and serum creatinine levels should not be allowed to increase above 30–50% of baseline value. The ultimate role of CsA in the treatment of MG, however, remains to be determined and further control studies are needed. Particular emphasis should be paid to drug toxicity, especially nephrotoxicity. Some of the side effects like hypertension, though, may be specifically related to other factors than the use of CsA per se (Scherrer *et al.*, 1990).

3. THE LAMBERT–EATON MYASTHENIC SYNDROME

The Lambert–Eaton myasthenic syndrome (LEMS) is a presynaptic disorder of neuro-muscular transmission often associated with small cell carcinoma of the lung, especially in men (Anderson et al., 1953; Lambert et al., 1956). It is characterized clinically by weakness of the shoulder and pelvic muscles and of proximal limb muscles, especially in the lower limbs. There is relative sparing of muscles innervated by cranial motor nerve nuclei. The myotatic reflexes are usually depressed or abolished, and autonomic features often occur (O'Neill et al., 1988). The fatigability is usually less pronounced than in MG. The diagnosis of LEMS is based on clinical and EMG findings. The EMG response shows a marked facilitation to repetitive nerve stimulation at rates above 10 Hz, due to a progressive increase in the amplitude of the end plate potential.

The neurophysiological abnormality is a reduced release of ACh quanta in response to a nerve impulse, causing reduced amplitude of the end plate potential with reduced safety margin of the neuromuscular transmission (Elmqvist and Lambert, 1968; Lambert and Elmqvist, 1971). More detailed studies with the passive transfer model have demonstrated a reduced number of voltage-gated calcium channels associated with the active zone parti-cles of the nerve terminal membrane (Lang et al., 1987). These channels become open when the terminal is depolarized. After entering the terminal calcium binds to the active zones and causes release of ACh.

The presence of LEMS in patients with other presumed autoimmune disorders (non-neoplastic LEMS) (Gutmann et al., 1972) and the association with the histocompatibility antigens HLA-B8 and -DRW3 suggest an autoimmune pathogenesis (Engel, 1986b). This is supported by the observation of characteristic clinical and EMG features of the human disease in mice after injection of the IgG fraction of LEMS plasma (Lang et al., 1981, 1983). Furthermore, freeze-fracture electron microscopy has demonstrated disorganization and a reduced number of active zone particles of the nerve terminal membrane after such IgG injection (Fukunaga et al., 1982; Fukuoka et al., 1987), and immuno-electron microscopy has localized the immunostaining to the active zone particles (Fukuoka et al., 1987). The presynaptic abnormality of neuromuscular transmission in LEMS thus seems to be IgG mediated. Recently, autoantibodies against presynaptic voltage-gated calcium channels have been found in many patients with LEMS and also in some patients with small cell carcinoma without LEMS symptoms (Sher et al., 1989; Leys et al., 1989). The autoantibodies interfere with the calcium channels (N, T, and L) in different ways. Patch clamp studies show a direct blockade of L-type channels by LEMS IgG (Peers et al., 1990). Antibodies may also reduce the number of calcium channels by cross-linking them, thereby causing antigenic modula-tion (Engel, 1986b). The autoimmune process seems not to involve complement activation (Engel, 1986b). In contrast to MG, anti-ACh-R antibodies do not occur in LEMS.

Only 3–6% of the patients with small cell carcinomas of the lung develops LEMS. These neoplasms probably share one or more common epitopes with nerve terminals (Engel, 1986b). LEMS may be present two to three years before the tumor can be detected. The finding that a human small cell carcinoma line has calcium channels (Roberts et al., 1985) may suggest an antigenic determinant of the tumor. However, since neoplastic LEMS has similar clinical expression as its nonneoplastic counterpart (O'Neill et al., 1988), more than one triggering factor of the disease may exist.

Anticholinesterase drugs have only a slight effect in LEMS (Lambert et al., 1961), while guanidine and 4-aminopyridine, which facilitate the calcium-dependent release of ACh from the nerve terminal, both have a beneficial effect (Engel, 1986b). Guanidine in a dosage of 10–35 mg/kg per day is most commonly used. In a recent study, the effectiveness of 3,4-diaminopyridine has been demonstrated in a placebo-controlled cross-over trial (McEvoy et al., 1989). Except for one seizure, side effects were minimal for doses up to 100 mg/day.

Both neoplastic and nonneoplastic LEMS may be improved by plasma exchange, corticosteroids and azathioprine (Streib and Rothner, 1981; Newsom-Davis and Murray, 1984; Engel, 1986b). A possible depression of the resistance to tumor growth may, however, limit the use of immunosuppressive drugs to nonneoplastic LEMS. In neoplastic LEMS, remission may follow when chemotherapy or radiotherapy induces tumor regression (Jenkyn et al., 1980), but symptoms recur when the tumor recurs.

REFERENCES

Anderson, H. J., Churchill-Davidson, H. C., and Richardson, A. T., 1953, Bronchial neoplasm with myasthenia prolonged apnoea after administration of succinylcholine, Lancet 2:1291–1293.
Bennett, W. M., and Pulliam, S. P., 1983, Cyclosporine nephrotoxicity, Ann. Intern. Med. 99:851–854.
Besinger, K. A., Toyka, K. V., Heininger, K., Fateh-Moghadan, A., Schumm, A., Sandel, P., and Birnberger, K. L., 1981, Long-term correlation of clinical course and acetylcholine receptor antibody in patients with myasthenia gravis, Ann. NY Acad. Sci. 377:812–815.
Blalock, A., Mason, M. F., Morgan, H. J., and Riven, S. S., 1939, Myasthenia gravis and tumors of the thymic region. Report of a case in which the tumor was removed, Ann. Surg. 110:544–560.
Borel, J. F., Feurer, C., Nagnee, C., and Stahelin, H., 1977, Effects of the new antilymphotic peptide cyclosporin A in animals, Immunology 32:1017–1027.
Burges, J., Wray, D. W., Pizzighella, S., Hall, Z., and Vincent, A., 1990, A myasthenia gravis plasma immunoglobin reduces miniature endplate potentials at human endplates in vitro, Muscle Nerve 13:407–413.
Carlsson, B., Wallin, J., Pirskanen, R., Matell, G., and Smith, C. I., 1990. Different HLA DR-DQ associations in subgroups of idiopathic myasthenia gravis, Immunogenetics 31:285–290.
Compston, D. A. S., Vincent, A., Newsom-Davis, J., and Batchelor, J. R., 1980, Clinical, pathological, HLA antigen and immunological evidence for disease heterogeneity in myasthenia gravis, Brain 103:579–601.
Connor, R. I., Lefvert, A. K., Benes, S. C., and Lang, R. W., 1990, Incidence and reactivity patterns of skeletal and heart (SH) reactive autoantibodies in the sera of patients with myasthenia gravis, J. Neuroimmunol. 26:147–157.
Elmqvist, D., and Lambert, E. H., 1968, Detailed analysis of neuromuscular transmission in a patient with the myasthenic syndrome sometimes associated with bronchogenic carcinoma, Mayo Clin. Proc. 43:689–713.
Engel, A. G., 1986a, Acquired autoimmune myasthenia gravis, in: Myology. Basic and Clinical (A. G. Engel and B. Q. Banker, eds.), McGraw-Hill Book Company, New York, pp. 1925–1954.
Engel, A. G., 1986b, Myasthenic syndromes, in: Myology. Basic and Clinical (A. G. Engel and B. Q. Banker, eds.), McGraw-Hill Book Company, New York, pp. 1955–1990.
Engel, A. G., Lambert, E. H., and Howard, F. M., 1977, Immune complexes (IgG and C3) at the motor end-plate in mysthenia gravis. Ultrastructural and light microscopic localization and electrophysiological correlations, Mayo Clin. Proc. 52:267–280.
Erb, W., 1879, Zur Casuistik der bulbaren Lahmungen. 3 über einen neuen, wahrscheinlich bulbaren Symptomencomplex, Arch. Psychiatr. Nervenkr. 9:336–350.
Fukunaga, H., Engel, A. G., Osame, M., and Lambert, E. H., 1982, Paucity and disorganization of presynaptic membrane active zones in the Lambert-Eaton myasthenic syndrome, Muscle Nerve 5:686–697.
Fukuoka, T., Engel, A. G., Lang, B., Newsom-Davis, J., and Vincent, A., 1987, Lambert-Eaton myasthenic syndrome: II. Immunoelectron microscopy localization of IgG at the mouse motor end-plate, Ann. Neurol. 22:200–211.
Guthrie, L. G., 1903, Myasthenia gravis in the seventeenth century, Lancet 1:330–331.
Gutmann, L., Crosby, T. W., Takamori, M., and Martin, J. D., 1972, The Eaton-Lambert syndrome and autoimmune disorders, Am. J. Med. 53:354–356.
Jenkyn, L. R., Brooks, P. L., Forcier, R. J., Maurer, L. H., and Ochoa, J., 1980, Remission of the Lambert-Eaton syndrome and small cell anaplastic carcinoma of the lung induced by chemotherapy and radiotherapy, Cancer 46:1123–1127.
Jolly, F., 1895, Uber Myasthenia gravis pseudoparalytica, Berl. Klin. Wochenschr. 32:1–7.
Komiya, T., and Sato, T., 1988, Long-term follow-up study of relapse in symptoms and reelevation of acetylcholine receptor antibody titers in patients with myasthenia gravis, Ann. NY Acad. Sci. 540:605–607.
Lambert, E. H., and Elmqvist, D., 1971, Quantal components of end-plate potentials in the myasthenic syndrome, Ann. NY Acad. Sci. 183:183–199.
Lambert, E. H., Eaton, L. M., and Rooke, E. D., 1956, Defect of neuromuscular conduction associated with malignant neoplasms, Am. J. Physiol. 187:612–613.
Lambert, E. H., Rooke, E. D., Eaton, L. M., and Hodgson, C. H., 1961, Myasthenic syndrome occasionally associated with bronchial neoplasm: Neurophysiologic studies, in: Myasthenia Gravis (H. R. Viets, ed.), C.C. Thomas, Springfield, Ill, pp. 362–410.

Lang, B., Newsom-Davis, J., Wray, D., Vincent, A., and Murray, N., 1981, Autoimmune aetiology for myasthenic (Eaton-Lambert) syndrome, *Lancet* 2:224–226.

Lang, B., Newsom-Davis, J., Prior, C., and Wray, D., 1983, Antibodies to motor nerve terminals: An electrophysiological study of a human myasthenic syndrome transferred to mouse, *J. Physiol.* (Lond.) 344:335–345.

Lang, B., Newsom-Davis, J., Peers, C., Prior, C., and Wray, D., 1987, The effect of myasthenic syndrome antibody on presynaptic calcium channels in the mouse, *J. Physiol.* 390:257–270.

Lefvert, A. K., 1981, The human acetylcholine receptor antibody: Studies of kinetic properties and the reaction with antiidiotypic antibodies, *Ann. NY Acad. Sci.* 377:125–141.

Leys, K., Lang, B., Wincent, A., and Newsom-Davis, J., 1989, Calcium channel autoantibodies in Lambert-Eaton myasthenic syndrome, *Lancet* 2:1107.

Limburg, P. C., The, H., Hummer-Tappel, E., and Oosterhuis, H. J. G. H., 1983, Anti acetylcholine receptor antibodies in myasthenia gravis. I. Their relation to the clinical state and the effect of therapy, *J. Neurol. Sci.* 58:357–370.

Lindstrøm, J. M., Seybold, M. E., Lennon, V. A., Whittingham, S., and Duane, D. D., 1976, Antibody to acetylcholine receptor in myasthenia gravis, *Neurology* 26:1054–1059.

McCarthy, M. P., Earnest, J. P., Young, E. F., Choe, S., and Stroud, R. M., 1986, The molecular neurobiology of the acetylcholine receptor, *Annu. Rev. Neurosci.* 9:383–413.

McEvoy, K. M., Windebank, A. J., Daube, J. R., and Low, P. A., 1989, 3,4-Diaminopyridine in the treatment of Lambert-Eaton myasthenic syndrome, *N. Engl. J. Med.* 321:1567–1571.

McIntosh, K., and Drachman, D. B., 1984, Suppressor-cell immunotherapy of experimental autoimmune myasthenia gravis, *Ann. Neurol.* 16:113.

Mertens, H. G., Hertel, G., Reuther, P., and Ricker, K., 1981, Effect of immunosuppressive drugs (azathioprine), *Ann. NY Acad. Sci.* 377:691–699.

Muraguchi, A., Butler, J. L., Kehrl, J. H., Falkoff, R. J. M., and Fauci, A. S., 1983, Selective suppression of an early step in human B cell activation by cyclosporin A, *J. Exp. Med.* 158:690–702.

Newsom-Davis, J., and Murray, N. M. F., 1984, Plasma exchange and immunosuppressive drug treatment in the Lambert-Eaton myasthenic syndrome, *Neurology* 34:480–485.

Nyberg-Hansen, R., and Gjerstad, L., 1985, Ciclosporin in the treatment of myasthenia gravis: Preliminary results from a pilot study, in: *Ciclosporin in Autoimmune Diseases* (A. Schindler, ed.), Springer Verlag, Berlin, pp. 96–99.

Nyberg-Hansen, R., and Gjerstad, L., 1988a, Myasthenia gravis treated with ciclosporin, *Acta Neurol. Scand.* 77:307–313.

Nyberg-Hansen, R., and Gjerstad, L., 1988b, Immunopharmacological treatment in myasthenia gravis, *Transplant. Proc.* 20(Suppl.4):201–210.

O'Neill, J. H., Murray, N. M. F., and Newsom-Davis, J., 1988, The Lambert-Eaton myasthenic syndrome, *Brain* 111:577–596.

Øst, L., 1984, Effects of cyclosporin on prednisolone metabolism, *Lancet* 1:451.

Ohta, M., Ohta, K., Mori, F., Itoh, N., Nishitani, H., and Hayashi, K., 1990, Improved radioassay of antiacetylcholine receptor antibody: Application for the detection of extremely low antibody titers in sera from patients with myasthenia gravis, *Clin. Chem.* 36:911–913.

Peers, C., Lang, B., and Newson-Davis, J., 1990, Selective action of myasthenic antibodies on calcium channels in a rodent neuroblastoma X glioma cell line, *J. Physiol.* 421:293–308.

Pestronk, A., Adams, R. N., Kuncl, R. W., Drachman, D. B., Clawson, L. L., and Cornblath, D. R., 1989, Differential effects of prednisone and cyclophosphamide on autoantibodies in human neuromuscular disorders, *Neurology* 39:628–633.

Roberts, A., Perera, S., Lang, B., Vincent, A., and Newsom-Davis, J., 1985, Paraneoplastic myasthenic syndrome IgG inhibits $^{45}Ca^{2+}$ flux in a human small cell carcinoma line, *Nature (Lond.)* 317:737–739.

Sahashi, K., Engel, A. G., Lambert, E. H., and Howard, F. M., 1980, Ultrastructural localization of the terminal and lytic ninth complement component (C9) at the motor end-plate in myasthenia gravis, *Neuropathol. Exp. Neurol.* 39:160–171.

Schalke, B. C. G., Kappos, L., Rohrbach, E., Melms, A., Kalies, I., Dommasch, D., and Mertens, H.-G., 1988, Ciclosporin A vs. azathioprine in the treatment of myasthenia gravis: Final results of a randomized, controlled double-blind clinical trial, *Neurology* 38(Suppl.1):135.

Scherrer, U., Vissing, S. F., Morgan, B. J., Rollins, J. A., Tindall, R. S., Ring, S., Hanson, P., Mohanty, P. K., and Victor, R. G., 1990, Cyclosporine-induced sympathetic activation and hypertension after heart transplantation, *N. Engl. J. Med.* 323:748–750.

Sher, E., Gotti, C., Canal, N., Scoppetta, C., Piccolo, G., Evoli, A., and Clementi, F., 1989, Specificity of calcium channel autoantibodies in Lambert-Eaton myasthenic syndrome, *Lancet* 2:640–643.

Shevach, E. M., 1985, The effects of cyclosporin A on the immune system, *Annu. Rev. Immunol.* 3:397–423.

Simpson, J. A., 1960, Myasthenia gravis: A new hypothesis, *Scot. Med. J.* 5:419–436.

Streib, E. W., and Rothner, A. D., 1981, Eaton-Lambert myasthenic syndrome: Long-term treatment of three patients with prednisone, *Ann. Neurol.* 10:448–453.

Tindall, R. S. A., 1981, Humoral immunity in myasthenia gravis. Biochemical characterization of acquired antireceptor antibodies and clinical correlations, *Ann. Neurol.* 10:437–447.

Tindall, R. S. A., Rollins, J. A., Phillips, J. T., Greenke, R. G., Wells, L., and Belendiuk, G., 1987, Preliminary results of a double-blind, randomized, placebo-controlled trial of cyclosporine in myasthenia gravis, *N. Engl. J. Med.* 316:719–724.

Tindall, R. S. A., Phillips, J. T., Rollins, J. A., Wells, L., Hall, K., and Belendiuk, G., 1988, A double-blind, randomized, and controlled trial to compare cyclosporine and prednisone in the treatment of myasthenia gravis, *Neurology* 38(Suppl. 1):135.

Vincent, A., and Newsom-Davis, J., 1980, Anti-acetylcholine receptor antibodies, *J. Neurol. Neurosurg. Psychiatry* 43:590–600.

Walker, M., 1934, Treatment of myasthenia gravis with physostigmine, *Lancet* 1:1200–1201.

Weigert, C., 1901, Pathologisch-anatomischer Beitrag zur Erbschen Krankheit (Myasthenia gravis), *Neurol. Zentralbl.* 20:597.

Willis, T., 1672, *De Amina Brutorum*, Theatro Sheldoniano, Oxford.

Chapter 26

IMMUNE THERAPY FOR AUTOIMMUNE UVEITIS

Robert B. Nussenblatt

1. INTRODUCTION

Intraocular inflammatory disease (uveitis) presents an ongoing challenge to ophthalmologists dealing with this problem. The term "uveitis" has been used since the last century, since it was felt that the problem stemmed from an inflammation of uvea. Today, it is clear that this limited definition is not the case, and the term denotes any intraocular inflammatory disease, no matter what the cause and no matter what portion of the eye is affected by the disorder. Ocular inflammation is commonly dealt with by all ophthalmologists, either as a primary or secondary problem. It is the cause of about 10% of the severe visual handicap in the United States and Great Britain (U.S. DHEW, 1976). The diseases that fall under the umbrella term "uveitis" generally strike children and young adults, and thus often have a major impact on the family structure. The disorders are grouped as to those affecting the anterior and posterior portions of the globe. The International Uveitis Study Group, made up of 26 ophthalmologists currently representing many nations, has developed guidelines for the classification of uveitis. The disease entities are divided into three broad categories: anterior uveitis, intermediate uveitis, and posterior uveitis. This simplified system permits a standardized system for the classification of these disorders.

The natural history of uveitis has recently been reviewed (Nussenblatt, 1990a). The exact cause of many of these disorders still remains to be clarified. However, it has become clear from empiric observation that immunosuppressive therapy favorably alters the course of these diseases, which are called endogenous uveitides. Additionally, particularly for many of the disorders involving the posterior portion of the globe, uveitogenic antigens isolated from the eye can possibly be incriminated in the disease process. Further, immune complexes have been associated with conditions involving the anterior segment. Immunoregulation of uveitis has been evaluated recently (Nussenblatt, 1990b).

Robert B. Nussenblatt • National Eye Institute, National Institutes of Health, Bethesda, Maryland 20892.

Immunopharmacology in Autoimmune Diseases and Transplantation, edited by Hans Erik Rugstad et al. Plenum Press, New York, 1992.

2. ANTERIOR UVEITIS

This appellation denotes that the examining physician finds the inflammatory disease localized in the main to the anterior chamber of the eye, with at times a small "spillover" into the anterior vitreous. The inflammatory disease is noted by the presence of cells and a Tyndall effect induced by increased protein in the anterior chamber (flare). These can be quantified according to published standards. It is this type of disease that is most often encountered by the nonophthalmologist since it is often associated with systemic disorders. Ankylosing spondylitis will often present with this type of inflammatory disease. This disease can be bilateral, but with unilateral exacerbations and typically there will be numerous, well-defined attacks. Pauciarticular arthritis in children will frequently manifest itself in the form of an anterior inflammatory episode, as can sarcoidosis.

The sequelae of ongoing inflammatory disease in the anterior segment are numerous, and include:

1. Corneal decompensation. Though rarely seen in the United States today, unabated severe inflammatory disease can cause the cornea to lose its normal turgidity, become opaque, and therefore lead to loss of vision. Band keratopathy, a deposition of calcium due to the ongoing inflammatory disease, is of particular import in children.
2. Glaucoma. Secondary glaucoma due to uveitis is one of the major problems confronting the ophthalmologist in this field, since the eye can easily become blind because of the glaucoma, while the uveitis has been controlled with immunosuppressive agents. In some cases, usually involving the posterior segment, uveitis patients will develop neovascular glaucoma, a diagnosis with an extremely ominous prognosis for the eye. A third type of glaucoma seen is that of acute angle closure glaucoma. The increased inflammatory activity causes the iris to stick to the lens, preventing normal egress of the aqueous produced in the posterior chamber to flow into the anterior chamber, from which it leaves the eye. This leads to an acute rise in ocular pressure and acute symptoms requiring an immediate intervention, frequently surgical.
3. Cataract. The frequent bouts of uveitis lead to a lens opacity and ultimately a drop in visual acuity. Though this may ultimately be remedied with surgical means, it is clear that it is in the patient's best interest to try to avoid this step, if possible.

2.1. Therapeutic Approaches

Until recently, the main therapeutic approach to anterior uveitis has been with the use of locally administered corticosteroids. The topical application of corticosteroids is an excellent way to treat this disorder. Though studies do show differences of corneal penetration between phosphate and acetate preparations of steroids, in our experience we have not noted a major difference in efficacy between the two preparations when dealing with an active inflammation. When the diagnosis is made, it is imperative to treat the uveitis aggressively. We will frequently ask the patient to take his or her drops every hour while awake. It has been our feeling that frequent "failures" of this therapy are due to infrequent dosaging schedules. Further, the longer the duration and chronicity of the disease, the more difficult it frequently will be to bring under control. Once a dosaging schedule has been found to be effective, as evidenced by a decrease in the flare and cells in the eye, we then see the patient often (every 2–3 days to once a week) and begin a very slow taper of the drops. A tapering schedule is tailored to each patient, but individuals who have had numerous attacks may need to take one or two drops a day for weeks or even months (though this is rare).

A second option the ophthalmologist has is to place the corticosteroid periocularly by injection. This method permits a relatively high concentration of material to be given rapidly, and is an effective way to treat particularly severe inflammatory conditions. There is the general choice between long-acting preparations (in a depot vehicle) and more short-acting soluble preparations. These injections can be given every one to two weeks for short periods. In addition to sever anterior segment disease in general, this is a useful approach in cases of unilateral disease, at time of surgery of an uveitic eye, and in cases where the systemic effects of systemic steroids are to be avoided. Several approaches to periocular injections have been suggested, and it probably is best to use the way one feels the most comfortable with. However, the approach from the temporal aspect of the globe as outlined in the handbook of the American Academy of Ophthalmology is an approach to be reviewed by the seasoned ophthalmologist and perhaps mastered by those beginning in the field.

2.2. Secondary Effects of Local Corticosteroid Therapy

In this section I would like to outline secondary effects that are expressly associated with the local application of steroids. The topical application of steroid will induce a rise in intraocular pressure in a significant number of individuals, which should be monitored closely. It has been our experience that some uveitis patients are exquisitely sensitive to steroid, with dramatic increases in intraocular pressure noted even when topical steroids are administered on a very modest schedule. The reactivation of corneal herpes simplex infection can occur with topical steroid therapy. This is even of greater import in those patients undergoing corneal grafts, since a large proportion of these individuals are undergoing this procedure because of corneal herpes.

The periocular injection of steroid has its unique secondary effects as well.

1. Though periocular steroid injections are an effective therapy for childhood uveitis, they do invariably require general anesthesia, with the potential side effects inherent with this.
2. Penetration of the globe with the needle is a constant concern to the ophthalmologist. It is hoped that the temporal approach in placing the needle will reduce this possibility considerably.
3. Continued periocular injections can induce orbital problems, such as proptosis of the globe and fibrosis of the extraocular muscles, inducing a tropia.
4. Severe, intractable glaucoma can arise after periocular injections. This can become particularly problematic when a depot injection has been used. In such cases, the surgical removal of the depot may need to be performed, which sometimes is a major undertaking.
5. Reactions to the vehicle in which the steroid injection has been placed can also occur.
6. The use of periocular injections is not indicated in cases of scleritis and ocular toxoplasmosis. In the former, the injections could potentially inhibit new collagen growth to a point that perforation of the globe may occur. In the case of toxoplasmosis, the acutely high intraocular steroid dose may effectively prevent the body's normal antitoxoplasma mechanisms, thereby causing an exacerbation of the ocular disease.

2.3. Other Approaches to Therapy

Nonsteroidal anti-inflammatory agents such as the prostaglandin inhibitors indomethacin and aspirin have been tried in the treatment of this entity. To date, this approach has not been particularly successful. Additionally, though some have proposed that the basis for the inflammatory response is an allergic one (type 1 hypersensitivity), there has been no evidence to suggest that desensitization injections are in any way helpful in curbing this cluster of disorders.

Recently, Hedner and Bynke (1985) reported their experience with the prolactin inhibitor, bromocriptine. Four patients with severe, recurrent iridocyclitis or anterior uveitis were in need of bromocriptine therapy for other medical reasons: hyperprolactinemia, galactorrhea, or Parkinson's disease. They noted that their ocular symptomatology was markedly alleviated while on bromocriptine. Further, when the medication was stopped, the ocular disease reoccurred. The authors could not find an explanation for their observations. However, it has recently been shown that lymphocyte responsiveness in rats appears to depend on serum prolactin levels (Hiestand et al., 1986). Blocking of the release of prolactin from the pituitary severely reduced lymphocyte reactivity in an in vitro mixed lymphocyte reaction and in vivo graft-versus-host reactions. Further, the work of Hiestand and colleagues would suggest that the capacity of lymphocytes to respond fully to antigenic stimulation is dependent on the presence of prolactin on their cell membranes.

We have recently seen that bromocriptine can have an immunomodulating effect on the retinal S-antigen-induced experimental autoimmune uveitis, a T-cell-mediated disease that has many characteristics of human disease (Palestine et al., 1987). Because of the original observation of Hedner and Bynke, as well as the results seen in animal models for human disease, we at the National Eye Institute have embarked on a double-blind randomized clinical trial in which we will test the effectiveness of bromocriptine in preventing recurrent episodes of anterior uveitis. It is our feeling that because of the variation in the number of attacks of anterior uveitis, open studies cannot provide any further information, and only within the scope of this randomized masked trial can a definitive answer be achieved.

3. DISEASES INVOLVING THE INTERMEDIATE AND POSTERIOR SEGMENT OF THE GLOBE

The diseases involving this portion of the globe are numerous and can take on several specific clinical appearances when in their classic form. The "intermediate" forms of these diseases all present with cellular activity in the vitreous due to the ongoing inflammatory disease. Changes include a breakdown of the normally impermeable retinal vascular barrier and the development of cystoid macular edema. These alterations can probably best be seen using fluorescein angiography.

Other alterations that can be seen with this group of diseases include neovascularization of the retina, optic nerve head, and the pars plana region peripheral retina. These neovascular tufts can led to vitreal hemorrhage and even retinal detachment. At times retinal holes may form just in the macula region, reducing vision dramatically. Vitreal opacities may be (though rarely) so numerous and thick as to be the cause of a decrease in vision. For the diseases involving the posterior segment directly, one can certainly see many alterations already noted. Additionally, one can see retinal vascular attenuation and retinal atrophy, as in Behçet's disease. An additional complication is that of subretinal neovascularization, a proliferation of new vessels that begin in the choroid and extend upward toward the retina. This will often result in a small detachment of the retina, and often leads to a subretinal hemorrhage, frequently causing a dramatic drop in visual acuity. Certain inflammatory conditions such as sarcoidosis, birdshot retinochoroidopathy, presumed ocular histoplasmosis, and the pseudohistoplasmosis syndrome all have a propensity to form these subretinal vascular nets.

All of the above problems can lead to severe alterations in visual acuity, some reversible and some not. A therapeutic strategy centers around treating the active inflammatory disease and attempting to prevent recurrences. This frequently means that the patient must be treated with an immunosuppressive agent for an extended period of time.

4. EVALUATION OF THE POSTERIOR UVEITIS PATIENT

In deciding whether a patient's ocular condition warrants intervention with an immunosuppressive agent, it is imperative for the physician to attempt to determine the degree of inflammatory activity and as well what specifically is causing the patient's altered visual status. These may seem to be rather obvious points, but they are frequently neglected by observers. A good, accurate, and reproducible visual acuity is imperative. We have arbitrarily decided not to treat patients with systemic agents if the visual acuity is 20/40 or better. We have seen many patients maintain good visual acuities for extended periods of time, in spite of obvious intraocular inflammatory disease. A thorough examination of the vitreous and retina is imperative. The determination as to why the vision may be poor should be determined at that time. An attempt should be made to determine whether the cause of the poor vision is reversible or not, such as cystoid macular edema versus a macular hole, or if it has a reasonable hope of responding to immunosuppressive therapy, such as a cataract or vitreal hemorrhage, as compared to severe vitreal inflammation. It is simply illogical to treat patients with immunosuppressive methods when the reasons for poor vision can be effectively treated in another manner. One useful evaluation is the determination of the laser interferometer visual acuity (Palestine *et al.*, 1985). This attenuated laser beam will project images onto the retina in spite of a hazy media.

It is known that "falsely good" visual acuities can be obtained in the presence of cystoid macular edema. We took advantage of this observation and measured the laser acuity as well as the standard acuity of patients about to undergo immunosuppressive therapy for their uveitis. If the laser acuity was three lines or more above the standard visual acuity, then the patient had an 86% chance of having an improvement in visual acuity with therapy. Additionally, fluorescein angiography is an extremely useful tool in determining the status of the macular and retinal vasculature.

5. THERAPEUTIC APPROACHES TO THE TREATMENT OF SEVERE BILATERAL ENDOGENOUS UVEITIS

Corticosteroids remain the initial drug of choice for most patients with severe endogenous uveitis. The striking exception to this rule would be patients with Behçet's disease, and this will be discussed later in this section. We generally find it necessary to begin at 1–1.5 mg/kg of prednisone per day. The relatively high dosage and daily therapy appears to increase the efficacy of this approach. The high dosages of corticosteroids should be maintained until one sees a clinical effect, but it is clear that the treating physician must set a reasonable time limit in order to decide whether this form of therapy is truly worthwhile. If the determination is made that the corticosteroids are having a beneficial effect, then a therapeutic dosing schedule in which there is a slow reduction schedule needs to be established. A too rapid reduction of systemic corticosteroid can lead to a recurrence. The slow tapering plan permits the treating physician to see if the reduction will cause a reactivation, which frequently manifests as a mild ocular inflammation and perhaps a minimal decrease in visual acuity.

5.1. Use of Cytotoxic Agents

Though a very large percentage of intermediate and posterior uveitis cases respond initially to corticosteroid therapy, a significant number will have either intolerable side effects, severe recurrences, or poor control of their disease at more modest dosages of steroid. Other agents have been used in an attempt to control this disease, including antimetabolites as well as the alkylating agents. Godfrey and colleagues (1974) reported the effectiveness of chlorambucil in treating several types of uveitis. It must be stressed that there have been no masked randomized trials that have evaluated the effectiveness of these agents in the treatment of sever uveitis. It appears, though, that alkylating agents have been used more frequently than other agents.

Investigators generally agree that corticosteroid therapy is not effective in the treatment of the ocular complications of Behçet's disease. Several reports have supported the notion that the ocular manifestations of this disease can be effectively treated with alkylating agents (Mamo and Azzam, 1970). The International Uveitis Study Group has published its recommendations for the use of cytotoxic agents in uveitis, with Behçet's disease being one of the clear indications. However, a more recent report by Tabbara (1983) would suggest that the long-term effectiveness of this therapy may not be as good as initially thought. Further, a recent report by Reeves and colleagues (1985) has demonstrated chromosomal damage after alkylating agent therapy of some duration. The question of the long-term effects of this therapy, particularly neoplasms, remain an ever-important question and may be seen as well in uveitis patients receiving cytotoxic agents (Robert Coles, personal communications).

To be complete, it should be added that colchicine, until recently, has been used as the drug of choice for Behçet's disease in Japan. This agent is thought to decrease the number of ocular attacks but is not used to treat active disease.

5.2. The Use of Cyclosporine in the Treatment of Severe Endogenous Uveitis

We have demonstrated the positive effects of cyclosporine in an animal model for autoimmune uveitis. This model is T-cell mediated and has many clinical characteristics that are seen in the human condition (Nussenblatt et al., 1981a). In our initial studies, cyclosporine given at 10 mg/kg per day effectively prevented 100% of the rats from experimentally induced uveitis (Nussenblatt et al., 1981b). We began a study in which we treated patients with severe endogenous uveitis who were considered either therapeutic failures on systemic corticosteroids and/or cytotoxic agents or they had intolerable side effects. The initial study began with cyclosporine 10 mg/kg per day as the sole immunosuppressive agent.

Using this therapeutic approach, we were able to achieve a clinical success in over three fourths of the patients at three months and nearly two thirds at one year (Nussenblatt et al., 1983a,b). The drop in the success rate indicates the secondary problem relating to nephrotoxicity. Particularly beneficial results were obtained in patients with Behçet's disease and intermediate uveitis, particularly those with macular edema. A masked randomized study comparing the effectiveness of cyclosporine to colchicine in the treatment of Behçet's disease demonstrated the superior efficacy of cyclosporine (Masuda and Nakajima, 1985).

When initially begun, the concept surrounding the nephrotoxicity of cyclosporine was that it was reversible. We had the opportunity to biopsy 17 cyclosporine-treated uveitis patients receiving the drug for at least one year. We have found that definite alterations attributable to cyclosporine could be seen when these biopsies were compared to age-matched controls in a masked fashion (Palestine *et al.*, 1986; Austin *et al.*, 1989). Therefore, we have attempted to find therapeutic regimens that would permit us to reduce the dosage of cyclosporine. An initial approach has been to use cyclosporine at a lower dosage (5–6 mg/kg per day) combined with a low dose of prednisolone (10–20 mg/day). To date, this approach has permitted us to use dosages of both agents that are in the main tolerable to the patient and to the clinician monitoring side effects.

In accordance with this, Diaz-Llopis *et al.* (1990) found a good response in 86% of 14 patients with Behçet's disease treated with cyclosporine 5 mg/kg per day. In patients who responded well, this dosage was reduced to a maintenance dosage of 2 mg/kg per day. Towler *et al.* (1990) treated 13 patients with chronic intraocular inflammation that had not been adequately controlled with oral prednisolone with low-dose cyclosporine (mean 4.1 mg/kg per day) combined when required with oral prednisolone. Visual acuity improved overall in ten patients and remained stable in three. The mean serum creatinine concentration had increased by 26% after six months and 32% after one year, but remained stable during the subsequent 18 months.

Guidelines have now been established to administer cyclosporine in such a way as to minimize the risk of irreversible functional or structural renal damage in patients treated for autoimmune disease. Initial doses of cyclosporine should not exceed 5 mg/kg per day. The dose should be reduced whenever serum creatinine increases by more than 30–50% over baseline (see Chapter 12, this volume).

An additional approach has been the combination of cyclosporine with bromocriptine, the prolactin inhibitor. In addition to its potential anti-inflammatory effects, prolactin appears to be an antagonist of cyclosporine. Prolactin may share a common receptor with cyclosporine, or their receptor may be situated closely one to the other. The reduction of prolactin levels therefore may effectively permit the use of lower dosages of cyclosporine, yet maintain the same therapeutic efficacy. This hypothesis is currently being tested in patients already being treated with cyclosporine at the National Eye Institute.

6. OTHER APPROACHES TO THERAPY

Alternative approaches to the treatment of endogenous uveitis make a long list, perhaps reflecting the fact that none have been found to be particularly efficacious and none to date have been studied in long-term clinical trials, let alone masked randomized trials. A few deserve further comment:

1. Immunostimulants. There has been no evidence to date to suggest that patients with endogenous uveitis are immunosuppressed. Indeed, the rare instances where systemic alterations have been noted suggest that a hyperactive immune state exists, as in the case of spontaneous interferon production by lymphocytes from patients with Behçet's disease (Ohno *et al.*, 1982). Therefore, the logic for the use of these agents is lacking. I have had the opportunity to see several patients who have received transfer factor without any effect on their ocular condition.

    It is certainly clear that a whole group of patients with immunodeficiency disorders, such as AIDS, will present with ocular inflammatory disease and agents augmenting the immune response seem quite justified.

2. Allergy. The notion that allergic reactions are the mediating force in uveitic eyes is an old one. Desensitization injections have been suggested by practitioners. Once again, serious studies are totally lacking. Further, experimental models suggest at best that immediate hypersensitivity reactions may play a secondary role by "opening the gates"

into the eye for T cells, which are the predominant cell in the eye during the height of the inflammatory process.

3. Infection. Some practitioners have suggested that the inflammation seen in endogenous uveitis is due to an infection of either difficult to isolate bacteria or virus. Numerous attempts have been made to support this concept, in general, without success. More recent work suggests a more complicated role for both bacterial and viral products, but not in the context of an active proliferation of the organism. Rather, it would seem that either an adjuvant effect or a secondary "molecular mimicry" response may be induced by these organisms.

4. Plasmapheresis. This interesting therapeutic mode has been tried in uveitis, with some claiming very positive effects (Saraux et al., 1982). Masked randomized studies in other fields have not been as promising (Lewis et al., 1979). Further, all studies have required the continued use of immunosuppressive agents to induce a positive therapeutic effect. Therefore, though positive short-term clinical improvements may have been noted, the long-term use of this modality in the treatment of uveitis still needs to be defined.

5. Surgery. I think it useful to include surgical intervention as a therapeutic approach. It has been suggested that intraocular surgery positively alters the course of the uveitis, with an improvement of macular edema and presumably visual acuity. Though surgery can certainly be performed safely in these patients, it has not been our impression that the uveitic response is fundamentally altered. There may be, however, an improvement in visual acuity because of the removal of a cataractous lens. Indeed, Limon et al., (1984) reported no improvement in uveitis eyes with macular edema after vitrectomy. This has been our experience as well.

The use of various immunosuppressive agents has permitted the uveitic patient to reasonably expect that his or her vision can be maintained. It is clear that newer agents and approaches, such as cyclosporine and prolactin inhibitors, have opened a new field in terms of therapeutics. The future seems bright that newer approaches will permit us to more specifically and effectively treat this cluster of most challenging diseases.

REFERENCES

Austin, H. A., III, Palestine, A. G., Sabnis, S. G., Balow, J.E., Preuss, H. G., Nussenblatt, R. B., and Antonovych, T. T., 1989, Evolution of cyclosporine nephrotoxicity in patients treated for autoimmune uveitis, Am. J. Nephrol. 9:392–402.
Diaz-Llopis, M., Cervera, M., and Menezo, J. L., 1990, Cyclosporin A treatment of Behçet's disease: A long-term study, Curr. Eye Res. 9(Suppl.):17–23.
Godfrey, W. A., Epstein, W. V., O'Connor, G. R., Kimura, S. J., Hogan, M. J., and Nozik, R. A., 1974, The use of chlorambucil in intractable idiopathic uveitis, Am. J. Ophthalmol. 78:415–428.
Hedner, L. P., and Bynke, G., 1985, Endogenous iridocyclitis relieved during treatment with bromocriptine, Am. J. Ophthalmol. 100:618–619.
Hiestand, P. C., Mekler, P., Nordmann, R., Grieder, A., and Permmongkol, C., 1986, Prolactin as a modulator of lymphocyte responsiveness provides a possible mechanism of action for cyclosporine, Proc. Natl. Acad. Sci. 83:2599–2603.
Lewis, R. A., Slater, N., and Croft, D. N., 1979, Exophthalmous and pretibial myxedema not responding to plasmapheresis, Br. Med. J. 11:390–391.
Limon, S., Bloch-Michel, E., and Furia, M., 1984, One hundred vitrectomies in uveitis, in: Uveitis Update (K. M. Saari, ed.), Excerpta Medica, Amsterdam, pp. 521–524.
Mamo, J. G., and Azzam, S. A., 1970, Treatment of Behçet's disease with chlorambucil, Arch. Ophthalmol. 84:446–450.
Masuda, K., and Nakajima, A., 1985, A double-masked study of ciclosporine in autoimmune diseases, in: Ciclosporin Treatment in Behçet's Disease (R. Schindler, ed.), Springer-Verlag, Berlin, pp. 162–164.
Nussenblatt, R. B., 1990a, The natural history of uveitis, Int. Ophthalmol. 14:303–308.
Nussenblatt, R. B., 1990b, Immunoregulation of uveitis, Int. Ophthalmol. 14:13–18.
Nussenblatt, R. B., Gery, I., Kuwabara, T., de Monasterio, F. M., and Wacker, W. B., 1981a, The role of the retinal S-antigen in primate uveitis, in: Immunology of the Eye. Workshop II: Autoimmune Phenomena and Ocular Disorders (R. J. Helmsen, A. A. Swan, I. Gery, and R. B. Nussenblatt, eds.), Information Retrieval Inc., Washington, D.C., pp. 49–65.

Nussenblatt, R. B., Rodrigues, M. M., Wacker, W. B., Cevario, S. J., Salinas-Carmona, M., and Gery, I., 1981b, Cyclosporin A: Inhibition of experimental autoimmune uveitis in Lewis rats, *J. Clin. Invest.* **67:**1228–1231.

Nussenblatt, R. B., Palestine, A. G., Rook, A. H., and Scher, I., 1983a, Cyclosporine therapy of intraocular inflammatory disease, *Lancet* **2:**235–238.

Nussenblatt, R. B., Palestine, A. G., and Chan, C. C., 1983b, Cyclosporine therapy in the treatment of intraocular inflammatory disease resistant to systemic corticosteroids or cytotoxic agents, *Am. J. Ophthalmol.* **96:**275–282.

Ohno, S., Kato, F., Matsuda, H., Fujii, N., and Minagawa, T., 1982, Detecting of gamma interferon in the sera of patients with Behçet's disease, *Infect. Immun.* **36:**202–208.

Palestine, A. G., Alter, G. J., and Chan, C. C., 1985, Laser interferometry and visual prognosis in uveitis, *Ophthalmology* **92:**1567–1569.

Palestine, A. G., Austin, H. A., III, Balow, J. E., Antonovych, T. T., Sabnis, S. G., Preuss, H. G., and Nussenblatt, R. B., 1986, Renal histopathologic alternations in patients treated with cyclosporine in uveitis, *N. Engl. J. Med.* **314:**1293–1298.

Palestine, A. G., Muellenberg-Coulombre, C. G., Kim, M. K., Gelato, M. C., and Nussenblatt, R. B., 1987, Bromocriptine and low dose cyclosporine in the treatment of experimental autoimmune uveitis in the rat, *J. Clin. Invest.* **79:**1078–1081.

Reeves, B. R., Casey, G., Harris, H., and Dinning, W. J., 1985, Long-term cytogenetic follow-up study of patients with uveitis treated with chlorambucil, *Carcinogenesis* **6:**1615–1619.

Saraux, H., Le Hoang, P., Audebert, A. A., Canuel, C., and Cavalier, J., 1982, Intérêt de la plasmapherise dans le traitement du syndrome de Behçet, *Bull. Soc. Ophthalmol. Fr.* **82:**41–44.

Tabbara, K. F., 1983, Chlorambucil in Behçet's disease: A reappraisal, *Ophthalmology* **90:**906–908.

Towler, H. M. A., Whiting, P. H., and Forrester, J. V., 1990, Combination low dose cyclosporin A and steroid therapy in chronic intraocular inflammation, *Eye* **4:**514–520.

U.S. DHEW: DHS, NIH, 1976, *Interim Report of the National Advisory Eye Council Support for Vision Research*, Washington, D.C., pp. 20–22.

Chapter 27

CYCLOSPORINE A IN THE TREATMENT OF DERMATOLOGIC DISEASES

Mark S. Fradin, Marc D. Brown, Charles N. Ellis, Kevin D. Cooper, and John J. Voorhees

1. INTRODUCTION

Systemic corticosteroids, used alone or in combination with cytotoxic drugs, have long been the mainstay of therapy for autoimmune-mediated dermatologic diseases. Since their introduction in 1949, corticosteroids have been used extensively in the treatment of diverse dermatologic disorders including systemic lupus erythematosus, dermatomyositis, bullous pemphigoid, pemphigus, herpes gestationis, erythema multiforme, scleroderma, sarcoidosis, and acute contact dermatoses. In general, systemic steroids are not used for the treatment of psoriasis since they may lead to rebound or even pustular flare when steroid therapy is discontinued.

Systemic steroids, when used for short periods of time, such as in the treatment of severe contact dermatitis, are generally safe and effective. Long-term corticosteroid use, however, is inevitably accompanied by the development of multiple undesirable side effects that may affect nearly every organ system, leading to glucose intolerance, sodium and water retention with resulting hypertension, proximal myopathy, osteonecrosis, glaucoma, cushingoid habitus, and suppression of the hypothalamic–pituitary–adrenal axis.

Various methods have been used to minimize the side effects of systemic steroids. Tapering the dose as soon as the desired clinical response has been achieved may decrease the incidence of toxicity. Use of an alternate-day dosing schedule may reduce the long-term toxicity of corticosteroids. Cytotoxic drugs such as azothioprine or cyclophosphamide may be added to the therapeutic regimen in an effort to decrease the total dose of systemic steroids or when steroids alone are ineffective in controlling the disease.

Azothioprine, an antimetabolite, inhibits both RNA and DNA synthesis. The drug is

Mark S. Fradin, Marc D. Brown, Charles N. Ellis, Kevin D. Cooper, and *John J. Voorhees* • Department of Dermatology, University of Michigan Medical Center, Ann Arbor, Michigan 48109.

Immunopharmacology in Autoimmune Diseases and Transplantation, edited by Rugstad *et al.* Plenum Press, New York, 1992.

well absorbed orally and can usually be used at relatively low maintenance dosages of 1–2 mg/kg per day. For dermatologic diseases, the drug is used primarily for its steroid-sparing effect in the treatment of pemphigus and bullous pemphigoid.

Cyclophosphamide is an alkylating agent that, through its ability to cause DNA damage and interfere with RNA synthesis, inhibits normal mitosis and cell division. Like azothioprine, cyclophosphamide is used primarily for its steroid-sparing effect in the treatment of bullous diseases. It is also effective in the treatment of Wegener's granulomatosis.

While cytotoxic drugs are very effective, their use is limited by their ability to induce profound myelosuppression (particularly leukopenia) and by their association with an increased risk of developing lymphoreticular malignancies.

Since its discovery in the early 1970s, the drug cyclosporine A (CsA) has been used primarily for the prevention and treatment of organ transplant rejection. Unlike other cytotoxic drugs, CsA has the advantage of being a potent immunosuppressive agent, without toxic effects on bone marrow. In recent years, the drug has begun to be used more widely and has become a promising therapeutic agent for the treatment of many autoimmune diseases. There have been encouraging trials in which CsA proved to be effective in the treatment of insulin-dependent diabetes mellitus, uveitis, rheumatoid arthritis, inflammatory bowel diseases, Grave's disease, myasthenia gravis, autoimmune anemias, and collagen vascular diseases. In addition, CsA has been used successfully in the treatment of many dermatologic diseases (Biren and Barr, 1986; Page *et al.*, 1986; Brown *et al.*, 1987, 1989; Fradin *et al.*, 1990a).

This chapter will review our experience and that of others in treating presumed autoimmune-mediated dermatologic diseases with CsA.

2. PHARMACOLOGY OF CYCLOSPORINE

The pharmacokinetics, mechanism of action, and side effects of CsA are discussed in detail elsewhere in this book (see Chapter 12). In general, the side effects seen in the treatment of dermatologic disease with CsA do not differ from those observed in the treatment of other diseases. The most commonly noted side effects are hypertension, headache, numbness and tingling of the extremities, hand tremors, increased temperature sensitivity of the hands and feet, hypertrichosis, and nausea (Fradin *et al.*, 1990b; Krupp and Monka, 1990). A rise in serum creatinine and/or a fall in creatinine clearance may be seen in up to 75% of patients. Most side effects are dose-dependent and can be minimized through the use of low dosages of CsA (usually under 5 mg/kg per day).

3. CLINICAL APPLICATIONS

3.1. Psoriasis

The beneficial effect of CsA on psoriasis was fortuitously discovered in 1979 by Mueller and Hermann (1979), who were using the drug for the treatment of psoriatic arthropathy. Four patients with psoriatic arthritis were noted to have near-complete clearing of their plaques of psoriasis within a week of treatment with CsA. All patients, however, had reappearance of their psoriasis after the drug was stopped. Harper *et al.* (1984) reported a case of a patient with severe psoriatic arthritis and chronic psoriasis who had failed to respond to methotrexate and etretinate. Treatment with CsA resulted in a dramatic improvement in both his psoriatic arthritis and psoriasis. Van Hooff *et al.* (1985) described another patient who had rapid clearing of her chronic plaques of psoriasis within days of receiving CsA, following a renal transplant.

The first controlled study to evaluate the efficacy of CsA in the treatment of psoriasis was performed by Ellis *et al.* (1986). Twenty-one patients with severe, chronic, plaque-type psoriasis were enrolled in a double-blind crossover study. All patients had psoriasis involving greater than 20% of their skin surface and had failed to respond adequately to standard and intensive psoriatic treatments, including ultraviolet B, oral psoralen and ultraviolet A, and methotrexate. Patients received either placebo or an oral dosage of CsA comparable to that used in the treatment of organ transplant patients (14 mg/kg per day). The results were rapid and striking. After a month of therapy, 20 of 21 patients given CsA showed significant to complete clearing. Placebo-treated patients, prior to crossover, had shown no response.

Side effects included the development of hypertension, tremor, paresthesias, gingival hypertrophy, and hypertrichosis. None of these, however, were severe enough to require early discontinuation of CsA. Elevations in serum BUN, creatinine, blood lipids, or bilirubin were seen in some patients. Clinical side effects and laboratory abnormalities all resolved on cessation of therapy. Unfortunately, when CsA was stopped, all patients had a gradual return of their psoriasis within 2 to 12 weeks. In an open trial we conducted, 11 additional patients were enrolled. All patients showed moderate improvement to complete clearing within four weeks while on CsA at 14 mg/kg per day.

Further studies have demonstrated the efficacy of lower dosages of CsA in the treatment of psoriasis. Marks (1986) treated ten psoriatic patients with CsA at a starting dosage of 1 mg/kg per day, increasing the dose biweekly, as needed, until a clinical response was noted, or a maximum dosage of 5 mg/kg per day was reached. Nine of ten patients cleared within 2 to 20 weeks. The tenth patient, with generalized pustular psoriasis, failed to respond. The average dosage required for clinical improvement was 3.3 mg/kg per day. No effects on blood pressure or renal function were noted at the dosages used. In a subsequent long-term follow-up study of seven of these patients, however, elevations in serum creatinine were noted in five patients after taking CsA for 36 to 68 weeks (Marks, 1988). The two youngest patients in the study (ages 36 and 42) had no change in serum creatinine after 84 and 64 weeks, respectively.

In an uncontrolled study, Griffiths *et al.* (1986) treated ten psoriatics who had failed to respond to conventional therapies. A maximum CsA dosage of 4 mg/kg per day was given for 12 weeks. Five patients cleared completely within two months. The remaining patients all showed significant clinical improvement. The minimal therapeutic dosage of CsA appeared to be 3 mg/kg per day. Hypertension, mild elevation in serum creatinine, hypertrichosis, and transient nausea were noted in this group. On withdrawal of drug, all side effects disappeared and all patients experienced a return of their psoriasis.

Fry *et al.* (1988) have followed eight patients receiving CsA for 32 to 66 weeks. They have been able to maintain near-complete remission of psoriasis in these patients using dosages as low as 1 to 4 mg/kg per day. Four patients developed hypertension. One required discontinuation of CsA, one was started on a diuretic, and two patients required dosage reduction of 1 mg/kg per day to reestablish normotension. Insignificant elevations in serum creatinine and mild hypertrichosis developed in three patients.

Van Joost *et al.* (1986) treated five patients with severe psoriasis with low dosages of CsA (average dosage 5 mg/kg per day) for four weeks. Clinical evaluation was performed using the Psoriasis Area and Severity Index (PASI), a scoring system that takes into account the total area of involved skin, as well as the degree of erythema, scaling, and induration in the plaques of psoriasis (Fredriksson and Patterson, 1978). The mean reduction in PASI score at the end of a month was 84%. Two patients cleared almost completely. Three patients noted a substantial improvement in their psoriatic nail lesions. Another reported a significant amelioration in his psoriatic arthropathy. In a double-blind study, conducted by the same investigators (Van Joost *et al.*, 1988), 20 patients were treated with placebo or CsA (mean dosage 5.6 mg/kg per day). Fifteen of 18 patients who completed the study showed a reduction in PASI of at least 75% within a month. An almost complete remission of psoriasis occurred in 22% of treated patients. Mild hypertension and elevated serum creatinine, both reversible, were the only significant side effects noted.

Harper *et al.* (1988) have also found low-dose CsA (2 to 5 mg/kg per day) to be effective in the treatment of the arthropathy that often accompanies severe psoriasis. They treated five patients with crippling arthritis who had failed to respond to methotrexate, etretinate, nonsteroidal anti-inflammatory drugs, and oral as well as intra-articular corticosteroids. CsA was administered at dosages of 2 to 5 mg/kg per day. Three of five patients experienced a dramatic improvement in their arthritis, which greatly improved their quality of life. The other two patients had little to no improvement. Of the patients who responded, one has received 2 mg/kg per day for three years, with good control of his psoriasis and arthropathy. He has required temporary dose reduction on two occasions due to elevations in serum creatinine. The second patient was maintained on 3 mg/kg per day for a year, but was then forced to stop CsA due to a rise in serum creatinine. The third patient has remained on the drug for two years with no adverse side effects. In an open study, Gupta *et al.* (1989) treated six patients with severe psoriatic arthritis with 6 mg/kg per day of CsA. Following two months of therapy, all patients noted clinical improvement in grip strength, joint tenderness, and duration of morning stiffness.

Picascia *et al.* (1987) treated four patients with severe psoriasis, two of whom had generalized erythroderma, with CsA at dosages of 7.5–8.5 mg/kg per day. All four responded rapidly and cleared completely within three weeks. Three of these patients have remained in remission for 14 months with CsA dosages of 1.7–3.5 mg/kg per day (Picascia *et al.*, 1988). Side effects seen in this group were hypertrichosis, leg cramps, fatigue, hand tremors, hypertension, and mild elevation in serum BUN. Meinardi *et al.* (1987) reported successful treatment of a patient who developed a generalized pustular flare of his psoriasis after being tapered off methotrexate. Treatment with CsA resulted in dramatic improvement in both his skin lesions and associated psoriatic arthritis. Zachariae and Thestrup-Pederson (1987) reported a case of a woman with incapacitating pustular psoriasis of the palms and soles who had been treated unsuccessfully with methotrexate, systemic steroids, etretinate, hydroxyurea, colchicine, and psoralen with UVA light (PUVA). Treatment with CsA, within three weeks, led to complete clearance of her disease for the first time in ten years. A maintenance dosage of 5 mg/kg per day has kept her in remission, without acute side effects. Fradin *et al.* (1990c) treated a patient with a 30-year history of generalized pustular psoriasis, starting with a CsA dosage of 7.5 mg/kg per day. Dramatic improvement was noted within a few days of therapy and the patient was completely clear by week 16. After a slow taper of the dosage, the patient was successfully maintained, without active disease, on 3.5 mg/kg per day.

Timonen *et al.* (1990) documented a dose response to CsA in 457 patients treated with CsA at 1.25, 2.5–3, or 5 mg/kg per day. Significant improvement was seen in 24%, 52%, and 88% of patients in each group, respectively. Ellis *et al.* (1991) conducted a 16-week double-blind trial of 85 patients with severe psoriasis and also found the response to be dose-dependent: After eight weeks of therapy, 36, 65, and 80% of patients receiving 3, 5, and 7.5 mg/kg per day of CsA, respectively, were rated as being clear or almost clear of psoriasis. 5 mg/kg per day was the dosage that proved to require the least dosage adjustments due to either toxicity or lack of efficacy.

Meinardi and Bos (1988) were able to induce remissions in 12 psoriatics with a mean CsA dosage of 6 mg/kg per day over a period of four to six weeks. On gradual tapering of the dose, each patient appeared to have a dose of CsA below which he could not go without beginning to flare. This "trigger dosage" ranged from 1.6 to 7 mg/kg per day and in several patients appeared to vary at different points in time. The use of interval therapy (in which patients received no drug during several days of each week) appeared to be unsuccessful in significantly reducing the incidence of hypertension or elevated serum creatinine. In addition, most patients needed to be converted back to daily therapy in order to maintain remission of their disease. The combination of etretinate (at dosages up to 1 mg/kg per day) and CsA did not seem to offer a major improvement over CsA monotherapy, nor did it allow dose reduction of CsA (Meinardi et al., 1990).

Combination therapy with a potent topical steroid and oral CsA, however, appeared to offer a benefit over CsA alone: In a trial comparing clearance and relapse rates of psoriasis, patients on combination therapy cleared faster than those on oral CsA alone. Relapse rates, once all medications were stopped, appeared to be equal in both groups (Griffiths et al., 1988; Meinardi et al., 1990). This suggests that combination therapy may provide a CsA-sparing effect that would allow usage of lower total doses of CsA. This, in turn, would provide a lower risk for the development of potential adverse effects.

Intralesional CsA can be effective in the treatment of plaque-type psoriasis. Ho et al. (1990), in a double-blind, vehicle-controlled study, treated discrete psoriatic plaques in six patients with intralesional CsA (17 mg/ml), vehicle, or saline. Injections were given three times per week for four weeks. Significant improvement to complete clearing was seen in all CsA-treated plaques in contrast to vehicle- or saline-treated plaques, which showed minimal to no improvement. Systemic absorption of CsA was negligible. Both CsA solution and vehicle caused significant pain on injection in all patients and a chemical cellulitis in one patient. These side effects were attributed to the drug vehicle rather than to CsA itself. Similar results using intralesional CsA were noted in a study of ten patients by Powles et al. (1988).

In contrast to intralesional therapy, topical CsA has, to date, been ineffective in the treatment of psoriasis. Griffiths et al. (1987) treated six patients with 2% CsA ointment twice a day for one month and noted no significant difference between active drug and placebo. In an open trial, we treated 15 patients with a 10% CsA solution and noted a comparable lack of efficacy (unpublished data). A report of six additional patients treated with 5% CsA solution also failed to demonstrate effectiveness of the drug topically (Gilhar et al., 1988). Ten percent CsA gel was no more effective (Bousema et al., 1990). This lack of clinical response to topical CsA appears to be due to the drug's impermeability through the skin in its present formulation. In vitro diffusion studies (Hermann et al., 1988) using CsA solution alone and in combination with two vehicles thought to increase percutaneous absorption failed to demonstrate passage of the drug through the skin. Future research will hopefully be directed toward finding a vehicle that will enhance CsA delivery through the skin, making it an effective topical preparation for the treatment of psoriasis.

3.2. Bullous Diseases

CsA has been reported to be effective in the treatment of bullous diseases. Thivolet et al. (1985) treated two patients with bullous pemphigoid and two cases of pemphigus vulgaris with CsA at a dosage of 6 mg/kg per day. Both patients with pemphigus and one of the bullous pemphigoid patients received CsA in addition to prednisone; the fourth patient received CsA alone. Healing was noted within two weeks in the pemphigus patients and within four weeks in the pemphigoid patients. Clinical improvement was accompanied by the disappearance of both fixed and circulating autoantibodies. The three patients given combination therapy were gradually tapered off their prednisone, and subsequently maintained on CsA alone. The authors noted no adverse side effects in this small treatment group.

Barthelemy and co-workers (Barthelemy and Thivolet, 1985; Barthelemy *et al.*, 1986) treated seven patients with bullous pemphigoid and eight patients with pemphigus vulgaris. All received CsA dosages of 6–8 mg/kg per day. Using CsA alone or in conjunction with low-dose steroids, remission was achieved in six of seven pemphigoid patients. Of these, two patients relapsed after stopping therapy, two remained in remission without treatment, and two patients continue to be followed on CsA. In the group of pemphigus patients, only one mild case could be adequately treated with CsA alone. Six other patients responded to treatment with both CsA and low-dose corticosteroids. Of the seven patients who responded, four patients did not relapse after stopping CsA. Side effects observed included elevated serum creatinine, hematuria, hypertrichosis, and hypertension. The authors concluded that CsA appeared to be a useful agent, in combination with low-dose steroids, for the treatment of both bullous diseases. However, it appeared to be more effective in pemphigus than in bullous pemphigoid. Boixeda *et al.* (1991) reported successfully treating two patients with bullous pemphigoid and psoriasis with CsA, 5 mg/kg per day, and was able to induce clearing of both dermatoses in four to six weeks.

CsA has been used in the treatment of two patients with epidermolysis bullosa acquisita (EBA) in whom systemic steroids and cytotoxic agents proved ineffective. Connolly and Sander (1987) treated a 54-year-old woman with prednisone and CsA at 9 mg/kg per day. After three weeks, only rare new bullae were reported and her antibasement membrane antibody titer had dropped from 1:640 to 1:160. Unfortunately, the drug needed to be discontinued after 24 days due to side effects. Zachariae (1987) treated a similar EBA patient with 7.5 mg/kg per day and noted significant remission of the disease within three weeks. After two and a half months, an elevation in serum creatinine and fluid retention necessitated withdrawal of the drug. Two months later, the patient still remained in partial remission. Merle *et al.* (1990) treated an EBA patient who had been unresponsive to conventional therapy for five years with CsA and low-dose prednisone and was able to induce clearing in six months, which persisted 36 months after all therapy was discontinued. Layton and Cunliffe (1990) also found CsA at a dosage of 6 mg/kg per day to be effective in the treatment of a patient with EBA who had been refractory to corticosteroids, sulfasalazine, and phenytoin.

3.3. Behçet's Disease

Nussenblatt *et al.* (1985) have reported excellent results with CsA in the treatment of Behçet's disease. Seven patients who had failed to respond to cytotoxic agents and/or systemic corticosteroids were treated with CsA at 10 mg/kg per day. All patients noted an increase in visual acuity as well as a reduction in the frequency of their attacks. The nonocular manifestations of their disease, including mucosal ulcerations, arthritis, and skin lesions improved as well. French-Constant *et al.* (1983), using the same dose of CsA, were able to induce a complete remission of disease, on two occasions, in a 44-year-old patient with Behçet's. Unfortunately, a rise in serum creatinine necessitated discontinuation of drug therapy. Muftuoglu *et al.* (1987) administered CsA at 10 mg/kg per day to eight patients with sight-threatening uveitis and Behçet's disease. Improvement was rapid, with increased visual acuity noted in most patients within a week. The associated mucocutaneous lesions improved in seven of eight cases; in six, the cutaneous manifestations of the disease cleared entirely. Cessation of therapy was accompanied by a marked rebound phenomenon in all patients that lasted several weeks. Ben Ezra et al. (1988) enrolled 40 patients in a study comparing the efficacy of CsA to corticosteroids or chlorambucil in the treatment of Behçet's disease. After three years of observation, they concluded that CsA was more effective than the other therapies in decreasing the ocular inflammatory process and arresting the deterioration of visual acuity. In contrast, however, they found that the extraocular symptoms had responded better to the more conventional therapies.

3.4. Dermatomyositis/Polymyositis

Bendtzen et al. (1984) treated two patients with polymyositis with CsA at dosages of 7.5–10 mg/kg per day. Both patients noted an improvement in muscle strength within a week of therapy. Serum CPK and aldolase levels dropped concurrently. Ejstrup (1984) treated a 42-year-old man with severe dermatomyositis that had been resistant to other therapies. Dramatic clinical improvement was achieved within a week of starting CsA. Van der Meer et al. (1986) noted that CsA had a steroid-sparing effect when used in combination with systemic corticosteroids. Borleffs (1988) successfully treated a 46-year-old woman with polymyositis that had become refractory to steroid therapy. Within several weeks of receiving 10 mg/kg per day of CsA, she noted clinical improvement and her CPK levels returned to normal. An unexplained exacerbation in her disease after 20 weeks of therapy required the addition of low-dose prednisone to her regimen.

Juvenile dermatomyositis also responds to oral CsA. Dantzig (1990) used CsA (2.5–3.5 mg/kg per day) as sole therapy for a 4-year-old girl with dermatomyositis and noted improved muscle strength, partial resolution of her rash, and resolution of her dysphagia and dysphonia within one month of therapy. Similar results were obtained in a study of 14 children with chronic active dermatomyositis (Heckmatt et al., 1989). All patients experienced an improvement in muscle strength and were able to either decrease or discontinue their corticosteroids after initiating CsA therapy.

In contrast to these reported cases, however, Jones et al. (1987) did not note success after brief courses of CsA in two patients with intractable polymyositis who had not responded to regimens that included high-dose steroids, azathioprine, methotrexate, cyclophosphamide, and plasma exchange.

3.5. Atopic Dermatitis

CsA appears to have at least a temporarily beneficial effect in atopic dermatitis. Van Joost et al. (1987) treated two patients with severe, recalcitrant atopic dermatitis with 5 mg/kg per day for one month. Both patients noted an improvement in their skin disease of 60–80% within ten days of starting CsA. At the end of four weeks, their disease was in near-complete remission. Both patients had a slow relapse of their disease following cessation of therapy. Taylor et al. (1989), in an open trial, treated six adult patients with 6 mg/kg per day. Four patients experienced greater than 50% clinical clearing within a month; the other two showed more modest improvement. Two patients were noted to flare within the eight-week trial, coincidentally with a rise in airborne pollen levels. All patients flared when CsA therapy was stopped. Wahlgren et al. (1990), in a double-blind, placebo-controlled study, found CsA decreased the itching, eczema, and dependency on corticosteroid creams in ten adults with atopic dermatitis. In an open study, Ross and Camp (1990) treated 13 atopic dermatitis patients with oral CsA for up to 31 months. Ten of thirteen patients had a good response, and two required discontinuation of drug after more than two years due to rise in serum creatinine.

3.6. Alopecia

CsA has been efficacious in temporarily inducing new hair growth in patients suffering from alopecia areata and alopecia universalis. The mechanism of action is presumed to be through immunomodulation of the abnormal peribulbar T lymphocytes. Gebhart *et al.* (1986) first noted this effect in a patient with a long history of alopecia areata who began to grow new scalp hair after he received CsA following a renal transplant. Topical application of a 0.25% solution resulted in partial localized hair growth in one patient (Parodi and Rebora, 1987). Thomson *et al.* (1986) treated seven men with topical 5% CsA applied daily to the scalp and noted new terminal growth in two patients after three months. Using the same concentration of CsA, Mauduit *et al.* (1987) reported new vellus or terminal hair growth in six patients after five months; however, eight patients failed to respond. In the largest trial conducted to date, de Prost *et al.* (1988) treated 43 patients with severe alopecia areata with a 10% solution of CsA or placebo. Mild, incomplete terminal hair regrowth was observed in seven patients in the CsA group; no regrowth was seen in the placebo-treated group. Gilhar *et al.* (1989) found 10% CsA topical solution to be ineffective in treating ten patients with alopecia areata or universalis.

Gupta *et al.* (1988) treated a 20-year-old patient with long-standing, refractory alopecia totalis with oral CsA at 6 mg/kg per day for a three-month period. At the end of one month, the patient noted dramatic growth of scalp and facial hair, and he began to need to shave again for the first time in two years. By five weeks of therapy, new vellus hairs were noted in the axilla and groin, as well as on the extremities. A small and completely reversible increase in serum creatinine was seen. Following discontinuation of therapy most of the newly grown hair was shed. Using the same dose of CsA, six additional patients who had alopecia areata, alopecia totalis, or alopecia universalis were successfully treated (Gupta *et al.*, 1990). All patients showed terminal hair regrowth within two to four weeks of therapy. The most dramatic response was seen in the regrowth of scalp hair.

CsA has also been used in the treatment of male pattern alopecia, which is not thought to be an immune-mediated process. In experiments involving the grafting of scalp skin samples taken from patients with alopecia areata to congenitally athymic mice, Gilhar and Krueger (1987) noted that CsA-treated mice grew more hairs per graft than did untreated mice. They attributed this to a direct effect of CsA on hair growth. Picascia and Roenigk (1988) report an ongoing study of 14 men enrolled in a six-month topical CsA study for the treatment of male-pattern baldness. After a month of therapy, three patients reported a decrease in hair loss. The authors are investigating the possibility that in addition to this effect, topical CsA, like minoxidil, may stimulate the conversion of vellus to terminal hairs. When compared to vehicle, 5% CsA was able to induce significant hair growth in two of eight patients after four months of treatment (Gilhar *et al.*, 1990).

3.7. Pyoderma Gangrenosum

CsA has been used successfully in the treatment of pyoderma gangrenosum, a destructive, necrotizing ulceration of the skin that often responds poorly to conventional therapies. Curley *et al.* (1985) treated a woman with a 14-year history of pyoderma gangrenosum who had failed to respond to systemic steroids, cytotoxic agents, and plasma exchanges. Within three weeks of beginning CsA at 10 mg/kg per day, she began to heal her ulcers. Over a four-month period, her dosage was gradually reduced to 4 mg/kg per day, and after a year of therapy no recurrence of her ulcers were noted. Mild hypertrichosis was the only side effect noted during this long-term treatment. Shelley and Shelley (1988) reported similarly impressive results in a 58-year-old woman with ulcerative colitis and a rapidly enlarging ulcerated lesion of pyoderma gangrenosum on her face. Multiple treatment modalities, including systemic antibiotics and corticosteroids, acyclovir, chloroquine, potassium iodide, and orthovoltage radiation, given over a period of two years, had failed to arrest the progression of her disease. The patient was then given CsA, 10 mg/kg per day. The lesions began to heal within days and were nearly gone within one month. CsA was gradually tapered to 2.5 mg/kg per day over three and a half months and was discontinued after seven months of therapy. After 14 months off medication, the patient has had no recurrence of her skin lesions. Her inflammatory bowel disease has remained in remission as well. Similarly impressive results were noted in a third case of recalcitrant pyoderma gangrenosum treated with CsA (Penmetcha and Navaratnam, 1988). We, too, have had excellent results using 6 mg/kg per day of CsA (unpublished data).

3.8. Systemic Lupus Erythematosus

The role of CsA in the treatment of systemic lupus erythematosus (SLE) remains a subject of debate. There is little evidence to support its use as monotherapy. Isenburg et al. (1981) treated five SLE patients with 10 mg/kg per day. Two patients reported improvement in their arthralgias, but all patients experienced side effects, including angioedema in three, which necessitated discontinuation of therapy. In the treatment of seven patients with life-threatening SLE, Halloran et al. (1985) noted moderate improvement in two patients but none in the other five. Four patients in the trial died. Heule et al. (1986) treated a patient with mutilating discoid LE with CsA. He noted neither clinical nor histological evidence of improvement after ten weeks of therapy.

The usefulness of CsA in the treatment of SLE appears to lie in its steroid-sparing effect. Bambauer et al. (1985) instituted low-dose CsA in the treatment of seven patients already on a regimen of immunosuppressive drugs and plasmapheresis. He found he was able to reduce the prednisone dose by up to 40% with this combination therapy. Only one of seven patients flared during the 25-week trial period. Feutren et al. (1987) treated 13 steroid-dependent SLE patients, all of whom showed the stigmata of chronic corticosteroid use. CsA was given at a dosage of 5–10 mg/kg per day. Three patients manifested CsA-related toxicity and were taken off the drug. Of the remaining ten patients, eight showed clinical improvement that was maintained despite slow taper of their steroids. Cessation of CsA therapy led to an exacerbation of disease in five patients. A reversible rise in serum creatinine, hypertension, and hypertrichosis were the most commonly reported side effects. No evidence of chronic nephrotoxicity was seen in successive renal biopsies of three patients. Despite clinical improvement, however, no decrease in antinuclear antibodies was noted. This finding is in agreement with the work of other authors (Bambauer et al., 1985). Miescher (Miescher, 1985; Miescher and Miescher, 1986) noted clinical improvement in 17 of 20 SLE patients treated with combination therapy of systemic steroids and CsA. No adverse side effects were noted and the investigators concluded that CsA was effective in permitting steroid dose reduction. This effect may be particularly important in the treatment of young patients with SLE in whom a reduction in steroid doses may permit resumption of normal growth.

3.9. Progressive Systemic Sclerosis

Knop and Bonsmann (1985) investigated the efficacy of CsA in the treatment of three patients with progressive systemic sclerosis (PSS). CsA was administered at a dosage of 10 mg/kg per day for the first month of the study. The drug was then given at half the initial dose for an additional eight to ten months. Neither significant clinical improvement nor laboratory evidence of decreased disease activity was noted. A softening of the skin sclerosis was seen in some patients as was a decrease in Raynaud's phenomenon. Zachariae and Zachariae (1987) reported improvement in two patients with PSS who had failed to respond to penicillamine or systemic steroids. One patient had significant softening of the sclerotic skin of her arms and the second noted increased mobility in his involved hands after treatment. No adverse side effects were seen in either patient. Using dosages of 1.5–7.5 mg/kg per day, Zachariae *et al.* (1990) treated ten patients with severe PSS. Two patients had marked improvement on the drug, with softening of the skin. One patient had only a slight improvement and two patients had no response. One patient experienced an initial benefit, but this was followed by a marked exacerbation of his disease.

4. CONCLUSION

CsA has proved to be an effective drug in the treatment of many cutaneous diseases known to have an immunologic basis, as well as in some diseases in which an immune etiology has yet to be clearly established, such as psoriasis. CsA's rapid onset of action and dramatic effectiveness in the treatment of a broad spectrum of diseases, many of which presently lack adequate treatments, make it an exciting and promising therapeutic agent. Its widespread use in dermatology, as in other fields of medicine, however, has been hampered by concerns about its toxicity. In most cases, toxicity can be minimized by using low-dose CsA and by careful monitoring of trough drug levels. However, potential side effects are sufficient to warrant cautionary use in the treatment of non-life-threatening diseases.

Topical CsA, unfortunately, has not yet proven to be an effective therapeutic modality. It is hoped that future research will provide oral analogues of CsA as well as topical preparations that maintain clinical efficacy but exert less toxicity. If this can be accomplished, CsA may well prove to be one of the most significant additions to the dermatologist's therapeutic agents since corticosteroids.

REFERENCES

Bambauer, R., Jutzler, G. A., Dans, H., Schoenenberger, H. J., Biro, G., and Keller, H. E., 1985, Ciclosporin and therapeutic plasma exchange in steroid-resistant SLE, in: *Ciclosporin in Autoimmune Diseases* (R. Schindler, ed.), Springer-Verlag, New York, pp. 346–355.

Barthelemy, H., and Thivolet, J., 1985, Ciclosporine in pemphigus and bullous pemphigoid, in: *Ciclosporine in Autoimmune Diseases* (R. Schindler, ed.), Springer-Verlag, New York, pp. 215–219.

Barthelemy, H., Biron, F., Claudy, A., Souterand, P., and Thivolet, J., 1986, Cyclosporine: New immunosuppressive agent in bullous pemphigoid and pemphigus, *Transplant. Proc.* **18:**913–914.

Bendtzen, K., Trede, N., Anderson, V., 1984, Cyclosporine for polymyositis, *Lancet* **1:**792–793.

Ben Ezra, D., Cohen, E., Chajek, T., Friedman, G., Pizanti, S., de Courten, C., and Harris, W., 1988, Evaluation of conventional therapy versus cyclosporine A in Behçet's syndrome, *Transplant. Proc.* **20:**(Suppl. 4):136–143.

Biren, C. A., and Barr, R. T., 1986, Dermatologic applications of cyclosporine, *Arch. Dermatol.* **122:**1028–1032.

Boixeda, J. P., Soria, C., Medina, S., and Ledo, A., 1991, Bullous pemphigoid and psoriasis: Treatment with cyclosporine, *J. Am. Acad. Dermatol.* **24:**152.

Borleffs, J. C. C., 1988, Cyclosporine as monotherapy for polymyositis? *Transplant. Proc.* **20:**(Suppl. 4):333–334.

Bousema, M. T., Tank, B., Heule, F., Naafs, B., Stolz, E., and van Joost, T., 1990, Placebo-controlled study of psoriasis patients treated topically with a 10% cyclosporine gel, *J. Am. Acad. Dermatol.* **22:**126–127.

Brown, M. D., Ellis, C. N., and Voorhees, J. J., 1987, Cyclosporine A: A review of its dermatologic applications, *Sem. Dermatol.* **6**:2–9.

Brown, M. D., Gupta, A. K., Ellis, C. N., Rocher, L. L., and Voorhees, J. J., 1989, Therapy of dermatologic disease with cyclosporine A, *Adv. Dermatol.* **4**:3–27.

Connolly, S. M., and Sander, H. M., 1987, Treatment of epidermolysis bullosa acquisita with cyclosporine (letter to editor), *J. Am. Acad. Dermatol.* **16**:890.

Curley, R. K., MacFarlane, A. W., and Vickers, C. F., 1985, Pyoderma gangrenosum treated with cyclosporine A, *Br. J. Dermatol.* **113**:601–604.

Dantzig, P., 1990, Juvenile dermatomyositis treated with cyclosporine, *J. Am. Acad. Dermatol.* **22**:310–311.

de Prost, Y., Teillac, D., Paqvez, F., Carrugi, C., Bachelez, H., and Touraine, R., 1988, Treatment of severe alopecia areata by topical applications of cyclosporine: Comparative trial versus placebo in 43 patients, *Transplant. Proc.* **20**:(Suppl. 4):112–113.

Ejstrup, L., 1984, Severe dermatomyositis treated with cyclosporine A, *Ann. Rheum. Dis.* **45**:612–613.

Ellis, C. N., Gorsulowsky, D. C., Hamilton, T. A., Billings, J. K., Brown, M. D., Headington, J. T., Cooper, K. D., Baadsgaard, O., Duell, E. A., Annesley, T. M., Turcotte, J. G., and Voorhees, J. J., 1986, Cyclosporine improves psoriasis in a double-blind study, *J. Am. Med. Assoc.* **256**:3110–3116.

Ellis, C. N., Fradin, M. S., Messana, J. M., Brown, M. D., Siegel, M. T., Hartley, A. H., Rocher, L. L., Wheeler, S., Hamilton, T. A., Parish, T. G., Ellis-Madu, M., Duell, E., Annesley, T. M., Cooper, K. D., and Voorhees, J. J., 1991, Cyclosporine for plaque-type psoriasis: Results of a multidose, double-blind trial, *N. Engl. J. Med.* **324**:277–284.

Feutren, G., Querin, S., Noel, L. H., Chatenoud, L., Beaurain, G., Tron, F., and Bach, J. F., 1987, Effects of cyclosporine in severe systemic lupus erythematosus, *J. Pediatr.* **111**:1063–1068.

Fradin, M. S., Ellis, C. N., and Voorhees, J. J., 1990a, Efficacy of cyclosporine A in psoriasis: A summary of the United States' experience, *Br. J. Dermatol.* **122**(Suppl. 36):21–25.

Fradin, M. S., Ellis, C. N., and Voorhees, J. J., 1990b, Management of patients and side effects during cyclosporine therapy for cutaneous disorders, *J. Am. Acad. Dermatol.* **23**(6):1265–1275.

Fradin, M. S., Ellis, C. N., and Voorhees, J. J., 1990c, Rapid response of von Zumbusch psoriasis to cyclosporine, *J. Am. Acad. Dermatol.* **23**:925–926.

Fredriksson, T., and Petterson, V., 1978, Severe psoriasis—oral therapy with a new retinoid, *Dermatologica* **157**:238–244.

French-Constant, C., Wolman, R., and James, P. G., 1983, Cyclosporine in Behçet's disease, *Lancet* **2**:454–455.

Fry, L., Griffiths, C. E. M., Powles, A. V., Baker, B. S., and Valdimarsson, H., 1988, Long-term cyclosporine in the management of psoriasis, *Transplant. Proc.* **20**(Suppl. 4):23–25.

Gebhart, W., Schmidt, J. B., Schemper, M., Spona, J., and Zezorˇnik, J., 1986, Cyclosporine A-induced hair growth in human renal allograft recipients and alopecia areata, *Arch. Dermatol. Res.* **278**:238–240.

Gilhar, A., and Krueger, G., 1987, Hair growth in scalp grafts from patients with alopecia areata and alopecia universalis grafted onto nude mice, *Arch. Dermatol.* **123**:44–50.

Gilhar, A., Winterstein, G., and Golan, D. T., 1988, Topical cyclosporine in psoriasis (letter to the editor), *J. Am. Acad. Dermatol.* **18**:378–379.

Gilhar, A,. Pillar, T., and Etzioni, A., 1989, Topical cyclosporin A in alopecia areata, *Acta. Derm. Venerol.* **69**:252–253.

Gilhar, A., Pillar, T., and Etzioni, A., 1990, Topical cyclosporine in male pattern alopecia, *J. Am. Acad. Dermatol.* **22**:251–253.

Griffiths, C. E. M., Powles, A. V., Leonard, J. N., and Fry, L., 1986, Clearance of psoriasis with low dose cyclosporine, *Br. Med. J.* **293**:731–732.

Griffiths, C. E. M., Powles, A. V., Baker, B. S., and Fry, L., 1987, Topical cyclosporine and psoriasis, *Lancet* **1**:806.

Griffiths, C. E. M., Powles, A. V., Baker, B. S., Fry, L., and Valdimarsson, H., 1988, Combination of cyclosporine A and topical corticosteroids in the treatment of psoriasis, *Transplant. Proc.* **20**(Suppl. 4):50–52.

Gupta, A. K., Ellis, C. N., Tellner, D. C., and Voorhees, J. J., 1988, Cyclosporine A in the treatment of severe alopecia areata, *Transplant. Proc.* **20**(Suppl. 4):105–108.

Gupta, A. K., Matteson, E. L., Ellis, C. N., Ho, V. C., Tellner, D. C., McCune, W. J., and Voorhees, J. J., 1989, Cyclosporine A in the treatment of psoriatic arthritic, *Arch. Dermatol.* **125**:507–510.

Gupta, A. K., Ellis, C. N., Ho, V. C., Chan, L. S., Cooper, K. D., Nickoloff, B. J., Tellner, D. C., and Voorhees, J. J., 1990, Oral cyclosporine for the treatment of severe alopecia areata, *J. Am. Acad. Dermatol.* **22**:242–250.

Halloran, P. T., Cole, E. A., and Bookman, A. A., 1985, Possible beneficial effect of cyclosporine in some cases of severe systemic lupus erythematosus, in: *Cyclosporin in Autoimmune Diseases* (R. Schindler, ed.), Springer-Verlag, New York, pp. 356–360.

Harper, J. I., Keat, A. C. S., and Staughton, R. C. D., 1984, Cyclosporine A for psoriasis, *Lancet* **2**:981–982.

Harper, J. I., Zemelman, V., Keat, A. C. S., and Staughton, R. C. D., 1988, Cyclosporine for psoriasis: Beneficial effect in refractory skin and joint disease, *Transplant. Proc.* **20**(Suppl. 4):63–67.

Heckmatt, J., Hasson, N., Saunders, C., Thompson, N., Peters, A. M., Cambridge, G,. Rose, M., Hyde, S. A., and Dubowitz, V., 1989, Cyclosporine in juvenile dermatomyositis, *Lancet* **1**:1063–1066.

Hermann, R. C., Taylor, R. S., Ellis, C. N., Williams, N. A., Weiner, N. D., Flynn, G. L., Annesley, T. M., and Voorhees, J. J., 1988, Topical cyclosporine A for psoriasis: *In vitro* skin penetration and clinical study, *Skin Pharmacol.* **1**:246–249.

Heule, F. H., Van Joost, T. V., and Benkers, R., 1986, Cyclosporine in the treatment of lupus erythematosus, *Arch. Dermatol.* **122**:973–974.

Ho, V. C., Griffiths, C. E. M., Ellis, C. N., Gupta, A. K., McQuaig, C. C., Nickoloff, B. J., and Voorhees, J. J., 1990, Intralesional cyclosporine A in the treatment of psoriasis: A clinical, immunologic and pharmacokinetic study, *J. Am. Acad. Dermatol.* **22**:94–100.

Isenberg, D. A., Snaith, M. L., Morrow, W. J., Al-Kahder, A. A., Cohen, S. L., Fisher, C., and Mowbray, J., 1981, Cyclosporine A for the treatment of systemic lupus erythematosus, *Int. J. Immunopharmacol.* **3**:163–169.

Jones, D. W., Snaith, M. L., and Isenberg, D. A., 1987, Cyclosporine treatment for intractable polymyositis (letter to editor), *Arthritis Rheum.* **30**:959–960.

Knop, J., and Bonsmann, G., 1985, Ciclosporine in the treatment of progressive systemic sclerosis, in: *Ciclosporin in Autoimmune Diseases* (R. Schindler, ed.), Springer-Verlag, New York, pp. 199–200.

Krupp, P., and Monka, C, 1990, Side-effect profile of cyclosporine A in patients treated for psoriasis, *Br. J. Dermatol.* **122**(Suppl. 36):47–56.

Layton, A. M., and Cunliffe, W. J., 1990, Clearing of epidermolysis bullosa acquisita with cyclosporine (letter), *J. Am. Acad. Dermatol.* **22**:535–536.

Marks, J., 1986, Psoriasis, *Br. Med. J.* **293**:509.

Marks, J., 1988, Low dose cyclosporine A in severe psoriasis, *Transplant. Proc.* **20**:68–71.

Mauduit, G., Lenvers, P., Barthelemy, H., and Thivolet, J., 1987, Treatment of severe alopecia areata with topical cyclosporine A, *Ann. Dermatol. Venereol.* **114**:507–510.

Meinardi, M. M., and Bos, J. D., 1988, Cyclosporine maintenance therapy in psoriasis, *Transplant. Proc.* **20**(Suppl. 4):42–48.

Meinardi, M. M., Westerhof, W., and Bos, J. D., 1987, Generalized pustular psoriasis (Von Zumbusch) responding to cyclosporine A, *Br. J. Dermatol.* **116**:269–270.

Meinardi, M. M. H. M., de Rie, M. A., and Bos, J. D., 1990, Oral cyclosporine A in the treatment of psoriasis: An overview of studies performed in The Netherlands, *Br. J. Dermatol.* **122**(Suppl. 36):27–31.

Merle, C., Blanc, D., Zultak, M., van Landuyt, H., Drobacheff, C., and Laurent, R., 1990, Intractable epidermolysis bullosa acquisita: Efficacy of cyclosporin A, *Dermatologica* **181**;44–47.

Miescher, P. A., 1986, Treatment of systemic lupus erythematosus, *Springer Semin. Immunopathol.* **9**:271–282.

Miescher, P. A., and Miescher, A., 1985, Combined ciclosporin-steroid treatment of systemic lupus erythematosus, in: *Ciclosporin in Autoimmune Diseases* (R. Schindler, ed.), Springer-Verlag, New York, pp. 337–345.

Mueller, W., and Hermann, B., 1979, Cyclosporine A for psoriasis, *N. Engl. J. Med.* **301**:555.

Muftuoglu, A. V., Pazarli, H., Yurdakul, S., Yazici, H., Ulku, B., Tuzun, Y., Serdaroglu, S., Altug, E., and Bahcecioglu, H., 1987, Short-term cyclosporine A treatment of Behçet's disease, *Br. J. Ophthalmol.* **71**:387–390.

Nussenblatt, R. B., Palestine, A. G., Chan, C., Mochizuku, M., and Yancey, K., 1985, Effectiveness of cyclosporine therapy for Behçet's disease, *Arthritis Rheum.* **28**:671–679.

Page, E. H., Wexler, D. M., and Guenther, L. C., 1986, Cyclosporine A, *J. Am. Acad. Dermatol.* **14**:785–791.

Parodi, A., and Rebora, A., 1987, Topical cyclosporine in alopecia areata, *Arch. Dermatol.* **123**:165–166.

Penmetcha, M., and Navaratnam, A., 1988, Pyoderma gangrenosum: Response to cyclosporine A, *Int. J. Dermatol.* **27**:253.

Picascia, D. D., and Roenigk, H. H., 1988, Effects of oral and topical cyclosporine in male pattern alopecia, *Transplant. Proc.* **20**(Suppl. 4):109–111.

Picascia, D. D., Garden, J. M., Freinkel, R. K., and Roenigk, H. H., 1987, Treatment of resistant severe psoriasis with systemic cyclosporine, *J. Am. Acad. Dermatol.* **17**:408–414.

Picascia, D. D., Garden, J. M., Freinkel, R. K., and Roenigk, H. H., 1988, Resistant severe psoriasis controlled with systemic cyclosporine therapy, *Transplant. Proc.* **20**(Suppl. 4):58–62.

Powles, A. V., Baker, B. S., McFadden, J., Rutman, A. J., Griffiths, C. E. M., and Fry, L., 1988, Intralesional injection of cyclosporine in psoriasis, *Lancet* **1**:537.

Ross, J. S., and Camp, R. D., 1990, Cyclosporin A in atopic dermatitis, *Br. J. Dermatol.* **122**(Suppl. 36):41–45.

Shelley, E. D., and Shelley, W. B., 1988, Cyclosporine therapy for pyoderma grangrenosum associated with sclerosing cholangitis and ulcerative colitis, *J. Am. Acad. Dermatol.* **18**:1084–1088.

Taylor, R. S., Cooper, K. D., Headington, J. T., Ho, V. C., Ellis, C. N., and Voorhees, J. J., 1989, Cyclosporine A therapy for severe atopic dermatitis, *J. Am. Acad. Dermatol.* **21**:580–583.

Thivolet, J., Barthelemy, H., Rigot-Muller, G., and Bendelac, 1985, Effects of cyclosporine on bullous pemphigoid and pemphigus, *Lancet* **1**:334–335.

Thomson, A. W., Aldridge, R. D., and Sewell, H. I., 1986, Topical cyclosporine in alopecia areata and nickel contact dermatitis, *Lancet* **2**:971–972.

Timonen, P., Friend, D., Abeywickrama, K., Laburte, C., von Graffenried, B., and Feutren, G., 1990, Efficacy of low-dose cyclosporine A in psoriasis: Results of dose-finding studies, *Br. J. Dermatol.* **122**(Suppl. 36):33–39.

Van der Meer, S., Inhof, J. W., and Borleff, J. C., 1986, Cyclosporine for polymyositis, *Ann. Rheum. Dis.* **45**:612.

Van Hooff, J. P., Leunissen, K. M. L., and Staak, W., 1985, Cyclosporine and psoriasis, *Lancet* **1**:335.

Van Joost, Th., Heule, F., Stolz, E., and Beukers, R., 1986, Short-term use of cyclosporine in severe psoriasis, *Br. J. Dermatol.* **114**:615–620.

Van Joost, Th., Stolz, E., and Heule, F., 1987, Efficacy of low-dose cyclosporine in severe atopic skin disease, *Arch. Dermatol.* **123**:166–167.

Van Joost, Th., Bos, J. D., Heule, F., and Meinardi, M. M., 1988, Low-dose cyclosporine A in severe psoriasis. A double-blind study, *Br. J. Dermatol.* **118**:183–190.

Wahlgren, C. F., Scheynius, A., and Hagermark, O., 1990, Antipruritic effect of oral cyclosporin A in atopic dermatitis, *Acta Derm. Venereol. (Stockh.)* **70**(4):323–329.

Zachariae, H., 1987, Cyclosporine A in epidermolysis bullosa acquisita (letter to editor), *J. Am. Acad. Derm.* **17**:1058–1059.

Zachariae, H., and Thestrup-Pedersen, K., 1987, Ciclosporin A in acrodermatitis continua, *Dermatologica* **175**:29–32.

Zachariae, H., and Zachariae, E., 1987, Cyclosporine A in systemic sclerosis (letter to editor), *Br. J. Dermatol.* **116**:741–742.

Zachariae, H., Halkier-Sorensen, L., Heickendorff, L., Zachariae, E., and Hansen, H. E., 1990, Cyclosporin A treatment of systemic sclerosis, *Br. J. Dermatol.* **122**(5):677–681.

Chapter 28

IMMUNOTHERAPY IN KIDNEY DISEASES

Knut J. Berg and *Tore Talseth*

1. INTRODUCTION

It is important to assess the effects of immunosuppressive therapy on experimental glomerulonephritis (GN) to evaluate the potential clinical effects of these drugs in human GN. Immunosuppressive agents have been used in many types of experimental GN. Cyclosporine A (CyA) inhibited the proteinuria and reduced glomerular proliferation in serum sickness models, but only for the time the drug was administered (Neild *et al.*, 1983, 1986). Methylprednisolone had no effect (Neild *et al.*, 1986). Rabbits with acute serum sickness treated with CyA, however, often developed glomerular capillary thrombi and symptoms resembling hemolytic uremic syndrome (Neild *et al.*, 1984). CyA also reduced proteinuria in active experimental glomerular basement membrane GN (anti-GBM-GN) if administered before preimmunization. The effect lasted only for the time the drug was administered (Tipping and Holdsworth, 1985). CyA was without effect on the passive, heterologous anti-GBM-GN (Tipping and Holdsworth, 1985; Schrijver *et al.*, 1988).

The lesions in Heyman nephritis (HN) are similar to those observed in membranous GN (MGN). The HN lesion can be modified by impairing antibody formation with conventional immunosuppressive agents (Fleuren and Hoedemaeker, 1980). CyA administered at the same time as the antigen blocked the production of free antibodies and immune complexes in HN and reduced proteinuria; the effect lasting only for the time CyA was given (Cattran, 1988). CyA increased azotemia in puromycin-induced glomerulosclerosis (Nahman and Cosio, 1990).

In summary, CyA seems to protect the development of GN in some experimental models, provided the drug is administered from the time of or before antigen stimulation. In other models, CyA is without effect on the immunological process. Proteinuria, however, is often reduced, irrespective of an effect on the morphological picture. In such cases, one cannot exclude that the effect of CyA is secondary to a reduction in the glomerular filtration rate (GFR).

Knut J. Berg and Tore Talseth • Section for Nephrology, Department of Medicine, The National Hospital, University of Oslo, 0027 Oslo 1, Norway.

Immunopharmacology in Autoimmune Diseases and Transplantation, edited by Hans Erik Rugstad *et al.* Plenum Press, New York, 1992.

2. IMMUNOSUPPRESSIVE TREATMENT OF GLOMERULONEPHRITIDES

In human disease, irrespective of the morphological classification or the presumed immunopathogenetic mechanisms involved, there is currently no well-documented benefit from the use of conventional immunosuppression in GN with slight or moderate proteinuria, that is, less than approximately 3 g/day. One notable exception is the syndrome of rapidly progressive GN. Neither in the group of mesangioproliferative disorders (among which IgA nephropathy is the most prevalent and most extensively studied), nor among those rather few instances where MGN or focal glomerular sclerosis may run a course with mild or moderate proteinuria, has a beneficial effect on long-term outcome been demonstrated. The course of the two latter disorders in cases without the nephrotic syndrome is not well defined, whereas the IgA glomerulonephritis with little proteinuria may have a close to 100% 5-year renal survival (D'Amico et al., 1986; Neelakantappa et al., 1988).

There are few documented reports on the effect of CyA in GN without nephrotic syndrome. Cattran et al. (1985) treated 28 patients with biopsy-proven GN, some of them with IgA nephropathy and mesangiocapillary GN without nephrotic syndrome with CyA 4–6 mg/kg for 4 months. No patient had a decline in creatinine clearance during this period. Lai et al. (1988, 1989) reported a trial with CyA in 24 patients with IgA nephropathy, 20 of them without nephrotic syndrome. Twelve of the patients were given CyA 5 mg/kg for 12 weeks and 12 placebo. CyA reduced proteinuria by more than 50% in 10 of 12 patients, but increased serum creatinine significantly. They concluded that patients with IgA nephropathy could be extremely sensitive to the nephrotoxic effect of CyA and that long-term treatment with CyA should be discouraged.

Thus, treatment of GN without nephrotic range proteinuria with a immunosuppressive drugs can therefore not be considered supported by the published experience.

2.1. Rapidly Progressive Glomerulonephritis

Rapidly progressive glomerulonephritis (RPGN) comprises a heterogenous group of disease processes, characterized by a rapid decline of renal function. RPGN may be associated with glomerular deposition of antibodies directed against defined elements of the glomerular basement membrane (anti-GBM-GN, Goodpasture's syndrome), with deposition of circulating immune complexes [as in systemic lupus erythematosus (SLE)] or there may be no well-defined immunological mechanism, such as in some of the vasculitic syndromes. The renal biopsy findings are usually either crescentic proliferation of the Bowman's capsule or necrotic lesions in the glomerular tuft.

2.1.1. Corticosteroids

All forms of RPGN require prompt and intense immunosuppression, including the use of corticosteroids. To administer corticosteroids as intravenous (IV) boluses of methylprednisolone is a rather novel treatment modality. However, its superiority over high-dose oral prednisolone has not been documented. The treatment of RPGN with steroids does not follow any fixed schedule. If therapy is initiated, as is often the case, with methylprednisolone 1 g IV three times during the first week, then oral prednisolone dosage may be limited to approximately 0.5 mg/kg per day. The duration of treatment will in part depend on the nature of the underlying disease. In anti-GBM disease, steroids may be stopped six months after the patient has become anti-GBM negative. In idiopathic RPGN, or RPGN as a part of a vasculitis syndrome, treatment will have to be continued for a prolonged time period, probably one to two years after clinical remission has been achieved.

2.1.2. Cytotoxic Drugs

These drugs are indicated in almost all forms of RPGN, irrespective of underlying disease. The published experience with treatment of Wegener's granulomatosis and current practice with anti-GBM disease have focused on cyclophosphamide as the drug of choice over azathioprine. A common dosage will be 1–3 mg/kg per day, adjusted to keep the WBC > 3500. The rather new practice to administer cyclophosphamide as monthly IV infusions in doses of 0.5–1 g in the treatment of SLE (Sessoms and Kovarsky, 1984; McCune et al., 1988) has currently no documentation in the treatment of RPGN.

2.1.3. Plasma Exchange

Certain forms of RPGN represent the most established indication for plasma exchange in nephrology (Rifle et al., 1990). However, the clinical experience with plasma exchange in SLE, as a prototype of immune complex disease, is disappointing, and the renal affection in SLE is not an accepted indication for plasma exchange. Plasma exchange can undoubtedly accelerate removal of anti-GBM, and anti-GBM disease is currently considered a solid indication for plasma exchange treatment. Anti-GBM nephritis with some residual renal function or with pulmonary hemorrhage does profit from plasma exchange (Savage et al., 1986). It is questionable whether idiopathic RPGN is an indication for apheresis (Glockner et al., 1988). Fuiano et al. (1988) concluded that prognosis of renal microscopic polyarteritis (including Wegener's granulomatosis) had improved since the introduction of aggressive immunosuppression comprising steroids, cyclophosphamide, and plasma exchange. The effect of plasma exchange could not be assessed separately, however. There are no clinical reports on the treatment of RPGN with CyA.

2.2. Glomerulonephritis with Nephrotic Syndrome

2.2.1. Conventional Immunosuppression

In this section we will discuss certain rather well-defined forms of GN that frequently occur with the nephrotic syndrome (NS). It may appear artificial to distinguish GN with NS syndrome from GN without NS, since apparently identical cases, based on renal biopsy, may or may not occur with NS. However, the treatment series reported is mainly limited to cases with NS.

2.2.1a.   Membranous Glomerulonephritis (MGN).   This is the most common cause for NS in adult patients. Between 60 and 80% occur with NS, and in 15–25% the condition may be part of a variety of systemic diseases or a consequence of treatment with gold salts or D-penicillamine (Honkanen, 1986; Donadio et al., 1988; Murphy et al., 1988). The immunopathogenesis is considered to be *in situ* formation of immune complexes in the subepithelial space. The nature of the antigen is unknown in the human disease (McCluskey, 1987; Wilson, 1987). Over an observation period of five to seven years, one can expect 20–40% of the patients to experience deteriorating renal function, and 40–60% may enter a remission of the NS (Noel et al., 1979; Davison et al., 1984; Honkanen, 1986;

Donadio *et al.*, 1988; Murphy *et al.*, 1988). The prognosis may be better in children (Ramirez *et al.*, 1982).

Corticosteroids. A collaborative study (Collaborative Study Group of the Adult Idiopathic Nephrotic Syndrome, 1979) concluded that there is a benefit from the use of prednisolone, 100–150 mg every other day over an eight-week period. The treated patients had a higher remission rate from the NS and also more stable renal function than the placebo-treated controls. In an earlier study, employing a lower steroid dosage (i.e., 40 mg/day), no effect of treatment was found (Black *et al.*, 1970). Cattran *et al.* (1989) also failed to find an effect of oral prednisone (45 mg/m^2 on alternate days for 6 months).

Cytotoxic Drugs. An Italian multicenter study (Ponticelli *et al.*, 1984) concluded that combination therapy with corticosteroids and chlorambucil over six months favors remission of the NS and preserves renal function (Ponticelli *et al.*, 1984, 1989). The notion that cytotoxic drugs may add to the beneficial effects of corticosteroids in this condition is supported by West *et al.* (1987).

Conclusions. The problem with both the Collaborative Study (1979) and that of Ponticelli *et al.* (1984) is a higher than expected rate of progression in the control groups. Schena and Cameron (1988) have recently reviewed the cumulative experience with MGN. They conclude that in all reported series combined, there is a significantly higher chance for a remission of the NS in treated than in untreated patients. The problem is to select those patients who can benefit from immunosuppressive treatment. Clearly they must be found among those with the most massive proteinuria, and also among those who exhibit deteriorating renal function over a few years of observation. The choice is between corticosteroids, as employed in the Collaborative Study, with alternate days on prednisolone for eight weeks and subsequent tapering. For unresponsive patients, the combined regimen employed by Ponticelli *et al.* (1984) may be used. Alternatively, one may use azathioprine together with prednisolone as employed by Williams and Bone (1989), who reported a favorable response in a small group of patients with predictably poor outcome.

2.2.1b. Minimal Change Nephrotic Syndrome (MCNS). This is most frequently encountered in childhood. In preschool age, MCNS represents 87% of new cases of idiopathic nephrotic syndrome, contrasting with only 15% in adults over the age of 35 years (Hoyer, 1982). The etiology of MCNS is unsettled. The prime event is thought to be altered glomerular permeability secondary to interference with the fixed anionic charge of the glomerular capillary wall. The clinical presentation is by definition the same as the nephrotic syndrome.

Corticosteroids. The view that MCNS should be treated with corticosteroids is almost universally held. Some authors include steroid responsiveness as a criterion for the diagnosis. The optimum steroid schedule and duration of steroid treatment is not fully standardized. For children, reference studies have been published (International Study of Kidney Disease in Children, 1978). On the order of 85–90% of children can be expected to respond to a two- to four-week course of corticosteroids (Koskimes *et al.*, 1982). In children who are relapsers, and where prolonged steroid treatment is required, steroid administration on alternate days (35 mg/m^2) is superior to sequential administration of 40 mg/m^2 per day (i.e., steroids on three successive days per week) (Arbeitsgemeinschaft fur Pediatrisches Nephrologie, 1981). Treatment of adult patients follows the same general guidelines as that of children (Coggins, 1981). By initiating treatment with IV methylprednisolone and there-after low-dose oral prednisolone, Imbasciati et al. (1985) retained the favorable effect of steroids, but apparently reduce side effects.

Cytotoxic Drugs.   Addition of alkylating drugs (chlorambucil or cyclophosphamide) can be expected to offer little in patients who are steroid-dependent (Brodehl, 1981). In patients who are frequent relapsers, an eight-week course of either drug (chlorambucil 0.1–0.2 mg/kg per day or cyclophosphamide 2–3 mg/kg per day) may prevent relapses and may also occasionally convert a primary nonresponder to a steroid responder. Azathioprine does not add to the beneficial effects of corticosteroids in this condition (Abramowicz et al., 1970).

Conclusions.   One should keep in mind that the aim of therapy in this condition is to relieve patients from the disabling symptoms that may be associated with the nephrotic syndrome. This condition does so rarely progress to renal failure that steroid treatment for avoiding this course is not warranted. Coggins (1981, 1988) recommends that adult patients who are mildly symptomatic should not be treated (as there is at least a 50% chance for spontaneous remission). Patients who are not steroid responsive should not receive prolonged treatment. Cytotoxic drugs should only be added when there is a strong clinical indication. The place for CyA in the treatment of MCNS is reviewed in Section 2.2.2.

2.2.1c.   *Focal Segmental Glomerulosclerosis (FSGS).*   As is the case with MCNS, the etiology and pathogenesis of FSGS is unknown. It is still questioned if FSGS represents a distinct disease entity. The morphological pattern, most often found in the deep juxta-medullary glomeruli, consists of sclerosing lesions, which may be focal and segmental in their distribution. The diagnosis of FSGS is made in approximately 20% of a population being evaluated for NS. FSGS can in some cases be secondary to rather nonspecific lesions of the kidney. Sixty to seventy percent have NS. The prognosis in adults is grave, as 50% will experience renal death ten years after diagnosis and 70% 15 years. The outlook is somewhat better among children. The degree of proteinuria in this condition may also have prognostic significance: certain subgroups with mild to moderate proteinuria may have 90% renal survival at ten years in spite of the typical lesion of FSGS in renal biopsy.

Treatment.   There are no controlled studies demonstrating effect of either steroids or cytotoxic drugs on the nephrotic syndrome. However, the recent experience published by the Toronto Glomerulonephritic Registry (Pei et al., 1987) may indicate some effect from steroid treatment, as one third of steroid-treated patients entered a complete remission from their NS.

Conclusions.   Presently FSGS is not an indication for steroid treatment, and no extra effect of cytotoxic drugs has been demonstrated. However, in severe cases, in particular when renal function is declining, a course of steroids may be indicated. The total dose and duration is not defined. It may be reasonable to employ treatment regimens as suggested for MGN. The effect of CyA is discussed separately (Section 2.2B).

2.2.2. Clinical Experience with CyA

As CyA has a selective action on T helper cells and inhibits the relapse of interleukin-2 and lymphokines, the drug might prevent the glomerular barrier dysfunction and thus induce remission of the NS. After encouraging results in some pilot studies, CyA was used in many controlled and uncontrolled studies, and several collaborative studies are now in progress. Data have been reported for 275 patients, 106 children and 169 adults with histologically verified NS treated with CyA (Table I). The morphological diagnosis was MCNS in 48%, FSGS in 30.9%, and unknown or other in 21.1% (Table II). One hundred twenty-three patients were considered steroid dependent and 152 patients were steroid resistant.

The definition of steroid dependence varies widely, and in some reports no definition is available. In this chapter the term "steroid dependence" includes both patients with relapse after reduction of the prednisolone dose to < 10–20 mg/day and frequent relapsers (> 2 relapses/6 months or > 4 relapses/12 months). The definition of "steroid resistance" varies even more. In most patients the term is defined as therapeutic failure after prednisolone 1 mg/kg per day for 6–12 weeks (adults) or 40–60 mg/m^2 per day for 6–8 weeks (children). In some reports, terms like "steroid and cytostatica resistant" or "steroid resistant" NS is used. Of the patients with MCNS, 72.7% were steroid dependent and 27.3% resistant (Table II). As expected, most of the patients with FSGS were resistant (89.4%), as were more than 75% of the patients with membranous or mesangiocapillary GN. The effect of CyA treatment in children and adults is shown in Table III. Of the steroid-dependent patients, 77.2% remitted completely on CyA and only 5.7% were CyA resistant. In the steroid resistant group, only 15.1% remitted completely. There was no difference in the effect of CyA between children and adults.

The initial CyA dosage varied from 3–10 mg/kg per day. In most reports the CyA dose was adjusted in order to get whole blood trough concentrations between 200–500 ng/ml (polyclonal radioimmunoassay).

2.2.2a.   Concomitant Therapy.   Prednisolone was not given in eight of the studies. In some patients prednisolone was withdrawn and the patients remitted on CyA; in three studies prednisolone 10 mg/day was administered concomitant with CyA. In the three largest studies, prednisolone was withdrawn after one to four months (Niaudet *et al.*, 1988), after 14 days (Tejani *et al.*, 1988), or not given (Meyrier *et al.*, 1988) during the CyA treatment.

TABLE I.   Trials with CyA in Patients with NS

Adults		Children	
Author	N^a	Author	N
Balcke *et al.* (1987)	5	Brandis *et al.* (1988)	9
Berthoux *et al.* (1987)	3	Brodehl *et al.* (1988)	14
Chan and Cheng (1987)	8	Capodicasa *et al.* (1986)	10
Clasen *et al.* (1988)	7	Garin *et al.* (1988)	8
DeSanto *et al.* (1987)	8	Niaudet *et al.* (1988)	45
Erbay *et al.* (1988)	18	Tejany *et al.* (1988)	20
Kühn *et al.* (1987)	16	Total	106
Lagrue *et al.* (1986)	13		
Maher *et al.* (1988)	15		
Meyrier *et al.* (1988)	51		
Millet *et al.* (1987)	3		
Sreepada Rao and Friedman (1987)	5		
Zietse *et al.* (1989)	17		
Total	169		

^{a}Number of patients in the trial.

TABLE II. Morphological Diagnosis in Patients with NS Treated with CyA

Effect of steroids	MCNS	FSGS	MGN	Mes. cap. GN	IgA GN	Other	Total
Dependent	96	9	5	3	2	8	123
	(72.7)[a]	(10.6)	(23.8)	(21.4)	(33.3)	(47.1)	
Resistant	36	76	16	11	4	9	152
	(27.3)	(89.4)	(76.2)	(78.6)	(66.7)	(52.9)	
Total	132	85	21	14	6	17	275

[a]Percent in parentheses.

Other cytostatic treatment or nonsteroidal anti-inflammatory drugs (NSAIDs) were not administered.

2.2.2b. Time to Induce Remission on CyA and Relapses after CyA.   The effect of CyA usually started within three to six weeks. In most cases the maximal effect of CyA was seen within eight weeks, and no remissions were induced later than three months after the start of CyA. Relapse of NS is seen frequently after CyA withdrawal in approximately two thirds of the children and even more frequently in adults. The time from withdrawal to relapse in children varied from 8–75 days (Niaudet *et al.*, 1988) to five months (Tejani *et al.*, 1988). In Tejani's study 40% of the children remained protein free more than 1 year after CyA withdrawal. The latency time before relapse seems to be the same as in adults. In one study (Zietse *et al.*, 1989), 11 of 12 patients relapsed within one month. Relapses also occurred when CyA blood levels were reduced to below 100–130 ng/ml.

2.2.2c. Effects of CyA on Renal Function.   S-creatinine or creatinine clearance was unchanged in most patients, as was also the case in many patients with MCNS and CyA-induced remission. S-Creatinine increased in approximately one third of the patients, and a more severe deterioration of renal function was reported in ten patients, five of whom were children. CyA treatment had to be withdrawn in three patients because of severe deterioration of renal function. In two cases renal function deteriorated after CyA withdrawal. Renal biopsy during or after CyA treatment was reported in two studies (Clasen *et al.*, 1988; Niaudet *et al.*, 1988). In one study interstitial fibrosis and tubular atrophy was reported in 11 of 22 of the rebiopsied patients. Other side effects were reported with a frequency comparable to CyA treatment in other studies. Increased blood pressure was seen in

TABLE III. Effect of CyA Treatment in Children and Adults with Steroid-Dependent or Steroid-Resistant NS

Effect of steroids	Patient group	Effect of CyA treatment				Total
		Remission	Part. rem.	Resistant	Unknown	
Dependent	Children	48 (77.4)[a]	4 (6.5)	3 (4.8)	7 (11.3)	62
	Adults	47 (77.0)	5 (8.2)	4 (6.6)	5 (8.2)	61
	Total	95 (77.2)	9 (7.3)	7 (5.7)	12 (9.8)	123
Resistant	Children	5 (11.4)	11 (25.0)	28 (63.6)	0	44
	Adults	18 (16.7)	41 (38.0)	37 (34.3)	12 (11.1)	108
	Total	23 (15.1)	52 (34.2)	65 (42.8)	12 (7.9)	152

[a]Percent in parentheses.

10–20%, and antihypertensive treatment had to be given in 3 of 5 patients in one study (Balcke *et al.*, 1987).

    2.2.2d. Conclusions. The studies reported show that CyA treatment can induce remission in most patients with steroid-dependent and frequent-relapsing MCNS. The effect of CyA in these cases seems to be independent of an effect on GFR, and it seems reasonable to conclude that immunological mechanisms are involved. This is in accordance with data that indicate that MCNS is an immune-mediated disease. It is, however, disappointing that so many patients have early relapses after CyA withdrawal. In this aspect CyA differs from alkylating agents, which can induce a more sustained remission in many cases. On the other hand, the effect of CyA is seen after a few weeks, and in a small group of patients this treatment will induce a sustained remission. In other CyA-dependent patients, it does not seem justified to continue long-term treatment with CyA in MCNS, a disease usually with an excellent long-term prognosis. In patients with FSGS the effect of CyA is disappointing in most cases. No doubt proteinuria can be diminished in many cases, but the patients usually relapse after discontinuation of CyA. In many reports GFR was reduced in parallel with the reduction in urinary protein excretion and one cannot exclude a hemodynamic effect on urinary albumin excretion. Complete and sustained remission, however, has been reported also in FSGS (Meyrier *et al.*, 1988; Meyrier, 1989) and a short-term trial with CyA seems justified in steroid-resistant patients with FSGS.

    In patients with NS syndrome in other forms of GN we have too few data to draw conclusions on the effect of CyA treatment. Controlled trials are needed.

3. EFFECT OF CyA IN POSTTRANSPLANT GLOMERULONEPHRITIS IN RENAL ALLOGRAFTED PATIENTS

    The recurrence rate of GN in transplanted kidneys is reported to be 5–8% on conventional immunosuppression with prednisolone and azathioprine (Cameron, 1982; Mathew, 1988). Certain diseases, such as FSGS, IgA nephropathy, Henoch-Schönlein purpura, and mesangiocapillary GN, show a particularly high recurrence rate. The clinical course of recurrent GN is benign in most cases, with a slow deterioration over many years. The recurrence of GN accounts for less than 2% of all graft failures. As the incidence of graft rejection is reduced by CyA treatment, the recurrence of the original disease will increase in relative importance.

    The studies of recurrent GN in transplanted kidneys is of great interest because of the insight it may give into the nature of glomerular diseases. Based on the experiences from experimental models of GN like active Heyman nephritis, where CyA seems to be most effective in the inductive phase of the immune response, CyA could theoretically protect against recurrent GN.

    The recurrence rate of immune-mediated glomerular diseases after renal transplantation on CyA was studied by Tomlanovich *et al.* (1988). They investigated 433 patients who were treated with CyA and prednisolone after renal transplantation from 1983 to 1987, 85% received a cadaveric transplant. In this material end-stage renal disease occurred secondary to biopsy-proven FSGS in 24 patients, to IgA nephropathy in 19 patients, and mesangio-capillary GN in 12 patients. Six patients (25%) had a recurrence of FSGS on biopsy; in all six, proteinuria recurred within three months and two patients developed graft failure. Three patients demonstrated recurrent IgA nephropathy (15.9%) and two patients recurrent mesangiocapillary GN. The recurrence rate in FSGS is comparable to the incidence reported in the literature on conventional immunosuppressive treatment. The same group (Vincenti *et al.*, 1989) discuss whether the signals mediating the sclerotic process in FSGS could be immune reactants that activate mesangial cells not sensitive to the effects of CyA.

The recurrence rat of IgA nephropathy was somewhat lower than that reported on azathioprine. Data on the recurrence of Henoch-Schönlein purpura in CyA-treated patients have not been reported. Morozumi *et al.* (1987) reported an incidence of posttransplant GN of 16.9% on CyA treatment, higher than usually reported on conventional therapy, but they do not report biopsies from the native kidneys. Other investigators (Voets *et al.*, 1986; Freedman *et al.*, 1989) also indicate that CyA does not prevent the development of recurrent GN. Specifically, a rapid recurrence of FSGS was typical for the CyA-treated patients.

One special group of posttransplant GN is *de novo* MGN, which seems to occur more frequently in patients with other native diseases than GN. *De novo* GN is seen in 1–2% of renal transplanted patients on conventional immunosuppressive therapy (Montagnino *et al.*, 1989). MGN can either recur or develop as a *de novo* GN after successful renal transplantation. CyA did not prevent either form of MGN; three of six patients with biopsy-proven MGN in the native kidneys recurred on CyA, and the frequency of *de novo* nephropathy was 5 of 321 CyA-treated patients (Montagnino *et al.*, 1989).

CyA is known to alter coagulation mechanisms, possibly also prostacyclin production in endothelial cells, and pathological lesions similar to the hemolytic–uremic syndrome (HUS) can be produced experimentally by CyA in rabbits with acute serum sickness (Neild *et al.*, 1984). There has been reported an increased recurrence rate of HUS in CyA-treated patients (Mathew, 1988) and it has been recommended not to use CyA in this condition (Hebert *et al.*, 1986). Mathew (1988) advocated not using CyA if there has been a rapid return of HUS in the first CyA-treated graft.

Conclusions. The protective effect of CyA against recurrent and *de novo* GN in renal allografted patients is disappointing. The incidence seems to be the same as in patients on conventional immunosuppressive treatment. Patients with HUS seem to be at especially high risk for recurrence on CyA treatment. Further studies, however, are required to assess the effects of CyA on posttransplant GN.

REFERENCES

Abramowicz, M., Arneil, G. C., Barnett, H. L., Barron, B. A., Edelmann, C. M., Gordillo, G., Greifer, I., Hallmann, N., Kobayashi, O., and Tiddens, H. A., 1970, Controlled trial of azathioprine in children with nephrotic syndrome, *Lancet* **1**: 959–961.

Arbeitsgemeinschaft für Pediatrisches Nephrologie, 1981, Alternate day prednisone is more effective than intermittent prednisone in frequently relapsing nephrotic syndrome, *Eur. J. Pediatr.* **135**:229–237.

Balcke, P., Derfler, K., Stockenhuber, F., Kopsa, H., and Sunder-Plassmann, G., 1987, Cyclosporintherapie bei Minimal-change-Nephritis, *Wien. Klin. Wschr.* **99**:242–245.

Berthoux, F. C., Guerin, C., Sabatier, J. C., Maret, J., and Genin, C., 1987, Cyclosporin A (CsA) treatment of steroid-resistant and persistent nephrotic syndrome in primary membranous glomerulonephritis, *Nephrol. Dial. Transplant.* **2**:412.

Black, D. A. K., Rose, G., and Brewer, D. B., 1970, Controlled trial of prednisone in adult patients with nephrotic syndrome, *Br. Med. J.* **3**:421–426.

Brandis, M., Burghard, R., Leititis, J., Zimmerhackl, B., Hildebrandt, F., and Helmchen, U., 1988, Cyclosporine A treatment of nephrotic syndrome, *Transplant. Proc.* **20**(Suppl.4):275–279.

Brodehl, J., 1981, Minimal change nephrotic syndrome in childhood, in: *Proceedings from the 8th International Congress of Nephrology* (W. Zurukzoglu, M. Papadimitreo, M. Pyrpasopolous, M. Sion, and C. Zamboulis, eds.), Karger, Basel, pp. 327–335.

Brodehl, J., Hoyer, P. F., Oemar, B. S., Helmchen, U., and Wonigeit, K., 1988, Cyclosporine treatment of nephrotic syndrome in children, *Transplant. Proc.* **20**(Suppl. 4):269–274.

Cameron, J. S., 1982, Glomerulonephritis in renal transplants, *Transplantation* **34**:237–245.

Capodicasa, G., De Santo, N. G., Nuzzi, F., and Giordano, C., 1986, Cyclosporin A in nephrotic syndrome of childhood—a 14 months experience, *Int. J. Pediatr. Nephrol.* **7**:69–72.

Cattran, D. C., 1988, Effect of ciclosporin on active Heymann nephritis, *Nephron* **48**:142–148.

Cattran, D. C., Dossetor, J., Halloran, P. F., Cardella, C., Stiller, C., Keown, P., and Clark, W. F., 1985, Ciclosporin in glomerulonephritis—a pilot study, in: *Ciclosporin in Autoimmune diseases, 1st International Symposium* (R. Schindler, ed.), Springer-Verlag, Berlin, pp. 311–315.

Cattran, D. C., Delmore, T., Roscoe, J., Cole, E., Cardella, C., Charron, R., and Ritchie, S., 1989, A randomized controlled trial of prednisone in patients with idiopathic membranous nephropathy, *N. Engl. J. Med.* 320:210–215.

Chan, M. K., and Cheng, I. K. P., 1987, Cyclosporine A in steroid-sensitive nephrotic syndrome with frequent relapses, *Postgrad. Med. J.* 63;757–759.

Clasen, W., Kindler, J., Mihatsch, M. J., and Sieberth, H. G., 1988, Long-term treatment of minimal change nephrotic syndrome with cyclosporin: A control biopsy study, *Nephrol. Dial. Transplant.* 3:.733–737.

Coggins, C. H., 1981, Minimal change nephrosis in adults, in: *Proceedings from the 8th International Congress of Nephrology* (W. Zurukzoglu, M. Papadimitriou, M. Pyrpasopolous, M. Sion, C. Zamboulis, eds.), Karger, Basel, pp. 336–344.

Coggins, C. H., 1988, Is idiopathic membranous nephropathy a treatable disease? in: *Proceedings of the Xth International Congress of Nephrology* (A. M. Davison, ed.), Balliere Tindall, London, pp. 695–700.

Collaborative Study Group of the Adult Idiopathic Nephrotic Syndrome, 1979, A controlled study of short-term prednisone treatment in adults with membranous nephropathy, *N. Engl. J. Med.* 301:1302–1306.

D'Amico, G., Minetti, L., Ponticelli, C., Fellin, G., Ferrario, F., Di Belgioioso, G. B., Imbasciati, E., Ragni, A., Bertoli, S., Fogazzi, G., and Duca, G., 1986, Prognostic indicators in idiopathic IgA nephropathy, *Q. J. Med.* 59:363–378.

Davison, A. M., Cameron, J. S., Kerr, D. N. S., Ogg, C. S., and Wilkinson, R. W., 1984, The natural history of renal function in untreated idiopathic membranous glomerulonephritic in adults, *Clin. Nephrol.* 22:61-67.

DeSanto, N. G., Capodicasa, G., and Giordano, C., 1987, Treatment of idiopathic membranous nephropathy unresponsive to methylprednisolone and chlorambucil with cyclosporin, *Am. J. Nephrol.* 7:74–76.

Donadio, J. V., Torres, V. E., Velosa, J. A., Wagoner, R. D., Holley, K. E., Okamura, M., Ilstrup, D. M., and Chu, C.-P., 1988, Idiopathic membranous nephropathy: The natural history of untreated patients, *Kidney Int.* 33:708–715.

Erbay, B., Karatan, O., Duman, N., and Ertug, A. E., 1988, The effect of cyclosporine in idiopathic nephrotic syndrome resistant to immunosuppressive therapy, *Transplant. Proc.* 20(Suppl. 4):288–292.

Fleuren, G. J., and Hoedemaeker, Ph. J., 1980, Triple-drug treatment of autologous immune complex glomerulonephritis, *Clin. Exp. Immunol.* 41:218–224.

Freedman, B. I., Graves, J. W., Burkart, J. M., Callahan, M. F., Tell, G. S., Heise, E. R., and Adams, P. L., 1989, The impact of different immunosuppressant regimens on recurrent glomerulonephritis, *Transplant. Proc.* 21:2121–2122.

Fuinao, G., Cameron, J. S., Raftery, M., Hartley, B. H., Williams, D., and Ogg, C. S., 1988, Improved prognosis of renal microscopic polyarteritis in recent years, *Nephrol. Dial. Transplant.* 3:383–391.

Garin, E. H., Orak, J. K., Hiott, K., and Sutherland, S., 1988, Cyclosporine therapy for steroid-resistant nephrotic syndrome, *Am. J. Dis. Child.* 142:985–988.

Glockner, W. M., Sieberth, H. G., Wichmann, H. E., Backes, E., Bambauer, R., Boesken, W. H., Bohle, A., Daul, A., Graben, N., Keller, F., Klehr, H., Kohler, H., Metz, U., Schultz, W., Thoenes, W., and Vlaho, M., 1988, Plasma exchange and immunosuppression in rapidly progressive glomerulonephritis: A controlled, multicenter study, *Clin. Nephrol.* 29:1–8.

Hebert, D., Sibley, R. K., and Mauer, S. M., 1986, Recurrence of hemolytic uremic syndrome in renal transplanted patients, *Kidney Int.* 30:S51–S58.

Honkanen, E., 1986, Survival in idiopathic membranous glomerulonephritis, *Clin. Nephrol.* 25:122–128.

Hoyer, J. R., 1982, Idiopathic nephrotic syndrome with minimal glomerular changes, in: *Contemporary Issues in Nephrology,* Volume 9: *Nephrotic Syndrome* (B. B. Brenner and J. H. Stein, eds.), Churchill Livingston, London, pp. 145–174.

Imbasciati, E., Gusmano, R., Edefonti, A., Zuchelli, P., Pozzi, C., Grassi, C., Della Volpe, M., Perfumo, F., Petrone, P., Picca, M., Claris Appiani, A., Pasquali, S., and Ponticelli, C., 1985, Controlled trial of methylprednisolone pulses and low oral prednisone for the minimal change nephrotic syndrome, *Br. Med. J.* 291:1305–1308.

International Study of Kidney Disease in Children, 1978, Nephrotic syndrome in children: Prediction of histopathology from clinical and laboratory characteristics at the time of diagnosis, *Kidney Int.* 13:159–165.

Koskimes, O., Vilska, J., Rapola, J., and Hallman, P., 1982, Long-term outcome of primary nephrotic syndrome, *Arch. Dis. Child.* 57:544–548.

Kühn, K., Futerova, M., Brunkhorst, R., Cullen, P. C., Koch, K. M., Wonigeit, K., and Helmchen, U., 1987, Cyclosporin A therapy in adult patients with minimal-change nephropathy and focal sclerosis, *Nephrol. Dial. Transplant.* 2:416.

Lagrue, C., Laurent, J., Belgheti, D., and Robeva, R., 1986, Cyclosporine and idiopathic nephrotic syndrome, *Lancet* 2:692–693.

Lai, K. N., Lai, F. M-M., and Vallance-Owen, J., 1988, A short-term controlled trial of cyclosporine A in IgA nephropathy, *Transplant. Proc.* 20(Suppl. 4):297–303.

Lai, K. N., Lai, F.M-M., Chui, S. H., Leung, K. N., and Lam, C. W. K., 1989, Effect of ciclosporin on lymphocyte subpopulations and immunoglobulin production in IgA nephropathy, *Nephron* 52:307–312.

Maher, E. R., Sweny, P., Chappel, M., Varghese, Z., and Moorhead, J. F., 1988, Cyclosporin in the treatment of steroid-responsive and steroid-resistant nephrotic syndrome in adults, *Nephrol. Dial. Transplant.* 3:728–732.

Mathew, T. H., 1988, Recurrence of disease following renal transplantation, *Am. J. Kidney Dis.* 12:85–96.

McCluskey, R. T., 1987, Immunopathogenetic mechanisms in renal disease, *Am. J. Kidney Dis.* 10:172–180.

McCune, W. J., Golbus, J., Zeldes, W., Bohlke, P., Dunne, R., and Fox, D. A., 1988, Clinical and immunological effects of monthly administration of intravenous cyclophosphamide in severe systemic lupus erythematosus, *N. Engl. J. Med.* 318:1423–1431.

Meyrier, A., 1989, Treatment of glomerular disease with cyclosporin A, *Nephrol. Dial. Transplant.* 4:923–931.

Meyrier, A., Condamin, M-C., and Simon, P., 1988, Treatment with cyclosporine of adult idiopathic nephrotic syndrome resistant to corticosteroids and other immunosuppressants, *Transplant. Proc.* 20(Suppl. 4):259–261.

Millet, V. G., Below, I., Oliet, A., and Praga, M., 1987, Cyclosporine (CyA) in minimal change nephrotic syndrome (MCNS), *Kidney Int.* **32**:614.

Montagnino, G., Colturi, C., Banti, G., Aroldi, A., Tarantino, A., and Ponticelli, C., 1989, Membranous nephropathy in cyclosporine treated renal transplanted recipients, *Transplantation* **47**:725–727.

Morozumi, K., Suganuma, T., Yoshida, A., Kobayashi, M., Shinmura, I., Kodera, K., Fyjinami, T., Uchida, K., Yamada, N., Tominaga, Y., Kano, T., and Takagi, H., 1987, Studies of post-transplant glomerulonephritis in patients immunosuppressed with cyclosporine A, *Transplant. Proc.* **19**:3707–3715.

Murphy, B. F., Fairley, K. F., and Kincaid-Smith, P. S., 1988, Idiopathic membranous glomerulonephritis: Long-term follow-up in 139 cases, *Clin. Nephrol.* **30**:175–181.

Nahman, Jr., N. S., and Cosio, F. G., 1990, The effects of ciclosporin in experimental glomerulosclerosis, *Nephron* **56**:414–420.

Neelakantappa, K., Gallo, G. R., and Baldwin, D. S., 1988, Proteinuria in IgA nephropathy, *Kidney Int.*, **33**:716–721.

Neild, G. H., Ivory, K., Hiramatsu, M., and Williams, D. G., 1983, Cyclosporine A inhibits acute serum sickness nephritis in rabbits, *Clin. Exp. Immunol.* **52**:586–594.

Neild, G. H., Ivory, K., and Williams, D. G., 1984, Glomerular thrombosis and cortical infarction in cyclosporine-treated rabbits with acute serum sickness, *Br. J. Exp. Pathol.* **65**:133–144.

Neild, G. H., Ivory, K., and Williams, D. G., 1986, Effect of cyclosporine on proteinuria in chronic serum sickness in rats, *Clin. Nephrol.* **25**(Suppl. 1):S186–188.

Niaudet, P., Tete, M-J., Broyer, M., and Habib, R., 1988, Cyclosporine and childhood idiopathic nephrosis, *Transplant. Proc.* **20**(Suppl. 4):265–268.

Noel, L. H., Zanetti, M., Droz, D., and Barbanel, C., 1979, Long-term prognosis of idiopathic membranous glomerulonephritis, *Am. J. Med.* **66**:82–90.

Pei, Y., Cattran, D., Delmore, T., Katz, A., Lang, A., and Rance, P., 1987, Evidence suggesting under-treatment in adults with idiopathic focal segmental glomerulosclerosis, *Am. J. Med.* **82**:938–944.

Ponticelli, C., Zucchelli, P., Imbasciati, E., Cagnoli, L., Pozzi, C., Passerini, P., Grassi, C., Limido, D., Pasquali, S., Volpini, T., Sasdelli, M., and Locatelli, F., 1984, Controlled trial of methylprednisolone and chlorambucil in idiopathic membranous nephropathy, *N. Engl. J. Med.* **310**:946–950.

Ponticelli, C., Zucchelli, P., Passerini, P., Cagnoli, L., Cesana, B., Pozzi, C., Pasquali, S., Imbasciati, E., Grassi, C., Redaelli, B., Sasdelli, M., and Locatelli, F., 1989, A randomized trial of methylprednisolone and chlorambucil in idiopathic membranous nephropathy, *N. Engl. J. Med.* **320**:8–13.

Ramirez, F., Brouhard, B. H., Travis, L. B., and Elli, E. N., 1982, Idiopathic membranous nephropathy in children, *J. Pediatr.* **101**:677–681.

Rifle, G., Dechelette, E, and the French Cooperative Group, 1990, Treatment of rapidly progressive glomerulonephritis by plasma exchange and methylprednisolone pulses. A prospective randomized trial of cyclophosphamide. Interim analysis, *Prog. Clin. Biol. Res.* **337**:263–267.

Savage, C. O. S., Pusey, C. D., Bowman, C., Rees, A. JH., and Lockwood, C. M., 1986, Antiglomerular basement membrane antibody mediated disease in the British Isles 180–4, *Br. Med. J.* **292**:301–304.

Schena, F. P., and Cameron, J. S., 1988, Treatment of proteinuric idiopathic glomerulonephritides in adults: A retrospective survey, *Am. J. Med.* **85**:315–326.

Schrijver, G., Wetzels, J. F. M., Robben, J. C. M., Assmann, K. J. M., Koene, R. A. P., and Berden, J. H. M., 1988, Antiproteinuric effect of cyclosporine A in passive antiglomerular basement membrane nephritis in the mouse, *Transplant. Proc.* **20**(Suppl. 4):304–308.

Sessoms, S. L., and Kovarsky, J., 1984, Monthly intravenous cyclophosphamide in the treatment of severe lupis erythematosus, *Clin. Exp. Rheumatol.* **2**:247–251.

Sreepada Rao, T. K., and Friedman, E. A., 1987, Prospective trial of cyclosporine (CyA) in refractory nephrotic syndrome in adults: Preliminary findings, *Kidney Int.* **31**:214.

Tejani, A., Butt, K., Trachtman, H., Suthanthiran, M., Rosenthal, C. J., and Khawar, M. R., 1988, Cyclosporine A induced remission of relapsing nephrotic syndrome in children, *Kidney Int.* **33**:729–734.

Tipping, P. G., and Holdsworth, S. R., 1985, Effect of cyclosporine A on antibody-induced experimental glomerulonephritis, *Nephron* **40**:201–205.

Tomlanovich, S., Vincenti, F., Amend, W., Biava, C., Melzer, J., Feduska, N., and Salvatierra, O., 1988, Is cyclosporine effective in preventing recurrence of immune-mediated glomerular disease after renal transplantation? *Transplant. Proc.* **20**(Suppl. 4): 285–288.

Vincenti, F., Biava, C., Tomlanovich, S., Amend, W. J. C., Garovoy, M., Melzer, J., Feduska, N., and Salvatierra, O., 1989, Inability of cyclosporine to completely prevent the recurrence of focal glomerulosclerosis after kidney transplantation, *Transplantation* **47**:595–598.

Voets, A. J., Hoitsma, A. J., and Koene, R. A. P., 1986, Recurrence of nephrotic syndrome during cyclosporine treatment after renal transplantation, *Lancet* **1**:266–267.

West, M. L., Jindal, K. K., Bear, R. A., and Goldstein, M. B., 1987, A controlled trial of cyclophosphamide in patients with membraneous glomerulonephritis, *Kidney Int.* **32**:579–584.

Williams, P. S., and Bone, J. M., 1989, Immunosuppression can arrest progressive renal failure due to idiopathic membranous glomerulonephritis, *Nephrol. Dial. Transplant.* **4**:181–186.

Wilson, C. B., 1987, Immune aspects of renal disease, *J. Am. Med. Assoc.* **258**:2857–2961.

Zietse, R., Wenting, G. J., Kramer, P., Mulder, P., Schalekamp, M. A., and Weimar, W., 1989, Contrasting response to cyclosporin in refractory nephrotic syndrome, *Clin. Nephrol.* **31**:22–25.

Chapter 29

MECHANISMS INVOLVED IN IMMUNOMODULATORY TREATMENT OF RHEUMATOID ARTHRITIS

Lars Klareskog

1. INTRODUCTION

Many inflammatory rheumatic diseases, including rheumatoid arthritis, appear to depend on a dysregulation of the immune system, that is, interference with pathogenetically important immune reactions can be expected to have beneficial or even direct curative effects on the respective diseases. Ideally, an adequate therapy would thus require knowledge of which immune reactions are critical for disease development and access to means whereby these but no other reactions could be down-regulated. Even if we are far from this situation both as to pathogenetic knowledge and access of practically working specific immunomodulatory treatment, our emerging knowledge on the immunopathogenesis of rheumatic joint diseases may be used both to reconsider the mode of action of currently used drugs and to critically approach some of the more experimental treatments that have recently been introduced.

This chapter will thus first touch briefly on some critical aspects of the immuno-pathogenesis of inflammatory joint disease, particularly rheumatoid arthritis (RA); second, deal with existing therapies with an emphasis on their effects on immunoregulation; and third, describe some results from the application of drugs primarily developed to interfere with immune activation.

2. ASPECTS ON THE IMMUNOPATHOGENESIS OF INFLAMMATORY JOINT DISEASE, PARTICULARLY RA

The immunopathogenesis in RA is characterized both by a T-cell activation, primarily within synovial tissue and synovial fluid of affected joints (Klareskog *et al.*, 1981, Burmester

Lars Klareskog • Department of Clinical Immunology, Uppsala University Hospital, S-751 85 Uppsala, Sweden.
Immunopharmacology in Autoimmune Diseases and Transplantation, edited by Hans Erik Rugstad *et al.* Plenum Press, New York, 1992.

et al., 1982), and by immune complex (IC) formation and rheumatoid factor (RF) production, also predominantly seen within the joints (Carson *et al.*, 1987). Cytokines from the activated T cells and effects of the immune complexes may subsequently cause the pronounced activation of macrophages and polymorphonuclear cells that, by their production of proteolytic enzymes (Krane *et al.*, 1982) and a variety of inflammatory mediators such as prostanoids (Klareskog *et al.*, 1985), are responsible for the actual tissue damage. All these processes, including RF and IC formation, are most probably dependent on initial major histocompatibility complex (MHC) class II-dependent T-cell activation, that is, a contact between an antigen-presenting cell (APC), often a macrophage, and a T cell. This process involves processing and binding of one (or several) as yet unknown antigens to the class II antigens of the APC, and a corecognition of the MHC class II antigen complex by the variable T-cell receptor. Additional molecular contacts between the T cell and the APC involving the so-called CD4 molecule also are necessary for T-cell activation, as well as production of cytokines such as interleukin-1 (IL-1) from the APC that can bind to appropriate receptor on juxtaposed T cells (for a review, see Klareskog and Wigzell, 1988). This scenario is rather well characterized concerning the local inflammation in the joints in RA. Less is so far known about the immunopathology of systemic inflammatory lesions; the subcutaneous nodules certainly contain both activated T cells and activated macrophages in their palisading layers (Ziff, 1990), and both skin and heart lesions contain many infiltrating inflammatory cells. Still, the sequence of events is less characterized than in the joints, and we do not know to which extent circulating immune complexes—as sometimes proposed—may play a relatively more important role for systemic lesions such as vasculitis, pleuritis, pericarditis, and so on compared to the situation in the joints.

Of interest in this context is that many of the extra-articular symptoms in RA, such as anemia, fatigue, muscle wasting, and metabolic changes, may be causatively related to the release of defined cytokines resulting from the immune activation described above. In many cases, these symptoms may not go parallel to joint destruction. As will be discussed in other sections of this book, many of the so-called remission-inducing drugs appear to interfere with early events in immune activation, thereby affecting not only local symptoms in joints but also a number of the generalized and often diffuse symptoms. Such considerations may be used as a further argument for early institution of remission-inducing drugs independent of whether signs of joint destruction have occurred or not.

3. POSSIBLE IMMUNOMODULATORY EFFECTS OF CURRENTLY ROUTINELY USED DRUGS IN RA

Although introduced very empirically, and without any primary objective to affect immune functions, there is evidence that most of our current slow-acting antirheumatic drugs (SAARD) may affect such immunologic events that from the description given above are essential for RA development. With the obvious precaution that the actual drugs may have multiple actions, and given the difficulties in extrapolating *in vitro* data to the *in vivo* situation, I will briefly summarize some possible immunological effects of SAARDs.

3.1. Antimalarials

These agents are *in vitro* among the most efficient and commonly used inhibitors of the intracellular processing of protein antigens, that is, in most cases needed before a peptide of this antigen can be appropriately presented to the T cell (Lee *et al.*, 1982; Nowell and

Quaranta, 1985). This inhibitory effect appears due to the fact that chloroquine compounds enter into the intracellular compartments where antigen processing normally takes place and here give rise to a local increase in pH that inactivates certain proteolytic enzymes with an acid pH working optimum (Homewood et al., 1972). This in vitro effect can also be corroborated in vivo in experimental animals, for example, in experimental arthritis where chloroquine phosphate both inhibits disease development and the development of strictly T-cell-dependent reactions, such as the delayed-type hypersensitivity reaction (Phadke et al., 1982). We conclude that antimalarials, at least under certain circumstances, can affect certain very early events in T-cell activation that involve antigen processing. That this inhibition of antigen processing must be all but complete is indicated by the fact that many other immune reactions are only marginally affected by antimalarial treatment (Papaio-annou et al., 1986; Maksymowych and Russell, 1987), but it is feasible that the minor effects achieved may nevertheless switch the balance in the immunologic dysregulation in RA quite considerably. Such generalized but weak effects on antigen presentation and T-cell activation would also be compatible with the presumed positive effects of antimalarials in other chronic inflammatory diseases, like SLE (see Maksymowych and Russell, 1987).

3.2. Gold Compounds

When administered to APC and T lymphocytes in vitro, colloidal gold can inhibit antigen processing and antigen presentation a swell as a number of other macrophage/monocyte functions (Lipsky and Ziff, 1977; Slameron and Lipsky, 1983). The gold compounds appear in these cases to work as inhibitors of certain enzymes, such as lysosomal hydrolases (Nechay, 1980), but they also exert certain other nonspecific anti-inflammatory actions such as inhibition of prostaglandin synthesis (Hassan et al., 1986). They also inhibit many monocyte functions such as phagocytosis and chemotaxis (Scheinberg et al., 1982). To which extent the effects of gold compounds affect synovial reactions more than immune reactions elsewhere is not known. From a theoretical standpoint, it is feasible, however, that gold particles may preferentially be picked up by the extremely activated macrophages of the joint (Klareskog et al., 1985), while also having some effect on RF and IC formation (Highton et al., 1980); such biases should be required to explain why the effects of gold compounds are mainly restricted to RA.

3.3. D-Penicillamine

This drug, like gold and chloroquine, can inhibit T-cell activation in vitro, but does, in contrast to the other two drugs, act directly on the T cell rather than on the antigen-presenting cell (Lipsky, 1984). How this effect on T-cell activation is achieved is not understood in detail, but it is possible that D-penicillamine in the presence of copper salts may damage the T cell by enhancing local hydrogen peroxide formation. In the case of penicillamine, many other observed in vitro functions have been considered for their possible relevance in vivo, such as the prevention of collagen cross-linking (Siegel, 1977) and a certain inhibition of DNA and protein synthesis (Chawalinska-Sodowska and Baum, 1976).

In neither of these three drugs, with theoretical similarities as to site of immunological action, have any convincing studies been carried out in vivo in RA patients that can definitely prove or disprove the above-mentioned hypothetical mechanisms of action. A certain decrease in number of peripheral $CD4^+$ T cells after treatment with antimalarials or D-penicillamine (Karlsson-Parra et al., 1986) may be taken as a circumstantial support for these ideas as is also the case for the observations of a decrease in numbers of MHC class II expressing cells within the synovial tissues of patients on gold therapy (Walters et al., 1987).

3.4. Sulfasalazine

This drug, initially introduced for use in RA by Nanna Svartz (Svartz, 1948), but for a long time used internationally mainly in ulcerative colitis, has during the last decade been reintroduced as a SAARD in RA as well as in other inflammatory joint diseases (Bird et al., 1980; Pinals, 1988). Its mechanisms of action, however, still precludes even the formation of plausible hypotheses. Thus, the unmetabolized drug, but not the cleavage products 5-ASA or sulfapyridine, has been shown to inhibit T-cell activation in vitro (Comer and Jasin, 1986; Klareskog et al., 1987), but only at those rather high concentrations that can be found in the intestine; no effects were seen in vitro with concentrations systemically present in sulfasalazine-treated patients. This observation may thus be taken as a support for the idea that sulfasalazine carries out much of its effect within the intestine. Such a notion is also supported by recent observations that mucosal IgA-responses appear to be rapidly affected by an institution of sulfasalazine treatment in RA patients (Feltelius et al., 1991).

The effects on the joint symptoms in RA patients would by this reasoning be due to hitherto not understood connections between events in the gut and development of inflammatory joint disease. A partially different explanation, still compatible with a main action within the intestine, would reside in the capacity of sulfasalazine to inhibit folate metabolism (Selhub et al., 1978), thereby making sulfasalazine similar to methotrexate, but exhibiting most of its actions locally in the gut.

4. CORTICOSTEROIDS AND NONSTEROIDAL ANTI-INFLAMMATORY DRUGS

4.1. Corticosteroids

Corticosteroids are well known to inhibit a great number of immunologic and inflammatory functions, among them macrophage functions that both govern the unspecific effector functions and immune activation, for example, production of cytokines like IL-1, which are necessary for T-cell activation (Gerrard et al., 1984; Bettens et al., 1984). Corticosteroids also affect multiple actions on cell migration. These multiple actions of corticosteroids may explain both why they are efficient in short-term therapy aimed at dampening immediate symptoms and in synergizing with other drugs in affecting potentially pathogenic immune reactions (Weiss, 1989). It is also worth mentioning that local administration of slow-release preparations of corticosteroids into inflamed joints may represent the most selective type of treatment currently available for inflammatory joint disease. More specific details on mechanisms of action of corticosteroids are provided in a separate chapter (see Chapter 8, this volume).

4.2. Nonsteroidal Anti-inflammatory Drugs

Although generally considered to be anti-inflammatory by entirely nonspecific mechanisms, that is, by inhibiting cyclo-oxygenase (for a review, see Abramson and Weissman, 1989), it appears that an inhibition of PGE_2 production within inflammatory lesions may also have effects on the immune system. Thus, enough high amounts of PGE_2 are produced by macrophages within the synovial tissue to allow an appreciable nonspecific down-regulation of local T-cell activation (Klareskog et al., 1985). As the down-regulation of T-cell responsiveness that is mediated by compounds like PGE_2 synthesized from pronouncedly activated macrophages may constitute part of an internal negative feedback loop in chronic inflammation, it is thus feasible that inhibition of PGE_2 synthesis may have dual effects on the local inflammation. To which extent this potential unwanted effect of nonsteroidal anti-inflammatory drugs is indeed effective in vivo or is overcome by other beneficial effects is, however, still dubious and under some debate (see Cush et al., 1990).

5. CYTOTOXIC DRUGS

The role of cytotoxic drugs in the treatment of RA and other inflammatory joint diseases is at present changing rapidly, particularly when it comes to methotrexate, which is increasingly introduced early in the treatment of disease (for a review, see Segal et al., 1990). Cyclophosphamide is still a drug of choice in certain serious cases of systemic manifestations of inflammatory joint disease, whereas the use of azathioprine is both less restricted and less efficient than cyclophosphamide (see Yunus, 1988).

5.1. Cyclophosphamide

The basic mechanisms of action of cyclophosphamide are described elsewhere in this volume (see Chapter 11). In brief, cyclophosphamide is an alkylating agent that interferes with DNA synthesis, thereby inhibiting proliferation of any type of cell in the treated patient. From this we conclude that cyclophosphamide works most efficiently in the initiation of an immune response, that is, while the lymphocytes are dividing. In later phases of an immune activation, where, for example, memory cells are repeatedly activated without necessarily proliferating, the effects of cyclophosphamide may be less pronounced. The frequent clinical use of a combination of cyclophosphamide and high-dose corticosteroids is thus warranted also from a theoretical point of view, since corticosteroids can also be supposed to down-regulate those ongoing immune reactions which may not be optimally controlled by cyclophosphamide.

5.2. Methotrexate

Being a folic acid antagonist, this drug inhibits DNA synthesis and cellular proliferation in a way that suppresses many immune functions, but—as discussed for cyclophosphamide— may leave certain reactions unaffected. As was the case for the classical SAARDs, the popularity of methotrexate in the clinic has grown mainly from tradition, that is, the knowledge of the exact mechanisms of action as well as the optimal dosage schemes are still incomplete (for a guidance, see Segal, 1990). A more extensive description of the mechanism of action of methotrexate is also given in Chapter 10, this volume.

5.3. Concluding Comment on Conventional Treatment

Apart from the treatment modalities discussed here, there are a number of treatments that have been in use for many years, being used on a small scale, but obviously deserving a place in the therapeutic arsenal. Included here is plasmapheresis, eventually combined with immunoglobulin or plasma administration. Efforts in dietary restrictions or complementations that may be beneficial in certain cases are also included (see, for example, Kremer et al., 1990). One additional conclusion from the discussion about the mechanisms of action of these drugs as they pertain to immunomodulation is that a scientific basis may now be built for the introduction of combinatorial therapies; that is, preferentially combining those drugs that appear to act on different events of an immune activation or an inflammatory response (for a more extensive discussion on combination therapy, see Paulus, 1990).

6. EXPERIMENTAL IMMUNOMODULATORY TREATMENTS

As mentioned initially, current knowledge on immunopathogenic events in RA should permit the introduction of more selective types of treatment than hitherto discussed. Whereas a large number of such possibilities have been tested in experimental animal systems for arthritis (for a review, see Klareskog, 1989), relatively few have hitherto reached practical clinical testing, the main one being cyclosporine A.

Concerning the principal questions, two main pathways exist as to immunomanipulation; one can be called immunologic blockade, that is, certain events are more or less specifically blocked by exogenously administered molecules. This form of therapy obviously demands continuous supply of the "drug" in question. The second possibility makes use of the fact that the immune system contains a memory, that is, long-lasting changes in behavior can be induced—typically through vaccination. In many cases, blocking therapy will also induce certain permanent changes, for example, in treatment against allograft rejection where treatment can be gradually diminished due to an increased "acceptance" of the transplanted organ by the host.

6.1. Cyclosporine A

Cyclosporine A (CyA) acts primarily on the immune system and so far has been used in RA within the framework of a few fairly large and well-controlled studies. The results show a positive effect both on inflammatory parameters and on symptoms such as arthritic index or morning stiffness in a large fraction of investigated patients (Förre et al., 1987; Weinblatt et al., 1987; Tugwell et al., 1990). Still, drastic "curativelike" effects were rare, and in the improved patients the CyA effects were comparable with those of conventional SAARDs and as with other SAARDs, some patients were not at all affected by the CyA therapy. Although the side effects from long-term therapy are still not fully evaluated with those relatively low doses of CyA now used (see also Berg et al., 1989), the conclusion from the first series of controlled CyA studies in RA is that at least for the next few years CyA should be reserved for further limited and well controlled studies, where side effects are carefully monitored.

Concerning mechanism of action, CyA appears to act mainly by an inhibition of IL-2 synthesis (Elliott et al., 1984; see also Chapter 12, this volume). Whereas this means that most IL-2-dependent T-cell activation and proliferation are inhibited, there is evidence both that residual IL-2 may contribute to some immune activation and that mechanisms independent of IL-2 may be activated during CyA therapy, possibly in a compensatory way. As to the situation in RA, very little IL-2 synthesis has actually been found in synovial biopsies of RA patients (Arend and Dayer, 1990), implicating mechanisms that are partially independent of IL-2 may be more important in RA than, for example, in allograft transplantation where large amounts of IL-2 are produced within the graft (Dallman *et al.*, 1991). This might obviously provide part of the explanation for the relative inefficacy of CyA in RA compared to transplantation. Another observation that may be of relevance concerning the relatively poor reproducibility of CyA effects between different RA patients is that CyA was found to be very efficient in preventing experimental arthritis when given from the administration of autoantigen (collagen type II) onward. In contrast, CyA was inefficient or even enhanced disease development when given only from the time of onset of disease and not before (Kaibara *et al.*, 1983). No clear-cut explanation has been provided concerning this observation, but it is possible that CyA may affect both disease-inducing and disease-controlling lymphocytes, and that the net effects therefore depend on at which phase of disease CyA therapy is instituted. If transferable to the human situation, this might both explain the varying efficacy of CyA in RA and suggest that better explain the varying efficacy of CyA in RA and suggest that better efficacy can be reached after an adequate monitoring of the disease and better understanding of when therapy should best be introduced.

6.2. Monoclonal Antibody Treatment

In a few as yet open studies, murine monoclonal anti-CD4 antibodies have been used in the treatment of RA (Herzog *et al.*, 1989; Walker *et al.*, 1989). Good results on symptoms, that is, arthritic index and morning stiffness, but less pronounced results on acute-phase reactants and sedimentation rates were reported. These studies should thus serve mainly as a reminder that we are now approaching the stage where similar treatments with monoclonal antibodies can be used in humans that have long proven to be efficient in experimental animal systems (Ranges *et al.*, 1985). The most interesting aspect of the current anti-CD4 antibody treatment is that such treatment in experimental animals under certain circumstances could include a long-lasting unresponsiveness against the immunogen(s) toward immune activation that was elicited at the time of anti-CD4 administration. This specific unresponsiveness (sometimes called immunologic anergy) is believed to be induced when a T cell recognizes a particular antigen but at the same time is unable to respond adequately due to a block of the CD4 coreceptor (for a discussion, see Benjamin and Waldmann, 1986). If transferable to the human situation, application of this principle would obviously open ways to specific immunotherapy even without knowing the specificity of the disease-inducing antigen(s).

7. CONCLUDING REMARK

This chapter has briefly discussed how increasing knowledge on the immunopathogenesis of RA might be used both in optimizing existing therapeutic principles and introducing new ones. What deserves particular emphasis in this context is the need to develop methods by which the local immunologic events can be closely followed during the disease course. As most dramatically illustrated by the opposite effects of cyclosporin A given at different phases of experimental arthritis (Berg *et al.*, 1989), efficient interferences with selected parts of the immune system may give rise to effects that are impossible to foresee from *in vitro* experiments or even from *in vivo* animal experience. Thus, it is feasible that development of methodologies for adequate monitoring of local immunologic events will grow in importance in parallel with the increasing possibilities of achieving selective immunomodulation. In this respect, rheumatic joint disease may well represent a model case for the evaluation of working principles for new immunomodulatory treatments since the inflamed synovium is more accessible to analysis than are target tissues in most other chronic inflammatory diseases.

REFERENCES

Abramson, S. B., and Weissman, G., 1989, The mechanisms of nonsteroidal antiinflammatory drugs, Arthritis Rheum. 32:1.

Arend, W., and Dayer, J. M., 1990, Cytokines and cytokine inhibitors or antagonists in rheumatoid arthritis, Arthritis Rheum. 33:305.

Benjamin, R. J., and Waldmann, H., 1986, Induction of tolerance by monoclonal antibody therapy, Nature 320:449.

Berg, K. J., Förre, Ö., Djöseland, O., Mikkelsen, M., Narverud, J., and Rugstad, H. E., 1989, Renal side effects of high and low cyclosporin A doses in patients with rheumatoid arthritis, Clin. Nephrol. 31:232.

Bettens, F., Kristensen, F., Walker, C., et al., 1984, Lymphokine regulation of activated lymphocytes. II Glucocorticoid anti-Tac induced inhibition of human T lymphocyte proliferation, J. Immunol. 132:261.

Bird, H. A., Dixon, J. S., Pickup, M. E., et al., 1980, A biochemical assessment of sulphasalazine in rheumatoid arthritis, J. Rheumatol. 9:36.

Burmester, G. R., Yu, D. T. Y., Irani, A. M., Kunkel, H. K., and Winchester, R. J., 1982, Ia+ T cells in synovial fluid and synovial tissue of patients with rheumatoid arthritis, Arthritis Rheum. 24:1370.

Carson, D. A., Chen, P. P., Fox, R. I., Kipps, T. J., Jirik, F., Goldfie, R. D., Silverman, G., Radoux, V., and Fong, S., 1987, Rheumatoid factors and immune networks, Annu. Rev. Immunol. 5:85.

Chawalinska-Sodowska, H., and Baum, J., 1976, The effects of D-penicillamin on polymorphonuclear leucocyte reactions, J. Clin. Invest. 58:871.

Comer, S. S., and Jasin, H. E., 1986, In vitro immunomodulatory effects of sulfasalazine and its metabolites, Arthritis Rheum. 29:79.

Cush, J. J., Jasin, H. E., Johnson, R., and Lipsky, P. E., 1990, Relationship between clinical efficacy and laboratory correlates of inflammatory and immunologic activity in rheumatoid arthritis patients treated with nonsteroidal anti-inflammatory drugs, Arthritis Rheum. 33:623.

Dallman, M. J., Montgomery, R. A., Larsen, C. P., Wanders, A., and Wells, A. F., 1991, Cytokine gene expression: Analysis using Northern blotting, polymerase chain reaction and in situ hybridization, Immunol. Rev. 119:5.

Elliott, J. F., Lin, Y., Mizel, S. B., Bleackley, R. C., Harnish, D. G., and Petkau, V., 1984, Induction of interleukin 2 mRNA inhibited by cyclosporin A, Science 226:1439.

Feltelius, N., Gudmundsson, S., Wennersten, L., Sjöberg, O., Hällgren, R., and Klareskog, L., 1991, Enumeration of IgA-producing cells by the ELISPOT technique in evaluation of sulphasalazine effects in inflammatory arthritides, Ann. Rheum. Dis. 50:369.

Förre, Ö., Bjerkhoel, F., Salvesen, C., Berg, K., Rugstad, H., Saelid, G., Mellbye, O., and Kass, E., 1987, An open, controlled, randomized comparison of cyclosporin and azathioprine in the treatment of rheumatoid arthritis: A preliminary report, Arthritis Rheum. 30:88.

Gerrard, T. L., Cupps, T. R., Jurgensen, C. H., et al., 1984, Hydrocortisone mediated inhibition of monocyte antigen presentation: Dissociation of inhibitory effects and expression of DR antigens, Cell. Immunol. 84:311.

Hassan, J., Hanley, J., Gresnihan, B., Feighery, C., and Whelan, C. A., 1986, The immunological consequences of gold therapy: A prospective study in patients with rheumatoid arthritis, Clin. Exp. Immunol. 63:614.

Herzog, C., Walker, C., Muller, W., Rieber, P., Reiter, C., Reithmuller, G., Wassmer, P., Stockinger, H., Madic, O., and Pichler, W. J., 1989, Anti-CD4 antibody treatment of patients with rheumatoid arthritis I. Effect on clinical course and circulating T cells, J. Autoimmun. 2:627.

Highton, J., Panayi, G. S., and Griffin, J., 1980, Cellular aspects of anti-rheumatic agents. Improvement in peripheral blood lymphocyte responses to concavalin A and pokeweed mitogen during gold treatment of rheumatoid arthritis, Agents Actions 7:508.

Homewood, C. A., Warhurst, D. C., Peters, W., et al., 1972, Lysosomes, pH and the antimalarial action of chloroquine, Nature 235:50.

Kaibara, N., Hotokebuchi, T., Tagahishi, K., and Katsuki, I., 1983, Paradoxical effects of cyclosporin A on collagen arthritis in rats, J. Exp. Med. 158:2007.

Karlsson-Parra, A., Svenson, K., Hällgren, R., Klareskog, L., and Forsum, U., 1986, Peripheral blood T-lymphocyte subsets in active rheumatoid arthritis patients—effects of different therapies on previously untreated patients, J. Rheumatol. 13:263.

Klareskog, L., 1989, What can we learn about rheumatoid arthritis from animal models? Springer Sem. Immunopathol. 11:315.

Klareskog, L., and Wigzell, H., 1988, Immune reactions in the rheumatoid synovial tissue, in: Immunopathogenic Mechanisms of Arthritis (J. Goodacre and D. W. Carson, eds.), MTP Press, London, pp. 143–156.

Klareskog, L., Forsum, U., Scheynius, A., Kabelitz, D., and Wigren, A., 1981, Appearance of anti-HLA-DR reactive cells in normal and rheumatoid synovial tissue, Scand. J. Immunol. 14:183.

Klareskog, L., Holmdahl, R., Rubin, K., Victorin, Å., and Lindgren, J. Å., 1985, Different populations of rheumatoid adherent cells mediate activation vs. suppression of T lymphocyte proliferation, Arthritis Rheum. 28:863.

Klareskog, L., Holmdahl, R., Goldschmidt, T., and Björk, J., 1987, Immunoregulation in arthritis. A review on synovial immune reactions in RA and in some experimental animal models for arthritis, Scand. J. Rheumatol. 64:7.

Krane, S. M., Dayer, J. M., and Goldring, S. R., 1982, Considerations of possible cellular events in the destructive synovial lesion of rheumatoid arthritis, Adv. Inflam. Res. 3:1.

Kremer, J. M., Lawrence, D. A., Jubiz, W., DiGiacomo, R., Rynes, R., Bartholomew, L. E., and Sherman, M., 1990, Dietary fish oil and olive oil supplementation in patients with rheumatoid arthritis, Arthritis Rheum. 33:810.

Lee, K. C., Wong, M., and Spitzer, D., 1982, Chloroquine as a probe for antigen processing by accessory cells, *Transplantation* **34:**150.

Lipsky, P. E., 1984, Immunosuppression by D-penicillamin *in vitro*. Inhibition of human T lymphocyte proliferation by copper or ceruloplasmin-dependent generation of hydrogen peroxide and protection of monocytes, *J. Clin. Invest.* **73:**53.

Lipsky, P. E., and Ziff, M., 1977, Inhibition of antigen- and mitogen-induced human lymphocyte proliferation by gold compounds, *J. Clin. Invest.* **59:**455.

Maksymowych, W., and Russell, A. S., 1987, Antimalarials in rheumatology: Efficacy and safety, *Sem. Arthritis Rheum.* **16:**206.

Nechay, B. R., 1980, Inhibition of adenosine triphosphatases by gold, *Arthritis Rheum.* **23:**460.

Nowell, J., and Quaranta, J., 1985, Chloroquine effects biosynthesis of Ia molecules by inhibiting dissociation of invariant chain from $\alpha\beta$ dimers in B cells, *J. Exp. Med.* **162:**1371.

Papaioannou, M., Fishbein, D. B., Dresen, D. W., Schwartz, I. K., Campbeu, G. H., Sumner, J. W., Patchen, L. C., and Brown, W. J., 1986, Antibody response to preexposure to human diploid-cell rabies vaccine given concurrently with chloroquine, *N. Engl. J. Med.* **314:**280.

Paulus, H. E., 1990, The use of combinations of disease-modifying antirheumatic agents in rheumatoid arthritis, *Arthritis Rheum.* **33:**113.

Phadke, K., Carroll, J., and Nanda, S., 1982, Effects of various anti-inflammatory drugs on type II collagen-induced arthritis in rats, *Clin. Exp. Immunol.* **47:**579.

Pinals, R. S., 1988, Sulfasalazine in the rheumatic disease, *Sem. Arthritis Rheum.* **17:**246.

Ranges, G., Sririam, S., and Cooper, S. M., 1985, Prevention of type II collagen-induced arthritis by *in vivo* treatment with anti-L3T4, *J. Exp. Med.* **162:**1105.

Scheinberg, M. A., Santos, L. M. B., and Finkelstein, A. E., 1982, The effect of auranofin and sodium aurothiomalate on peripheral blood monocytes, *J. Rheumatol.* **9:**366.

Segal, R., Yaron, M., and Tartakovsky, B., 1990, Methotrexate: Mechanisms of action in rheumatoid arthritis, *Sem. Arthritis Rheum.* **20:**190.

Selhub, J., Dhra, G. J., and Rosenberg, I. H., 1978, Inhibition of folate enzymes by sulphasalazine, *J. Clin. Invest.* **61:**221.

Siegel, R. C., 1977, Collagen cross-linking. Effect of D-penicillamin on cross-linking *in vitro*, *J. Biol. Chem.* **252:**254.

Slameron, G., and Lipsky, P. E., 1983, Modulation of human immune responsiveness *in vitro* by auranofin, *J. Rheumatol.* **9:**30.

Svartz, N., 1948, The treatment of rheumatic polyarthritis with acid azo compounds, *Rheumatism* **4:**56.

Tugwell, P., Bombardier, C., Gent, M., Bennett, K. J., Bensen, W. G., Carette, S., Chalmers, A., Esdaile, J. M., Klinkhoff, A. V., Kraag, G. R., Ludwin, D., and Roberts, R. S., 1990, Low-dose cyclosporin versus placebo in patients with rheumatoid arthritis, *Lancet* **335:**1051.

Walker, C., Herzog, C., Riber, P., Riethmuller, G., Muller, W., and Pichler, W. J., 1989, Anti CD4 antibody treatment of patients with rheumatoid arthritis II. Effect of *in vivo* treatment on *in vitro* proliferative response of CD4 positive cells, *J. Autoimmun.* **2:**643.

Walters, M. T., Smith, J. L., Moore, K., Evans, P. R., and Cawley, M. I. D., 1987, An investigation of the action of disease modifying antirheumatic drugs on the rheumatoid synovial membrane: Reduction in T lymphocyte subpopulations and HLA-DP and DQ antigen expression after gold or penicillamine therapy, *Ann. Rheum. Dis.* **46:**7.

Weinblatt, M. E., Coblyn, J. S., and Fraser, P. A., 1987, Cyclosporin A treatment of refractory rheumatoid arthritis, *Arthritis Rheum.* **30:**11.

Weiss, M., 1989, Corticosteroids in rheumatoid arthritis, *Sem. Arthritis Rheum.* **19:**9.

Yunus, M., 1988, Investigational therapy in rheumatoid arthritis. A critical review, *Sem. Arthritis Rheum.* **17:**163.

Ziff, M., 1990, The rheumatoid nodule, *Arthritis Rheum.* **33:**761.

Part IV

IMMUNOTHERAPY IN ORGAN AND BONE MARROW TRANSPLANTATION

Chapter 30

IMMUNOTHERAPY IN ORGAN TRANSPLANTATION

Luis Mieles, Robert L. Kormos, Leonard Makowka, and *Thomas E. Starzl*

1. INTRODUCTION

Surgical techniques for organ transplantation were developed as early as the first half of the century by surgeons such as Carrel, Jaboulay, Voronoy, and several other pioneers in the field (Cannon, 1956; Groth, 1972; Edwards, 1979). However, all of these early attempts at homografting and heterografting failed, and transplantation as a practical endeavor had to await developments during the second half of the century, mainly in the areas of immunosuppression and organ preservation.

Identifying the process of rejection as a cause of organ failure was the first step toward the development of immunosuppression. Sir Peter Medawar in his classic studies demonstrated the existence of an immunological phenomenon that he called rejection as the biological barrier to the successful engraftment of foreign tissue (Medawar, 1944). The realization that control or abrogation of the response of the immune system could enhance acceptance of a transplanted organ led to the first trials of immunosuppression, which consisted of total body irradiation, 6-mercaptopurine, adrenal cortical steroids, and azathioprine (Dempster *et al.*, 1950; Billingham *et al.*, 1950; Lindley *et al.*, 1955; Hamburger *et al.*, 1959; Merril *et al.*, 1960; Murray *et al.*, 1960; Schwartz and Dameshek, 1959; Calne, 1960; Starzl *et al.*, 1963; Hume *et al.*, 1963).

Complete control of rejection with a single agent was rarely successful without lethal side effects in both animals and humans. Relatively successful immunosuppression was achieved when combined therapy with azathioprine and prednisone was demonstrated to have an additive and possibly synergistic effect with decreased toxicity (Starzl *et al.*, 1963). The group of agents to be used in immunosuppressive protocols grew with the subsequent addition of antilymphocyte globulin (ALG) (Woodruf and Anderson, 1963; Starzl *et al.*,

Luis Mieles, Robert L. Kormos, Leonard Makowka, and *Thomas E. Starzl* • Department of Surgery, University Health Center of Pittsburgh, University of Pittsburgh, and the Veterans Administration Medical Center, Pittsburgh, Pennsylvania 15213. *Present address* of L. Makowka: Department of Surgery, Cedars Sinai Medical Center, Los Angeles, California 99048.

Immunopharmacology in Autoimmune Diseases and Transplantation, edited by Hans Erik Rugstad *et al.* Plenum Press, New York, 1992.

1967) and was revolutionized with the more recent introduction of cyclosporine (Calne *et al.*, 1978, 1979; Starzl *et al.*, 1980, 1981) and the murine monoclonal antibody OKT3 (Kung *et al.*, 1979; Cosimi *et al.*, 1981; Ortho Multi-Center Transplant Study Group, 1985). Promising new pharmacological agents such as FK-506 and 15-deoxyspergualin are now being tested for their immunosuppressive properties (Dickneite *et al.*, 1986; Swada *et al.*, 1987; Zeevi *et al.*, 1987; Todo *et al.*, 1988a,b). In fact, clinical trials evaluating FK-506 in organ transplantation have recently been initiated at the University of Pittsburgh with very encouraging results (Starzl *et al.*, 1989b). Finally, more specific and potent monoclonal antibodies such as antiinterleukin receptors are now being developed (Cantarovich *et al.*, 1989; Kirkman *et al.*, 1989).

2. IMMUNOSUPPRESSION IN LIVER TRANSPLANTATION

Before the introduction of cyclosporine in 1981, azathioprine and prednisone were the standard form of immunosuppression (first 170 liver transplants). With this regimen the one-year survival was only 33%. After the introduction of cyclosporine in 1981, the one-year survival increased significantly to 74% (Fig. 30.1) (Iwatsuki *et al.*, 1988). Thereafter and up until June 1989, the standard immunosuppressive regimens at our institution consisted of cyclosporine and prednisone therapy, with additional azathioprine in approximately one third of the patients. In March 1989, human trials with FK-506 were started at the University of Pittsburgh. Since initial results with the drug were very encouraging, by the end of the summer of 1989, the mainstay immunosuppression in about 80% of our liver transplant recipients consisted of FK-506 and small amounts of steroids. Human trials with FK-506 in cadaveric kidney transplant recipients are now being conducted.

With the exception of FK-506, for which an entire section will be devoted at the end of the chapter, a brief discussion of the way we use each one of the pharmacological agents in our organ transplant unit will follow.

2.1. Cyclosporine

Initially the liver transplant recipient is started on 6 mg/kg body weight, divided in two doses and administered intravenously. The dosage is adjusted in order to maintain TDX

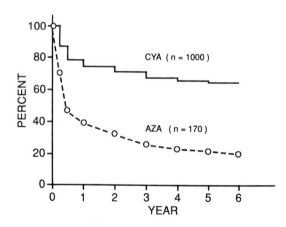

FIGURE 30.1. Overall actuarial survival rates of 1000 patients treated with cyclosporine–steroid therapy in comparison with overall actuarial survival rates of 170 patients treated with azathioprine–steroid therapy. Reprinted from Iwatsuki *et al.* (1988).

(12-hr trough) whole blood levels of greater than 1000 and less than 1900 ng/ml. As soon as the patient is able to tolerate oral intake, cyclosporine is started orally at 17.5 mg/kg body weight given in two divided doses. Intravenous cyclosporine is then tapered and eventually stopped once adequate intestinal absorption of the drug is assured. During the ensuing weeks, there is a significant increase in the intestinal absorption of the drug, which usually dictates a downward adjustment of the dosage. The reasons accounting for the increased absorption of cyclosporine are a progressive improvement in the oral intake and GI tract function, and clamping of the T tube around the tenth postoperative day. Further decrease in cyclosporine dosage is also required in cases in which impaired metabolism of the drug results in high blood levels. This usually happens in patients with severe ischemic injury of the allograft or in patients with good functioning allografts who are also receiving agents that inhibit the cytochrome P-450 enzymatic system (i.e., erythromycin, diltiazem, etc.).

Upward adjustment of the cyclosporine dose is required in patients with impaired intestinal absorption of the drug due to diarrhea, biliary fistulae, intestinal fistulae, or intestinal malabsorption. Patients metabolizing the drug in an accelerated fashion due to agents that enhance the cytochrome P-450 enzymatic system (phenobarbital, phenytoin) also require a higher cyclosporine dose. Table I discloses some of the most frequent medications used in clinical transplantation, with a well-documented interaction with cyclosporine. A more detailed list of drug interactions are found in other sections of the book and in literature reviews (Lake, 1988).

Patients are usually discharged three to five weeks postoperatively on a dose of cyclosporine that is required to maintain a blood level of approximately 1000 ng/ml TDX. Although adjusting the cyclosporine dose to maintain a particular blood level is the most frequent practice, this is by no means the only way of following the cyclosporine dose. As a matter of fact, very often patients will become toxic with relatively low cyclosporine levels or will have a rejection episode with what seemed to be an adequate blood level. Clinical evidence of toxicity such as shakiness, hirsutism, gum hypertrophy, postnasal drip, seizures, hypertension, hyperkalemia, and increasing azotemia almost always call for either a dose reduction or an increased interval between doses. If the levels drop too low and rejection becomes a threat, then azathioprine can be introduced as a third drug. Another alternative is FK-506 "rescue" therapy (Fung et al., 1990).

TABLE I.   Agents of Frequent Use in Clinical Transplantation
That Interact with Cyclosporine

Action	Agents
Increased cyclosporine Metabolism, decreased Blood level	Carbamazepine (Lele et al., 1985)
	Phenobarbital (Carstensen et al., 1986)
	Phenytoin (Keown et al., 1984)
	Isoniazid (Coward et al., 1985)
	Rifampin (Coward et al., 1985; Cassidy et al., 1985)
Impaired cyclosporine Metabolism, increased Blood level Enhanced nephrotoxicity	Erythromycin (Ptachcinski et al., 1985)
	Ketoconazole (Dieperink and Moller, 1982)
	Diltiazem (Grino et al., 1986; Kohlhaw et al., 1988)
	Amphotericin B (Kennedy et al., 1983)
	Sulfamethoxazole trimethoprim (Thompson et al., 1983)
	Furosemide (Whiting et al., 1984)
	Amymoglycosides (Hows et al., 1983)
	Vancomycin (Hows et al., 1983)

On the other hand, if patients are tolerating relatively high levels well with no clinical evidence of toxicity, then there should not be an automatic move to lower the cyclosporine dose. Thus it is clear that even though the majority of patients will require less cyclosporine as time passes, no exact dosage or drug level can be recommended. Good clinical judgment must replace rigid schedules in order to achieve adequate levels of immunosuppression and to avoid dangerous over immunosuppression and the toxic side effects of cyclosporine. Nothing can replace the clinical experience that one develops with repeated use of the drug. Pediatric patients are started on 6 mg/kg of body weight divided in three doses. When oral intake is reestablished, patients are given 20 mg/kg of body weight divided in two doses. Because of increased metabolism of the drug, pediatric patients when compared to adults require more cyclosporine per kilogram of body weight and a shorter administration interval in order to maintain adequate blood levels of the drug (Burckart *et al.*, 1986). Although not completely understood, it is believed that this is due to a more active cytochrome P-450 enzyme system.

2.2. Cyclosporine Concentration Monitoring

The technique of whole blood TDX cyclosporine and metabolites fluorescent polarization immunoassay was recently adopted at our institution for monitoring cyclosporine levels in our transplant recipients. This method has proved to be as reliable and as sensitive as the radioimmunoassay (RIA) and the high-performance liquid chromatography (HPLC) methods, with the added benefits of having a more rapid turnaround time, making it easer to have same-day results (Schroeder *et al.*, 1989). Since there is a good correlation with the RIA method (previously used in our institution), adopting this new assay has not been a problem. However, the TDX uses an antibody different from that employed in the RIA method provided by Sandoz and certain cyclosporine metabolites show a stronger cross-reaction in the TDX method.

2.3. Steroids

One gram of methylprednisolone is given intravenously at the time of unclamping the vessels. Subsequently, the patient is placed on a steroid recycle. Methylprednisolone, 200 mg, is given on the first day and this is rapidly tapered to the equivalent of 20 mg of prednisone by the fifth postoperative day. Table II shows the steroid recycle used in both pediatric and adult recipients. At the time of discharge, adult patients are usually on 15 mg of

TABLE II.   Steroid[a] Recycle Used in Organ Transplantation at the University of Pittsburgh

Day	Adults and Children > 30 kg	Children between 5–30 kg	Children < 5 kg
1	200 mg	100 mg	50 mg
2	160 mg	80 mg	40 mg
3	120 mg	60 mg	30 mg
4	80 mg	40 mg	20 mg
5	40 mg	20 mg	10 mg
6	20 mg	10 mg	5 mg

[a]Dosages are for prednisone. If parenteral route is needed, an equivalent dose of methylprednisolone is used.

prednisone a day and by the sixth month posttransplant this has been further lowered to 10 mg a day. The corresponding doses for pediatric recipients are roughly one half of the adult doses for patients with more than 5 kg of body weight and one fourth of the adult doses for patients with less than 5 kg of body weight. Lower doses of steroids are desirable if patients can tolerate good levels of cyclosporine since the side effects of steroids are not always reversible and are more difficult to manage (i.e., aseptic necrosis of the hip, glaucoma, etc.). Diabetic patients, obese patients, and patients with severe bone disease will also benefit from a lower steroid dosage.

2.4. Azathioprine

This drug is used early in the posttransplant period in patients with severe renal impairment. In such cases patients are started on doses of 3–4 mg/kg body weight and rapidly tapered during the first week posttransplant to 1–2 mg/kg body weight. Cyclosporine is simultaneously reduced or in rare circumstances it is completely stopped in order to avoid dangerous overimmunosuppression. This group of patients is usually discharged on triple therapy with the usual amount of prednisone, 1–1.5 mg/kg of azathioprine, and doses of cyclosporine that maintain slightly lower blood levels. Close monitoring of white blood cell count is required, and other myelosuppressants such as doxorubicin or allopurinol are avoided if possible or judiciously added if the clinical situation absolutely warrants it.

3. IMMUNOSUPPRESSION IN RENAL TRANSPLANTATION

Since the introduction of cyclosporine in clinical transplantation in 1978, most centers in the United States and around the world use double or triple drug regimens in renal transplantation. Cyclosporine continues to be the mainstay of these polypharmacological immunosuppressive protocols. At the University of Pittsburgh during 1987, half of the renal transplant patients were treated with cyclosporine and prednisone and the other half with cyclosporine, azathioprine, and prednisone (Shapiro et al., 1989). Although patient survival was similar in both groups, graft survival was significantly improved in the triple drug therapy group (Figs. 30.2 and 30.3). Since 1987, we have been using triple drug therapy in all of our cadaveric kidney transplants. This has permitted us to use less cyclosporine, which has resulted both in better initial and late renal function.

3.1. Cyclosporine

Just before the operation, patients receive a single dose of 17.5 mg/kg body weight orally. The same amount, divided in two daily doses, is used subsequently. The dosage is then adjusted to maintain a 12-hr trough level of cyclosporine > 700 and < 1000 ng/ml TDX. Lower cyclosporine doses are used in cases of primary nonfunction. Occasionally, in cases of patients with high panel reactive antibody (PRA) and with delayed graft function, cyclosporine may be given in very small doses or withheld completely for a few days. In such cases, OKT3 in combination with azathioprine and prednisone is introduced at the outset.

Although the same general principles outlined for the use of cyclosporine in liver transplantation are applicable in kidney transplantation, there are certain differences that should be emphasized. Lower cyclosporine levels can be used in kidney transplant. Opportunistic infection and other complications of overimmunosuppression must be avoided in the case of kidney transplantation, where dialysis is a reasonable and life-saving alternative to a

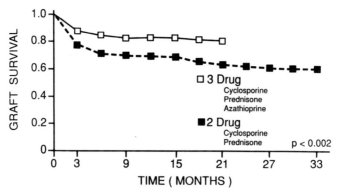

FIGURE 30.2. Overall graft (kidney) actuarial survival with two- and three-drug immunosuppression at the University of Pittsburgh. Redrawn from Shapiro *et al.* (1989).

failed graft. It is also important to remember that since cyclosporine is nephrotoxic, the clinical and even pathological differentiation between rejection and cyclosporine toxicity often becomes a diagnostic dilemma.

3.2. Azathioprine

Azathioprine 3 mg/kg body weight in a single daily dose is used initially and this is slowly tapered to 1–1.5 mg/kg body weight by the time the patient is discharged. Similarly, the white blood cell count is closely monitored and the oral dosage is reduced or stopped if leukopenia becomes a problem.

3.3. Prednisone

The same regimen is used as previously mentioned for adult and pediatric liver transplant patients. In diabetic patients who have good renal function and who can tolerate it, we aim for a higher cyclosporine level and a lower prednisone dose. The steroid recycle used in pediatric recipients is the same as depicted in Table II.

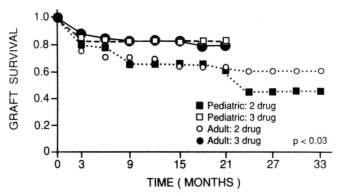

FIGURE 30.3. Pediatric and adult graft (kidney) survival with two and three-drug immunosuppression at the University of Pittsburgh. Redrawn from Shapiro *et al.* (1989).

4. IMMUNOSUPPRESSION IN MULTIORGAN TRANSPLANTATION

The following multivisceral transplants are being performed at the present time at the University of Pittsburgh: heterotopic kidney and pancreas transplantation, orthotopic liver and heterotopic kidney transplantation, orthotopic liver and heterotopic pancreas transplantation, orthotopic liver–pancreas transplantation en bloc (organ cluster transplant), and orthotopic liver–pancreas and intestinal transplantation en bloc (multivisceral transplant).

The immunosuppressive management of patients with simultaneous kidney and pancreas transplants does not differ much from the management of patients with kidney transplants alone. On the other hand, the immunosuppressive management of patients with simultaneous liver and kidney and orthotopic liver and heterotopic pancreas transplantation does not differ much from the management of patients with liver transplantation alone. Patients who receive multivisceral transplants en bloc such as orthotopic liver–pancreas or liver–pancreas and intestine generally receive higher doses of immunosuppressants. The threat of graft versus host disease in such patients who receive a large donor load of lymphatic tissue has warranted the higher doses of immunosuppressants. Furthermore, rejection must be avoided due to the more sophisticated and difficult nature of such transplants (Starzl et al., 1989a,c).

5. TREATMENT OF ACUTE REJECTION

Elevation of the liver function tests in liver transplant recipients and of the creatinine and BUN in kidney transplant recipients demand a careful clinical evaluation. If technical complications are ruled out, the differential diagnosis of elevated liver function tests in liver transplant recipients or of elevated BUN and creatinine in kidney transplant recipients is then limited to infection, rejection, and drug toxicity. Careful assessment of the patient plus a percutaneous needle biopsy when indicated almost always lead to the correct diagnosis.

Diagnosing rejection in pancreas transplant recipients is more troublesome. The reason is that hyperglycemia is almost always a late sign of rejection and that tissue diagnosis is rarely if ever available. In patients with multiorgan transplants on which the other allograft serves as a telltale for rejection or in patients with exocrine drainage into the bladder, rejection may be easier to detect (Sollinger et al., 1987; Groth, 1989).

Regardless of the organ or organs involved, the same drugs are used in the management of rejection.

5.1. Steroids

Boluses of 1 gm of intravenous methylprednisolone and/or a full steroid recycle are our first choice for the treatment of acute rejection. Almost all rejection episodes will respond to steroid treatment if they are mild. The corresponding doses used for pediatric patients are the same as those in Tables II.

5.2. OKT3

This monoclonal antibody directed to the CD3 receptor of the mature T lymphocyte is a powerful immunosuppressant and a very effective antirejection medication (Cosimi et al., 1981; Ortho Multi-Center Transplant Study Group, 1985; Fung et al., 1987). We reserve this drug for the treatment of steroid-resistant rejection, although it can be the first choice in some patients with serious rejection. In this case the efficacy of the drug has to be weighed against the increased incidence of opportunistic infections, especially cyto-megalovirus (CMV) infections. Ninety to ninety-five percent of the rejection episodes will respond to this drug. In carefully selected patients with recurrent rejection, a second course of the drug can be given, provided that the antimurine antibodies are negative and the CD3 receptor levels are monitored.

5.3. ALG

This nonspecific lymphocyte killer, first developed by Starzl in 1967 (Starzl *et al.*, 1967), is rarely used in our institution for the treatment of acute rejection, since OKT3, a more specific antilymphocyte agent, is now available.

6. IMMUNOSUPPRESSION IN CARDIAC TRANSPLANTATION

Developments in immunosuppressive therapy in extrathoracic organs have made immuno-suppression possible in cardiac, pulmonary, and cardiopulmonary transplantation. Following the introduction of cyclosporine in 1980, the mainstay of immunosuppressive therapy in thoracic transplantation at the University of Pittsburgh, has been based on triple therapy, with cyclosporine as the foundation and azathioprine and prednisone being used to augment therapy. More recently, antilymphocyte therapy has been used for induction therapy in the early postoperative period.

6.1. Cyclosporine

Between 1980 and 1985, patients undergoing cardiac transplantation received a loading dose of cyclosporine, 17.5 mg/kg body weight orally. Cyclosporine was then continued posttransplantation at a dose of 2.5–5 mg orally twice a day and adjusted to maintain a trough whole blood level of approximately 800–1000 ng/ml TDX for the first month following transplantation. Subsequently, the whole blood levels were maintained at approx-imately 500–750 ng/ml with adjustments being made for a creatinine greater than 2.5 mg/dl. In 1985, azathioprine was substituted preoperatively for cyclosporine and cyclosporine was started only postoperatively. The effect of this was a reduction in the incidence of the cyclosporine nephrotoxicity seen following cardiopulmonary bypass. Although improve-ments were seen in renal function for up to a year following transplantation, the incidence of serum creatinine elevation above 2 mg/dl beyond one year after transplantation did not appear to be affected.

6.2. Azathioprine

Guidelines for the use of azathioprine in cardiac transplantation follow those of the extrathoracic organs. The use of azathioprine preoperatively has prevented a higher inci-dence of cyclosporine-induced renal failure perioperatively. Again, the use of azathioprine permits acceptance of a lower serum trough level of cyclosporine. Azathioprine is given preoperatively intravenously at a dose of 4 mg/kg. Subsequent to transplantation, the dose is continued at 2 mg/kg a day either intravenously or orally as tolerated. Adjustments are made for leukopenia.

6.3. Steroids

Steroids in the form of methylprednisolone are given at the time of removal of the aortic cross-clamp during cardiac transplantation. Although the absolute value has varied, the current dosage is 500 mg intravenously. Immediately postoperatively, the dose has also varied; however, our current practice is to use 125 mg every 8 hr for the first 24 hr. Following this, 20 mg of prednisone are given orally every day. In the past three to four years, an effort has been made to reduce the amount of steroid intake by cardiac transplant recipients. This has been mainly instigated by the development of steroid complications such as glaucoma, diabetes, and osteoporosis as well as obesity. Most patients tolerate reduction from 20 mg to a maintenance dose of 5–10 mg/day. It is our current practice to begin reduction of steroid use approximately three to six months following cardiac transplantation. Patients who are more than a year following transplantation may have steroids discontinued altogether as dictated by the ability to maintain adequate cyclosporine levels, good tolerance to azathioprine, and a low incidence of late rejection.

6.4. Rabbit Antithymocyte Globulin and OKT3

The use of antilymphocyte globulin has become popular in the past three years as induction therapy following cardiac transplantation. The only commercially available product at present is OKT3, which is a powerful lympholytic agent having drastic effects on the CD3 subset of lymphocytes. Although OKT3 has enjoyed recent popularity as an adjunct to triple therapy, it is accompanied by a slight increase in the incidence of viral infections and is associated with several systemic side effects, especially after the administration of the first dose. Cardiac transplant recipients are particularly prone to a positive fluid balance following cardiopulmonary bypass and are at some risk of developing severe systemic side effects from the administration of OKT3, including fever, rigors, severe peripheral vasodilatation, severe shortness of breath, and in some circumstances aseptic meningitis.

Rabbit antithymocyte globulin (RATG) is a polyclonal immunoglobin effective across many subsets of lymphocytes but especially the CD4 subset. This agent is not commercially available and is made within the laboratories of the University of Pittsburgh Department of Surgery and was developed by Dr. Charles Beiber at Stanford. Since 1982, this agent has been effective as a rescue agent following steroid-resistant cardiac rejection. In 1985, we began using RATG for induction therapy perioperatively. This agent had the capacity to reduce the incidence of early rejection significantly to the extent that cardiac rejection is extremely rare in the first four to five weeks following transplantation. Rabbit antithymocyte globulin is given intramuscularly at a dose of 1.5 mg/kg for approximately five days following transplantation compared to 14 days of OKT3 therapy. In a recent randomized trial using RATG and OKT3 prophylaxis, RATG clearly reduced the actuarial and absolute incidence of moderate cardiac rejection in the first 90 days (Kormos *et al.*, 1990).

6.5. Monitoring for Rejection

Cardiac rejection is monitored using a endomyocardial biopsy as the gold standard. A modified Billingham scale is currently used at the University of Pittsburgh with biopsy scores of grade 3 (severe lymphocytic infiltrate with myocyte necrosis) as an indication for augmented immunosuppression. Treatment of rejection centers around giving extra steroid in the form of intravenous methylprednisolone at a dose of 1 gm either as a single bolus or during three successive days. In some cases, the maintenance prednisone dose is taken up to 100 mg/day and tapered over a 10- to 14-day period back to the maintenance dose of 20 mg. Finally, in steroid-resistant rejection, either OKT3 or RATG may be given in a course similar to one used during induction therapy.

7. IMMUNOSUPPRESSION IN PULMONARY AND CARDIOPULMONARY TRANSPLANTATION

Immunosuppression again is triple therapy based and is managed the same as cardiac transplantation except for the use of steroids. After the original steroid taper in the first 24 hr, the use of prednisone is avoided until approximately two weeks following pulmonary or cardiopulmonary transplantation. This is primarily to avoid the tracheal dehiscence that has a high incidence in the presence of steroid therapy.

Monitoring for rejection is based on a number of functional and histological studies. Pulmonary function studies appear to be a very sensitive indicator of pulmonary rejection and a 20% drop in the FEV 1 or FEF 25-75 is an indication for either open lung or transbronchial biopsy. The presence of bronchial or pulmonary vascular infiltration by active lymphocytes is an indication for augmented immunosuppression using either steroids or RATG. In cardiopulmonary transplantation, the cardiac biopsy is rarely positive and is, therefore, a poor indicator of the presence of rejection in the heart–lung block. Indeed, it is not uncommon to see pulmonary rejection in the absence of cardiac rejection.

8. COMPLICATIONS OF IMMUNOSUPPRESSION

In transplantation, one must constantly balance the danger of overimmunosuppression with that of rejection in order to realize a successful immunosuppressive regimen in a particular patient. This delicate balance can only be achieved with individualization of therapy, meticulous patient care, and continuous monitoring of organ function and drug side effects. Multiple drug therapy has evolved in order to minimize drug toxicity; however, this does not ensure that overimmunosuppression with subsequent opportunistic infections and/ or *de novo* neoplasia formation will be prevented. Toxic side effects should alert the physician to the probability of overimmunosuppression in its attendant complications.

8.1. Opportunistic Infections

The most frequent opportunistic infections in the transplant population are *Pneumocystis carinii* pneumonitis, cytomegalovirus infections, and invasive fungal infections (mainly *Candida albicans* and *Aspergillus fumigatus*), although the incidence of the first one has been steadily decreasing because of the widespread use of prophylactic trimethroprim-sulfa. The basic management of these and other opportunistic infections consists of the use of the appropriate therapeutic agent (trimethroprim-sulfa, ganciclovir, amphotericin, etc.) and a decrease or on occasion, depending on the severity of the illness, a complete cessation of the immunosuppressant agents. When to stop immunosuppression in a patient with opportunistic infection is a matter of good clinical judgment that comes with experience and close monitoring of the patients. Although the guidelines are variable, we feel that central nervous system infections, rapidly progressive pulmonary infiltrates, and, in general, any life-threatening infections warrant complete cessation of immunosuppression as the first step in the management of these patients.

8.2. *De Novo* Cancers

Since the first case described by Starzl in 1968 (Starzl *et al.*, 1968), there have been numerous reports on the incidence, pathophysiology, and management of posttransplant neoplasia, especially as it relates to lymphoproliferative disease. As described in our most recent publication, the majority of cases of lymphoproliferative disorder respond to a decrease or complete cessation of immunosuppression (Nalesnik *et al.*, 1988). In general, we approach this problem with a 50% reduction in immunosuppression. If no response is observed, then we will stop all immunosuppressive agents. If remission of the lesion is complete, we then resume immunosuppression at slightly lower levels. Chemotherapy should be reserved for those patients with monoclonal and monomorphous tumors who do not respond to a reasonable trial of reduced or discontinued immunosuppression. Acyclovir should be administered in all cases since the Epstein–Barr virus has been implicated as an etiologic factor for such tumors.

9. DONOR PRETREATMENT

Extensive research is being conducted on organ pretreatment in an attempt to modify donor immunogenicity and increase allograft survival. Overall, these modes of pretreatment (allograft irradiation, electrical, chemical, and pharmacological manipulation, etc.) have not yet demonstrated prolonged graft survival. Presently, the only situations in which we condition the donor with an immunosuppressive agent are when there is an increased risk for a graft versus host disease (GVHD) reaction, such as in patients receiving multivisceral transplants, and, rarely, in patients receiving orthotopic liver transplants across ABO blood groups. In such cases the donor is treated with 15 cc of OKT3 one hour prior to cross-clamping in an attempt to purge the donor organ of lymphocytes.

10. NEW DEVELOPMENTS IN IMMUNOSUPPRESSION

New immunosuppressive drugs are constantly being developed. More powerful and specific monoclonal antibodies are now under extensive testing in several laboratories around the world. Some of the most promising are a group of monoclonal antibodies directed against the interleukin-2 receptor of the T cells, such as the 33B3.1 and the anti-TAC 3 (Cantarovich *et al.*, 1989; Kirkman *et al.*, 1989).

Immunotoxins are a new fascinating field in the immunotherapy of transplantation. This pharmacological approach uses monoclonal antibodies as probes to deliver toxic substances to specific cell types. In the case of xomazyme-H65, an antibody to the CD.5 receptor of mature T lymphocytes is conjugated to the toxic ricin-A chain. This experimental drug has thus far only been used to treat GVHD in bone marrow transplant recipients, with encouraging results (Jansen *et al.*, 1982; Kernan *et al.*, 1988). Plans are underway to begin clinical trials for the treatment of rejection in solid organ transplantation at our institution.

Currently, one of the major limitations in renal transplantation involves the large number of sensitized dialysis patients. These highly sensitized patients, who have antibodies to most or all HLA antigens, are rendered immunologically untransplantable because they are at high risk to develop hyperacute rejection. At present there are no effective means of dealing with this problem, and these patients can spend years on transplant waiting lists.

One potential solution to these problems utilizes the ability of the staphylococcal protein A to bind selectively the Fc receptor of IgG. A novel technology has been developed whereby plasma can be passed over a column of protein A–Sepharose, and the IgG can be adsorbed. This technique of immunodepletion can decrease the level of preformed antibodies and thus should be potentially helpful in the abrogation of the hyperacute rejection response.

In the United States, a multicenter trial of immunodepletion is currently underway. If successful, the protein A column may be used in the future to immunodeplete the highly sensitized recipient prior to transplantation.

11. FK-506

In 1986, Dr. Thomas Starzl at the University of Pittsburgh, a pioneer in many fields of transplantation, noted the properties of a novel immunosuppressive agent called FK-506. This agent, a macrolide produced by *Streptomyces tsukubaenisis* (Swada *et al.*, 1987), was discovered in 1984 in Japan during a search for new immunosuppressive and cancer chemotherapeutic agents. Intensive animal research was conducted at the University of Pittsburgh with this agent (Todo *et al.*, 1987, 1988b; Nalesnik *et al.*, 1987) before human trials were begun in the spring of 1989. Although still not the ideal immunosuppressive agent, the initial results, which were recently presented at the Congress of the European Organ Transplant Society, have shown FK-506 to be a major breakthrough in immunosuppression (Starzl *et al.*, 1990). If long-term results prove to be as good as the initial results, no doubt FK-506 will become the mainstay of immunosuppression for organ transplantation in the near future.

The most prominent qualities of this new agent and a brief outline of some of the basic aspects of its use in liver transplant patients are presented below.

11.1 Advantages of FK-506 over Other Immunosuppressive Regimens

11.1.1. Low Dose or No Steroid Maintenance Therapy

Liver transplant recipients placed on FK-506 require 50% less steroid maintenance therapy compared to patients on cyclosporine at the end of one month following transplantation (Todo *et al.*, 1990). We estimate that roughly between one third to one half of our liver transplant recipients are completely weaned from steroid maintenance therapy by the fourth month posttransplant. Being able to release some of the patients from the complications of long-term steroid therapy is definitely a great accomplishment.

11.1.2. Treatment of Chronic Rejection

The first patient ever placed on FK-506 was a 28-year-old female who had lost her first two liver allografts to chronic rejection and was showing evidence of rejecting her third liver. In addition, she had severe hypertension and rising BUN and creatinine secondary to cyclosporine toxicity. In March 1989, she was switched to FK-506. Although her kidney (one was removed at the time of her third orthotopic liver transplant) could not be saved, her liver function became normal. Twenty-seven days later, she received a kidney transplant that is working well under FK-506. In addition to this patient, there had been several patients whose liver allografts were "rescued" from ongoing rejection when switched from cyclosporine to FK-506. Overall, 70% of the liver transplant recipients with chronic rejection have had clinical and histological improvement after FK-506 rescue (Starzl et al., 1989b; Fung et al., 1990). This is the only agent so far that has been capable of halting chronic rejection in liver transplant recipients.

11.1.3. Prevention of Acute Rejection

The incidence of acute rejection in liver allograft recipients receiving FK-506 was reported to be 15% at the meeting of the European Society of Organ Transplantation in Barcelona, Spain. This low incidence of rejection unravels a cascade of benefits that consist of less use of OKT3 and steroid boluses, lesser incidence of opportunistic infections early after transplantation, shorter hospital stay, and a decrease in hospital costs (Todo et al., 1990; Allesiani et al., 1990; Staschak et al., 1990).

11.1.4. Low Toxicity

Although not devoid of toxicity, preliminary trials have shown the drug to be relatively less toxic than cyclosporine. As with cyclosporine, the main problems so far have been nephrotoxicity, neurotoxicity, and diabetogenicity. The nephrotoxicity and neurotoxicity are less than that observed with cyclosporine (McCauley et al., 1990; Shapiro et al., 1990), while diabetogenic effects do not seem to be worse than cyclosporine itself (Mieles et al., 1990). Other less important side effects of the drug are listed in Table III.

11.1.5. Easy Handling and Dosing of the Medication

Dosages and blood levels are not yet fully delineated for all organ transplant systems. The recommended schedule reported here is the one that is currently being used at our institution for liver transplant recipients. Other guidelines may develop since this drug is still experimental. Nevertheless, we start liver allograft recipients on 0.15 mg/kg a day intravenously, divided in two doses. When oral intake is resumed, patients are given 0.3 mg/kg a day orally, divided in two doses. At 24-hr overlap of the oral and intravenous routes is done to assure adequate blood levels. At the time of discharge, most patients are taking 0.15 mg/kg twice a day, but by the second month the dosage is reduced to 0.15 mg/kg once a day in about half of the patients.

TABLE III. Most Frequent Side Effects Observed in Patients Receiving FK-506

Intravenous FK-506	Oral FK-506
Headaches	Headaches
Diarrhea	Tremors
Nausea	Photophobia
Vomiting	Blurred vision
Psychosis	Anorexia
Paresthesias	
Tremors	
Blurred vision	
Photophobia	

In general, FK-506 compared to cyclosporine requires fewer dosage adjustments since it has a wider therapeutic range. Twelve-hour trough levels that ranged from 0.2 to as high as 6 ng/ml have been observed without detectable evidence of toxicity (plasma concentrations are measured by the two-step monoclonal enzyme immunoassay technique of Tamura *et al.*, 1987).

Routine steroid recycle is started immediately postoperatively in addition to the FK-506. A rapid tapering of the steroids is done in such a way that at the time of discharge patients are receiving just 5–10 mg a day of prednisone and about one third to one half of the patients are completely weaned from steroids by the fourth month following transplantation.

ACKNOWLEDGMENTS. The work was supported by research grants from the Veterans Administration and project grant No. DK29961 from the National Institutes of Health, Bethesda, Maryland.

REFERENCES

Allesiani, M., Kusne, S., Martin, M., Fung, J. J., Jain, A., Todo, Simmons, R., and Starzl, T. E., 1990, Infections under FK 506 immunosuppression: Preliminary results with primary therapy, *Transplant. Proc.* **22**(Suppl. 1):44–46.

Billingham, R. E., Kuhn, P. L., and Medwar, P. B., 1950, Effect of cortisone on skin homotransplants in the rabbit by irradiation of the host, *Br. J. Exp. Pathol.* **21**:670–679.

Burckart, G. J., Ventkataramanan, R., Ptachcinski, R. J., Starzl, T. E., Gartner, J. C., Jr., Zitelli, B. J., Malatack, J. J., Shaw, B. W., Iwatsuki, S., and Van Thiel, D., 1986, Cyclosporine absorption following orthotopic liver transplantation, *J. Clin. Pharmacol.* **26**:647–651.

Calne, R. Y., 1960, The rejection of renal homografts: Inhibition in dogs by 6-mercaptopurine, *Lancet* **1**:417–418.

Calne, R. Y., White, D. J. G., Thiru, S., Evans, D. B., McMaster, P., Dunn, D. C., Craddock, G. N., Pentlow, B. D., and Rolles, K., 1978, Cyclosporine A in patients receiving renal allografts from cadaver donors, *Lancet* **2**:1323–1327.

Calne, R. Y., Rolles, K., White, D. J. G., Thiru, S., Evans, D. B., McMaster, P., Dunn, D. C., Craddock, G. N., Henderson, R. G., Aziz, S., and Lewis, J., 1979, Cyclosporine A initially as the only immunosuppressant in 34 recipients of cadaveric organs: 32 kidneys, 2 pancreases and 2 livers, *Lancet* **2**:1033–1036.

Cannon, J. A., 1956, Brief report, *Transplant Bull.* **3**:7.

Cantarovich, D., LeMauff, B., Hourmant, M., Giral, M., Denis, M., Jacques, Y., and Soulillou, J. P., 1989, Anti-1L2 receptor monoclonal antibody (33B3.1) in prophylaxis of early kidney rejection in humans: A randomized trial versus rabbit antithymocyte globulin, *Transplant. Proc.* **21**:1769–1771.

Carstensen, H., Jacobsen, N., and Dieperink, H., 1986, Interaction between cyclosporine A and phenobarbitone, *Br. J. Clin. Pharmacol.* **21**:550–611.

Cassidy, M. J., Van Zyl-Smit, R., Pascoe, M. D., Swanepoel, C. R., and Jacobson, J. E., 1985, Effect of rifampicin on cyclosporine A blood levels in a renal transplant recipient, *Nephron* **41**:207–208.

Cosimi, A. B., Burton, R. C., Colvine, R. B., Boldstein, G., Delmonico, F. L., LoQuoelia, M. P., Tolkhoffrubin, N., Rubin, R. H., Herrin, J. T, and Russel, P. S., 1981, Treatment of acute renal allograft rejection with OKT3 nomoclonal antibody, *Transplantation* **32**:535–539.

Coward, R. A., Raftery, A. T., and Brown, C. B., 1985, Antituberculous therapy, *Lancet* **1**:1342–1343.

Dempster, W. J., Lennox, B., and Bogg, J. W., 1950, Prolongation of survival skin homotransplants in the rabbit by irradiation of the host, *Br. J. Exp. Pathol.* **31**:670–679.

Dickneite, P. K., Schorlemmer, H. V., Walter, P., and Sedlacek, H. H., 1986, Graft survival in experimental transplantation could be prolonged by the action of the antitumoral drug 15-deoxyspergualin, *Transplant. Proc.* **18**:1295–1296.

Dieperink, H., and Moller, J., 1982, Ketoconazole and cyclosporine (letter), *Lancet* **2**:1217.

Edwards, W. S., 1979, Alexis Carrel, 1873–1944, *Contemp. Surg.* **14**:65–79.

Fung, J. J., Demetris, A. J., Porter, K. A., Iwatsuki, S., Gordon, R. D., Esquivel, C. O., Jaffe, R., Shaw, B. W., Jr., and Starzl, T. E., 1987, Use of OKT3 with cyclosporine and steroids for reversal of acute kidney and liver allograft rejection, *Nephron* **46**:19–33.

Fung, J. J., Todo, S., Jain, A., McCauley, J., Alessiani, M., Scotti, C., and Starzl, T. E., 1990, Conversion of liver allograft recipients with cyclosporine related complications from cyclosporine to FK 506, *Transplant. Proc.* **22**:6–12.

Grino, J. M., Sebate, I., Castelao, A. M., and Alsina, J., 1986, Influence of diltiazem on cyclosporine clearance, *Lancet* **1**:1387.

Groth, C. G., 1972, Landmarks in clinical renal transplantation, *Surg. Gynecol. Obstet.* **134**:323–328.

Groth, C. G., 1989, Is there an indication for pancreatic transplantation? *Transplant Proc.* **21**(1):2757–2758.

Hamburger, J., Vaysse, J., Crosmier, J., Tubiana, M., Lalanne, C. M., Antoine, B., Auvert, J., Soulier, J. P., Dormont, J., Salmon, C. H., Maisonnet, M., and Amiel, J. L., 1959, Transplantation d'un rein entre jumeaux non monozijotes apres irradiation du receveur, *Presse Med* **67**:1771–1775.

Hows, J. M., Chipping, P. M., Fairhead, J., Smith, J., Baughan, A., and Gordon Smith, E. C., 1983, Nephrotoxicity in bone marrow transplant recipients treated with cyclosporine A, *Br. J. Haematol.* **54**:69–78.

Hume, D. M., Magee, J. H., Kauffman, H. M., Rittenbury, M. S., and Prout, G. R., Jr., 1963, Renal transplantation in man in modified recipients, *Ann. Surg.* **158**:608–644.

Iwatsuki, S., Starzl, T. E., Todo, S., Gordon, R. D., Esquivel, C. O., Tzakis, A. G., Makowka, L., Marsh, J. W., Koneru, B., Stieber, A., Klintmalm, G., and Husberg, B., 1988, Experience in 1000 liver transplants under cyclosporine–steroid therapy: A survival report, *Transplant. Proc.* **20**:498–504.

Jansen, F. K., Blythman, H. E., Carriere, D., Casellas, P., Gros, O., Gros, P., Laurent, J. C., Paolucci, F., Pau, B., Poncelet, P., Richer, G., Vidal, H., and Voisin, I. A., 1982, Immunotoxin: Hybrid molecules combining high specificity and potent cytotoxicity, *Immunol. Rev.* **62**:185–216.

Kennedy, M. S., Deeg, H. J., Siegel, M., Crowley, J. J., Storb, R., and Thomas, E. D., 1983, Acute renal toxicity with combined use of amphotericin B and cyclosporine after marrow transplantation, *Transplantation* **35**:211–215.

Keown, P. A., Laupacis, A. Carruthers, G., Stawecki, M., Koegler, J., McKenzie, F. N., Wall, W., and Stiller, C. R., 1984, Interaction between phenytoin and cyclosporine following organ transplantation, *Transplantation* **38**:304–306.

Kernan, N. A., Byers, V., Scannon, P. J., Mischak, R. P., Brochstein, J., Flomenberg, N., Dupont, B., and O'Reilly, R. J., 1988, Treatment of steroid resistant acute graft-versus-host disease by *in vivo* administration of an anti-T-cell ricin A chain immunotoxin, *J. Am. Med. Assoc.* **259**:3154–3157.

Kirkman, R. L., Shapiro, M. E., Carpenter, C. B., Milford, E. L., Ramos, E. L., Tilney, N. L., Waldmann, T. A., Zimmerman, C. E., and Strom, T. B., 1989, Early experience with anti-Tac in clinical renal transplantation, *Transplant. Proc.* **21**(1):1766–1768.

Kohlhaw, K., Wonigeit, K., Frei, U., Oldhafer, K., Neumann, K., and Pichlmayr, R., 1988, Effect of the calcium channel blocker diltiazem on cyclosporine A blood levels and dose requirements, *Transplant. Proc.* **20**(Suppl. 2):572–574.

Kormos, R. L., Herlan, D. B., Armitage J. M., Stein, K., Kaufman, C., Zeevi, A., Duquesnoy, R., Hardesty, R. L., and Griffith, B. P., 1990, Monoclonal versus polyclonal antibody therapy for prophylaxis against rejection after heart transplantation, *J. Heart Transplant.* **9**(1):1–10.

Kung, P. C., Goldstein, G., Reinherz, E. L., and Schlossman, S. F., 1979, Monoclonal antibodies defining distinctive human T cell surface antigens, *Science* **206**:347–349.

Lake, K. D., 1988, Cyclosporine drug interactions. A review, *Cardiac Surg.* **2**(4):617–630.

Lele, P., Peterson, P., Yang, S., Jarrel, B., and Burke, J. F, 1985, Cyclosporine and tegretol; another drug interaction, *Kidney Int.* **27**:344.

Lindley, D. L., Odell, T. T., Jr., and Tausche, F. G., 1955, Implantation of functional erythropoietic elements following total body irradiation, *Proc. Soc. Exp. Biol.* **90**:512–515.

McCauley, J., Fung, J. J., Jain, A., Todo, S., and Starzl, T. E., 1990, The effects of FK 506 upon renal function after liver transplantation, *Transplant. Proc.* **22**(Suppl. 1):17–20.

Medawar, P. B., 1944, The behavior of skin autografts and homografts in rabbits, *J. Anat.* **78**:176–199.

Merril, J. P., Murray, J. E., Harrison, J. H., Friedman, E. A., Dealy, J. B., Jr., and Dammin, G. J., 1960, Successful homotransplantation of the kidney between monozygotic twins, *N. Engl. J. Med.* **262**:1251–1260.

Mieles, L., Todo, S., Fung, J. J., Jain, A., Furukawa, H., Susuki, M., and Starzl, T. E., 1990, Oral glucose tolerance test in liver recipients treated with FK 506, *Transplant. Proc.* **22**(Suppl. 1):41–43.

Murray, J. E., Merril, J. P., Dammin, G. J., Dealy, J. B., Jr., Walter, C. W., Brooke, M. S., and Wilson, R. E., 1960, Study on transplantation immunity after total body irradiation: Clinical and experimental investigation, *Surgery* **48**:272–284.

Nalesnik, M. A., Todo, S., Murase, N., Gryzan, S., Demetris, A. J., Lee, P., and Starzl, T. E., 1987, Toxicology of FK-506 in the Lewis rat, *Transplant. Proc.* **19**(Suppl. 6):89–92.

Nalesnik, M. A., Makowka, L., and Starzl, T. E., 1988, The diagnosis and treatment of post-transplant lymphoproliferative disorders, in: *Current Problems in Surgery*, Vol. 25 (N. Ravitch, ed.), Year Book Medical Publishers, Chicago, pp. 367–472.

Ortho Multi-Center Transplant Study Group, 1985, A randomized clinical trial of OKT3 monoclonal antibody for acute rejection of cadaveric renal transplants, *N. Engl. J. Med.* **313**:337–342.

Ptachcinski, R. J., Carpenter, B. J., Burckart, G. J., Venkataramanan, R., and Rosenthal, J. T., 1985, Effect of erythromycin on cyclosporine levels, *N. Engl. J. Med.* **313**:1416–1417.

Schroeder, T. J., Brunson, M. E., Pesce, A. J., Hindenlang, L. L., Mauser, P. A., Ruckrigl, D. I., Weibel, M. L., Wadih, G., and First, M. R., 1989, A comparison of the clinical utility of the radioimmunoassay, high-performance liquid chromatography, and TDX cyclosporine assays in outpatient renal transplant recipients, *Transplantation* **47**:262–266.

Schwartz, R., and Dameshek, W., 1959, Drug induced immunological tolerance, *Nature* **183**:1682–1683.

Shapiro, R., Tzakis, A. G., Hakala, T. R., Lopatin, W., Mitchell, S., Koneru, B., Stieber, A., Gordon, R. D., and Starzl, T. E., 1989, Cadaveric renal transplantation at the University of Pittsburgh: A two and one half year experience with the point system, in: *Clinical Transplantation 1988* (P. Terasaki, ed.), UCLA Tissue Typing Lab, Los Angeles, pp. 181–187.

Shapiro, R., Fung, J. J., Jain, A., Parks, P., Todo, S., and Starzl, T. E., 1990, The side effects of FK 506 in humans, *Transplant. Proc.* **22**(Suppl. 1):41–43.

Sollinger, H. W., Stratta, R. J., Kalayoglu, M., Pirsch, J. D., and Belzer, F. O., 1987, Pancreas transplantation with pancreatico-cystostomy and quadruple immunosuppression, *Surgery* **102**:674–679.

Starzl, T. E., Machioro, T. L., and Waddell, W. R., 1963, The reversal of rejection in human renal allografts with subsequent development of homograft tolerance, *Surg. Gynecol. Obstet.* **117**:385–395.

Starzl, T. E, Machioro, T. L., Porter, K. A., Iwasaki, Y., and Cerilli, B. J., 1967, The use of heterologous antilymphoid agents in canine renal and liver homotransplantation and in human transplantation, *Surg. Gynecol. Obstet.* **124**:301–318.

Starzl, T. E., 1968, Discussion of Murray, J. E., Wilson, R. E., Tilney, N. L., *et al.*, Five years' experience in renal transplantation with immunosuppressive drugs: Survival, function, complications and the role of lymphocyte depletion by thoracic duct fistula, *Ann. Surg.* **168**:416–435.

Starzl, T. E., Weil, R., III, Iwatsuki, S., Klintmalm, G., Schroter, G. P. J., Koep, L. J., Iwaki, Y., Terasaki, P. I., and Porter, K. A., 1980, The use of cyclosporine A and prednisone in cadaver kidney transplantation, *Surg. Gynecol. Obstet.* **151;**17–26.

Starzl, T. E., Iwatsuki, S., Klintmaln, G., Schroter, G. P. J., Weil, R., III., Koep, L. J., and Porter, K. A., 1981, Liver transplantation, 1980, with particular reference to cyclosporine A, *Transplant. Proc.* **13:**281–285.

Starzl, T. E., Todo, S., Tzakis, A., Podesta, L., Mieles, L,. Demetris, A., Teperman, L., Selby, R., Stevenson, W., Stieber, A., Gordon, R., and Iwatsuki, S., 1989a, Abdominal organ cluster transplantation for the treatment of upper abdominal malignancies, *Ann. Surg.* **210:**374–386.

Starzl, T. E., Todo, S., Fung, J., Demetris, A. J., Venkataramanan, R., and Jain, A., 1989b, FK-506 for human liver, kidney and pancreas transplantation, *Lancet* **2:**1000–1004.

Starzl, T. E., Rowe, M., Todo, S., Jaffe, R., Tzakis, A., Hoffman, A., Esquivel, C., Porter, K., Venkataramanan, R., Makowka, L., and Duquesnoy, R., 1989c, Transplantation of multiple abdominal viscera, *J. Am. Med. Assoc.* **26:**1449–1457.

Starzl, T. E., Todo, S., Fund, J. J., and Groth, C., 1990, Second International Workshop on FK 506, Barcelona, Spain, *Transplant. Proc.* **22**(Suppl. 1)**:**5–113.

Staschak, S., Wagner, S., Block, G., Van Thiel, D., Jain, A, Fung, J. J., Todo, S., and Starzl, T. E., 1990, A cost comparison of liver transplantation within FK 506 or cyclosporine as the primary immunosuppressive agent, *Transplant. Proc.* **22**(Suppl. 1)**:**47–49.

Swada, S., Susuki, G., Kanase, Y., and Takaku, F., 1987, Novel immunosuppressive agent, FK 506: *In vivo* effects on cloned T cell activation, *J. Immunol.* **139:**1797–1803.

Tamura, K., Kobayashi, M., Hashimoto, K., Kojima, K., Nagase, K., Iwasaki, K., Kaizu, T., Tanaka, H., and Niwa, M., 1987, A highly sensitive method to assay FK 506 levels in plasma, *Transplant. Proc.* **19:**23–29.

Thompson, J. F., Chalmers, D. H. K., Hunnisett, A. G. W., Wood, R. F. M., and Morris, P. J., 1983, Nephrotoxicity of trimethoprim and cotrimoxazole in renal allograft recipients treated with cyclosporine, *Transplantation* **36:**204–206.

Todo, S., Podesta, L., Chapchap, P., Kahn, D., Pan, C. E., Ueda, Y., Okuda, K., Imventarza, O., Casavilla, A., Demetris, A. J., Makowka, L., and Starzl, T. E., 1987, Orthotopic liver transplantation in dogs receiving FK 506, *Transplant. Proc.* **19**(Suppl. 6)**:**64–67.

Todo, S., Murase, N., Kahn, D., Pan, C. E., Okuda, K., Cemaj, S., Casavilla, A., Mazzaferro, V., Ghalab, A., Rhoe, B. S., Yang, M., Taniguchi, K., Nalesnik, M., Makowka, L., and Starzl, T. E., 1988a, Effect of 15-deoxyspergualin on experimental organ transplantation, *Transplant. Proc.* **20**(Suppl. 1)**:**233–236.

Todo, S., Ueda, Y., Demetris, J. A., Imventarza, O., Nalesnik, M., Vekataramanan, R., Makowka, L., and Starzl, T. E., 1988b, Immunosuppression of canine, monkey and baboon allografts by FK 506, with special reference to synergism with other drugs and to tolerance induction, *Surgery* **104:**239–249.

Todo, S., Fung, J. J., Demetris, A. J., Jain, A., Venkataramanan, R., and Starzl, T. E., 1990, Early trials with FK 506 as primary treatment in liver transplantation, *Transplant. Proc.* **22**(Suppl. 1)**:**13–16.

Whiting, P. A., Cunningham, C., Thomson, A. W., and Simpson, J. G., 1984, Enhancement of high dose cyclosporine A toxicity by furosemide, *Biochem. Pharmacol.* **33:**1075–1079.

Woodruf, M. F. A., and Anderson, N. F., 1963, Effect of lymphocyte depletion by thoracic duct fistula and administration of antilymphocyte serum on the survival of skin homografts in rats, *Nature* **200:**702.

Zeevi, A., Duquesnoy, R., Eiras, G., Rabinowich, H., Todo, S., Makowka, L., and Starzl, T. E., 1987, Immunosuppressive effect of FK 506 on *in vitro* lymphocyte alloactivation: Synergism with cyclosporine A, *Transplant. Proc.* **19**(Suppl. 6)**:**40–44.

Chapter 31

BONE MARROW TRANSPLANTATION

Dagfinn H. Albrechtsen

1. INTRODUCTION

Bone marrow transplantation (BM tx) is increasingly being used for the treatment of malignancy (i.e, leukemia), congenital immunodeficiency (i.e., severe combined immunodeficiency (SCID), genetic metabolic disorders (i.e., mucopolysaccharidosis), and hematologic diseases (i.e, aplastic anemia, thalassemia) (Deeg *et al.*, 1988). Bone marrow transplantation allows for the use of greatly intensified and otherwise lethal cytoreductive treatment of malignancies, since the eradication of immunohemopoietic competence is corrected by the transplantation of healthy immunohemopoietic stem cells. These bone marrow-derived cells are procured either from a healthy genetically disparate donor (allogeneic BM tx) or harvested from the patient prior to the cytoreductive therapy (autologous BM tx). Occasionally a genetically identical donor (homozygous twin) is available (syngeneic BM tx).

In nonmalignant disorders the patient's diseased immunohemopoietic tissues are eradicated by an immunomyeloablative regimen and substituted by healthy bone marrow stem cells from an allogeneic donor. Allogeneic BM tx requires the successful integration of several procedures:

1. Pretransplant cytoreductive therapy to eradicate diseased cells in the bone marrow and elsewhere in the body.
2. Peritransplant immunotherapy to abrogate host versus graft alloimmunity and prevent graft rejection.
3. Transplantation of donor bone marrow stem cells.
4. Posttransplant life support during a period of immunohemopoietic aplasia, which lasts for weeks until immunohemopoietic functions are restored by the developing graft.
5. Posttransplant immunotherapy to modulate the alloimmune competence of the graft and prevent graft versus host disease (GVHD).

Dagfinn H. Albrechtsen • Surgical Department, The National Hospital, University of Oslo, 0027 Oslo 1, Norway.
Immunopharmacology in Autoimmune Diseases and Transplantation, edited by Hans Erik Rugstad *et al.* Plenum Press, New York, 1992.

In autologous and syngeneic BM tx, alloimmune reactivity does not interfere with engraftment and recovery, and immunotherapy (steps 2 and 5) is not required. Since autologous grafts may be contaminated by neoplastic cells present in the marrow at the time of procurement, *in vitro* treatment of autografts are often performed to purge contaminating tumor cells.

2. CYTOREDUCTIVE THERAPY TO ERADICATE DISEASE

2.1. Malignant Disease

Various cytoreductive regimens are presently used to eradicate neoplastic cells prior to transplantation. For hematologic malignancies a combination of total body irradiation (TBI) and cytotoxic drugs is often employed (Thomas *et al.*, 1975).

TBI, delivered by a radioisotope (^{90}Co) or by a high-voltage x-ray machine, is given at a total dose of 750–1600 cGy, either in one single fraction (lower doses) or fractionated over three to seven days. An optimal TBI protocol has not been agreed upon and various centers use irradiation regimens differing as to source, total dose, fractionation (1–12 fractions), dose rate (2–26 cGy/min), and lung shielding (lung dose 7–14 Gy) (van Bekkum, 1984; Santos, 1987; O'Reilly, 1987). Usually, TBI is employed in combination with cyclophosphamide, which is given intravenously at a dosage of 60 mg/kg per day × 2 before or after TBI (Thomas *et al.*, 1975; O'Reilly, 1987).

Alternatively, some centers use a combination of busulfan (oral dose 4 mg/kg per day × 4) and cyclophosphamide (given as above or at a dose of 50 mg/kg per day × 4) (Santos *et al.*, 1983; Tutschka *et al.*, 1989, 1991). Additional therapy aiming at leukemic sanctuary sites are often included: intrathecal injections of methotrexate and additional field irradiation (against testes, central nervous system, spleen costae) (Deeg *et al.*, 1988). A number of alternative cytotoxic drug combinations are also being explored, particularly for lymphoma and other nonleukemic malignancies, such as BCNU (carmustine), arabinosyl cytosine, thioguanine, VP-16 (etoposide), and melphalan (O'Reilly, 1987; Santos, 1987; Ash *et al.*, 1990).

All presently known cytoreductive regimens have limited antineoplastic efficacy and significant toxicity. Recurrence of malignancy is observed in 5–70% of the patients, predominantly depending on the stage of the disease (Santos, 1987; Sullivan, 1989). A reduced rate of recurrence is observed in patients experiencing GVHD, the "graft versus leukemia" effect, while a higher relapse rate is seen following syngeneic and autologous BM tx (Storb and Thomas, 1985).

Effective cytoreductive regimens cause irreversible damage of the immunohemopoietic system, resulting in complete bone marrow aplasia, profound immunodeficiency, and severe susceptibility to infection. Extramedullar toxicity includes dermatitis and alopecia, nausea, mucositis (orally, enterally, in the bladder), hepatic injury (sometimes causing veno-occlusive liver disease), cardiomyopathy, and interstitial pneumonia (Deeg *et al.*, 1988). Although usually transient and manageable by appropriate therapy, toxicity is severe and may be fatal. Of particularly concern are long-term sequelae of TBI, such as cataract, sterility, premature menopause, and in children suboptimal growth and sexual maturation.

Unfortunately, antineoplastic efficacy and toxicity of presently known cytoreductive regimens are closely correlated. Attempts at escalating potency to avoid tumor recurrence have incurred the price of enhanced toxic mortality. Clearly, more selective cytoreductive strategies need to be explored, that is, radionucleoids or toxins conjugated to carrier molecules specifically reactive with neoplastic cells.

2.2. Nonmalignant Disease

Pretransplant ablation of the bone marrow also is required when BM tx is performed for nonmalignant disorders. Host versus graft alloimmunity must be abrogated, and proliferatively normal, but qualitatively pathological myelopoiesis (i.e, metabolic disease, thalassemia) must be eradicated to make space for the allograft and preclude disease recurrence (Hobbs, 1985).

Ablation of aplastic anemia is accomplished by giving cyclophosphamide intravenously at a dose of 50 mg/kg per day × 4 (Storb et al., 1982). Some centers use additional total lymphoid (or thoracoabdominal) irradiation (TLI, TAI) at a dose of 200–800 cGY (in one or several fractions) or a combined busulfan–cyclophosphamide regimen to enhance immunosuppression (Champlin, 1987).

These latter, more potent regimens are required when BM tx is performed for genetic disorders (i.e., metabolic disease, thalassemia, Wiskott Aldrich disease) (Hobbs, 1985; Lucarelli et al., 1985; Fischer et al., 1986a). BM tx for classical SCID, however, is usually successfully performed from an HLA-identical donor without prior cytoreductive therapy (Fischer et al., 1986a; O'Reilly, 1987).

3. PREVENTION OF GRAFT REJECTION

3.1. Immunobiology of Rejection

Bone marrow grafts from genetically nonidentical donors are invariably rejected by immunocompetent recipients. Allograft rejection is triggered by and directed against certain cell membrane molecules in the graft dissimilar to the patient's own—the transplantation (or histocompatibility) antigens. These are genetically determined by the HLA chromosomal complex (HLA antigens) and by other genes (minor antigens), some of which are sex-linked, but generally remain unidentified. The greater the genetic disparity between the donor and the recipient, particularly for HLA, the stronger the alloimmune response. Rejection is associated with the posttransplant appearance in the circulation of host cells expressing T-cell markers (O'Reilly, 1987).

Although the cytoreductive regimens used to eradicate the patients' disease cause profound host immunodeficiency, allowing for the transplantation of unmanipulated bone marrow grafts from HLA-compatible donors the nonsensitized patients, host alloimmunity is not completely abrogated (O'Reilly, 1987; Storb, 1989). Residual immunity, mediated by radioresistant and/or alloimmunized ("sensitized") T cells [and possibly natural killer (NK) cells] account for a rejection rate of 10–60% in (1) sensitized patients, (2) recipients of HLA-mismatched grafts, and (3) recipients of T-cell-depletion grafts (O'Reilly, 1987; Butturini and Gale, 1989; Storb, 1989).

Sensitization is usually caused by previous transfusions given to immunocompetent transplant candidates, that is, patients with aplastic anemia or thalassemia (Storb et al., 1982). Why T-cell-depleted grafts are more susceptible to rejection is not clear. Conceivably, the manipulation may reduce the number and/or the quality of transplanted stem cells, trophic supportive cells (stromal cells, hemopoietic growth factors), or graft immune cells (T cells, NK cells) capable of suppressing residual host alloimmunity.

3.2. Prevention of Rejection

Several strategies are employed to influence the balance between host immunocompetence and graft susceptibility to rejection in favor of engraftment.

3.2.1. Histocompatibility

Because of the risk of GVHD, only HLA-compatible donors, or related donors mismatched for no more than one HLA-A, -B, -C, -D, or -DR antigen are routinely accepted. Rejection of unmanipulated grafts are then rarely seen in nonsensitized patients (Storb, 1989).

3.2.2. Allograft Growth Potential

Grafts containing few progenitor cells tend to engraft less well. A cell dose exceeding 2×10^8 nucleated donor cells per kilogram patient weight is aimed for (Deeg et al., 1988). The use of hemopoietic growth factors (G-CSF, GM-CSF, IL-3) given to the patient after transplantation to enhance engraftment is being explored (Metcalf, 1989; Asano et al., 1991).

3.2.3. Sensitization

This should be avoided by using leukocyte-depleted blood products for immunocompetent transplant candidates. Family members should not be used as blood donors before transplantation (Storb et al., 1982).

3.2.4. Immunosuppression of the Host

The cytoreductive transplant regimens used to eradicate the disease provide adequate immunosuppression of nonsensitized patients to allow for allografting of unmanipulated bone marrow from an HLA-compatible donor. Rejection of such grafts rarely (< 1%) occurs (Storb, 1989). More powerful immunosuppression is required for sensitized patients and for recipients of T-cell-depleted and/or HLA-mismatched grafts (Ash et al., 1990). There is no firm evidence that the administration of steroids or cyclosporine given to abrogate GVHD reduces the risk of rejection in clinical bone marrow allografting.

3.3. Prevention of Rejection in High-Risk Patients

3.3.1. Sensitized Patients with Aplastic Anemia

The risk of rejection is reduced by giving buffy coat transfusions procured by leukapheresis of the donor for five days posttransplant (Storb et al., 1982). Although GVHD may be provoked by this procedure, overall survival is improved. An alternative and equally successful approach is to use more powerful immunosuppression of the host, by adding either busulfan or TLI (or TAI) to the cytoreductive regimen (see Section 2.2).

3.3.2. HLA-Mismatched Grafts and T-Cell-Depleted Grafts

Various methods are presently being explored to overcome the problem of rejection of HLA-mismatched and/or T-cell-depleted grafts. First, the procedure used for T-cell depletion is not inconsequential to graft susceptibility to rejection. Although effective (i.e., GVHD preventive) pan-T-cell depletion incurs a high risk of rejection, this may not be the case if the depletion is less complete, or if NK cells are spared, or if only some T-cell subpopulation(s) are depleted (O'Reilly, 1987; Butturini and Gale, 1989). Second, the problem of rejection may be overcome by more powerful immunosuppression of the host, that is, intensified chemotherapy (Ash et al., 1990) or intensified irradiation, either by high-dose rate (26 cGy/min) single fraction TBI, hyperfractionated high-dose (1.2 Gy × 12) TBI, or by adding TLI (2 Gy × 3–4) (Prentice et al., 1984; O'Reilly,1987; Slavin et al., 1987; Champlin et al., 1987). Additional immunosuppression by antilymphocyte antibodies given to the host for some days before and after transplantation is also being explored, that is, monoclonal antibodies reactive with lymphocytes (Campath I), T cells (OKT 3), or leukocytes (anti-LFA$_1$) (Fischer et al., 1986b; O'Reilly, 1987).

4. PREVENTION OF GRAFT VERSUS HOST DISEASE

4.1. Immunobiology of GVHD

Following engraftment of allogeneic bone marrow, the patient's own nonfunctioning immunohemopoietic system is replaced by donor-derived immunocompetent cells. Mature donor T cells transplanted with the graft are challenged by incompatible transplantation antigens present in host tissues, HLA antigens in mismatched transplantations, and minor antigens in all allogeneic transplantations (Gale, 1985; O'Reilly, 1987; Storb, 1989). The ensuing graft versus host alloimmune reaction causes damage to cells expressing incompatible antigens, notably in skin, gut, and liver. If no preventive measures are taken, this reaction invariably causes acute GVHD, manifested by fever, malaise, exanthema, liver dysfunction, and/or enteritis with diarrhea within a few weeks, even in HLA-identical transplantations (Storb and Thomas, 1985).

Acute GVHD may by itself cause death by liver failure or gastrointestinal hemorrhage, GVHD also suppresses the function and development of the evolving graft-derived immunohemopoietic system immune defense mechanisms, already severely compromised by pretransplant cytoreductive therapy, which may not recover, and lethal infections are common (Storb and Thomas, 1985).

No GVHD is observed in patients receiving bone marrow grafts depleted of mature donor T cells by in vitro manipulation prior to transplantation (Prentice et al., 1984; O'Reilly, 1987; Ash et al., 1990). There is, however, no agreement as to which T-cell subpopulations are responsible for GVHD.

Less GVHD has been reported in patients transplanted for aplastic anemia and treated by special techniques to prevent infection (Storb and Thomas, 1985). Microbial antigens may mimic (incompatible) transplantation antigens, and infection may potentiate the expression of transplantation antigens.

Most cases of GVHD respond to immunosuppressive therapy and may even resolve spontaneously (Gale, 1985; Storb and Thomas, 1985). A state of stable chimerism between host tissues and graft immunocompetence evolves in most patients within six months, with no evidence of an ongoing alloimmune reaction and no need for long-term immunosuppressive therapy (in contradistinction to organ allografting) (Storb and Thomas, 1985; O'Reilly, 1987). The reason for this may be (1) graft-versus-host-mediated eradication of susceptible host target cells (dendritic cells, etc.), (2) gradual depletion of anti-host-reactive donor-derived T cells, and (3) evolution of graft-derived T cells tolerized in the thymus of the host. Some of these cells may suppress the anti-host reactivity of surviving donor-derived immunocytes (Tutschka, 1987).

A chronic form of GVHD develops in approximately one third of the patients, characterized in severe cases by skin discoloration, scleroderma, contractures, bronchiolitis, intestinal mucosal atrophy and diarrhea, liver dysfunction, conjunctivitis sicca, and immunodeficiency with infections (Storb and Thomas, 1985). The clinical picture mimics autoimmune disease and autoantibodies are frequently found. Although sometimes occurring in patients with no previous acute GVHD, chronic GVHD is probably initiated by the same mechanisms and propagated as a consequence of any aberration in the evolution of graft tolerance as described above (Tutschka, 1987).

Of major interest is the observed correlation between GVHD and a reduced incidence of recurrence of malignancy in leukemic patients (Ringden and Horowitz, 1989). The risk of relapse after transplantation for early-phase leukemia is at least 50% in patients transplanted from a syngeneic donor (where no GVHD occurs), 15–30% in allograft recipients experiencing no or minimal GVHD, and less than 10% in patients surviving significant GVHD (Sullivan, 1989). The protective effect of GVHD, probably a consequence of alloimmune killing of residual host cancer cells surviving pretransplant cytoreductive therapy, offers appealing perspectives in oncological therapy.

4.2. Prevention of GVHD

Several avenues of intervention are taken to prevent GVHD.

4.2.1. Histocompatibility

Because fulminant GVHD is frequently observed after HLA mismatched bone marrow allografting, transplantations are routinely performed only from HLA-identical siblings or HLA-haploidentical relatives mismatched for no more than one HLA-A, -B, -D, or -DR antigen (Hansen et al., 1987). Recent experience has demonstrated similar success rates in transplantations from unrelated donors identical for HLA-A, -B, -D, or -DR (Beatty et al., 1989; Hows et al., 1989; Ash et al., 1990). Large national and international registries of potential volunteer bone marrow donors are presently being organized to increase the possibility of finding a suitable donor for patients lacking an acceptable family donor. Since male recipients of allografts from female donors have increased risk of GVHD, presumably because of Y-linked minor transplantation antigens, male donors should be selected for male patients when possible (Gale, 1985).

4.2.2. In Vitro Depletion of T Cells from the Bone Marrow Allograft

Clinical experience indicates that allografts containing fewer than 10^5 T cells per kilogram recipient weight do not provoke GVHD (O'Reilly, 1987; Butturini and Gale, 1989). This requires the selective removal of approximately 99% of T cells present in the unmanipulated graft. Several methods have been developed for this purpose, such as cytolysis with T-cell antibodies and complement (Prentice et al., 1984; Slavin et al., 1987;

Herve et al., 1985; Ash et al., 1990), cell toxin conjugated to T-cell antibodies (Filipovich et al., 1984), or physical separation by soybean agglutination and sheep red cell rosetting (Reisner et al., 1983), counterflow centrifugation (DeWitte et al., 1986), or microbeads coated with T-cell antibodies (Vartdal et al., 1987).

Although effective in preventing GVHD, most of these methods have been found to cause a high rate of graft rejection and leukemic relapse, and T-cell depletion has so far not proved beneficial for malignancy (Goldman et al., 1988; Butturini and Gale, 1989). More encouraging results have been reported in congenital disorders (O'Reilly, 1987; Fischer et al., 1986a). Since the biology of engraftment, rejection, GVHD, and malignant relapse has not been fully elucidated, new methods may change the picture in the future.

4.2.3. Selective Stem Cell Stimulation and/or Transplantation

The availability of immunohemopoietic growth factors provides the possibility of selective stimulation of progenitor cell proliferation, thus accelerating the recruitment of graft-derived T cells to be tolerized in the host thymus and capable of preventing GVHD. Another intriguing possibility is the transplantation of purified stem cells.

4.2.4. Immunosuppressive Drugs

Several studies have proved the efficacy of posttransplant immunosuppressive therapy of the host in suppressing donor T-cell anti-host reactivity and preventing GVHD (Gale, 1985; Storb and Thomas, 1985; Deeg et al., 1987). Methotrexate, cyclosporine, steroids, cyclophosphamide, and anti-T-cell antibodies, and combinations thereof, are presently being used for GVHD prophylaxis.

4.2.4a. Methotrexate (MtX). An incidence of acute GVHD (grades II–IV) of 25% was reported in recipients of HLA-identical grafts treated with a "standard course" of MtX, 61% with a "short course" of MtX, and 100% without posttransplant immunosuppression (Storb and Thomas, 1985). Standard MtX consisted of MtX 15 mg/m^2 IV on days 3, 6, 11 and then biweekly until day 105; short MtX consisted of similar doses given on days 1, 3, 6, and 11. Bone marrow toxicity is a concern even at low doses in bone marrow recipients, and MtX should not be given to patients having progressive liver or renal dysfunction, ascites, or edema.

4.2.4b. Cyclosporine (Csp). This drug has been found to be equally effective as standard MtX in preventing GVHD and promoting patient survival (Powles et al., 1980; Gluckman et al., 1983; Gale, 1985; Forman et al., 1987; Santos et al., 1987; Storb et al., 1987). There is no bone marrow toxicity, engraftment is faster, and time and costs of hospitalization are reduced. Renal toxicity is a significant problem, however, and some studies suggest a somewhat higher incidence of leukemia relapse (IBMT, 1989; Sullivan, 1989). Thus, while Csp immunosuppression has greatly improved results in organ transplantation, similar major gains have not materialized in BM tx.

This may largely be a consequence of difficulties in handling the drug in bone marrow transplant patients whose intestinal, renal, hepatic, and general metabolic functions fluctuate rapidly and frequently fail and who require intensive treatment with drugs that interfere with Csp metabolism or potentiate Csp toxicity (i.e., dilantine, rifampicin, aminoglycosides, amphotericin B) (Kennedy et al., 1983; Atkinson et al., 1984; Kahan,

1989). Careful drug monitoring and dose adjustments to avoid insufficient or toxic levels are probably crucial (Gratwohl et al., 1983; Kennedy et al., 1983; Lindholm et al., 1987; Kahan, 1989). Clinically useful methods (HPLC or RIA detecting parent drug levels) have only recently become available for routine drug monitoring (Kahan, 1989).

Thus, no consensus has yet evolved as to how Csp should be administered, or at which dose. Intravenous medication is usually required for the first weeks because of erratic gastrointestinal function, while oral medication is started as soon as possible thereafter. Opinions vary as to the merit of continuous infusion versus infusions given over 1–8 hr once or twice daily (Tallman et al., 1988).

The drug is usually started the day before transplantation at a dose of 2.5–5 mg/kg per day IV, in some centers individually tailored according to pretransplant pharmacokinetic studies (Gluckman et al., 1983; Kennedy et al., 1983; Gratwohl et al., 1983; Storb, 1989). Higher doses (by 25–50%) are required in children. Later on, dosage is modified by signs of renal toxicity (i.e, allowing for no more than a doubling of serum creatinine levels) and/or adjusted according to drug levels (Powles, 1980; Yee et al., 1988a,b). Whether whole blood or plasma levels should be monitored is controversial. There is no agreement on which levels provide adequate immunosuppression and which are excessive (toxic, overimmunosuppression provoking infection).

Blood and plasma trough levels (of parent drug) should probably be in the range of 100–300 and 50–150 ng/ml, respectively, with high levels during the first month and declining levels as time passes and GVHD problems resolve. Monitoring of levels is particularly important when switching from intravenous to oral administration. Oral doses required may range from 1 to 15 mg/kg per day, frequently 6–10 mg/kg per day for maintenance, and are usually given twice daily (Gluckman et al., 1983; Gratwohl et al., 1983; Atkinson et al., 1984; Yee et al., 1988a,b; Bacigalupo et al., 1990).

Csp treatment is usually slowly tapered and discontinued 6–12 months after transplantation in patients without signs of GVHD. Some centers favor earlier (3–6 months posttransplant) cessation of medication to facilitate early immune reconstitution, but a flare-up of GVHD may occur in approximately 25% (Storb and Thomas, 1985). Prolonged medication, even for years, may be required in patients with chronic GVHD (Bacigalupo et al., 1990).

4.2.4c. Csp plus Short MtX. Csp combined with a short course of MtX (as given above) has been shown to be more effective than either treatment modality alone and today is widely used for GVHD prevention (Storb et al., 1987). A GVHD (grades II–IV) rate of 15–30%, lowest in children, is still observed, however (Deeg et al., 1987). Bone marrow toxicity is negligible.

4.2.4d. Csp plus Corticosteroids. Favorable results have been reported using a combination of Csp and prednisone, given at an initial dose of 10–15 mg/m^2 per day starting on day 15 after BM tx and slowly tapered and discontinued after three months (Forman et al., 1987; Santos et al., 1987). Whether this combination is better than Csp plus short MtX is not known, nor if a combination of all three drugs is advantageous.

4.2.4e. Antilymphocyte Preparations. These preparations given intravenously from the day of transplantation and daily for 1–2 weeks are presently being studied (Deeg et al., 1987). Polyclonal (ATG) and monoclonal (i.e., Campath, OKT3, BMA 031, etc.) antibodies with various specificities, including T cells, have been reported to be effective in preliminary studies, often in combination with Csp and steroids. Clinical benefits have not yet been documented. Marrow toxicity, engraftment failure, thrombocytopenia, and serum sickness are potential side effects.

5. TREATMENT OF GRAFT VERSUS HOST DISEASE

5.1. Acute GVHD

When significant GVHD (grades II–IV) develops despite prophylaxis, treatment with additional immunosuppression is required. Many transplant teams do not consider slight GVHD (grate I) an indication for treatment, since spontaneous resolution may occur (Storb and Thomas, 1985).

The choice of immunosuppressive therapy for acute GVHD depends partly on the regimen used for GVHD prophylaxis. If that regimen did not include Csp or if GVHD evolved subsequent to intentional or accidental Csp tapering or discontinuation, cyclosporine therapy (see Section 4.2.4) is instituted or intensified (Kennedy et al., 1985; Deeg et al., 1988). Most cases respond, although additional corticosteroids may be required as secondary therapy (Sullivan et al., 1990).

Corticosteroids are generally used as primary GVHD therapy in (adequately) Csp-treated patients (Deeg et al., 1987). There is no consensus as to dosage, and several regimens of prednisone, prednisolone, or methylprednisolone are in use. A total of 3–6 infusions of 0.25–0.5 g prednisolone have been given for 1–2 weeks by some groups (Bacigalupo et al., 1983). A daily dose of 2–2.5 mg/kg IV is more commonly utilized (Doney et al., 1981; Kennedy et al., 1985). The dose is halved weekly or biweekly, and maintained at approximately 20 mg/day until the clinical situation allows for further tapering and withdrawal several weeks later. A response rate of 30–50% is generally reported (Deeg et al., 1987). The continued use of (high doses of) steroids renders BM allograft recipients, already severely immunocompromised by cytotoxic drugs, Csp, and GVHD, exceedingly susceptible to infection. The usual steroid side effects are also seen.

A number of antilymphocyte preparations have been tested in mostly small studies: (1) polyclonal anti-T-cell immunoglobulins produced from horse or rabbit (ATG), that is, "Atgam" (Doney et al., 1981); (2) monoclonal murine or rat antibodies with various specificities, usually including T cells, that is, CD 3 (OKT3), T-cell receptor (BMA 031), lymphocyte (Campath), or IL-2 receptor (on activated T cells, Tac, LFA-1, etc.) (Deeg et al., 1987; Sullivan, 1989). Daily infusions are given for one to two weeks.

Antilymphocyte preparations have mostly been used as secondary therapy for steroid-resistant cases. Although peripheral blood cells carrying the relevant target antigen are effectively removed, response rates are often less than 30%. The use of these preparations as primary GVHD treatment may prove more effective, but clinical experience is limited. Side effects vary slightly for various preparations, are generally modest, and may include allergic events, thrombocytopenia, and leukopenia. More problematic is their immunogenicity (mouse protein, idiotype), which precludes effective long-term (> 2 weeks) use. Engineering of human monoclonal antibodies and coupling of a cytotoxin to the antibody offer promise of future advances.

5.2. Chronic GVHD

Therapy is usually not required for patients with limited chronic GVHD (Deeg et al., 1988). Extensive GVHD causes significant morbidity and mortality, and immunosuppressive therapy should be instituted as early as possible (Sullivan et al., 1987).

Cyclosporine (see Section 4.2.4) is the mainstay of treatment. Oral medication is usually sufficient, but gastrointestinal and hepatic dysfunction caused by the disease mandate monitoring of Csp levels and renal function for appropriate dose adjustments. Treatment is continued for at least 6–12 months, before slow tapering is attempted (Sullivan et al., 1987, 1990).

Corticosteroids (see Section 4.2.4) are either instituted in combination with Csp or added to Csp for patients not responding well to Csp monotherapy (Deeg et al., 1987). Some centers administer the drugs on alternate days. The prednisone dose is tapered to a minimal effective one; in children, it is frequently given on alternate days only. Duration of treatment is as for Csp, but the drugs should be discontinued sequentially.

Treatment by Csp plus steroids is quite effective in controlling GVHD, and has generally replaced the previously used combination of azathioprine plus steroids, which resulted in a 75% disease-free survival (Deeg et al., 1987; Sullivan et al., 1987, 1990). Whether the combination of Csp plus azathioprine plus steroids (triple therapy used in organ transplantation) may further improve results is not known. Recently, thalidomide has shown effect in treatment of resistant cases (Deeg et al., 1987).

Other treatment options include psoralen and ultraviolet irradiation (PUVA) for skin lesions, sunblocking local steroids creams (dexamethasone 0.25% solution) for mucosal disease, prophylactic antibiotics, artificial saliva and tears, and antacids (Deeg et al., 1988).

REFERENCES

Asano, S., Masako, T., and Takaku, F., 1991, Beneficial effect of recombinant human granulocyte stimulating factor in marrow transplanted patients: Results of multicenter phase II studies, Transplant. Proc. 23:1701.

Ash, R. C., Casper, J. T., Chitambar, C. C., Hansen, R., Bunin, N., Truitt, R. L., Lawton, C., Murray, K., Hunter, J., Baxter-Lowe, L. A., Grottschalli, J. L., Oldham, K., Anderson, T., Camitta, B., and Menitove, J., 1990, Successful allogeneic transplantation of T cell depleted bone marrow from closely HLA matched unrelated donors, N. Engl. J. Med. 322:485.

Atkinson, K., Biggs, J. C., Britton, K., Short, R., Mrongoverus, R., Concannon, A., and Dodds, A., 1984, Oral administration of cyclosporin A for recipients of allogeneic marrow transplants, Br. J. Haematol. 56:223.

Bacigalupo, A., van Lint, M. T., Frassoni, F., Podesta, M., Veneziano, G., Avanzi, G., Vitale, V., and Marmont, A. M., 1983, High dose bolus methylprednisolone for the treatment of acute graft versus host disease, Blut 46:125.

Bacigalupo, A., Maiolino, A., van Lint, M. T., Occhini, D., Gualandi, F., Clavio, M., Lamparelli, T., Tong, J., and Marmont, A. M., 1990, Cyclosporin A and chronic graft versus host disease, Bone Marrow Transplant. 6:341.

Beatty, P. G., Hansen, J. A., Anasetti, C., Sanders, J., Buckner, C. D., Storb, R., and Thomas, E. D., 1989, Marrow transplantation from unrelated HLA matched volunteer donors, Transplant. Proc. 19:2993.

Butturini, A., and Gale, R. P., 1989, T-cell depletion in bone marrow transplantation, Clin. Transplant. 3:122.

Champlin, R., 1987, Treatment of aplastic anemia: Current role of bone marrow transplantation and immunomodulatory therapy, in: Progress in Bone Marrow Transplantation (R. P. Gale and R. Champlin, eds.), Alan R. Liss, New York, pp. 37–52.

Champlin, R. E., Ho, W. G., Mitsuyasu, R., Burnison, M., Greenberg, P., Holly, G., Winston, D. W., Ferg, S. A., and Gale, R. P., 1987, Graft failure and leukemia relapse following T lymphocyte depleted bone marrow transplants: Effects of intensification of immunosuppressive conditioning, Transplant. Proc. 19:3516.

Deeg, H. J., Doney, K., Sullivan, K. M., Witherspoon, R. P., Appelbaum, F. R., Storb, R., 1987, Prevention and treatment of graft-versus-host disease with drugs, in: Progress in Bone Marrow Transplantation (R. P. Gale and R. Champlin, eds.), Alan R. Liss, New York, pp. 265–276.

Deeg, H. J., Klingemann, H. G., and Phillips, G. L., 1988, A Guide to Bone Marrow Transplantation, Springer Verlag, Berlin.

DeWitte, T., Hoogenhout, J., Wessels, J., van Daal, W., Hustinx, T., and Haanen, C., 1986, Depletion of donor lymphocytes by counterflow centrifugation successfully prevents acute graft-versus-host disease in matched allogeneic marrow transplantation, Blood 67:1302.

Doney, K. C., Weiden, P. L., Storb, R., and Thomas, E. D., 1981, Treatment of graft-versus-host disease in human allogeneic graft recipients: A randomized trial comparing antithymocyte globulin and corticosteroids, Am. J. Hematol. 11:1.

Filipovich, A. H., Vallera, D. A., Youle, R. J., Quinores, R. R., Neville, D. M., and Kersey, J. H., 1984, Ex vivo treatment of donor bone marrow with anti-T cell immunotoxins for prevention of graft-versus-host disease, Lancet 1:469.

Fischer, A., Freidrich, W., Levinsky, R., Vossen, J., Griscelli, C., Kubanek, B., Morgan, G., Wakemaker, G., and Landais, P., 1986a, Bone marrow transplantation for immunodeficiencies and osteopetrosis: European survey, Lancet 2:1080.

Fischer, A., Blanche, S., Veber, F., Delaage, M., Mawa, C., Gricelli, C., Le Deest,F., Lopez, M., Olive, D., and Janossy, G., 1986b,

Prevention of graft failure by an anti-HLFA-1 monoclonal antibody in HLA-mismatched bone-marrow transplantation, *Lancet* 2:1058.

Forman, S. J., Blume, K. G., Krance, R. A., Muner, P. J., Metter, G. E., Hill, L. R., O'Donrell, M. R., Nademanee, A. P., and Snyder, D. S., 1987, A prospective randomized study of acute graft-versus-host disease in 107 patients with leukemia: Methotrexate/prednisone v. cyclosporine A/prednisone, *Transplant. Proc.* 19:2605.

Gale, R. P., 1985, Graft-versus-host disease, *Immunol. Rev.* 88:193.

Gluckman, E., Devergie, A., Poirier, O., and Lobiec, F., 1983, Use of cyclosporine as prophylaxis of graft-versus-host disease after human allogenic bone marrow transplantation, *Transplant. Proc.* 15:412.

Goldman, J. M., Gale, R. P., Horowitz, M. M., Biggs, J. C., Champlin, R. E., Gluckman, E., Hoffmann, R. G., Jacobsen, S. J., Marmont, A. M., McGlave, P. B., Messner, H. A., Runin, A. A., Rozman, C., Speck, B., Tura, S., Weerer, R. S., and Bortin, M. M., 1988, Bone marrow transplantation for chronic myelogenous leukemia in chronic phase. Increased risk for relapse with T-cell depletion, *Ann. Intern. Med.* 108:806.

Gratwohl, A., Speck, B., Wenk, M., Forster, I., Muller, M., Osterwalder, B., Nissen, C., and Follath, F., 1983, Cyclosporine in human bone marrow transplantation: Serum concentration, graft-versus-host disease, and nephrotoxicity, *Transplantation* 36:40.

Hansen, J. A., Beatty, P. G., Anasetti, C., Clift, A. C., Martin, P. J., Sanders, J., Sullivan, K., Buchner, C. D., Storb, R., and Thomas, E. D, 1987, Treatment of leukemia by marrow transplantation from donors other than HLA genotypically identical siblings, in: *Progress in Bone Marrow Transplantation* (R. P. Gale and R. Champlin, eds.), Alan R. Liss, New York, pp. 667–675.

Herve, P., Flesch, M., Cahn, J. Y., Rocadot, E., Plouvier, E., Lamy, B., Rosenbaum, A., Noir, A., LesFloris, R. L., and Peters, A., 1985, Removal of marrow T cells with OKT3–OKT11 monoclonal antibodies and complement to prevent graft versus host disease, *Transplantation* 39:138.

Hobbs, J., 1985, Correction of 34 genetic diseases by displacement bone marrow transplantation, *Plasma Ther. Transfus. Technol.* 6:221.

Hows, J., McKinnon, S., Brookes, P., Kaminski, E., and Bidwell, J., 1989, Matched unrelated donor transplantation, *Transplant. Proc.* 21:2973.

IBMT (International Bone Marrow Transplant Registry) 1989, Effect of methotrexate on relapse after bone-marrow transplantation for acute lymphoblastic leukemia, *Lancet* 1:535.

Kahan, B. D., 1989, Cyclosporine, *N. Engl. J. Med.* 321:1725.

Kennedy, M.S ., Deeg, H. J., Storb, R., and Thomas, E. D., 1983, Cyclosporine in marrow transplantation: Concentration dependent toxicity and immunosuppression *in vivo*, *Transplant. Proc.* 15:471.

Kennedy, M. S., Deeg, H. J., Storb, R., Doney, K., Sullivan, K. M., Witherspoon, R. P., Appelbaum, F. R., Sterwart, P., Sanders, J., Buckner, C. D., Martin, P., Werden, P., and Thomas, E. D., 1985, Treatment of acute graft-versus-host disease after allogeneic transplantation. Randomized study comparing corticosteroids and cyclosporine, *Am. J. Med.* 78:978.

Lindholm, A., Ringden, O., and Lønnqvist, B., 1987, The role of cyclosporine dosage and plasma levels for efficacy and toxicity in bone marrow transplant recipients, *Transplantation* 43:680.

Lucarelli, G., Galimberti, M., Polchi, P., Delfini, C., Giardini, C., Baronciani, D., Politi, P., Manenti, F., and Angeluci, E., 1985, Bone marrow transplantation for thalassemia, *Lancet* 1:1355.

Metcalf, D., 1989, Hemopoietic growth factors and marrow transplantation: An overview, *Transplant. Proc.* 21:2932.

O'Reilly, R. J., 1987, Current development in marrow transplantation, *Transplant. Proc.* 19:92.

Powles, R. L., Clink, H. M., Spence, D., Morgenstern, G., Watson, J. G., Selby, P. J., Woods, M., Barret, A., Jameson, B., Sloane, J., Lawler, S. D., Kay, H. E. M., Lawson, D. E, McEbvain, T. J., and Alexander, D., 1980, Cyclosporine A to prevent graft-versus-host disease in man after allogeneic bone marrow transplantation, *Lancet* 1:327.

Prentice, H. G., Blacklock, H. A., and Janossy, G., 1984, Depletion of T lymphocytes in donor marrow prevents significant graft-versus-host disease in matched allogenic leukemic marrow transplant recipients, *Lancet* 1:472.

Reisner, Y., Kapoor, N., Kirkpatric, D., Polback, M. S., Dupont, B., and O'Reilly, R. J., 1983, Transplantation for severe combined immunodeficiency with HLA-A, B, C, DR incompatible parental marrow cells fractionated by soybean agglutinin and sheep red blood cells, *Blood* 61:341.

Ringden, O., and Horowitz, M. M., 1989, Graft-versus-leukemia reactions in humans, *Transplant. Proc.* 21:2989.

Santos, G. W., 1987, Workshop summary: preparative regimens for allogeneic bone marrow transplantation in leukemia, in: *Progress in Bone Marrow Transplantation* (R. P. Gale and R. Champlin, eds.), Alan R. Liss, New York, pp. 113–119.

Santos, G. W., Tutschka, P., Brookmeyer, R., Saral, R., Beschorner, W. E., Biss, W. E., Bias, W. B., Braire, H. G., Burns, W. H., Elfenbein, J., and Kaizer, H., 1983, Marrow transplantation for cute nonlymphocytic leukemia after treatment with busulfan and cyclophosphamide, *N. Engl. J. Med.* 309:1347.

Santos, G. W., Tutschka, P. J., Brookmeyer, R. I., Saral, R., Beschorner, W. E., Bias, W. B., Braine, H. G., Burns, W. H., Farmer, E. R., Hess, A. D., Kaizer, H., Mellits, D., Sensenbrenner, L. L., Stuart, R., and Yeager, A. M., 1987, Cyclosporine plus methylprednisolone versus cyclophosphamide plus methylprednisolone as prophylaxis for graft-versus-host disease: A randomized double-blind study in patients undergoing allogeneic transplantation, *Clin. Transplant.* 1:21.

Slavin, S., Or, R., Naparstek, E., Weiss, L., Mumcuoglu, M., Weshler, Z., Brautbar, H., Civadalli, G., Glikson, M., Hale, G., and Waldmann, H., 1987, Allogeneic bone marrow transplantation without graft-versus-host disease: True tolerance of graft against the host through depletion of donor T lymphocytes pregrafting in malignant and non-malignant disorders, *Transplant. Proc.* 19:2614.

Storb, R., 1989, Graft rejection and graft-versus-host disease in marrow transplantation, *Transplant. Proc.* 21:2915.

Storb, R., and Thomas, E. D., 1985, Graft-versus-host disease in dog and man: The Seattle experience, *Immunol. Rev.* 88:215.

Storb, R.. Dorey, K. C., Thomas, E. D., Appelbaum, F., Buckner, C. D., Clift, R. A., Deeg, H. J., Goodell, B. W., Hackman, R.,

Hansen, J. A., Sanders, J., Sullivan, K., Weiden, P. L., and Witherspoon, R. P., 1982, Marrow transplantation with or without donor buffy coat cells for 65 transfused aplastic anemia patients, *Blood* **59**:236.

Storb, R., Deeg, H. J., Whitehead, J., Farewell, V., Appelbaum, F. R., Beatty, P., Benserger, W., Buckner, C. D., Clift, R. A., Doney, K., Hansen, J. A., Hill, R., Lum, L. G., Martin, P., McGriffin, R., Sanders, J., Singer, J., Stewart, P., Sullivan, K. M., Witherspoon, R. P., and Thomas, E. D., 1987, Marrow transplantation for leukemia and aplastic anemia: Two controlled trials of a combination of methotrexate and cyclosporine v. cyclosporine alone or methotrexate alone or methotrexate alone for prophylaxis of acute graft-versus-host disease, *Transplant. Proc.* **19**:2608.

Sullivan, K. M., 1989, Current status of bone marrow transplantation, *Transplant. Proc.* **21**(Suppl. 3):41.

Sullivan, K. M., Witherspoon, R., Deeg, H. J., Doney, K., Appelbaum, F., Sanders, J., Liem, L., Loughran, T., Hill, R., Anasetti, C., Shields, A., Nuns, J., Shulman, H., Storb, R., and Thomas, E. D., 1987, Chronic graft-versus-host disease in man, in: *Progress in Bone Marrow Transplantation* (R. P. Gale and R. Champlin, eds.), Alan R. Liss, New York, pp. 473–487.

Sullivan, K. M., Siadak, M. F., and Witherspoon, R. P., 1990, Cyclosporine treatment of chronic graft-versus-host disease, *Transplant. Proc.* **22**:1336.

Tallman, M. S., Nemunatis, J. J., McGuire, T. R., Yee, G. C., Hughes, T. E., Almgren, J. D., Appelbaum, F. R., Higano, C. S., McGuffin, R. W., Singer, J. W, and Thomas, E. D., 1988, Comparison of two intravenous cyclosporine infusion schedules in marrow transplant recipients, *Transplantation* **45**:810.

Thomas, E. D., Storb, R., Clift, R. A., Fefer, A., Johnson, F. L., Neiman, P. E., Lee, K. G., Glucksberg, H., and Buckner, C. D., 1975, Bone marrow transplantation, *N. Engl. J. Med.* **292**:832.

Tutschka, P. J., 1987, Mechanisms of chronic GVHD, in: *Progress in Bone Marrow Transplantation* (R. P. Gale and R. Champlin, eds.), Alan R. Liss, New York, pp. 457–472.

Tutschka, P. J., Copelan, E. A., and Kapoor, N., 1989, Replacing total body irradiation with busulfan as conditioning with leukemia for allogenic marrow transplantation, *Transplant. Proc.* **21**:2952.

Tutschka, P. J., Coplan, E. A., Kapnoor, N., Avalos, B. R., and Klein, J. P., 1991, Allogeneic bone marrow transplantation for leukemia using chemotherapy as conditioning: 6-year results of a single institution trial, *Transplant. Proc.* **23**:1709.

van Bekkum, D, 1984, Conditioning regimens for marrow grafting, *Semin. Hematol.* **21**:81.

Vartdal, F., Kvalheim, G., Lea, T. E., Bosnes, V., Gaudernack, G., Uglestad, J., and Albrechtsen, D., 1987, Depletion of T lymphocytes from human bone marrow. Use of magnetic monosized polymer microspheres coated with T lymphocyte-specific monoclonal antibodies, *Transplantation* **43**:366.

Yee, G. C., McGuire, T. R., Gmur, D. J., Lennon, T. P., and Deeg, H. J., 1988a, Blood cyclosporine pharmacokinetics in patients undergoing marrow transplantation, *Transplantation* **46**:399.

Yee, G. C., Self, S. G., McGuire, T. R., Carlen, J., Sanders, J. E., and Deeg, H. J., 1988b, Serum cyclosporine concentration and risk of acute graft-versus-host disease after allogeneic marrow transplantation, *N. Engl. J. Med.* **319**:65.

INDEX